D1397146

Stuttering Intervention

Stuttering Intervention

A Collaborative Journey
to Fluency Freedom

David Allen Shapiro

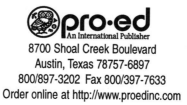

pro·ed
An International Publisher

8700 Shoal Creek Boulevard
Austin, Texas 78757-6897
800/897-3202 Fax 800/397-7633
Order online at http://www.proedinc.com

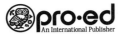

© 1999 by PRO-ED, Inc.
8700 Shoal Creek Boulevard
Austin, Texas 78757-6897

Library of Congress Cataloging-in-Publication Data

Shapiro, David A. (David Allen), 1954–
    Stuttering intervention : a collaborative journey to fluency freedom / David Allen Shapiro.
        p.   cm.
    Includes bibliographical references and index.
    ISBN 0-89079-740-4 (alk. paper)
    1. Stuttering—Treatment. I. Title.
RC424.S553   1999
616.85′5406—dc21   97-31307
                                     CIP

This book is designed in New Century Schoolbook and Frutiger Bold.

Printed in the United States of America

5 6 7 8 9 10   09 08 07 06 05 04

To Kay, Sarah, and Aaron Shapiro, who are the light of my life and the finest friends anyone could ever have;

To all comrades—people who stutter, families, clinicians, and others—who are willing to work with and learn from each other; and

To my grandparents, Hattie and Joseph Lyman, in whose memory I find inspiration to dream, to journey, and to try to make a difference.

Contents

◆ ◆

Foreword ◆ *xvii*

Preface ◆ *xix*

Acknowledgments ◆ *xxiii*

Unit I
Stuttering in Relief:
A Foundation for Intervention

Chapter 1
The Nexus of Stuttering: An Introduction ◆ *2*

The Face of Stuttering ◆ *3*

About This Book ◆ *4*

Definitions ◆ *6*

    Fluency ◆ *6*

    Disfluency Vs. Dysfluency ◆ *8*

    Stuttering ◆ *9*

    Other Terms ◆ *14*

More Than Just Terminology ◆ *15*

    Stutterer Vs. Stuttering ◆ *15*

    Categorical Vs. Noncategorical Behaviors ◆ *16*

    Fluency Facilitating Controls Vs. Tricks ◆ *16*

    Negative Stereotypes, Bias, and Misinformation: Implications for the Clinician ◆ *20*

    The Impact of Stuttering ◆ *24*

Chapter Summary and Discussion ◆ *27*

Chapter 1 Study Questions ◆ *29*

Chapter 2
The Onset, Development, and
Nature of Stuttering ♦ *32*

Knowledge and Assumptions Ground Understanding ♦ *34*

The Onset and Development of Stuttering ♦ *35*

    Bluemel ♦ *37*

    Froeschels ♦ *37*

    Van Riper ♦ *37*

    Bloodstein ♦ *42*

    Summary and Extension—Onset and Development of Stuttering ♦ *44*

The Nature of Stuttering ♦ *46*

    Types of Disfluency ♦ *46*

    Symptoms, Prevalence, and Incidence ♦ *46*

    Differences Between People Who Stutter and Those Who Do Not ♦ *49*

    Variability and Predictability of Stuttering ♦ *51*

    Treatment ♦ *52*

    Summary—Nature of Stuttering ♦ *53*

Chapter Summary ♦ *53*

Chapter 2 Study Questions ♦ *56*

Chapter 3
Etiology and Treatment of Stuttering:
Past and Present ♦ *58*

History of Stuttering: The Past ♦ *60*

    "If You Stutter, You're Not Alone" ♦ *60*

    Stuttering in Egyptian Hieroglyphics ♦ *61*

    Stuttering in the Bible ♦ *63*

    Stuttering in Professional Literature ♦ *64*

    Summary—History of Stuttering ♦ *69*

Etiology of Stuttering: The Present ♦ *70*

    Etiology Defined: Three Ps ♦ *70*

    Theoretical Explanations ♦ *73*

    Summary and Synthesis—Etiology of
    Stuttering and Theoretical Explanations ♦ *82*

A Personal Postscript on Theory ♦ *86*

Chapter Summary ♦ *91*

Chapter 3 Study Questions ♦ *93*

Chapter 4
Other Fluency Disorders ◆ *96*

Cluttering ◆ *97*

Neurogenic Disfluency ◆ *99*

    Stroke ◆ *104*

    Head Trauma ◆ *104*

    Extrapyramidal Diseases ◆ *105*

    Dementia and Tumors ◆ *106*

    Drug Usage ◆ *106*

    AIDS ◆ *106*

    Other ◆ *107*

Psychogenic Disfluency ◆ *108*

Malingering ◆ *109*

Adductor Spasmodic (i.e., Spastic) Dysphonia ◆ *110*

Acquired Disfluency Following Laryngectomy ◆ *110*

Tourette Syndrome ◆ *111*

Linguistic Disfluency ◆ *113*

Normal Developmental Disfluency ◆ *114*

Other Forms of Disfluency ◆ *115*

    Disfluency in Manual Communication ◆ *115*

    Disfluency During the Playing of a Wind Instrument ◆ *115*

Chapter Summary ◆ *116*

Chapter 4 Study Questions ◆ *116*

Unit II
Central and Guiding
Intervention Assumptions

Chapter 5
Personal Constructs and Family Systems:
Intrafamily Considerations ◆ *118*

Personal Construct Theory ◆ *120*

    Personal Constructs Defined ◆ *120*

    Personal Constructs Applied to Intervention ◆ *120*

    Case Example ◆ *123*

Summary and Extension—Personal Construct Theory ♦ *124*

Family Systems Theory ♦ *125*

A Paradigm Shift ♦ *125*

Family Based Treatment—Families
and Professionals as Partners ♦ *127*

Family Based Treatment—Modeling
Characteristics of Optimal Families ♦ *128*

Family Based Treatment—Modeling
Characteristics of Successful Families ♦ *129*

Family Based Treatment and Heightened Effectiveness ♦ *130*

Family Based Treatment and Fluency Disorders ♦ *132*

Family Diversity ♦ *134*

Family Characteristics ♦ *134*

Family Interactions ♦ *138*

Family Functions ♦ *142*

Family Life Cycle ♦ *145*

Summary—Family Based Treatment ♦ *149*

Chapter Summary ♦ *150*

Chapter 5 Study Questions ♦ *151*

Chapter 6
Interdisciplinary Teaming and Multicultural Awareness:
Extrafamily Considerations ♦ *154*

Interdisciplinary Practice ♦ *155*

Interdisciplinary Practice Defined ♦ *156*

Case Example ♦ *157*

Background and Justification for Interdisciplinary Teaming ♦ *158*

Models of Team Practice ♦ *159*

Conceptual Foundation and Necessary
Competencies for Interdisciplinary Practice ♦ *160*

Summary—Interdisciplinary Practice ♦ *163*

Multicultural Awareness ♦ *163*

A Context for Multicultural Appreciation ♦ *163*

Background Related to Multicultural Awareness ♦ *166*

Multicultural Considerations in Research on Stuttering ♦ *168*

Multicultural Considerations in Intervention ♦ *169*

Cultural Sensitivity and the Clinical Process ♦ *172*

Summary—Multicultural Awareness ♦ *175*

Chapter Summary ♦ *175*

Chapter 6 Study Questions ♦ *177*

Chapter 7
Stuttering Modification and Fluency Shaping: Psychotherapeutic Considerations ♦ *180*

General Definitions ♦ *182*

    Stuttering Modification ♦ *182*

    Fluency Shaping ♦ *183*

Significant Differences ♦ *184*

    Premise ♦ *184*

    Behavioral Treatment Goals ♦ *184*

    Affective Treatment Goals ♦ *186*

    Treatment Procedures ♦ *187*

    Treatment Structure ♦ *188*

Advantages and Disadvantages ♦ *188*

    Stuttering Modification ♦ *188*

    Fluency Shaping ♦ *189*

Differential Diagnostic Indicators for Treatment Design ♦ *189*

    Stuttering Modification ♦ *190*

    Fluency Shaping ♦ *191*

    Combined Stuttering Modification and Fluency Shaping Approaches ♦ *192*

Exemplar Treatments ♦ *192*

    Stuttering Modification ♦ *193*

    Fluency Shaping ♦ *203*

Chapter Summary ♦ *209*

Chapter 7 Study Questions ♦ *211*

Unit III
Assessment and Treatment Strategies with People Who Stutter: A Life Span Perspective

Chapter 8
Preschool Children: Assessment and Treatment ♦ *214*

General Precepts About Preschool Children ♦ *217*

Preassessment Procedures ♦ *218*

    Case History Form ♦ *218*

Audio- or Videotape Recording ◆ *218*

A Preliminary Phone Call ◆ *223*

Assessment Procedures ◆ *223*

General Considerations ◆ *223*

Parent Interview ◆ *224*

Parent–Child Interaction ◆ *227*

Child–Clinician Interaction ◆ *229*

Trial Management ◆ *235*

Post-Assessment Procedures ◆ *236*

Normal Disfluency and Incipient Stuttering ◆ *236*

Speech Analysis ◆ *239*

Diagnosis ◆ *257*

Prognosis and Recommendations ◆ *258*

Post-Assessment Parent Interview ◆ *259*

Treatment ◆ *262*

Parent Intervention ◆ *263*

Direct Intervention ◆ *272*

Clinical Portrait: Amy Stiles ◆ *280*

Selected Background Information ◆ *280*

Abbreviated Speech–Language Analysis ◆ *280*

Recommendations ◆ *281*

Follow-Up ◆ *281*

Treatment Snapshot ◆ *281*

Follow-Up and Epilogue ◆ *283*

Central and Guiding Intervention Assumptions ◆ *284*

Chapter Summary ◆ *285*

Chapter 8 Study Questions ◆ *287*

Chapter 9
School-Age Children Who Stutter: Assessment and Treatment ◆ *290*

General Precepts About School-Age Children Who Stutter ◆ *294*

Preassessment Procedures ◆ *295*

Assessment Procedures ◆ *296*

General Considerations ◆ *296*

Parent Interview ◆ *296*

Teacher Interview ◆ *297*

Child Interview ♦ *298*

Trial Management ♦ *305*

Post-Assessment Procedures ♦ *307*

Speech Analysis ♦ *308*

Diagnosis ♦ *309*

Prognosis and Recommendations ♦ *310*

Post-Assessment Interview with the Parent, Teacher, and Other Participants ♦ *311*

Treatment ♦ *312*

Goals ♦ *312*

Objectives ♦ *312*

Rationale ♦ *312*

Procedures ♦ *315*

Working with School-Age Children Who Stutter and
Have Concomitant Language or Phonological Impairment ♦ *340*

Concomitant Disorders ♦ *340*

Effects of Concomitant Disorders ♦ *340*

To Treat or Not To Treat? ♦ *341*

If *Yes,* Where Do I Begin? ♦ *341*

Sequential Vs. Concurrent Intervention ♦ *342*

Blended Intervention Approaches ♦ *343*

General Principles ♦ *343*

Working with Parents ♦ *344*

Access to Parents ♦ *344*

Respecting the Primary Role of Parents ♦ *345*

Meeting Parents' Needs ♦ *346*

Working with Teachers and Other School Personnel ♦ *348*

Build Rapport and Establish Colleagueship with Teachers ♦ *348*

Banish Elitism—All Colleagues in Education Are Equal ♦ *349*

Provide Teachers with Strategies To Facilitate Fluency in the Classroom ♦ *351*

Clinical Portrait: Thomas Wells ♦ *355*

Selected Background Information ♦ *355*

Abbreviated Speech–Language Analysis ♦ *355*

Recommendations and Objectives ♦ *356*

Treatment Snapshot ♦ *356*

Follow-Up and Epilogue ♦ *358*

Central and Guiding Intervention Assumptions ♦ *358*

Chapter Summary ♦ *359*

Chapter 9 Study Questions ♦ *362*

Chapter 10
Adolescents, Adults, and Senior Adults Who Stutter: Assessment and Treatment ◆ *364*

General Precepts About Adolescents, Adults, and Senior Adults Who Stutter ◆ *367*

    Precepts Common Across These Three Groups ◆ *368*

    Precepts About Adolescents ◆ *368*

    Precepts About Adults ◆ *370*

    Precepts About Senior Adults ◆ *371*

Preassessment Procedures ◆ *375*

    Case History Form, Audio- or Videotape Recording, Preliminary Phone Call ◆ *375*

    Preassessment Conference ◆ *376*

Assessment Procedures ◆ *382*

    General Considerations ◆ *382*

    Client and Family Interview ◆ *383*

    Trial Management ◆ *392*

Post-Assessment Procedures ◆ *394*

    Speech Analysis ◆ *395*

    Diagnosis ◆ *397*

    Prognosis and Recommendations ◆ *397*

    Post-Assessment Interview ◆ *405*

Treatment ◆ *407*

    Goals ◆ *407*

    Objectives ◆ *407*

    Rationale ◆ *408*

    Procedures ◆ *410*

Clinical Portrait: Bill Rice ◆ *434*

    Selected Background Information ◆ *434*

    Abbreviated Speech–Language Analysis ◆ *434*

    Trial Management ◆ *435*

    Recommendations, Goals, and Objectives ◆ *436*

    Treatment Snapshot ◆ *438*

    Follow-Up and Epilogue ◆ *440*

    Central and Guiding Intervention Assumptions ◆ *441*

Chapter Summary ◆ *442*

Chapter 10 Study Questions ◆ *445*

Unit IV
The Clinician: A Paragon of Change

Chapter 11
The Clinician and the Client–Clinician Relationship ♦ *448*

Importance of Clinicians to the Change Process ♦ *450*

Interpersonal Factors of Effective Clinicians ♦ *452*

Clinician Behaviors ♦ *452*

Clinician Attributes and Manner of Interaction ♦ *452*

Clinician Language ♦ *460*

Intrapersonal Factors of Effective Clinicians ♦ *460*

Clinician Thoughts, Feelings, and Beliefs ♦ *460*

Clinician Needs ♦ *464*

Clinician Satisfaction and Rewards ♦ *466*

The Clinician as Guardian Angel ♦ *468*

Chapter Summary ♦ *470*

Chapter 11 Study Questions ♦ *472*

Chapter 12
Professional Preparation and Lifelong Learning:
The Making of a Clinician ♦ *474*

Professional Preparation of Clinicians
Who Work with People Who Stutter ♦ *476*

Academic Process ♦ *477*

Clinical Process ♦ *480*

Supervisory Process ♦ *487*

Maintenance of Professional Competence ♦ *505*

Knowing and Internalizing the Desire To Learn ♦ *505*

Learning as a Lifelong Process ♦ *507*

Maintaining Parallels: Different Trees, Same Forest ♦ *508*

Chapter Summary ♦ *510*

Chapter 12 Study Questions ♦ *512*

Appendixes

Appendix A—Reprinted Publications ◆ *513*

Appendix A.1. Clinical Supervision in Speech-
Language Pathology and Audiology (ASHA, 1985) ◆ *514*

Appendix A.2. Code of Ethics (ASHA, 1994a) ◆ *520*

Appendix A.3. Guidelines for Practice in Stuttering
Treatment (ASHA, 1995) ◆ *524*

Appendix A.4. Scope of Practice in Speech-
Language Pathology (ASHA, 1996b) ◆ *536*

Appendix B—Resources: Materials and Organizations ◆ *541*

References ◆ *549*

Author Index ◆ *573*

Subject Index ◆ *577*

About the Author ◆ *591*

Foreword

♦ ♦

Fortunately for those who stutter and their families, as well as for those who treat those who stutter, there has been a proliferation in recent years of texts devoted to defining and refining treatment processes for fluency disorders that warrant the label of stuttering. Seldom, however, has there been such a comprehensive review of the treatment literature as is included in this text. Even more unique is the text's tone of placing each diagnostic and treatment procedure in the context of collaborative efforts on the part of all those concerned for the client's welfare. Written from the perspective of one who stuttered severely until the age of 25 and who has devoted his professional life to serving those who stutter, *Stuttering Intervention* is filled with personal anecdotes illuminating the processes being described with passion and compassion, without forsaking professional objectivity. Such writing is rare. In this text, it is combined with a disciplined and scholarly approach, thus providing the reader with an exceptionally balanced and frequently touching account. Highlighted in this book are the efforts of those who help people who stutter to live rewarding and joyful lives—whether as normally fluent speakers or as ones for whom coping with stuttering remains a lifelong challenge. Concern for the client's point-of-view is present throughout the text, as is a sensitivity to the challenges confronting clinicians. Clinicians are not only required to be understanding and sagacious counselors; they also must be skilled technicians in addressing the affective, behavioral, and cognitive components of stuttering syndromes. Anyone having spent a lifetime in the "vineyards of fluency," as our beloved Van Riper was wont to say (and his wisdom is cited frequently herein), knows and feels the enormity of the challenge one takes on in accepting the role of primary caregiver to individuals who stutter. Dr. Shapiro's text is an outstanding testament to that challenge and an invaluable resource for those seeking to increase their understanding of coping with the enigma of stuttering syndromes. Finally, Dr. Shapiro's text is a testament of hope for those who now and for those who one day will experience, undeniably, one of life's most frustrating and potentially debilitating conditions.

Eugene B. Cooper
Professor and Chair Emeritus
University of Alabama, Tuscaloosa

Coordinator
ASHA Special Interest Division
for Fluency and Fluency Disorders

Distinguished Professor
Nova Southeastern University
Fort Lauderdale, Florida

Crystal S. Cooper
Past Curriculum Associate
Speech, Language, Hearing Services
Tuscaloosa City Schools

Past Vice President
Professional Practices in
Speech–Language Pathology, ASHA

Adjunct Instructor
Nova Southeastern University
Fort Lauderdale, Florida

Preface

The word *therapist* rarely is used today in speech–language pathology and audiology. I like that word. It comes from the Greek root *therapeuein,* meaning "comrade in a common struggle." This book is designed for all comrades, including student clinicians and professional speech–language pathologists, who are committed to understanding stuttering and people who stutter. Stuttering continues to be one of the most perplexing communication disorders. People who stutter and their families are the beneficiaries of our best clinical and scientific efforts to unveil the mysteries of stuttering, as well as our source of motivation to approach the challenge of informed and effective intervention with insight and vigor.

Over the past 2 decades alone, more than 1,400 articles and 30 books have been written about stuttering (Culatta & Goldberg, 1995). Some present a compendium of knowledge to date about stuttering. Others emphasize precise measurements of stuttering and related behaviors. Still others transform these data into intervention strategies based on a particular clinical philosophy. The purpose of this book is to present a specific point of view—i.e., a unique approach to intervention with people who stutter, based on what is known about learning and communication, speech and language fluency, stuttering, and people who stutter. You might say, "Aha! This book presents a recipe." It does not. It shares with you some of my ideas and what I do. I am convinced that as clinicians, we have an obligation to share with each other what we do, the rationale for what we do, and accountability for what we do, in order to ensure the highest quality of service for our clients and maximum growth for our profession. The procedures presented are what I find successful. You, the reader, are free to sift through, select, change, or even drop any of the procedures according to the strengths and needs of your individual clients or your own theoretical orientation, as long as what you do, why, and your accountability are clear. This book tells a story. Every good story has a moral. This story has two. First, design and implementation of intervention with people who stutter are not arbitrary events. Assessment and treatment are based on decision rules that are guiding principles to effective and reliable intervention. Second, the future for people who stutter is and must be sincerely viewed as bright and optimistic. This interpretation is based on promising clinical data and an understanding of the impact that the clinician's attitude has on the success of the treatment experience.

You might have noticed that this is not a traditional textbook. It has had no less than a 20-year gestation. Over this period of time, my professional motivation has been maintained by working continuously as a speech–language pathologist providing assessment and treatment services to people of all ages who stutter and their families. Also, teaching undergraduate and graduate courses in communication disorders (including stuttering), supervising clinical practica required for professional preparation of speech–language pathologists, and providing workshops for literally thousands of professional clinicians in the field, I continue to address a series of predictable questions, including:

(a) What is stuttering? (b) What is known and not known about stuttering and people who stutter? (c) How do I distinguish stuttering from normal speech disfluencies? (d) How do I assess people who stutter? (e) How do I treat people who stutter? and (f) How do I work with the families and significant others of people who stutter? Such families, teachers, and allied service providers, among others, continue to ask: (g) What can I do to facilitate the process of intervention and development of long-term communication independence by the person who stutters? This book is intended to address these and other questions. Specifically, the book addresses, outlines, and accounts for an individualized, collaborative approach to assessment and treatment (within the framework of communication systems) across the life span *with* (i.e., not for) people who stutter. This is done from an interdisciplinary perspective and with sensitivity toward multicultural and otherwise diverse realities.

It is said that lightening does not strike twice. It should be said, however, that magic in fluency intervention strikes at least three times. Magic, used here, is the overpowering quality within the process of effective interpersonal communication (i.e., clinical intervention) that distinguishes and enchants the event as a quintessential human experience. The first time magic strikes is when a clinician first experiences the gestalt, the "aha!," the predictable shift in a clinician's focus from oneself (i.e., What do I do if the parent begins to cry? What should I do if my behavior management techniques don't work for the young child? What do I do if the adult client asks me something I don't know?) to the client (i.e., When the child denies that he stutters, is this child unaware or emotionally unprepared to address the issue? When the client fails to complete her assignment, does this mean that she truly forgot, as reported, or is this client unmotivated? What is the clinical significance of what the client is not saying?). This shift in focus from oneself to the client typically is built upon a foundation of academic and clinical knowledge and successful clinical experience and renders the process of intervention to be thoroughly enjoyable and rewarding. Magic strikes a second time when, within a supportive and open clinical relationship, the client experiences, perhaps for the first time, either controlled or spontaneous fluency. As will be seen, fluency shaping—i.e., more behaviorally oriented techniques (e.g., choral reading with slower, gentler, and more natural sounding speech)—will render all people who stutter to be temporarily fluent. This experience can offer a client a glimmer of fluency freedom that can be powerfully motivating. From this experience, I have seen clients laugh and cry with mixed emotions of joy, fear, and wonderment of one's fluency future.

Magic strikes a third time when the families of people who stutter feel that they are sincerely cared for and understood, actively involved in the process of intervention, and contributing meaningfully to communication improvement of their family member who stutters. Expressions of thanks are frequent, and family bonds within a communication system are strengthened. When magic has struck three times, it strikes a fourth. At this point, clinicians, clients who stutter, and their families are communicating and learning with and from each other. At an earlier time, my colleague and I described the ability to shift perspective as "the hallmark of communication" (Shapiro & Moses, 1989). This type of communication is professionally gratifying, if not exhilarating. I have found these experiences to be communicatively intimate, rendering the dialogue among the participants within the clinical interaction to seem both time-less and placeless. It has not been uncommon for me to lose track of the time and place because of my focus on and communication with a person who stut-ters and the family. I continue to be intrigued by and concerned about the num-ber of clinicians who have completed programs of graduate study, yet fail to experience this magic. While the printed word has limitations in conveying the multidimensionality of the clinical experience, I hope this book helps impart the magic of fluency intervention to you.

To this point, it might seem that my motivation for writing this book is strictly professional. That is a major part, but not the whole story. This book also has a personal motivation. I was anything but communicatively indepen-dent for nearly a quarter of a century. I stuttered miserably for many years and experienced frequent disappointments in scheduled treatment. I have enjoyed fluency freedom for nearly 20 years and perhaps am making up for lost time. In a way, I feel it is unfortunate that I must credit myself for most of my own progress. My commitment to write such a book is in part the settlement of a debt—to myself. I inform my many clients that I will expect them to return the favor, in a way of their own design, to the field or to an individual who might not have been as fortunate and who is still in pursuit of the fluency that seems so elusive. I have always been one to put my actions where my mouth is, and to lead by example so that others may do as I do, rather than do only as I say. Indeed I know firsthand what it is like to be unable to speak, only to dream of enjoying the freedom of speech enjoyed by so many others. More than a free-dom, I have come to believe that fluent speech is one's natural right. I have become convinced from the many clients and their families I have worked with, as well as the feedback I received from former students, that my ideas need to be written. I remain positive by nature and believe that every experience, par-ticularly the most challenging, becomes meaningful and instructive. So, this book is my way of integrating my academic and clinical training; my experi-ences (i.e., both professional and, as appropriate, personal); my own positive, collaborative, whole-person, systematic and systems-based approach to indi-vidualized and interdisciplinary intervention with persons who stutter; and yes, my way of saying thanks. I believe that ultimately our legacy will be our caring for and dialogue with others who also are seeking to improve the human condition and to make even better the communicative world in which we all live.

As you begin reading *Stuttering Intervention: A Collaborative Journey to Fluency Freedom,* and thereby your own journey to understanding stuttering and people who stutter, it is helpful to know what to expect along the way. As I indicated earlier, this book is intended for all student clinicians and profes-sional speech–language pathologists who are interested in and committed to designing and implementing effective intervention with people who stutter. This book may be used in upper-level undergraduate or graduate-level courses addressing disorders of speech fluency including stuttering. It may be used in one semester or across a two-semester sequence. Furthermore, the book may serve as a clinical guide for practitioners who are looking for a clinical method that is practical, directly applied, reliable, and accountable, while based upon theoretical concepts and research across human service disciplines. The con-cepts and content in the book are presented developmentally in such a way that earlier chapters serve as the instructional foundation for later chapters.

The book contains four units. Unit I contains Chapters 1 through 4 and provides the reader with a conceptual foundation for clinical intervention. Chapter 1 introduces the reader to the uniqueness of this book and to concepts that are critical for understanding stuttering and people who stutter. Chapter 2 addresses the onset, development, and nature of stuttering and reviews related literature. Chapter 3 covers the etiology of stuttering from past and present perspectives and conveys how present thinking relates to ideas we once believed to be true. Chapter 4, the last in Unit I, helps clinicians distinguish and differentially diagnose stuttering from other disorders of fluency, some of which are not mentioned in any other book to date in speech–language pathology. Unit II contains Chapters 5 through 7 and addresses central and guiding assumptions that are critical to the design of effective intervention. Chapter 5 addresses intrafamily considerations (i.e., personal constructs and family systems); Chapter 6, extrafamily considerations (i.e., interdisciplinary teaming and multicultural perspectives); and Chapter 7, psychotherapeutic considerations (i.e., stuttering modification and fluency shaping) including exemplar forms of treatment. Unit III, the largest and most substantive of the book, contains Chapters 8 through 10, which address assessment and treatment across the life span with people who stutter. Chapter 8 focuses on intervention with preschool children; Chapter 9 with school-age children; Chapter 10 with adolescents, adults, and senior adults. Finally, Unit IV contains Chapters 11 and 12, which address the clinician from multiple perspectives. Chapter 11 focuses on the clinician and the client–clinician relationship. Chapter 12 discusses the roles of professional preparation and lifelong learning as critical processes for developing and maintaining effective speech–language pathologists.

One additional point of information is necessary. Ease of reading was one of the principles guiding the design and writing of this book. For this and other reasons, the book is as gender-neutral as possible. When it was not possible—and to avoid use of cumbersome pronoun constructions such as *she or he* and *her or his*—people who stutter are referred to as *he* and student clinicians and professional speech–language pathologists are referred to as *she*. This rationale is based on the documentation that the majority of people who stutter are male; the majority of speech–language pathologists are female.

As you begin your own journey, I encourage you to dialogue with your colleagues in speech–language pathology who, like yourself, are working to understand stuttering and people who stutter. Talk about what you are learning—the excitements, the challenges, the fears. In our shared commitment to providing the best intervention services possible, I would love to hear your reactions, as well as those of your clients and their families, to the material presented here. Feel free to contact me. I can be reached at Western Carolina University, Department of Human Services, Communication Disorders Program, Cullowhee, NC 28723-9043. Good luck.

Acknowledgments

◆ ◆ ◆ ◆ ◆ ◆ ◆ ◆ ◆ ◆ ◆ ◆ ◆ ◆ ◆ ◆ ◆ ◆ ◆

This book represents the support of many good people. First, I am grateful to the administration at Western Carolina University, which awarded me a Scholarly Development Assignment during the fall of 1995 to begin writing this book and provided me with the necessary institutional resources to complete it. Particularly, I want to thank Drs. Gurney Chambers, Dean, and A. Michael Dougherty, Associate Dean, of the College of Education and Allied Professions, and Billy Ogletree, Head of the Department of Human Services, for their support and encouragement. I am thankful also for the support of and ongoing interest in this work among the faculty and students in the Communication Disorders Program and the Department of Human Services. Thanks to a number of graduate assistants, particularly Julie Herman Taylor, and Machelle Cathey and Theresa Rudy, for help in locating and gathering many professional reprints. Thanks to Barbara Parris for computer generating Figure 9.2. Thanks to Drs. Lynda Miller and Nelson Moses for valuable editorial suggestions on an earlier version of the manuscript. Thanks to the good folks at PRO-ED, including James Patton, Annie Koppel, Robin Spencer, and Chris Anne Worsham, for believing in and encouraging this project from the beginning.

Second, a project such as this becomes a family affair at some point. Thanks to my parents, Alice and Sidney Shapiro, and my parents-in-law, Esther and Calvin Slattery, for being available when I was not. Thanks to the two finest children ever, Sarah and Aaron, who are my best teachers and of whom I am so proud. And thanks to my best friend for life, Kay, who, more than anyone else, has understood and encouraged my need to write this book, all the while putting up with me. Thanks to friends including Dr. Jane Schulz, Professor Emeritus, Naomi King, and Bill and Karen Clarke for ongoing support and expressions of kindness.

Last, I owe a debt of gratitude to the many people who stutter and their families who have contributed to our knowledge of fluency disorders and who put their confidence in our hands to help guide their collaborative journey to fluency freedom. May we always be deserving of their confidence; may we always nurture their dreams; and may we always help each other work toward improved communication and thereby global understanding and world peace.

Unit I

◆ ◆ ◆ ◆ ◆ ◆ ◆ ◆ ◆ ◆ ◆ ◆ ◆ ◆ ◆ ◆ ◆ ◆

Stuttering in Relief:
A Foundation
for Intervention

Chapter 1
The Nexus of Stuttering: An Introduction

Chapter 2
The Onset, Development, and Nature of Stuttering

Chapter 3
Etiology and Treatment of Stuttering: Past and Present

Chapter 4
Other Fluency Disorders

Chapter 1

The Nexus of Stuttering:
An Introduction

◆　◆　◆　◆　◆　◆　◆　◆　◆　◆　◆　◆　◆　◆　◆　◆　◆　◆　◆　◆

The Face of Stuttering　3

About This Book　4

Definitions　6

　Fluency　6

　Disfluency Vs. Dysfluency　8

　Stuttering　9

　　Descriptive Definitions of Stuttering　10

　　Explanatory Definitions of Stuttering　11

　　Combined Descriptive/Explanatory Definitions of Stuttering　11

　　Stuttering Defined　13

　Other Terms　14

More Than Just Terminology　15

　Stutterer Vs. Stuttering　15

　Categorical Vs. Noncategorical Behaviors　16

　Fluency Facilitating Controls Vs. Tricks　16

　Negative Stereotypes, Bias, and Misinformation: Implications for the Clinician　20

　　Interaction Between Clinicians' Attitude and Treatment Outcome　21

　　Misinformation Begets Misinformation　23

　　Pervasiveness of Negative Stereotypes, Bias, and Misinformation　23

　The Impact of Stuttering　24

　　Stuttering and Articulation　25

　　Stuttering and Language　25

　　Stuttering and Voice　26

　　Stuttering and Functioning in Society　26

　　Stuttering and Interpersonal Relationships　27

Chapter Summary and Discussion　27

Chapter 1 Study Questions　29

*It is difficult for those who have not possessed or been possessed by
the disorder to appreciate its impact on the stutterer's self-concepts,
his roles, his way of living.*

(VAN RIPER, 1982, P. 1)

THE FACE OF STUTTERING

Picture a young boy preparing to make his first phone call to a girl he has
become fond of at school. You, the reader, can recall your own similar experiences. He waits until his family is out of earshot. To a young boy, this experience is so significant that he wishes not to offer explanation to his surely disbelieving parents and siblings. Boys are supposed to think that girls have
cooties. Not this boy. He dials her phone number, but hangs up the receiver
before the ring begins because he is not quite ready yet. Regaining his composure, all the while rehearsing, "Hello, this is . . . ," he redials. "This time I really
am going to do it," he thinks to himself. "I am ready." Before he can change his
mind, the phone begins to ring. It seems to the boy an eternity between the end
of the first ring and the beginning of the second. Finally, a voice answers,
"Hello." This voice is very important to the boy. It could be the girl's father,
mother, brother, or sister. Or it could be a wrong number. To the boy, the bearer
of the voice represents someone important to the girl. The voice again says,
"Hello." The boy begins to say the first sound in *H*ello. He says, "H. H. H." Try
as he might, all that result are little inaudible puffs of air. "Hello! Hello! Hello!"
the voice repeats with increasing impatience. While the boy continues his
valiant attempts, he hears, "Oh, these damn pranks!" The phone goes dead.
This is stuttering.

The same boy, some years later, prepares at great length for his turn to
recite a poem in eighth grade English class. He knows the poem well. He mem-
orizes it and recites it alone and with his family. He always does his best and is
a serious student. He particularly wants to do well on this day because Nancy
is in his class. He likes Nancy a lot. He thinks she knows it, although he has
never told her. When she recited her poem the day before, the boy smiled at her
and told her that she did great. The boy feels relatively confident, although
knows that he never can seem to predict his speech fluency. He takes his place
at the front of the room. The teacher says, "Begin." "There once was . . . a . . .
a . . ." Oh, dread! Horror! "Why does this have to happen now?" the boy thinks.
"Why always to me?" After several attempts, the boy hears some students
chuckling; others move uncomfortably in their seats. The teacher interrupts,
"You do know your poem, don't you?" "Yes sir," the boy responds. "Now let's all
be patient," the teacher continues. "We know that our presenter today tries as
hard as the rest of us. We need to show him that we are listening and that we
are interested." The boy wishes that he could be somewhere else, anywhere else.
Time seems to stand still. The boy feels that he is taking too long. Everybody is
waiting. He sees Nancy looking away. "She can't even look at me," he thinks.
This is stuttering.

The boy now is a young man in high school who rarely speaks because of
embarrassment frequently associated with his stuttering. After much fore-
thought and measured anticipation, he collects his courage and asks a young

woman if she would accompany him to the basketball game on Friday evening. His speech is so disfluent. He tries to relax, but his face contorts. He speaks haltingly. He knows that his speech sounds more like a growl. He sees her beautiful face first tense, then turn into an amused, uncomfortable grin. She tells him she is busy. "Thanks all the same." Both look down, anywhere but at each other, with only fleeting eye contact. This is stuttering.

The man and his wife now are expecting their second child whom they know will be a boy. They agree that the name Aaron is their favorite, although they joke that they selected it because, with so little time, it was the first on the name list. The name Aaron has an additional significance to the man because of its Biblical association, particularly to the book of Exodus. As will be reviewed in Chapter 3, Moses stuttered and brought his brother Aaron with him as his spokesperson. The point is that their son's name clearly is to be Aaron. But the man knows that the initial vowel (*A*) occasionally will be difficult for him to say. Even before the boy is born, the man pictures himself introducing his son and blocking on his name. He rehearses over and over, "Aaron. Aaron Joseph. This is my son, Aaron." Joseph is to be the son's middle name in honor of the man's grandfather. "Maybe I should name him Joseph Aaron," he thinks, "since Joseph would be easier for me to say, and Joseph provides a transition to say Aaron, unlike saying Aaron Joseph. Or maybe I should just replace the name Aaron with another containing an initial consonant. Who would ever know?" But how could he raise his son, knowing fully that his given name was to be Aaron, but his father decided to call him Kevin, or Seth, or Robert? That would be the ultimate avoidance, if not a permanent penalty, for a boy and his father. This is me. This is stuttering.

This is the face of stuttering. Stories such as these are relived daily by people who stutter. Communication is a uniquely human experience. Stuttering, a significant disorder of communication, reminds people who stutter of their particularly human limitations. Van Riper (1982) captured the significance of the impact stuttering has on one's life:

> Once it has taken hold, after a period of insidious growth, almost every aspect of the person's existence is colored by his communicative disability. Ease in verbal communication is a vital prerequisite for more than marginal existence in any modern culture such as ours. Stuttering is not merely a speech impediment; it is an impediment in social living. (pp. 1–2)

Stuttering, as we will see, potentially influences all aspects of one's communication and one's life, and the lives of others who communicate with people who stutter.

ABOUT THIS BOOK

This book is based on the conviction that stuttering is both a multidimensional and manageable composite of behaviors, thoughts, and feelings. Successful intervention must take into account not only the individual who stutters, but virtually all persons within that individual's communication system. This collaborative enterprise requires that the person who stutters be actively engaged in all aspects of the intervention process, and be treated as whole and able. The communication environment becomes the object of study as does the communication itself. Overt (i.e., directly observable behaviors) and covert (i.e., internalized thoughts and feelings) manifestations of communication are considered, if not addressed, equally. The primary focus of intervention, and the source of ongoing motivation, is success—what the person who stutters can, rather than cannot, do. The approach is tailored to each individual's unique communication strengths and needs; is consistent with what we know about communication, learning, change, and the role of the communicator in the change process; is committed to an interdisciplinary perspective; and results in positive change by speakers of all ages within communication systems. This approach is in immediate and direct contrast to traditional forms of intervention in which people who stutter are only passively engaged, are the sole focus of treatment, and are treated as disabled or disordered. Such a narrow and negative focus results in treatment that is lacking in its relatedness to one's real communication strengths and needs (i.e., lacking in ecological validity) and therefore does not generalize to contexts outside of the clinical environment. Selected features that distinguish the method presented in this book include:

- The person who stutters is viewed as a whole person who communicates within a communication system, a meaningful context for communication and intervention, rather than as a disabled person in isolation.

- The intervention process is treated as multidimensional and collaborative, necessarily involving the client, clinician, members of the communication system, and allied professionals, rather than as unidimensional and solely an interaction between the clinician and client.

- The clinician is guided in how to involve directly other members of the interdisciplinary team, thus facilitating the necessary integration across participants, rather than focusing nearly exclusively on the client–clinician relationship.

- The client is viewed as an active and critical member of the interdisciplinary team, necessarily involved in all aspects of intervention planning, implementation, evaluation, and follow-up, rather than as a passive participant who follows the direction of the clinician.

- The methodology focuses on the fluent aspects of one's communication, not only the disfluency. While numbers do not tell the whole story, 15% or 20% disfluency typically renders a speaker significantly disfluent (i.e., independent of severity, for illustration only). That also means that 80% to 85% of the individual's speech is fluent. This method first addresses the fluent component, and instructs the client in how to do more of what he already is doing right (i.e., facilitative of fluency). Only then are the remaining disfluencies targeted and eliminated. This process (i.e., facilitation) is in contrast to a preliminary and primary focus on disfluency (i.e., and the resulting perspective of rehabilitation).

- Transfer (i.e., generalization) is begun from the first contact with the client. This is in contrast to the traditional focus on transfer toward the end of scheduled treatment.

- Relapse is treated as clinically inevitable, so clients are prepared to handle it productively and with fluency facilitating control. This is in contrast to ignoring its existence, which results in the client's surprise and communicative defenselessness.

- Change is treated as realistic, desirable, and possible at any age across the life span within communication systems.

- Stuttering (i.e., behaviors, thoughts, and feelings) reflects in part the consequence of active and alternative choices.

- Early intervention with young children is seen as a form of prevention.

- Regular assignments designed with, not for, the clients are viewed as a critical form of treatment that occurs between scheduled sessions.

- Multicultural considerations in assessment and treatment, particularly with persons who stutter, are addressed.

- Intervention with senior adults who stutter is viewed as providing a positive, inviting, and enlightening opportunity.

The objectives of this book, therefore, are to address, outline, and account for individualized assessment and treatment across the life span *with* (i.e., not for) people who stutter within communication systems. The book takes an interdisciplinary perspective, and has particular awareness of and sensitivity toward multicultural and otherwise diverse realities. There are at least two additional overriding objectives. One is to excite you, the reader, to want to know even more about stuttering and to feel a professional calling to work with people who stutter. Another is to highlight a number of clinical methods that you might already be using, so as to encourage their use. Blood (1995b) noted, "Sometimes validation of the techniques people are using already is as important as the creation of new techniques" (p. 177). You will see that this last objective is parallel to a procedure that I will be recommending for intervention (i.e., highlighting what a client is already doing right that is conducive to fluency or fluency facilitating control, so as to help him know how to do more of what he is already doing right).

DEFINITIONS

Fluency

There seems to be little disagreement that when people stutter, they are not talking fluently. Listeners tend to be reliable and accurate in distinguishing individuals as belonging to categories of stutterers or nonstutterers (Bloodstein, 1995). Defining stuttering and identifying with precision individual instances of stuttering, however, prove to be more difficult and less reliable.

Because of our agreement in categorizing speakers on the basis of their relative speech fluency, Starkweather (1984) suggested that we have assumed erroneously the definition that fluency is the absence of stuttering. He indicated several problems that arise with such a temptingly simple definition. First, stuttering behaviors vary in how fluent they are. People who stutter demonstrate different degrees of fluency at different times and when compared to each other. Furthermore, the therapy goal referred to as *fluent stuttering* seeks to achieve a less effortful, less abnormal, less disruptive, and more brief form of disfluency. Therefore, defining fluency as the absence of stuttering is counterintuitive. Instead, fluency should be defined in terms of effort and temporal duration. Second, people who stutter do not stutter all of the time. In fact, most of their speech is free of stuttering. However, this nonstuttered speech varies in its degree of fluency. People who stutter tend to speak more slowly than people of the same age and sex who do not stutter. People who stutter have the same normal nonfluencies as people who do not stutter. The nonstuttered speech of people who stutter also is less fluent when they expend effort and time on fluency tricks such as circumlocution (i.e., word changing) to avoid stuttering. Finally, people who do not stutter demonstrate times of increased and decreased fluency for reasons of health, fatigue, perceived stress, level of conviction, etc. Their nonfluency is characterized by varying degrees of filled pauses, hesitations, false starts, and repetitions of sounds, words, and phrases. The point is that defining fluency as the absence of stuttering is insufficient. Furthermore, fluency is a continuous rather than dichotomous variable. In other words, the speech of people who stutter and those who do not stutter can be more or less fluent, demonstrating differences in relative effort or ease with which speech is produced.

Starkweather indicated that, in our own speech, we recognize fluency by the ease and rapidity with which words are produced and disfluency by production that is slowed down by unexpected effort. In the speech of others, however, we cannot directly feel how easy or difficult speech production is. We must infer this ease of speech fluency from observable events, including the rate (i.e., units per time) at which speech is produced and the continuity (i.e., smoothness) of its output. Both speech rate and continuity are influenced by the information load of the utterance. Information load refers to the "level of uncertainty associated with a transition from one location in an utterance to the next" (Starkweather, 1984, p. 34). Because of the influence of information load on speech fluency and the influence of syntactic structure and word frequency on information load, one must consider a distinction between speech fluency (i.e., motor speech production) and language fluency (i.e., word finding and sentence formulation) (Starkweather, 1984, 1985, 1987). Semantic fluency refers to the ease of retrieving from a large pool of lexical items (i.e., vocabulary words) for reference to many different concepts. Syntactic fluency is the ease with which speakers construct complex sentences containing linguistically complex structures. Pragmatic fluency refers to both knowing and demonstrating what one wants to say within and in response to a variety of situational constraints. Phonologic fluency refers to the ease of producing long and complex strings of sounds within meaningful and complex language units.

The location of stuttering and normal disfluency is influenced by language. For example, stuttering is more likely to occur at clause boundaries, on longer and less frequently used words, and within the context of greater information load. Other influences of language on stuttering are reviewed elsewhere (Starkweather, 1987; Wall & Myers, 1995; Williams, 1978). The point is that speech fluency and language fluency are different, and that most people who stutter demonstrate language fluency. Such people can stutter severely (i.e., demonstrate deficient speech fluency) and still have and use a large repertoire of productive vocabulary (semantic fluency), the ability to construct complex sentences (syntactic fluency), knowledge of what sentences are appropriate given the uniqueness of specific conversational and situational constraints (pragmatic fluency), and knowledge of how sounds are produced and combined in meaningful sentences (phonological fluency). So stuttering is not a disorder of language fluency.

Starkweather (1985, 1987) decried the traditional practice of evaluating stuttering only by counting the frequency of disfluent words and by observing qualitative characteristics including associated struggle. He recommended that the assessment of stuttering should contain an analysis of speech fluency including rate, rhythm, and ease with which the person speaks, as well as the continuity of the speech. An implicit challenge here is to determine when a fluency deviation becomes stuttering. Ham (1990) offered the following definition (revised from Starkweather, 1985):

> Fluency is deviant when planning and/or execution effort is excessive, when discontinuities occur at a frequency and/or to a degree inappropriate for speaker age, or when speech rhythm is atypical or occurs in such a way as to impede or disrupt the speech production. (p. 8)

A closer look at disfluency follows.

Disfluency Vs. Dysfluency

Disfluency and dysfluency are terms that have been used to refer to breaks in the forward flow of speech. Some have referred to disfluency as the nonfluent speech of people who do not stutter, and the nonstuttered yet nonfluent speech of people who do stutter. Dysfluency has referred to the stuttered speech of people who stutter, and the stuttered speech of people who do not usually stutter (Ham, 1990). Making these distinctions, however, has resulted in theoretical encampment of limited practical utility. Starkweather (1987) argued that speech fluency consists of more than just continuity (i.e., smoothness), including effort and rate as well. Disfluency and dysfluency are inadequately descriptive because they do not specify the dimension by which fluency is disrupted. Furthermore, such terms suggest that speech fluency is a dichotomous variable (i.e., that speech either is or is not fluent), rather than the continuous variable that it is (i.e., speech varies in its degree and nature of fluency, as noted earlier). Cooper (1993c) aptly stated:

> Time and effort are being wasted speculating on whether a discrete behavior is a stuttering behavior on the basis of data obtained in assessments of behaviors devoid of any consideration of the affective and cognitive milieu in which the behavior occurs. I am hopeful we have seen the last of studies concerned with differentiating a "disfluency" from a "dysfluency" on the basis of a series of sophisticated psychoacoustical measurements of vocalizations made without respect to the subjects' histories and their affective and cognitive states at the moment of assessment. (pp. 377–378)

For these and other reasons, superficial distinctions between disfluency and dysfluency are avoided in this book. Rather, all events relating to stuttering and people who stutter will be identified, to the extent possible, with terms that generate molecular descriptions.

Stuttering

As noted earlier, there is no universally accepted definition of stuttering. Culatta and Goldberg (1995) concluded that if 10 speech–language pathologists were put in a room, 11 definitions of stuttering would emerge. The divergence of definitions reflects at least a lack of agreement in the attributes considered significant by the definers, and differing hypotheses about the etiology of stuttering upon which the definitions are based (Silverman, 1996). Each definition reflects the kernels of truth considered to be most salient to the author. Wingate (1988) indicated that the reason stuttering is so poorly understood is precisely that so much has been written about it; "the intrinsic mystery of the disorder has been embellished by the many efforts to explain it" (p. 3).

Bloodstein (1990) summarized that traditionally there have been three alternative types of definitions. The first is the observer's perceptual definition—that is, stuttering is whatever observers or conversational partners hear or see it to be. The second is a standard, or dictionary, definition that defines stuttering by other words (e.g., repetition, prolongation, struggle, etc.), each of which is defined by other words. The third is the perceptual definition of people who stutter—that is, stuttering is whatever people who stutter feel their own stuttering to be. Each definition is significant in its impact on the conversational experience. However, Bloodstein acknowledged that speech–language pathologists, in their frequent attempts to count stuttering blocks, have ignored the significance of what the person who stutters perceives to be his own stuttering and have concluded that people who stutter are not as accurate observers of their own stuttering. Furthermore, clinicians and researchers have assumed that stuttering must be reliably countable and that if it is not, something must be wrong. Bloodstein indicated "it may be that stuttering is inherently indeterminate, uncertain, and relative. If so, it should not surprise us that we have not been able to find a definition that allows us to identify unequivocally when or whether a person stutters" (p. 393). It seems obvious that the acoustic event (i.e., the listener perception) allows for greater precision in measurement than the personal or subjective experience of the person who stutters. Perkins (1990b) concurred and questioned, "But does that warrant continued use of listener judgments as valid, or even useful, when the acoustical signal has been demonstrated incontrovertibly to be all but devoid of information about what the stutterer considers to be stuttering?" (p. 404).

So the purpose here in defining stuttering is more than a semantic exercise. The significance of a definition and the process of its construction become clear when one considers the extent to which such a definition establishes the foundation for and generates relevant theories, therapies, and research. Perkins (1990a) indicated that "a definition of stuttering should not only be an explicit reflection of assumptions about the disorder, it should define one's understanding of its basic nature" (p. 370). He expressed concern that invalid definitions generate invalid therapy, theory, and research that are based upon that definition. He stated:

> Definitions, theories, therapies, and research all have underlying assumptions, albeit sometimes obscure. When assumptions are shared, then definitions, research, theories, and therapies are unified in a common conception. Each is logically related to the others. Although each is necessarily predicated on some

> assumption, these assumptions are not always the same. When they are not, as is currently the case for stuttering, then definitional, investigatory, theoretical, and therapeutic domains become unrelated in ways that impair, if not nullify, progress in all domains. Being conceptually disconnected from each other, advances in one domain are not likely to generalize readily to the others. (p. 370)

An example illustrates the significance of a definition and the nature of concern when such a definition is unrelated to its subsequent application. Perkins (1990a) stated:

> The therapies currently in vogue are all related to stuttering as learned, or at least modifiable, behavior. Conversely, research into the nature of stuttering almost entirely reflects the conviction that it is a biologically based disorder with probable genetic origin. This research has not only become disconnected from theory for the most part, but it also now has little relation to therapy. (p. 371)

Others have built similar arguments for the importance of coherent definitions and theories as a foundation to integrated research and treatment efforts (Johnston, 1983; Kent, 1989–1990; Klein & Moses, 1994; Shapiro & Moses, 1989). We will address the importance of theory as a practical guide to fluency intervention and the importance of identifying and understanding the assumptions of all participants in the intervention process. For now, let us return to the task of defining stuttering.

Having said what I have to this point, it would seem futile to attempt to characterize a definition of stuttering. Each definition in existence represents the author's own description of salient characteristics and assumptions about its nature, cause, or both. Definitions must supply the criteria by which similar-appearing items can be included or excluded on the basis of differentiation by characteristics of the definitions (Ham, 1990). Reviewing definitions over history reveals the evolution of our professional thinking about stuttering. Having completed such a review, it seems to me that definitions roughly fall into one of three different categories—descriptive, explanatory, and combined descriptive/explanatory. The word *roughly* is used deliberately. Few definitions are purely descriptive or explanatory. Most contain elements of both. The categories, descriptive and explanatory, might be viewed as anchor points at the two ends of a continuum with most definitions falling somewhere in between. Some definitions are more heavily descriptive, some more heavily explanatory. A few examples are given for illustration.

Descriptive Definitions of Stuttering

Descriptive definitions respond to the question, "What does a person do when he stutters?" These definitions tend to list a variety of audible and occasionally visible behaviors. However, most definitions mention repetitions of sounds and syllables and prolongations of speech sounds (Silverman, 1996). The following is an example of a definition that is more heavily descriptive:

> For introductory purposes stuttering can be defined as a higher frequency of sound, syllable, and one-syllable word disfluency (more irregular in rhythm and averaging two to four repetitions per instance) and prolonged sounds or

postures of the speech mechanism. There may be a disruption of air flow or phonation between repetitions, or a schwa-sounding vowel may be substituted for
the correct one in the repetition of a syllable. There may be other signs of
increased tension in the lips, jaw, larynx, or chest as well as accessory movements of bodily parts not closely associated with speaking. A covert feature of
stuttering includes expectation of difficulty and frustration, which lead to
avoidance and inhibitory behaviors—reactions that can be described by older
children and adults and that may be mentioned by a preschool child. In the latter we can only assume that covert reactions accompany the development of
overt behaviors and are more likely to be present the longer the problem exists.
In keeping with the social nature of speaking, as stuttering persists, the person's self-concept is influenced by the speaking problem, and unadaptive attitudes develop. (Gregory, 1986b, p. 5)

Explanatory Definitions of Stuttering

Other definitions tend to be more explanatory in nature. That is, they address
the question, "Why does a person stutter?" They attempt to provide etiological
justification for the composite of behaviors, feelings, and thoughts. When such
definitions have an etiological basis, they tend to limit the objectivity of
speech–language pathologists' observational skills (Culatta & Goldberg, 1995)
and run the risk of prejudicing the study of stuttering through presumption of
a known cause (Wingate, 1988). Wingate stated directly:

> The fact of the matter remains that the cause of stuttering—its essential
> nature—is unknown. Efforts made toward understanding the nature of stut-
> tering are only obstructed by investigations mounted from a motivation to sup-
> port conjectures. Unfortunately, a considerable amount of stuttering research
> bears this onus. (p. 5)

Culatta and Goldberg (1995) expressed concern that definitions with initial
biasing statements such as, "stuttering is a learned disorder which . . . " or
"stuttering is an emotional disorder which . . . " or "stuttering is a neurologically based disorder which . . . " might lead clinicians to force clients into categories inappropriately. Furthermore, Culatta and Goldberg advised that clinicians cannot, and perhaps should not, escape from their beliefs, but should
avoid prejudgment. The following are examples of explanatory definitions:

- Stuttering is a symptom in a psychopathological condition classified as a
  pregenital conversion neurosis. (Glauber, 1958, p. 78)

- Stuttering, then, is a child's conscientious effort to speak acceptably despite
  a deep conviction that he cannot do so . . . . We may call stuttering a severe
  form of speech consciousness. (Bloodstein, 1958, p. 38)

- Stuttering is the consequence of the young child speaking with his mother
  and father. In his words he sought their appraisal of him. In his utterances
  he asked to be known and to be understood. In their reply they told of his
  unacceptability in his current verbalized form. (Travis, 1971, p. 1009)

Combined Descriptive/Explanatory Definitions of Stuttering

The third category of definitions contains both descriptive and explanatory elements. For example, Van Riper (1982) indicated that "Stuttering occurs when

the forward flow of speech is interrupted by a motorically disrupted sound, syllable, or word or by the speaker's reactions thereto" (p. 15). This definition highlights the audible or otherwise directly visible aspects of stuttering, emphasizes the reactions of the person who stutters, and implies that the cause of stuttering is a disruption in the motor sequence required to produce speech.

Another definition with both descriptive and explanatory elements was proposed by Wingate (1964):

> The term "stuttering" means :
>
> 1. (a) Disruption in the fluency of verbal expression, which is (b) characterized by involuntary, audible or silent, repetitions or prolongations in the utterance of short speech elements, namely: sounds, syllables, and words of one syllable. The disruptions (c) usually occur frequently or are marked in character and (d) are not readily controllable.
>
> 2. Sometimes the disruptions are (e) accompanied by accessory activities involving the speech apparatus, related or unrelated body structures, or stereotyped speech utterances. These activities give the appearance of being speech-related struggle.
>
> 3. Also, there are not infrequently (f) indications or report of the presence of an emotional state, ranging from a general condition of "excitement" or "tension" to more specific emotions of a negative nature such as fear, embarrassment, irritation, or the like. (g) The immediate source of stuttering is some incoordination expressed in the peripheral speech mechanism; the ultimate cause is presently unknown and may be complex or compound. (p. 488)

This definition characterizes stuttering as a disruption of speech fluency taking the form of audible or silent repetitions or prolongations that are frequent or marked in character and not readily controllable. Sometimes the disruption is accompanied by unusual movements of the speech mechanism or other body structure. People who stutter report negative emotional reactions to their disfluent speech. This definition is particularly significant in its specificity, in introducing the concept of "involuntariness" (i.e., being out of control) of the speaker, and in acknowledging that the cause is unknown. The involuntary aspect of disfluency again was addressed as a critical diagnostic aspect by the World Health Organization (1977) and Perkins (1990a, 1990b), among others.

A third illustrative definition of stuttering containing descriptive and explanatory elements was presented by Nicolosi, Harryman, and Kresheck (1996):

> 1. Disturbance in the normal fluency and time patterning of speech. Primary characteristics include one or more of the following: (a) audible or silent blocking; (b) sound and syllable repetitions; (c) sound prolongations; (d) interjections; (e) broken words; (f) circumlocutions; or (g) words produced with an excess of tension. Associated behaviors or secondary characteristics include the habitual use of speech musculature or of other body parts which a stutterer employs along with the primary characteristics; thought to be initiated to release, conceal, or modify the dysfluency. The disturbance may be at the level of neuromuscular, respiratory, phonatory, or articulatory mechanisms.

Dysfluencies are so numerous that they exceed the normal number or degree for the individual's age, sex, or speaking situation.

2. Involuntary repetition and prolongation of speech sounds and syllables, and fluency interruptions, that the individual struggles to end. (p. 261)

This definition presents highly specific behavioral components and introduces the etiology as a timing disturbance. Furthermore, reference is made to events occurring at and involving functions within the neuromuscular, respiratory, phonatory, or articulatory mechanisms.

Stuttering Defined

So, what is stuttering? A frugal response would be "all of the above." Indeed, any current definition of stuttering borrows heavily from present and past comrades (refer back to the Preface for an explanation of *comrades* as used here) in assessment and intervention of speech fluency and stuttering. Two definitions to which I align most closely are those presented by Peters and Guitar (1991) and Cooper (1993c).

Peters and Guitar (1991) defined stuttering as follows:

Stuttering is characterized by an abnormally high frequency and/or duration of stoppages in the forward flow of speech. These stoppages usually take the form of (a) repetitions of sound, syllables, or one-syllable words, (b) prolongations of sounds, or (c) "blocks" of airflow and/or voicing in speech. Individuals who stutter are usually aware of their stuttering and are often embarrassed by it. Moreover, they often use abnormal physical and mental effort to speak. (p. 9)

Peters and Guitar, using terminology from Van Riper (1982), distinguished between core behaviors and secondary behaviors. Core behaviors are the basic, involuntary, observable behaviors of stuttering, including part-word and whole-word repetitions, sound prolongations, stoppage of air, etc. Secondary behaviors are the learned reactions to the core behaviors. Secondary behaviors include escape behaviors (i.e., attempts to exit the stutter and finish the word, such as eye blinks, head nods, interjection of sounds, etc.) and avoidance behaviors (i.e., attempts to prevent stuttering, such as pauses, word changes, hand movements, etc.). Also addressed are the feelings and attitudes of people who stutter. Peters and Guitar made the point that negative feelings may precipitate stuttering and stuttering may precipitate negative feelings (e.g., shame, embarrassment). Therefore, the feelings related to stuttering may be as much a part of the disorder as the observable behaviors. This definition is highly descriptive and inclusive without offering prejudgment about etiology.

Cooper (1993c) captured the essence of stuttering when he stated, "Stuttering is a diagnostic label referring to a clinical syndrome characterized most frequently by abnormal and persistent dysfluencies in speech accompanied by characteristic affective, behavioral, and cognitive patterns" (p. 382). Cooper indicated that the stuttering syndromes (i.e., developmental, remediable, and chronic perseverative) result from multiple coexisting and interacting physiological, psychological, and environmental factors. Cooper stated that stuttering syndromes are multifaceted and consist of characteristic *affective, behavioral,* and cognitive components (the ABCs of stuttering). The significance of any one of these components to an individual who stutters varies over time. Assessment and treatment of people who stutter, therefore, must address the affective, behavioral, and cognitive components. Cooper noted the following:

> While disfluent speech behavior is the most frequently observed characteristic of stuttering syndromes, an individual's affective and cognitive states, irrespective of the presence or lack thereof of observably disfluent speech, may warrant the use of a stuttering syndrome diagnostic label. (p. 383)

For our purposes, stuttering refers to individualized and involuntary interruptions in the forward flow of speech and learned reactions thereto interacting with and generating associated thoughts and feelings about one's speech, oneself as a communicator, and the communicative world in which we live. Etiology, yet unknown, is conceptualized to relate to the interaction of physiological, psychological/psychosocial, psycholinguistic, and environmental factors. Stuttering occurs within the context of communication systems, thus affecting and being affected by all persons who communicate with the person who stutters. Stuttering is a diagnostic label referring to a complex, multidimensional composite of behaviors, thoughts, and feelings of people who stutter. Whether for clinical or research purposes, stuttering should not be studied and cannot be understood without consideration of the person who stutters, the social contexts within which the person communicates, and the interaction of communicative demands and individualized capacities for speech fluency. The implications of this brief definition and its elements will unfold in the pages to follow. The nature of stuttering will be addressed in Chapter 2; etiology and theoretical explanations in Chapter 3; and thoughts and feelings of people who stutter and the significance of communication systems in Chapter 5. Suffice it now to note that understanding the assumptions underlying the thoughts, feelings, and behaviors of people who stutter and of the members of their communication systems is critical. Stuttering does not occur in a communicative vacuum. It must be understood and addressed, therefore, within an individualized, social, and communicatively meaningful context.

Other Terms

A number of other terms often are used when describing aspects of fluency, disfluency, and stuttering. These include, among others, frequency, duration, severity, disfluency type, and associated or secondary behaviors (Conture, 1990a). Frequency of stuttering refers to the number of instances of stuttering per unit of speech (e.g., 100 words of reading or conversational speech). Duration of stuttering refers to the temporal length, usually in seconds for clinical purposes, of an instance of stuttering, often averaged over a randomly selected sample of several instances of stuttering within a speaking context (e.g., reading or conversational speech, word or sentence repetition, etc.). Severity of stuttering is a judgment based on objective measurement of the degree of stuttering demonstrated by a person who stutters. When terms such as *mild, moderate,* or *severe* are used to refer to the severity of a stuttering instance or to the nature of the stuttering observed as a whole, such terms should be defined or qualified to the limits possible. Type of speech disfluency refers to any within-word or between-word hesitations, interruptions, pauses, prolongations, repetitions, and stoppages that are observed in one's speech. Associated or secondary behaviors are those speech (e.g., filler expressions ["Let me see"] or circumlocutions [word changes]) and nonspeech (e.g., pitch changes, eye blinks, head shakes and turns, or hand movements) behaviors that occur with relative consistency during and in learned response to instances of stuttering.

MORE THAN JUST TERMINOLOGY

Stutterer Vs. Stuttering

Our frequent references to people who stutter as *stutterers* in our clinical and research contexts is of considerable concern to me. You might say, "What's wrong with that word?" Some might assume that my concern is merely of semantic origin. It is not. The word *stutterer* equates the person with the disorder. When a person who stutters is asked to describe himself by sharing his personal story (Kent, 1989–1990) or point of view (Williams, 1957), his most frequent responses are, "I stutter" or "I am a stutterer." Indeed, people who stutter come to view themselves as a disorder, focusing more on the DISorder than the disORDER, or the DISability than the disABILITY. I maintain that clinicians prematurely and too often narrowly focus more on the DISfluency than the disFLUENCY. Even more worrisome to me is when professionals share a negative and fractured view of people who stutter. The point is that referring to a person as a stutterer establishes that the disorder captures the essence of the person. The person who stutters is a boy or girl, man or woman, son or daughter, father or mother, boyfriend or girlfriend, spouse, friend, person who goes to school or work, a valued member within a family system and larger community, not just a person who stutters. This is not to minimize the impact that stuttering has on the perceptions and experiences of one who stutters. However, we need to understand how a person who stutters views himself as a person and as a communicator in order to facilitate his understanding, acceptance, and growth in these areas leading to improved and independent communication skills.

When we professionals refer to our clients in spoken or written word as *stutterers,* we tend to acknowledge only one aspect of the person and enable or facilitate maintenance of a narrow view of and by the person who stutters. How often do we say about a client to professional colleagues, "He is a stutterer," or "I've got to get downstairs now to the clinic. My stutterer is coming in"? I maintain that our choice of words reflects our assumptions and attitudes about ourselves, our work, and the people we serve. It might be a valuable and instructive exercise to take note of how you and others refer to each other in the language we use. Later, we will address the significance of hearing and understanding how a person who stutters refers to himself in expressing his point of view (Williams, 1957). Furthermore, we will address the dangers of using a "deficit ledger" (Kent, 1989–1990) in our approach to assessment and intervention with people who stutter. Kent warns that "increasing fragmentation of our clinical perspective—specialization is one word for it—can make the disorder come into focus even as the person goes out of focus" (p. 5). More respectful and empathic use of language views the whole person with dignity (Rush &

The League of Human Dignity, n.d.) and is consistent with recent legislation mandating accommodations and guaranteeing rights for people with exceptionalities (e.g., Federal Rehabilitation Act of 1973, Section 504; Americans with Disabilities Act of 1990 [ADA], P.L. 101-336).

A few simple equations might help remind us of our assumptions and the language we use. A person who stutters is an individual with a unique past, present, and future. Stuttering is a composite of behaviors, feelings, and attitudes defined earlier. You might say that stuttering = disorder; stutterer (i.e., more appropriate description is *person who stutters*) = person. Therefore, stutterer ≠ disorder. For the reasons outlined here, we will deliberately put the whole and able person first by referring to *people who stutter* rather than *stutterers*.

Categorical Vs. Noncategorical Behaviors

When defining fluency above, we distinguished between dichotomous (i.e., categorical, discrete) and continuous (i.e., noncategorical, nondiscrete) variables. We tend to think of speech as fluent or stuttered, incorrectly assuming that these represent categorical behaviors. In fact, both represent noncategorical or continuous variables, which more appropriately should be represented along continua. It may be tempting to think of the following as categorical variables: fluency/disfluency, stuttered speech/nonstuttered speech, normalcy/abnormalcy, order/disorder, ability/disability, truth/falsehood, hot/cold, etc. In reality, however, each set reflects multiple continuous variables, each of which contain numerous points along continua. We will experience a parallel challenge when we attempt to categorize and represent behaviors, thoughts, and feelings of people who stutter. At best, we will define each as molecularly and scientifically possible. However, professional judgment cannot and should not be ignored in the clinical context. Conture (1990a) reminded us that:

> (a) there are no known objective, listener-independent criteria for identifying instances of stuttering or classifying children as stutterers versus normally fluent speakers and (b) there is no consensus among experienced clinicians and researchers regarding behavioral definitions of stuttering in childhood or classification of children as stutterers. (p. 3)

What this means in practical terms is that all clinical interpretations, to a certain extent, are necessarily tentative. This does not mean that we must be reluctant to exercise informed professional judgment. On the contrary, our judgment indeed must be fully informed, yet must demonstrate the flexibility necessary to invite and respond to incoming information and alternative and challenging perspectives.

Fluency Facilitating Controls Vs. Tricks

It is instructive to note that stuttering is variable and intermittent. Van Riper (1982) noted:

> The very intermittency of the disorder compounds the problem. One of our clients said it well: "I can't get used to it. I can't get used to it. I wish I were blind

or deaf or crippled. Then I'd always be that way and though it would be hard I could finally accept it. But the way it is, I talk all right for a bit and then get clobbered. I hope I can talk; I fear I can't; sometimes I can; sometimes I can't. I'm always torn." (p. 2)

People who stutter learn that stuttering varies by time, situation, and language factors. For this discussion, however, I want to note that there are special conditions that immediately eliminate, or at least significantly reduce, stuttering. These include, among others:

- *choral reading*—reading the same text at the same time with a speaker who is fluent

- *lipped speech*—speaking without voicing

- *whispered speech*—speaking with greatly reduced volume

- *prolonged speech with or without Delayed Auditory Feedback*—speaking with an increase in segment duration

- *rhythmic speech*—speaking with a regularly recurring cadence in response to a rhythmic stimulus, such as the beat of a metronome or finger tapping

- *shadowing*—repeating what someone else is saying immediately but not in chorus

- *singing*—replacing the suprasegmentals, or pitch, juncture, intonation, etc., of speech with that of song

- *slowed speech*—reducing the rate by increasing pause time

- *other speech conditions*—speaking in the presence of a loud bilateral masking noise (i.e., 90 dB), with altered pitch (i.e., increased or decreased fundamental frequency), or alone or with a nonhuman listener (Andrews et al., 1983; Williams, 1978)

We will address how such observations can be used in the clinical setting to differentially diagnose stuttering from other disorders of fluency and to facilitate an experience of success that generates motivation among people who stutter. However, the point is that precisely because we know stuttering to be variable (changing based on special conditions), individualized (nonidentical, no two people demonstrate the same stuttering), and intermittent (not consistent), yet predictable (people who stutter report knowing when they are going to stutter), we need to distinguish between fluency facilitating controls and tricks.

In Chapters 8, 9, and 10, which address assessment and treatment with people across the life span who stutter, we will discuss specific fluency facilitating controls. These are clinical procedures used to alter the fluency of one's speech that are communicatively reliable and useful, based on what we know about communication and the role of the communicator, and intended to foster independent communication skills. These might include cancellations, pull-outs, and preparatory sets (Peters & Guitar, 1991; Van Riper, 1973), analysis and facilitation of fluency, speech with soft articulatory contacts and slight prolongation, among other controls.

In contrast to fluency facilitating controls are fluency tricks. I will identify them for your information, but do not recommend them as a centerpiece of treatment. These are behavioral adjustments that temporarily improve fluency, are communicatively unreliable, and potentially form communicative dependence. Such tricks are based on expediency and are not consistent with what we know about communication and the role of the communicator. As noted, they improve fluency only temporarily and often become part of the learned reactions referred to as associated or secondary behaviors. These might include an alteration in one's nature of speaking (e.g., demonstrating a more proper or formal presentation), accent (e.g., sounding British, French, or as though from another country), pitch (e.g., raising or more typically lowering the fundamental frequency of one's voice), etc. These changes are not only temporary; they have secondary risks including damage to the vocal cords (e.g., nodules, contact ulcers, etc.). Other tricks might include interjecting to feign the temporary loss of thought (e.g., "Let me see," "How do you say it," etc.) or movements of the body (e.g., hand, head, foot, whole body, etc.) associated with the anticipation of disfluency. Such tricks have the potential of reducing communicative effectiveness of the message being conveyed. A few examples will illustrate how communication tricks can detract from the effectiveness of the communication message.

Many years ago, I moved to Connecticut to begin my career as a speech–language pathologist. In search of fluency facilitating controls, I still occasionally resorted to tricks for expediency. When talking with a gentleman from England who was to become my landlord, my fluency seemed out of control and I attempted circumlocution (i.e., avoiding certain words by selecting others), phrase insertion to feign lapse of thought (e.g., "Now what was I saying?"), and word retrieval difficulty (e.g., "Let me see. What is that word?"). Circumlocution is a challenging task for a speaker. Not only are lesser feared words substituted for greater feared words, there is an eye-for-an-eye condition (i.e., a noun must be substituted for a noun, a verb for a verb, and so on). Van Riper (1982) indicated that such word selection facilitates the development of very large vocabularies as a result of habitual substitution, and that the speech of people who circumlocute is "so tortuous and strangely imprecise that a listener must work hard to comprehend its meaning" (p. 132). I cannot recall my exact words today, but I do remember responding in an awkward manner when the landlord asked me, "What do you do professionally?" Having some expertise in working with people who stutter, I tried not to blow my cover and stutter all over the well-meaning soul. I tried to convey that I was new in my career, hence the gentleman should be merciful in his determination of the monthly rent. After responding to this man's questions, while trying my best to manage my fluency and his impression, I remember what seemed like an interminable silence. The man furrowed his brow, pulled with one hand on his gray beard and wiped his balding head with the other, looked at me sadly, and said, "Young man, what you just said was remarkably cryptic." He was right. Such tricks, without intervention, often have a snowball effect and become part of an individualized behavioral repertoire.

Some years later, a college student came to me to assess his stuttering. His speech was remarkably fluent with a pronounced southern accent and he demonstrated outstanding interpersonal and social skills. He later revealed that his fluency was dependent upon the accent, one that he had affected to perfection. He referred to this speech as "hillbilly speech." When demonstrating this pattern of speaking, his vowels were lengthened into diphthongs, consonants were produced with gentle articulatory contacts, pitch had tremendous variation, and juncture was so minimized as to approximate the melody of song. His speech was only fluent as long as he maintained this pattern. He expressed that a fluency trick such as this was limiting to him in certain conversational contexts and that he felt like an impostor. He desired, and eventually achieved, more reliable and versatile fluency facilitating controls.

In an advanced stage of stuttering, the associated sequence of secondary behaviors may seem to the untrained observer to be simply bizarre, if not haphazard. However, longitudinal or retrospective analysis of such behaviors indicates their development to be highly systematic and somewhat strategic. The following scenario illustrates this pattern. Some years ago, when working as a speech–language pathologist in the public schools, I met with Alan, a 17-year-old in his junior year of high school. When asked a direct question about his classroom activity, Alan tightly closed then opened his eyes, turned his head abruptly to the left, violently threw his head back again closing his eyes tightly, and rapidly opened and closed his mouth without any audible sounds, all the while demonstrating significant eye, jaw, facial, and neck tension. Bringing his head forward and opening his eyes, still rapidly opening and closing his mouth, Alan then alternated raising his left and right arms, slightly raising himself from his chair while maintaining a seated position, turning himself in the opposite direction of the hand raised. Arm movements became increasingly abrupt with his hand each time, barely missing the back of his head. Verbalizations were rapid when fluent and punctuated by rapid interjection of *schwa* (i.e., *uh*) preceding monosyllable sentence initial words (e.g., uh–uh–uh–uh–uh–I) and repetition of subsequent consonant–vowel combinations (e.g., wuh–wuh–wuh–wuh–wuh want). Intermittent verbalization on inhalation was less disfluent, yet strained and monotone. On the surface, Alan indeed demonstrated a bizarre behavioral repertoire. At an earlier time, closing his eyes was likely to prevent a disfluent episode. When the novelty of that relatively discrete behavior (closing his eyes) and its effect ended, he revised the behavior (tensing then opening his eyes) to achieve the desired outcome. Because the effect of this revised behavior again was temporary, he then chained (i.e., added on) another slightly more noticeable, yet still relatively discrete, behavior (turning his head to the left) to prevent the anticipated experience and consequence of disfluency. This cycle of behavior revision and acquisition continues (e.g., tilting the head back, moving and tensing his mouth, lifting his arms, turning his body) until, in this case, Alan seemed to most conversational partners virtually to be dancing, if not thrashing, in his chair. This story does have a happy ending. Before Alan graduated from high school the following year, he successfully completed the two highest objectives on his personalized hierarchy. Specifically, he demonstrated reliable yet controlled fluency facilitating techniques in two new contexts, without exhibiting the overt associated behaviors. These contexts were working for a political representative in his home state and establishing a dating relationship with a young woman. In addition to achieving heightened communication independence, the impact of the intervention process effected improvements in academic success, personal hygiene, personal motivation, professional aspiration, social adeptness, and interpersonal family and school relationships. How such changes are achieved will be addressed in Chapters 9 and 10.

While the behaviors of people who stutter might seem superficially alike and generally bizarre, they are uniquely sequenced, synchronized, and executed, almost like the wind-up of a professional pitcher. Van Riper (1982) clarified the development of such behaviors as follows:

> Most adult stutterers pass through a whole series of different reaction patterns before they develop the final set which is as unique as their fingerprints. At four years of age, the stutterer may have only syllabic repetitions; at five, postural fixations. By his 11th birthday he could be retching and gasping; by his 16th, his speech may also be punctuated by long pauses. When he is 30, all of these behaviors may be in his stuttering repertoire, and there may also be some head-jerks. But some of these behaviors may also be suddenly discarded or replaced by others less abnormal. We knew one man, at the age of 70, who stopped the struggling and avoiding of many years, and began to stutter easily and with the syllabic repetition of his childhood. He told us he was too tired and too old to stutter so hard any longer. (p. 112)

Van Riper (1982) analyzed further the hierarchical development of such behaviors and described why one behavior is used first and another second or third. He stated:

> We have been able to watch this aspect of the disorder develop in only a few cases, but it is our impression that there are two factors determining the sequence of the various behaviors. First, the final hierarchy often reflects the order in which the coping behaviors were acquired. Those the stutterer adopted first are those that occur first in the sequence; those developed last are the final ones to be tried out as he struggles to utter the word. Second, the behaviors may occur in the order of their social visibility or listener wince-value. Thus the stutterer may use the least conspicuous coping behavior first. If this fails, he uses one that is just a bit more visible or abnormal, and so on until finally he gives up trying to hide his difficulty. It is then that he shows his most bizarre struggle. (p. 113)

Negative Stereotypes, Bias, and Misinformation: Implications for the Clinician

While volumes have been written about stuttering and people who stutter, negative stereotypes, bias, and misinformation continue to be held by classroom teachers, principals, pediatricians, the general public, and most woefully, certified speech–language pathologists (Cooper & Rustin, 1985; Crowe & Walton, 1981; Lass et al., 1992, 1994; Ragsdale & Ashby, 1982; Ruscello, Lass, & Brown, 1988; Silverman, 1982; St. Louis & Lass, 1981; Turnbaugh, Guitar, & Hoffman, 1979; Woods & Williams, 1971, 1976; Yairi & Carrico, 1992; Yairi & Williams, 1970; Yeakle & Cooper, 1986). Typically, people who stutter are stereotyped as submissive, nonassertive persons who are tense, insecure, and fearful. Attribution of such negative personality traits tends to increase with greater degrees of observed stuttering behavior. Since listeners play a major role in shaping the attitudes of people who stutter about themselves as people and communicators, Peters and Guitar (1991) indicated that changing the negative attitudes of people who stutter can be a major focus in treatment. This conclusion is not disputable. Equally urgent, it seems, is to identify the rampant misinformation and bias among potential conversational partners, particularly speech–language pathologists, and to effect change among these persons (Cooper & Cooper, 1985a, 1996; Manning, 1996).

Interaction Between Clinicians' Attitude and Treatment Outcome

Andrews et al. (1983) reported as a statement of fact that "the speech–language pathology profession entertains negative views about stutterers as persons and holds pessimistic views about the benefits of therapy" (p. 234). They indicated the following:

> This research refers to the U.S. speech–language pathology profession, but it is our impression that speech–language pathologists in England, Canada, and Australia have similar views. For 20 years there has been good evidence that stutterers, as people, are no different from anybody else. For 10 years there has been good evidence that a planned and disciplined approach to therapy is effective. Yet these negative stereotypes persist, unsupported by empirical evidence. The authors of this review are neither stutterers nor speech–language pathologists and are at a loss to understand how such negative stereotypes can continue to be believed. We can only surmise that some academics who teach speech–language pathologists have not assimilated the new knowledge and have continued to teach the diagnosogenic/mental health approach to stuttering that was current 30 years ago. (p. 234)

I share the concern expressed by others regarding the negative stereotypes about people who stutter and misinformation about stuttering. Indeed, the level of misinformation about stuttering became all too clear to me when a graduate student of mine conducted a systematic survey of freshmen, sophomores, juniors, and seniors (not studying speech–language pathology) at a regional comprehensive university (Nichols, 1987). She discovered that 30% of the respondents believed that stuttering can be contracted from intimate sexual contact. I am most concerned when I learn of speech–language pathologists' negative biases and stereotypes toward stuttering and people who stutter, along with overall pessimism about the potential benefits of treatment (Cooper & Cooper, 1985a; Manning, 1996; St. Louis & Durrenberger, 1993). Over many years in the workshops I present, I have frequently heard sincere frustration and discouragement from speech–language pathologists regarding the outcomes of their best treatment efforts with people who stutter. Speech–language pathologists report feeling otherwise well trained, yet uncomfortable addressing all of the needs faced by people who stutter and lacking in the necessary clinical and interpersonal (i.e., counseling) skills. When I hear and learn of the negative bias and persistent stereotypes, I become concerned about what we are accomplishing in university training programs, particularly if we only are affecting clinicians' knowledge (i.e., cognitive domain) and behaviors (i.e., behavioral domain) to the exclusion of feelings and attitudes (i.e., affective domain).

Stuttering, it seems, presents unique challenges and confusion. As will be seen, stuttering necessitates that a clinician feel confident and competent to address clients' communication past, present, and future from multiple perspectives (i.e., cognitive, affective, social, academic, professional, etc.). I am concerned also when I see published recommendations, albeit well meaning, that the client be given "a realistic if not pessimistic perception of how successful therapy is going to be" (Starkweather, 1993, p. 163). While a realistic perspective is essential for all participants to embark on effective and individualized treatment, a measure of sincere optimism must be foremost. I do not dispute that our profession must be mindful of how we present ourselves to the public and, in so doing, must avoid explicit and implicit guarantees of the results of treatment (ASHA, 1994a; see Appendix A.2). Nevertheless, a critical ingredient for successful treatment is lacking when the clinician does not sincerely feel good about what she is doing and the potential benefits of treatment.

In discussing three critical variables (in addition to client motivation in the therapy process) for successful treatment with people who stutter, Daly (1988) listed the attitudes and expectations of the clinician as primary. He underscored that "the clinician's attitudes toward stuttering and people who stutter have as much to do with the successful treatment of this disorder as the methods selected for therapy" (p. 34). The clinician must believe in the client, just as the client must believe in the clinician. He supported his statements from the literature on terminally ill cancer patients indicating that a positive attitude toward treatment was a better predictor of treatment outcome than the severity of the illness. Daly urged clinicians to be positive, patient, and persistent with clients who stutter, and err in the direction of optimism rather than pessimism. After years of working with clients who stutter, he concluded, "Clinical experience repeatedly demonstrates that intelligent persons will expend effort and energy in treatment only when they expect substantial results" (pp. 34–35). The clinician must not take lightly the responsibility to manage the client's attitude as well as observable symptoms of disfluency. Surely the clinician's attitude affects that of the client.

The impact of the clinician's attitude on the client's success was eloquently and powerfully conveyed by a former speech–language pathologist, Joysa Gale Post, who became a client after incurring a cerebral vascular accident at age 29 (Post & Leith, 1983). Ms. Post's article should be required reading for all student clinicians and practicing speech–language pathologists. After regaining her communication skills, she conveyed the frequent disappointment that she had experienced with her speech–language pathologists and, in so doing, constructed a number of valuable suggestions. These included conveying sincerity, empathy, caring, enthusiasm, and patience; possessing and demonstrating requisite knowledge in clinical competence and confidence; dressing professionally; maintaining a sense of humor; designing informed, meaningful, and purposeful treatment; and respecting the dignity of the client as a valuable and whole person; among many others. Ms. Post concluded that, "Many clinicians just do not realize how much clients like me depend on them for moral support as well as professional treatment. We want you to care about us as well as care for us" (p. 26). Our attitude and knowledge about stuttering and people who stutter is at least as critical as the services we provide. We can facilitate the process of communication intervention and the development of communication competence by our attitudes, aspirations, and actions, or we can impede such an endeavor. Negative bias about stuttering and people who stutter and pessimism regarding the value of treatment is incisive. Let us not become another obstacle for people who stutter. Rather, in our knowledge, beliefs, and actions, let us lead the way, realistic and sincerely optimistic, to facilitate fluent futures.

Misinformation Begets Misinformation

Another instance in which misinformation seems persistent is in the frequent advice given by professionals in education and allied medical services to concerned parents of children beginning to stutter. The advice usually takes the form of, "Don't worry about it. He will outgrow it." First, telling a parent not to worry is futile, if not insensitive and inappropriate. When you read the fine print, indeed worry is within every parent's job description! Second, while the odds are in favor of those giving the advice that the child will "outgrow it," my concern nevertheless continues to be with those children who become disfluent and develop stuttering, perhaps unnecessarily. Ignoring the issue has proven to be an ineffective yet significant clinical decision. Managing the communication of a young child within the child's communication system through relatively indirect intervention procedures (i.e., knowledgeably facilitating fluency while not drawing attention to the disfluency, as will be discussed in Chapter 8) is not the same as ignoring the issue. Many well-meaning people intending to ignore the disfluency have exacerbated the problem by establishing the child's awareness of fluency breakdown and related feelings. Guy, a man of 63 years with whom I worked clinically for 2 years, spoke during a televised broadcast about having received similar advice. He said:

> My parents shielded me, like any parent would do. And I had seen doctor after doctor and they had always said, "Leave him alone. He'll get over it. Just don't worry with it." Well, I got to be 60 years old and I never had gotten over it. So, I began to think, "When in the world am I supposed to get over this thing?"

During the course of treatment, Guy achieved controlled, reliable fluency and met his objectives of being able to order dinner for his wife, introduce himself on the golf course, and lay read in church. His level of fluency was maintained during the follow-up period of 2 years. The type of intervention Guy received in his later years after a half century of unsuccessful treatment will be discussed in Chapter 10.

Pervasiveness of Negative Stereotypes, Bias, and Misinformation

Why such negativity persists about stuttering and people who stutter is not easily explained and certainly not justified. Likewise, negative interpretations are not confined to the professional literature or service delivery. One needs only to look at the arts and literature within and across cultures to determine that negative stereotypes, bias, and misinformation about stuttering are pervasive. Silverman (1996) noted that, "One way to gain a little insight into how stutterers are viewed in a particular culture is to observe how they are portrayed in the arts and literature of that culture" (p. 26). For example, representations of stuttering and people who stutter depicted in children's literature, novels, movies, dramas, opera, and newspaper headlines have been analyzed (Anderson, 1995; Benecken, 1995; Bushey & Martin, 1988).

Bushey and Martin reviewed 20 works of children's fiction in which a character stutters. They found that stuttering typically was represented as severe with visible struggle (i.e., frequent behavioral symptoms described with words such as speechless, choking, painful, rocking on feet, hopping, and squinting), increasing with emotional upset and nervousness (e.g., talking with strangers, in class, and authority figures), and learned primarily in an unhealthy home and parental environment (e.g., parental separation or divorce, distant or uninterested parents, or death of a parent). Of most concern, however, was that in not a single book was the child being seen or recommended to be seen by a speech–language pathologist. Only one depicted a child receiving professional services (that of a psychiatrist). In others, the stuttering disappeared when the character achieved physiological maturity, gained inner strength, began to think about or help other people, or gained moral strength or courage. In other words, stuttering was not depicted as treatable. About stuttering in children's literature, Bushey and Martin (1988) concluded the following:

> The appearance of these nonspecific, unsystematic, and highly improbable "cures" for stuttering reflected in children's fiction suggests that many people may not view stuttering as a routinely "treatable" problem, and further, that many people may harbor the view that when the unhealthy psychological milieu surrounding stuttering is made healthy, the stuttering will disappear. (pp. 249–250)

Similarly, Benecken (1995) reviewed 19 movies, 23 novels, and 13 children's books. Results indicated that people who stutter are portrayed as unattractive males, neurotic or even psychopathologic, and in subordinate roles, characterized by the following:

> a rather soft, unattractive, rather frail, pinched, subordinating, perhaps thinking about murdering somebody, sexually deprived, possibly perverted man with pimples or nibbled fingernails, if of a tall build, then with a baby face. Mostly he is not married or still as a mother's darling in unsolved symbiosis. . . . Not as I actually expected, the clown or the idiot. His bondage is the central issue, he subordinates himself, and normally he isn't acknowledged, but gets beaten. Almost never you find a stuttering man in a happy leading position, as father and husband, to say nothing of a hero. (p. 548)

Presenting a somewhat contrasting perspective, Anderson (1995) reviewed historical perceptions of stuttering as reflected in the arts, specifically films, operas, and novels, and concluded the following:

> It cannot be denied that stuttering has been associated with comedy over the centuries. Interpretation is often up to the reader or to the audience, but most of the characters discussed are comic characters, not buffoons. It is striking that these authors, and their societies, do not depict stutterers as members of some societal "underclass": they are a lawyer, a trusted advisor to an aristocrat, a humble but well-loved sailor, and a respected and erudite musician. . . . Perhaps these fictional portrayals argue that the often encountered stereotype of the stutterer may be held more by stutterers themselves than by society. (pp. 569–570)

The Impact of Stuttering

Stuttering and intervention with people who stutter potentially can have a global impact. Spoken communication is a complex, dynamic experience between no less than two conversational partners. Both published and anecdotal records indicate that stuttering, a significant and universal disorder of communication, continues to intrigue and fascinate, if not elude, student clinicians, professional speech–language pathologists, and clinical researchers. In light of the other human problems including poverty, hunger, disease, and war, among others, one might question why so much time and energy should be devoted to the alleviation of an individual's communication disorder. The answer is not as simple as might be suggested in a brief response. It has to do with heightening one's communication competence within a communicative milieu and strengthening the effectiveness of communication within and between all potential conversational partners. Another part of the response has to do with social consciousness, feeling in part responsible for the ills that afflict others—being committed to search for solutions, realizing in a communicative sense that we might be our brother's keeper. Perhaps such an influence on individuals and those with whom we communicate could reduce the human problems of intolerance and injustice, thus impacting those noted above.

Then one is likely to question why, of all the communication disorders, should so much effort be devoted to understanding and addressing stuttering. After all, while an instance of stuttering is a temporal and temporary interruption, it does not last forever. It is intermittent and inconsistent, not permanent. Van Riper (1972) pointed out that no one ever dies from a moment of stuttering. Understanding stuttering is difficult. I do not believe that "those who have not possessed or been possessed by the disorder" (Van Riper, 1982, p. 1) cannot work effectively with people who stutter. As will be seen, personal experience can sensitize, but it also can bias. Above all, we need to come to understand the uniqueness of each person who stutters as a person and as a communicator, a member of a communicative network. The potential complexity and unique magnitude of stuttering might lie in its impact on individual speakers and all people with whom they communicate. Stuttering potentially affects all communicative and psychoemotional aspects of a person.

Stuttering and Articulation

Stuttering can affect the articulation of one's speech. A person who stutters might demonstrate inappropriate articulatory targets—that is, forming a posture with the articulators that is not appropriate for the target sound within the target word. For example, if a person who stutters is trying to say the *b* in "The *boy* is . . . ," the appropriate target would be the voiced bilabial plosive (*b*). If this person were observed to be blocked with an open mouth and the back of the tongue raised, this back, velar position (*g, k*) would be considered inappropriate. It is noteworthy that people who stutter often do not realize that they are blocking on the wrong sound. If they are going to block, block on the right sound! Most people who do not stutter repeat syllables by retaining the correct vowel within the repetition (*bo, boat*). People who stutter tend to repeat an inappropriate vowel (*buh, buh, boat*).

Stuttering and Language

Another impact is seen in the reciprocal relationship between stuttering and language. In other words, stuttering affects language and language affects stuttering. We already noted the tendency for word substitution, or circumlocution, resulting from the ability of people who stutter to predict the words on which they will and will not stutter (as well as the people with whom and situations within which they will and will not stutter). Van Riper (1982) discussed how people who stutter develop word fears and indicated that because of their need for synonyms, "some stutterers have developed supervocabularies" (p. 154). This is an influence of stuttering on language. Language also influences stuttering (Starkweather, 1987; Williams, 1978), as seen in the following paragraph.

Stuttering occurs more often at the beginnings of sentences; on words positioned early in a sentence than on words positioned later; on nouns, verbs, adjectives, and adverbs (lexical words) than on function words for adults; on conjunctions and pronouns than on nouns and interjections for children; on longer than shorter words; on words beginning with consonants than with those beginning with vowels—a pattern hypothesized to relate more with the nature of the English language than with stuttering; on the first syllable of the word than on later syllables; on less frequently used words, but only when the sentences are syntactically more simple; on stressed than on unstressed syllables; at points of high information load—that is, propositional value; on words toward the beginning of long sentences than on the same words when they are at the beginning of short sentences; on emotionally loaded material than on emotionally neutral material; at locations where language formulation is occurring, etc. The point is that stuttering and language affect each other.

Stuttering and Voice

Stuttering also affects voice. Consider the strain observed in the voice of a person who stutters trying to say the *a* in *apple* or the *h* in *hello*. The voice cracks and bursts of air are audible, sounding like frying bacon. This is vocal fry. Or consider the increase in pitch that accompanies vocal strain, rendering a prolongation with rising pitch. Just like a guitar string that tightens or shortens, the vocal cords tense and/or shorten, causing the pitch increase. Clearly the suprasegmental aspects of speech (rate, pitch, juncture, melody, etc.) are affected as well. This is vocal tension.

Stuttering and Functioning in Society

Stuttering affects one's participation within socially and culturally determined roles. The boy who must cope after the caller hangs up the phone because he cannot say hello; the woman who must cope after she is passed over for promotion because she cannot speak fluently to her subordinates; the man who must cope with the fact that he has chosen factory work to avoid having to speak with people; the girl who must cope with ordering a vanilla ice cream because she knows she will be unable to say strawberry in front of her boyfriend; the child who must cope after responding "I don't know" to a question from the teacher because he knows he cannot say fluently the answer that he does know well; the young man who must cope when the young woman turns him down for a date after he struggled valiantly with the invitation, and so on. Stuttering rallies coping skills and potentially affects the psychological and emotional makeup, educational achievement, and professional aspiration of people who stutter. Guy ordered dinner for his wife in a restaurant for the first time in their 40-year marriage after 2 years of fluency treatment. He reported for the first time feeling in control. "For the first time in my life, I feel like I can wear the pants in this family." While this statement would raise more than an eyebrow in this time of gender equity (Shapiro, 1994b) and heightened awareness and appreciation of nonsexist language, its sentiment conveys the impact of stuttering on a person's functioning within society.

Stuttering and Interpersonal Relationships

Stuttering also affects the emotions and dreams of all members of the communication system within which a person who stutters communicates. Mothers and fathers ask, if not plead (by their questions and silence), to be reassured that they did not cause their child's stuttering and that there is hope for their child's fluency future. Guy's wife, a most dignified and polite woman, tearfully expresses concern that she is being misjudged as bold, while in fact she is terribly shy, because she speaks for Guy rather than watching him struggle. The wife of a new client candidly expresses her desire to help the process of her husband's fluency enhancement, but is fearful that once he becomes communicatively independent, "he won't find me attractive any longer." Interestingly, her feelings of perceived attractiveness were related to the extent and contexts in which she felt needed. Stuttering affects interpersonal relationships and reminds us that intervention is not just with a person who stutters, but with all people within the communication network. This might involve spouses, boyfriends, girlfriends, young and adult children and siblings, relatives, parents, teachers, coworkers, and allied educational (counselors, music directors, coaches, etc.) and medical (physicians, nurses, counselors, therapists, etc.) personnel. Working with people who stutter is a responsibility of considerable magnitude.

CHAPTER SUMMARY AND DISCUSSION

This chapter introduced the nexus (i.e., the essence or core) of stuttering and the perspective that stuttering represents a multidimensional and manageable composite of behaviors, thoughts, and feelings. Implications for intervention include that the person who stutters should be viewed as a whole, unique person and communicator functioning within a communication system. Intervention should involve actively not only the client, but other members of the communication system and the interdisciplinary team. Assessment and treatment emphasize communication strengths rather than weaknesses and focus on facilitation rather than rehabilitation. Clinicians must understand their clients' assumptions about communication and themselves as communicators because these represent filters through which the clients interpret and anticipate interactions within their communication world.

While there seems to be general agreement that people are not talking fluently when they stutter, actual definitions of fluency and stuttering are based inherently on the individual's assumptions about the nature and etiology of stuttering. Fluency is viewed along continua reflecting the ease with which speech is produced, rather than as a dichotomy reflecting the presence or absence of stuttering. In addition, fluency can be divided into both speech fluency and language fluency, with the latter including semantic, syntactic, pragmatic, and phonologic fluency. Most people who stutter exhibit language fluency, but have deficits in the area of speech fluency. A brief historical review of definitions of stuttering reveals that most definitions describe stuttering, explain why stuttering occurs, or fall somewhere in between, containing both descriptive and explanatory elements. For the purposes presented in this book, stuttering was defined as referring to individualized and involuntary interruptions in the forward flow of speech and learned reactions thereto interacting with and generating associated thoughts and feelings about one's speech, oneself as a communicator, and the communicative world in which we live. Etiology, yet unknown, was conceptualized to relate to the interaction of physiological, psychological, psychosocial, psycholinguistic, and environmental factors.

Concern was expressed over the use of the word *stutterer* rather than the phrase *person who stutters. Stutterer* reduces the individual person to a simple description of the disorder, rather than recognizing each as a whole person functioning within many roles in today's society who also happens to stutter. As professionals, we need to be aware of our assumptions and associations connected to the terms we use to refer to others. These terms may be indicative of negative stereotypes and bias, which can have a detrimental effect on intervention. In particular, a pessimistic view of the outcome of therapy may be communicated to the client. Instead, clinicians must hold and communicate a sincerely optimistic view and be ready to provide moral support and encouragement as a part of skillful and sensitive intervention.

Because stuttering potentially affects every aspect of a person's life, intervention *with* (not for) the person who stutters should encompass all areas of speech–language and communication. For example, stuttering may affect articulation when the person shapes the articulators into a posture that is inappropriate for the sound he is targeting on which he is experiencing a block. Tendencies toward circumlocution may result in the development of "supervocabularies." Stuttering also may affect voice as the person tenses the vocal cords while trying to utter a sound. In addition, stuttering may affect the individual's functioning in society and interpersonal relationships. People who stutter make choices based on their perceived relative ability to handle certain social situations, thereby affecting professional aspirations and educational achievements. Because interpersonal relationships are affected, intervention does not just impact the person who stutters, but others within his communicative network as well.

Stuttering, although defying explanation, defines who a person is and has a profound impact on one's life. Johnson (1930) articulated the impact of stuttering on his life:

> I am a stutterer. I am not like other people. I must think differently, act differently, live differently—because I stutter. Like other stutterers, like other exiles, I have known all my life a great sorrow and a great hope together, and they have made me the kind of person that I am. An awkward tongue has molded my life. (p. 1)

Before looking further at stuttering and people who stutter, Van Riper's (1972) words continue to present an inspiration and challenge to speech–language pathologists today:

> When we deal with speech, we deal with the essence of man. Only human beings have mastered speech. It is what sets us apart from all other species. Because we can speak, we can think symbolically; and it is this which has enabled man to conquer the world and space and every other creature. Dimly we believe or at least hope that someday it may enable us to master ourselves. (p. 5)

Chapter 1 Study Questions

1. Many definitions exist for stuttering. How would you answer the question, "What is stuttering?" when asked by a client, parent, or another professional?

2. Stuttering potentially impacts the communicative exchange with a variety of communication partners. How might stuttering affect not only a person who stutters, but his communicative partners? Consider a broad range of partners, social settings, and communication contexts, in addition to your own personal experiences with people who stutter.

3. Negative attitudes toward stuttering and people who stutter continue to exist among the general population, allied health and education professionals, and woefully, student clinicians and professional speech–language pathologists. Why do you believe such negative attitudes persist and what can be done about this situation? What can you do as a speech–language pathologist, and how do such a situation and potential strategies relate to ASHA's Code of Ethics (ASHA, 1994a; see Appendix A.2) and Scope of Practice in Speech–Language Pathology (ASHA, 1996b; see Appendix A.4)?

4. Clinical intervention is a multidimensional experience involving a variety of key participants. In what ways might the thoughts, feelings, and attitudes of each impact each other and the process and outcome of treatment?

5. People who stutter develop a variety of techniques to cope with stuttering. What are some of these techniques? How do they impact the behavioral, cognitive, and affective domains? How are such techniques addressed in intervention? Why is it important for clinicians and clients to understand the difference between fluency facilitating controls and communication tricks?

Unit I

◆ ◆ ◆ ◆ ◆ ◆ ◆ ◆ ◆ ◆ ◆ ◆ ◆ ◆ ◆ ◆ ◆ ◆ ◆

Stuttering in Relief:
A Foundation
for Intervention

Chapter 1
The Nexus of Stuttering: An Introduction

Chapter 2
The Onset, Development, and Nature of Stuttering

Chapter 3
Etiology and Treatment of Stuttering: Past and Present

Chapter 4
Other Fluency Disorders

Chapter 2

The Onset, Development, and Nature of Stuttering

◆ ◆ ◆ ◆ ◆ ◆ ◆ ◆ ◆ ◆ ◆ ◆ ◆ ◆ ◆ ◆ ◆ ◆ ◆

Knowledge and Assumptions Ground Understanding   34

The Onset and Development of Stuttering   35

Bluemel   37

Froeschels   37

Van Riper   37

Track 1 Onset   37

Track 1 Development   40

Track 2 Onset   40

Track 2 Development   40

Track 3 Onset   41

Track 3 Development   41

Track 4 Onset   41

Track 4 Development   42

Bloodstein   42

Phase 1   42

Phase 2   42

Phase 3   42

Phase 4   44

Summary and Extension—Onset and Development of Stuttering   44

The Nature of Stuttering   46

Types of Disfluency   46

Symptoms, Prevalence, and Incidence   46

What do we know about the speech of young children and particularly the symptoms of stuttering at its onset?   46

When does stuttering develop?   47

How prevalent is stuttering and what is the likelihood of recovery?   47

What about the male:female ratio for stuttering and how widespread is stuttering?   48

Does stuttering result from one's environment?   48

What is stuttering like in its developed form?   49

Differences Between People Who Stutter and Those Who Do Not   49

What is known about the intelligence of people who stutter?   49

Do people who stutter have a different personality?   50

Do children who stutter show a different pattern of speech and language development?   50

Does the central nervous system of people who stutter work differently?   50

Variability and Predictability of Stuttering   51

What commonalities are there among people who stutter?   51

Treatment   52

What does the clinical literature tell us about designing effective treatment?   52

Summary—Nature of Stuttering   53

Chapter Summary   53

Chapter 2 Study Questions   56

The possibilities of exercising creativity in refining our understanding of the problem of stuttering are far from exhausted, and therefore there are kinds of disagreement among those seeking to comprehend the problem that can hardly be other than reassuring to the duly perceptive. They are evidence of continuing investigation, even, in certain instances, of the outcroppings of constructive ingenuity. So long as this continues to be true, there would seem to be cause for glad anticipation of the future, and so for present joy within reason.

(JOHNSON, 1958A, P. XXIV)

KNOWLEDGE AND ASSUMPTIONS GROUND UNDERSTANDING

An understanding of stuttering—of how it begins and develops, its nature, how it has been viewed historically, and current theoretical explanations regarding its etiology—is a critical foundation for a clinician to develop confidence and competence in designing and implementing effective intervention with people who stutter. In Chapter 1, we emphasized the importance of cohesion within and across assumptions underlying stuttering-related domains including definitions, theories, therapies, and research. A lack of such cohesion impedes the treatment process and the extent to which advances in one domain generalize to others. A clinician's understanding of stuttering is necessary to develop and refine such assumptions.

These assumptions form a clinician's personal construct, a dynamic and generative perspective or point of view on communication, stuttering, and people who stutter. All clinicians have a personal construct about their profession and the roles and responsibilities of the participants within it. In fact, all people have, albeit often implicitly, personal constructs regarding all aspects of life. More to the point, not all clinicians are explicitly aware of their own assumptions, thus risking the relatedness between what they know, or assume to be true, and what they do, or how they design and implement assessment and treatment. For example, many clinicians assume that stuttering must be understood on the bases of overt (i.e., observable behaviors) and covert (i.e., internalized thoughts, feelings, and beliefs) phenomena, that the person who stutters should and is able to participate actively in the change process, and that stuttering occurs within communication in social settings. Add to these assumptions a person who stutters and who demonstrates negative, if not destructive, feelings and attitudes toward himself as a communicator. It makes little clinical sense in such a case to embark on a program of strict fluency shaping, in which speech behaviors are addressed to the exclusion of feelings and attitudes, the person who stutters is only passively engaged in the treatment process, and all activities focus on the treatment setting. This is lacking in ecological validity with respect to the person being served and inhibiting transfer to meaningful communicative contexts.

I am concerned that the treatment just described is frequently implemented. My concern is that the design of such treatment is unrelated to the unique strengths and needs of the person who stutters and the assumptions held by the clinician and the client. One's knowledge and assumptions are the bases for interpreting events and planning and implementing assessment and treatment. Williams (1957) indicated the centrality of clients' and clinicians' assumptions when he stated, "It is recognized that one cannot discuss a 'way of thinking' about a particular problem such as stuttering without implying, either implicitly or explicitly, certain assumptions about the nature of that problem" (p. 390). Amplifying the clinical importance of these assumptions, Johnson (1939) stated, "So long as an individual retains and operates on assumptions regarding stuttering and speech, which are characteristic of stutterers, he will not become the sort of individual we refer to as a normal speaker" (p. 172).

Therefore, an understanding of stuttering is a necessary foundation for approaching the challenge and privilege of working with people who stutter. Silverman (1996) warned that clinicians who remain unaware of how stuttering has been treated in the past (i.e., I add how stuttering begins and develops, its nature, and theories about its etiology) are more likely to use intervention strategies that have been shown repeatedly to be of little long-term value. These strategies, he cautioned, may produce rapid reduction in stuttering severity, "but the vast majority of clients on whom they are used are likely to relapse within five years following termination of therapy" (p. 10). So, the purpose of this and subsequent chapters in Unit I is to provide a foundation for such an understanding. To do so, the onset, development, and nature of stuttering are covered in this chapter; etiology and treatment from past and present perspectives in Chapter 3; and other fluency disorders in Chapter 4.

THE ONSET AND DEVELOPMENT OF STUTTERING

There is little debate that stuttering behaviors often change and develop over time. Yet still defying adequate explanation is the observation that a large number of children who begin to stutter cease to do so without treatment. Estimates of such cases vary considerably (23% to 80%—Andrews et al., 1983; 36% to 79%—Bloodstein, 1995; 50% to 80%—Peters & Guitar, 1991; 17.8% to 94%—Van Riper, 1982). The differences in the rates of spontaneous recovery are explained by several factors. Many studies are based on retrospective self-reports of people who stutter. These people may have been told by their parents that they stuttered, but in actuality were no more disfluent than children who do not stutter (Peters & Guitar, 1991). Van Riper (1982) indicated that retrospective reports regarding the child's age and related conditions at the time of stuttering onset contain error because of parents' lapse in memory, need to respond to frequent questions about what caused the disorder, and erroneous assumption that correlation infers causality (i.e., assuming that one event causes another because they occur at the same time). Furthermore, there are differences in the size of the group studied and methodology within the investigations (self-reports vs. longitudinal investigations) (Peters & Guitar, 1991) and ambiguities in the defining characteristics of *stuttering* and *spontaneous recovery* (Bloodstein, 1995). The remainder of this section, however, addresses those who continue to stutter.

Stuttering itself is a dynamic composite of behaviors, thoughts, and feelings. Van Riper (1982) indicated that new behaviors replace or join the original ones. The new behaviors can be understood only within the context of how they developed. Ham (1990) stated that changes in stuttering behavior are affected by altered motor skills, self-awareness, reactions to the disfluency, and reactions to the responses of others. Many attempts have been made to describe the evolution of stuttering on the basis of developmental stages. While such attempts provide valuable descriptions of behavior, they all fail inevitably because there are clients whose speech behavior and development of stuttering cannot be classified neatly into predetermined categories. Developmental classification systems suggest an oversimplification of behavior, that the variables to be considered are unidimensional and dichotomous in nature. We noted in Chapter 1 that this simplification is unrealistic and fails to represent adequately the multidimensionality inherent to human communicative behavior. Van Riper indicated his discomfort with existing classification schemes, including his own, and described attempts to design such systems as "sheer folly" (1982, p. 92). Trying to account for all people who stutter and the uniqueness of communication behaviors, developers of classification schemes could result in an infinite number of minimally differentiated categories. Van Riper (1982) cautioned, however, as follows:

> This does not mean that the beginning stutterer should be treated in the same way we would treat him after he has learned to struggle or avoid. It means that our treatment should fit his needs as shown by his current behaviors, including their history; it should not be a prescribed treatment appropriate only to the child's classification in a developmental category. (p. 92)

Having cautioned to the limitations in classifying the development of stuttering, such systems nevertheless provide valuable descriptions for building understanding among professional clinicians. In other words, it is essential to know how stuttering frequently develops in order to have a point of comparison for detecting the uniqueness in each client's experience. The categories must not be interpreted as confining or rigid; they provide a general picture that might serve as a point of departure. Emerick and Haynes (1986) underscored this point and warned against the "recent article syndrome" (p. 13) and "hardening of the categories" (p. 66). In both of these errors, clinicians attempt to fit people into categories, rather than maintaining clinical flexibility, addressing each person on the bases of individual strengths and needs.

Several examples of classification systems are summarized below in order to suggest what we know about the development of stuttering. Most of our knowledge has resulted from cross-sectional investigations. Our understanding would be heightened considerably by longitudinal investigations of how stuttering behavior begins and develops over time (Bloodstein, 1995; Van Riper, 1982; Wall & Myers, 1995). For the time being, you will notice similarities yet different areas of emphasis across the different descriptions. Again, these are provided to build an understanding of how stuttering emerges and how your client's behavior might relate to the patterns presented.

Bluemel

Bluemel (1932, 1935, 1957), a medical doctor, introduced the terms "primary" and "secondary" stuttering, still heard today, to distinguish two stages of the disorder. Primary stuttering refers to the most incipient stage, consisting of easy, effortless repetitions of the first word or syllable of a sentence, behaviors that are intermittent yet recurring. Secondary stuttering begins after a period of no observed disfluency for several years or after the child is made aware of or embarrassed by the stuttering. Secondary behaviors are more forceful and consistent and contain learned fears and motor behaviors, characterized by physical effort, use of starters and synonyms, attempts to conceal stuttering, and observed fear of letters, words, people, and related speech contexts. Bluemel viewed stuttering as a habit learned as a consequence of conditioning. Intervention to discover the answer to "the riddle of stuttering" (1957) was to be found in psychotherapy.

Froeschels

In a series of papers, Froeschels (1956, 1964) indicated that the onset and development of stuttering can be observed as a consistent progression from initially effortless syllable and word repetitions that become more rapid, irregular, tense, and inhibited. Speech rate increases at first and then decreases as the disfluency worsens, generating avoidance reactions and deliberateness from the child. Froeschels distinguished between tonic and clonic types of stuttering. Namely, tonic stuttering is characterized by hard pressure and tension (i.e., sustained contraction of the speech muscles), often resulting in breathing interruption, grimaces, and clenching; clonic stuttering is more repetitive and oscillatory, resulting in syllable and sound repetitions.

Van Riper

Van Riper (1982) expanded on Bluemel's (1932, 1935) work, adding a transitional stage between primary and secondary stuttering, and eventually adding an entire fourth category. After reviewing client folders, Van Riper (1982) reported that 41 of the 44 longitudinal cases (93%) followed from onset of stuttering to maturity and 187 of the 256 shorter term cases (73%) fell roughly into one of these four tracks of development. For each track, he described the onset and patterns of subsequent development (pp. 94–108). See Tables 2.1 and 2.2, as well as the paragraphs that follow, for a summary.

Track 1 Onset

This was the most frequent pattern of development (48% of the longitudinal histories—21 of 44; 55% of the shorter observations—141 of 256). Children in this track begin speech development with normal sounding and integrated speech fluency, rate, and articulation. Stuttering begins gradually between 2.5 and 4.0 years of age with long periods of remission. These children demonstrate the greatest inconsistency in development, showing a behavior characteristic of the

Table 2.1. Onset Characteristics

Track 1	Track 2
Begins 2½ to 4 years.	Often late. At time of first sentences.
Previously fluent.	Never very fluent.
Gradual onset.	Gradual onset.
Cyclic.	Steady.
Long remissions.	No remissions.
Good articulations.	Poor articulations.
Normal rate.	Fast; spurts.
Syllabic repetitions.	Gaps, revisions, syllable, and word repetitions.
No tension; unforced.	No tension.
No tremors.	No tremors.
Loci: First words, function words.	Loci: First words, long words; scattered throughout sentence; content words.
Variable pattern.	Variable pattern.
Normal speech is well integrated.	Broken speech with hesitation and gaps even when no disfluency.
No awareness.	No awareness.
No frustration.	No frustration.
No fears; willing to talk.	No fears; willing to talk.

Track 3	Track 4
Any age after child has consecutive speech.	Late, usually after 4 years.
Previously fluent.	Previously fluent.
Sudden onset, often after trauma.	Sudden onset.
Steady.	Erratic.
Few short remissions.	No remissions.
Normal articulation.	Normal articulation.
Slow, careful rate.	Normal rate.
Unvoiced prolongations.	Unusual behaviors.
Laryngeal blockings.	
Much tension.	Variable tension.
Tremors.	Few tremors.
Beginning of utterance after pauses primary.	First words; rarely on function words; content words especially.
Consistent pattern.	Consistent pattern.
Normal speech is very fluent.	Normal speech is very fluent.
Highly aware.	Highly aware.
Much frustration.	No frustration.
Fears speaking; situation and word fears.	No evidence of fear; willing to talk.

Note. From *The Nature of Stuttering* (2nd ed.) (p. 106), by C. Van Riper, 1982, Englewood Cliffs, NJ: Prentice-Hall. Copyright 1982 by Allyn & Bacon. Reprinted with permission.

most advanced form one day, then returning to gentle syllabic repetitions or normal disfluency the next. Behaviors characteristic of this track include frequent gentle syllabic repetitions (without schwa, averaging 3 to 5 per word) on initial and function words. The repetitions occur in clusters, followed by considerable normal fluency. No tension or tremors are noted. The child demonstrates no awareness of or frustration over the disfluency and no speech-related fears. Therefore, the child talks without any perceived interference.

Table 2.2. Developmental Characteristics

Track 1	Track 2
Repetitions of syllables increase in frequency and speed and become irregular.	Behaviors remain the same but the speed increases; their number also increases.

Then:

Repetition of syllables begin to end in prolongations.	Little change in form.

Then:

Prolongations show increased tension, tremors, struggle. Evidence of frustration.	Little change; little awareness; little frustration.

Then:

Overflow of tension; facial contortions; retrials; speech output decreases; signs of concern.	Duration of nonfluencies increases; more syllabic repetitions; little awareness.

Then:

Word fears and avoidance occur. Fears of certain sounds arise. Then situation fears develop. Repetitions and prolongations turn into silent fixations with struggle (blocking). Poor eye contact and tricks to disguise the difficulty are observed. Shows hesitancy, embarrassment.	Occasional fears of situations, not of words or sounds. Long strings of syllabic repetitions at fast speed are added to other behaviors. Some fears of situations. Good eye contact. No disguise. Output of speech increases. Little avoidance. Primarily repetitive. Unorganized.

Track 3	Track 4
An increase in the frequency but the behavior at first changes little. Signs of frustration.	The number of instances increases, and they are shown in more situations.

Then:

More retrials are seen; lip protrusions, and tongue fixations appear; prolongations of initial sounds.	Little change in form; monosymptomatic and symbolic.

Then:

Tremors; struggling; facial contortions; jaw jerk, gasping; marked frustration.	Little change.

Then:

Interruptor devices become prominent; rate slows; more hesitancy; more refusals to talk.	Little change in type but duration and visibility increase; no interruptors or new forcings; increased output of speech.

Then:

Intense fears of words and sounds; many avoidances; patterns change in form and grow more bizarre; much overflow; output of speech decreases; will cease trying to talk. Poor eye contact; the normal speech becomes hesitant. Nonvocalized blockings are frequent. Primary tonic blocks with multiple closures.	Very few avoidance or release behaviors. Not much evidence of word fears. Few consistent loci. Very aware of stuttering. Stutters very openly. Good eye contact. Little variability in the stuttering behavior. Normal speech very fluent. Talks a lot. Consistent pattern; few silent blockings. Either tonic or clonic.

Track 1 Development

Syllable repetitions increase in rate and frequency and their rhythmic pattern becomes less regular. Prolongations start to appear at the end of the repetitions and begin to demonstrate increased disruption (i.e., tension, tremor, struggle). Vowels within the syllables being repeated begin to be prolonged. Pitch increases indicative of laryngeal tension during prolongation are often observed. Prolongations move forward, from the final repeated syllable of a series to the initial syllable. Frustration and concern become evident and there is a general overflow of tension indicated by facial contortion, retrials, and decreased speech output. As this pattern develops, word fears and avoidance occur. These fears lead to sound fears, then situation fears. Repetitions and prolongations increase in frequency and complexity, becoming silent fixations with associated struggle behavior. Breathing during speech is interrupted, and rate of speech slows considerably. Eye contact is noticeably interrupted and avoidance tactics are observed as a consequence of fear. The child shows embarrassment over speaking and therefore develops reluctance. Ultimately, patterns of stuttering behavior, both overt and covert, become stabilized and stereotyped. Stuttering enters into the child's self-concept, affecting personality factors and establishing defenses.

Track 2 Onset

This track is the second most frequent pattern of development of stuttering (25% of the longitudinal histories—11 of 44; 12% of the shorter observations—31 of 256). The onset of stuttering is gradual but occurs later, coinciding typically with a delayed and disorganized onset of connected speech (phrases or sentences are not observed until between 3 and 6 years of age). Development of stuttering is more steady, without remission. Unlike the child in Track 1, the child in this track was never very fluent, demonstrating irregular and rapid rate of speech and relatively poor articulation. Syllabic repetitions are hurried and irregular, and monosyllabic word repetitions constitute the majority of the repetitions. Later, there are more silent gaps and hesitations, revisions, and interjections. Disfluencies tend to occur on first words, longer words, and generally distribute throughout the sentence and on content words. The pattern of speech is more variable, typically demonstrating broken speech with hesitation and gaps even when there is no disfluency. Prolongation and fixation are rare, but children demonstrating this pattern of development may silently preform or prepost an initial sound, particularly a vowel, occurring in the first word in a sentence. Children demonstrating this pattern seem to be free of frustration, tension, and tremor. Awareness, fear, struggle, and avoidance develop more slowly than in Track 1.

Track 2 Development

Disfluent behaviors remain relatively the same, but their rate and frequency increase. Long strings of syllabic and whole-word repetitions of increasing rate develop. The child's awareness of disfluencies increases slowly and there is little development of situation fears, avoidance behaviors, sound or word fears, or loss of eye contact. When fears are present, situation fears are more likely than word or sound fears. Overall speech output tends to increase, albeit disorganized, with primarily repetitive, arrhythmic forms of disfluency. In a later stage, compulsive and perseverative (i.e., runaway) repetitions increase in rate, tension, and pitch, resulting in overall unintelligibility. The speaker seems unable to terminate the repetitions until the exhalation is finished. The eyes appear fixed or glazed, and the speaker reports a clear awareness that something dreadful and involuntary is happening to him. Others have described the speech behavior in this stage as *cluttering*.

Track 3 Onset

Only 11% of Van Riper's 44 longitudinal cases (5 of 44) and 5% of his shorter observations (13 of 256) demonstrated this pattern of development. At any age after establishment of connected, fluent speech, a child in this track demonstrates a sudden, acute onset of disfluency often following a traumatic experience. The pattern of development tends to be steady with few remissions. Articulation is normal. At first, stuttering is confined to the beginning of an utterance after a pause, and takes the form of tense prolonged fixation of an articulatory posture. Struggle ensues, usually at the level of the larynx. Breathing during speech is interrupted, and vocal fry (bubbling, cracking type of low-pitched phonation) is common combined with struggling and forcing. Tense musculature tremors and awareness and frustration develop almost immediately. General speaking fear and specific situation and word fears develop rapidly, as does speech-related frustration. Speaking rate tends to slow. Non-stuttered speech sounds quite fluent.

Track 3 Development

The frequency and complexity of forms of disfluency increase and are accompanied by observed frustration and retrials. Lip protrusions and tongue fixations appear, as do prolongations of initial sounds. Repetitions follow prolongations; each repetition begins with a slight prolongation of the first sound. As tension and tremors increase, facial contortions, jaw jerking, and gasping are observed. Frustration and interruptor devices become prominent. Overall rate of speech slows and speech reluctance increases. At this point, the child develops avoidance patterns and intense fears of words and sounds. Severity increases, resulting in bizarre forms of disfluency. Eye contact is interrupted and nonstuttered speech becomes irregular and hesitant. Nonvocalized tense blockings become frequent.

Track 4 Onset

Only 9% (4 of 44) of Van Riper's longitudinal cases and less than 1% (2 of 256) of the briefer observations fell into this track. Stuttering usually begins later in this track than in the other three tracks. As in Track 3, stuttering begins suddenly, after several years of fluency. Initial disfluencies often are repetitions of whole words and phrases, rather than syllables that later become observed. Lengthy repetition of words already spoken normally is a characteristic of this group. Some children initially demonstrate gaps and pauses. Remissions are rare, and the behaviors acquired early change little over time. Articulation and rate essentially are normal. These children seem aware of their stuttering and listener reactions. Stuttering occurs most frequently on first words and content words but rarely on function words. The child demonstrates little evidence of fear or frustration and remains talkative.

Track 4 Development

The frequency of stuttering increases, but the pattern remains stable. Unlike those in other tracks who pass through phases and develop a repertoire of different avoidance and release reactions, those in this track tend to be "monosymptomatic." Avoidance and release reactions, therefore, are not common. Stuttering seems to be undisguised with few consistent loci. While the child demonstrates keen awareness of stuttering behavior, there is little evidence of fear. Eye contact remains uninterrupted. These children are talkative and open with their stuttering. Van Riper indicated that these people talk about their speech disorder and related experiences, but do not demonstrate being negatively affected by it.

Bloodstein

Bloodstein (1995) reported an earlier investigation (1960) in which he reviewed case records of 418 people who stuttered and were 2 to 16 years of age. In this review, he proposed four phases in the development of stuttering. These phases, according to Bloodstein, are to be viewed as reference points along a continuum. Thus, the development of stuttering is a continuous and gradual process. Many people who stutter correspond to one of the four phases; others might be in transition between two of the phases. The phases are summarized in Table 2.3 and in the paragraphs that follow.

Phase 1

During the preschool period, typically between 2 and 6 years of age, the following characteristics are observed: Disfluency is highly episodic, being observed for weeks or months between intervals of normal speech, and most noticeable under conditions of communicative pressure or emotional arousal. The dominant form of disfluency is whole-word repetition at the beginning of sentences, clauses, and phrases and on content and function words. Evidence of concern or frustration by the child is infrequent, yet brief, and it is fleeting when present.

Phase 2

Children in this phase tend to be of elementary school age, but such patterns have been observed in children as young as 4 years and in people who have reached adulthood. The disfluencies become chronic with few intervals of normal speech, thus affecting the child's self-concept. The disfluency occurs mainly on the content words. However, there is less tendency to stutter on initial and whole words. There is little evidence of concern (i.e., no evidence of avoidance tactics or word, sound, or situation fears). Stuttering worsens under conditions of excitement or during rapid or demanding speech.

Phase 3

This phase typically is observed in late childhood and early adolescence (approximately 8 years to adulthood). The stuttering becomes more specific to

Table 2.3. Four Phases in the Development of Stuttering

Phase 1

- The disfluency tends to be episodic.
- The child stutters most when excited or upset or under other conditions of communicative pressure.
- Repetition is the dominant symptom.
- Stuttering tends to occur at the beginning of the sentence, clause, or phrase.
- In contrast to more advanced stuttering, disfluencies occur not only on content words, but also on the function words of speech (i.e., pronouns, conjunctions, articles, and prepositions).
- The child shows little evidence of concern about the interruptions in his speech.

Phase 2

- The disorder becomes chronic.
- The child develops a self-concept as a "stutterer."
- The stuttering occurs primarily on the content words (i.e., nouns, verbs, adjectives, and adverbs).
- Despite the evolving self-concept as a "stutterer," the child usually demonstrates little or no concern about the speech difficulty.
- The stuttering worsens under conditions of excitement or when the child is speaking rapidly.

Phase 3

- Stuttering severity varies with specific situations.
- Certain words or sounds are regarded as more difficult than others.
- Substitutions and circumlocutions are observed to varying degrees.
- There is minimal, if any, avoidance of speech situations or evidence of fear or embarrassment.

Phase 4

- Vivid, fearful anticipation of stuttering is apparent.
- Word, sound, and situation fears are observed.
- Word substitutions and circumlocutions are frequent.
- Speech situations are avoided and fear and embarrassment are evident.

Note. Adapted from *A Handbook on Stuttering* (5th ed.) (pp. 53–56), by O. Bloodstein, 1995, San Diego, CA: Singular.

situations, words, or sounds. Circumlocutions and substitutions emerge as an escape to impending frustration. Avoidance of speech situations is not observed. Little or no evidence of fear or embarrassment is apparent. Bloodstein emphasized that the distinguishing feature of this phase is that the person speaks freely, despite the advanced development of stuttering. Reactions tend to be more of irritation than shame or anxiety.

Phase 4

Although typically seen in later adolescence and adulthood, this phase may be recognized in later childhood (i.e., 10 years). In this last phase, stuttering is characterized by fearful anticipation of stuttering; feared sounds, words, and situations; frequent word substitutions and circumlocutions; and avoidance of speech situations and other indications of fear and embarrassment. This phase is particularly characterized by the emotional reactions and the extent to which the stuttering has become a personal problem. Sensitivities and disguises are a significant cause of impairment in social relationships and avoidance of social interaction.

Summary and Extension—Onset and Development of Stuttering

The foregoing pictures of stuttering's onset and development represent snapshots to generate clinicians' understanding of how it begins and progresses. What we do know is that stuttering usually begins gradually during the preschool years and only infrequently in adults. When stuttering persists, the behaviors, thoughts, and feelings that characterize stuttering change and develop with the passage of time and interaction within a social context. Typically, stuttering begins with repetitions of sounds and syllables or prolongations. Most people who stutter develop struggle or avoidance reactions as a consequence of frustration, embarrassment, and fear.

There are risks in sharing snapshots, however. Namely, in presenting this information, some will adhere strictly to the stage or phase concept, attempting to fit clients into categories that do not fit them (like square pegs into round holes), failing to realize the uniqueness of each person who stutters and the stuttering experience itself. We must not abandon current developmental representations of stuttering, yet we must not become prisoners to them. Wall and Myers (1995) concurred and indicated that implicit in a stage approach to developmental stuttering is the tenet that stuttering, particularly in children, gets worse when left untreated. They verified this premise in "a good many" (p. 84) clinical cases. They cautioned, however, that holding too rigidly to a stage approach excludes other possibilities. They urged readers to remember that stuttering can remain unchanged or show great periodicity and fluctuation, that symptoms can remit spontaneously, that stuttering may be severe at onset, even at early childhood, and that stuttering may be mild in adults. Others have offered similar cautions. Bloodstein (1995) indicated that the presence of secondary symptoms does not mean that the child is habitually fearful of speaking; and that childhood disfluency, anticipatory preparation, and emotional reaction are inevitable, yet not sufficient, to define stuttering behavior. Recall the caution (discussed in Chapter 1) not to misinterpret continuous variables, such as stuttering, as though they are dichotomous. Wingate (1976) also indicated that progression concepts only present stuttering as becoming worse and do not provide for conditions of no change, fluctuation, or improvement. Furthermore, he objected to the assumed yet unsubstantiated positive correlation between age and severity (cf. Schwartz, Zebrowski, & Conture, 1990), and suggested abandonment of developmental labels or stages in favor of precise description of simple or complicated patterns. Wingate argued: "In fact, we have absolutely no grounds for predicting either course or destination for any case of stuttering" (1976, p. 67). Van Riper (1982) also emphasized the benefits of "molecular" description, which is defined both qualitatively and quantitatively, over "molar" identifications, which he called "gross categories" and "wastebasket phrases" (pp. 14–17). Furthermore, Van Riper reminded clinicians and researchers to exercise caution in interpreting developmental patterns of stuttering that are based on cross-sectional data. Longitudinal investigation of the onset and development of stuttering continues to be a critical need facing our field.

Promising inroads are being made in such longitudinal investigations as those by Yairi and Ambrose (1992a, 1992b). These authors found: (a) that 75% of the risk for stuttering onset occurred before the age of 3 years, 5 months, with the greatest risk occurring before 3 years of age; (b) that the relationship between age of onset and prognosis may be significant; and (c) that there are subgroups of people who stutter whose onset is rapid and directly observable. Furthermore, Yairi (1997) expressed concern that developmental profiles such as those reviewed earlier incorrectly perpetuate the belief that disfluencies most often increase in frequency and severity over time. Rather, several longitudinal investigations negate, or reverse, such beliefs, indicating that remission rates are high, especially during the first 12 to 18 months after onset. Yairi and Ambrose (1992a) followed 27 children who stutter, and found: (a) that without intervention total disfluency reduced significantly during the first 2 years (most occurred within the first 14 months of onset), (b) that 65% of these children recovered within 2 years of onset, and (c) that recovery climbed to 85% by the end of the study. This recovery was so complete that judges could not distinguish the speech of these children from their normally fluent peers (Finn, Ingham, Yairi, & Ambrose, 1994; Yairi, 1997). Similarly, Yairi, Ambrose, and Niermann (1993) followed 16 children and reported that severe stuttering and high disfluency levels during the first 2 or 3 months of onset were followed by quick, sharp reductions in disfluency without intervention. There was a tendency for boys' stuttering to persist longer than that of girls. Yairi (1997) noted that these longitudinal data indicating substantial reduction in disfluency and eventual recovery of 65% to 85% of the children studied within 2 years of onset, particularly for girls, "should be carefully considered when developing a case-selection strategy for treatment and in assessing treatment efficacy of early childhood stuttering" (p. 73). Yairi (1997) described clinicians' decisions to initiate or delay treatment as presenting "a difficult, double-edged ethical dilemma" (p. 73). Recognizing that this controversy represents an ongoing professional debate, he recommended that clinicians making such decisions consider that we do not know why some children experience spontaneous recovery (recovery without treatment), that some children persist in stuttering, and that disfluency tends to lessen after 2 or 3 months of onset, followed by an increase in chronicity from 14 to 18 months after onset. Yairi (1997) recommended that all young children who are beginning to stutter receive a thorough communication evaluation and subsequent reevaluations combined with parent education about childhood stuttering, and that those children who have stuttered for more than 14 to 18 months without exhibiting substantial improvement receive a priority for direct fluency intervention.

THE NATURE OF STUTTERING

While interacting with people who stutter and their families, clinicians are asked many questions. Being able to distinguish between what is known and not known about stuttering and people who stutter is pivotal to sensitive and accurate responding, as well as to competent planning, implementing, and interpreting clinical interactions. This section presents another snapshot, this time of the nature of stuttering. Others have presented more complete portraits (Andrews et al., 1983; Bloodstein, 1995; Curlee & Perkins, 1984; Curlee & Siegel, 1997; Van Riper, 1982) and their works are primary sources for the material in this section. The literature is vast indeed and the knowledge base is ever expanding. An exhaustive review of current knowledge is beyond the scope of the purposes stated here. What is presented here are frequently asked questions and research-based findings in response, selected on the bases of clinical relevance and applicability and representative of people who stutter as a group. Therefore, caution again must be exercised when interpreting this section because each individual client who stutters may or may not exhibit any of these characteristics.

Types of Disfluency

Providing examples for types of disfluency will prove helpful to the new clinician reading this section. Williams, Darley, and Spriestersbach (1978) presented a classification system containing eight types of overt forms of disfluency. They included: interjections of sounds, syllables, words, or phrases (for example, *uh, er, hmmm, well, you know*); part-word repetitions (*buh–boy, guh–guh–girl*); word repetitions (*I–I–I, was–was–was*); phrase repetitions (*I was—I was going*); revisions (*I was—I am going*); incomplete phrases (*She was—and after she got there he came*); broken words (*g—oing, b—oy*); prolonged sounds (*sssssssee sssssssaw*). Williams et al. (1978) invited use of two categories, dysrhythmic phonation in words and tension pause, to replace that of broken words and prolonged sounds, respectively.

Symptoms, Prevalence, and Incidence

What do we know about the speech of young children and particularly the symptoms of stuttering at its onset?

First of all, we know that preschool children typically demonstrate speech disfluencies including word and phrase repetitions, interjections, and revisions. In other words, disfluency is the norm for young children. However, being able to distinguish between normal disfluencies of childhood and incipient stuttering is an essential skill for speech–language pathologists. This distinction will be addressed directly in Chapter 8. Children who stutter demonstrate more within-word disfluencies (e.g., sound or syllable repetitions, sound prolongations, broken words, etc.) than children who do not. In fact, disfluencies that fragment the word (within-word disfluencies) are more likely to be perceived as stuttering than those that do not (i.e., between-word disfluencies; e.g., whole-word repetitions, revisions, incomplete phrases) (Bjerkan, 1980; Guyette & Baumgartner, 1988). This is what Van Riper (1982) meant when he said, "It is the broken word that characterizes the majority of the stutterer's difficulty. Stuttering interruptions to the forward flow of speech are primarily intra-morphemic; normal disfluencies are primarily supra-morphemic" (p. 13). We know that repetitions are most often the first indication of stuttering in children and that associated or secondary features follow. Nevertheless, the onset, development, and features of the stuttering are unique to each individual.

When does stuttering develop?

The majority of children who stutter begin stuttering between speech onset and puberty; most between ages 2 and 5 years (Conture, 1990a, 1990b). A person can begin to stutter at any age, however. Stuttering begins in adulthood only in rare cases. When it does, its onset typically is sudden and represents a distinct subtype of the disorder (e.g., subsequent to emotional trauma, intracranial trauma, etc.) (Attanasio, 1987a; Haynes, Pindzola, & Emerick, 1992; Mahr & Leith, 1992; Wingate, 1983). Andrews (1984) summarized that, "On the basis of data presently available, half the risk of ever stuttering is passed by Age 4, three quarters by Age 6, and virtually all by Age 12" (p. 8).

How prevalent is stuttering and what is the likelihood of recovery?

The prevalence of stuttering (total number of cases at or during a specified time, determined from cross-sectional retrospective studies and surveys) in prepubertal school children is 1% and generally drops in postpubertal school children. No reliable prevalence figures are available for adults who stutter. However, if prevalence continues to decline after puberty, the figure for adults would be less than 1% (i.e., 0.8%) (Andrews et al., 1983; Guyette & Baumgartner, 1988; Ham, 1990; Moscicki, 1984; Peters & Guitar, 1991). The incidence of stuttering (total number of people who have stuttered at some point in their lives) lasting longer than six months is approximately 5%. The difference between incidence (5%) and prevalence (1%) indicates that most people who stutter recover from it (Peters & Guitar, 1991). Certain special conditions resulting from perinatal brain damage including mental retardation, epilepsy, cerebral palsy, and other syndromes reveal a higher than expected prevalence of stuttering. Deafness is the only condition revealing a lower than expected prevalence of stuttering (Andrews et al., 1983; Peters & Guitar, 1991; Van Riper, 1982). However, as will be discussed in Chapter 4, there is a literature addressing disfluencies in manual communication including repetitions, hesitations, interjections, and extraneous movements found in signing and finger spelling (Silverman & Silverman, 1971).

Generally, some people who stutter recover spontaneously, others recover after minimal therapy, and others require extended treatment. Recovery by age 16 years is 78%. When the probability of recovery is related to age, the following emerges: By 16 years, 75% of those stuttering at age 4 years will improve, as will 50% of those stuttering at age 6 years and 25% of those stuttering at age 10 years (Andrews et al., 1983). A corollary is that stuttering recovery is almost always a gradual process (Wingate, 1983). Furthermore, these data argue for the importance of early intervention with preschool- and school-age children who stutter.

What about the male:female ratio for stuttering and how widespread is stuttering?

The ratio of males who stutter to females who stutter is approximately 3:1. This ratio increases with age (Guyette & Baumgartner, 1988; Peters & Guitar, 1991). Although age of onset interpreted from retrospective and cross-sectional data continues to be controversial (Andrews et al., 1983, reported age of onset to be the same for both sexes; Yairi, 1993, reported onset for girls to be 6 months earlier than for boys), it appears that girls recover more frequently and quickly than boys. Some have suggested that this tendency might reflect a genetically controlled and milder form of stuttering in girls (Kidd, 1984; Yairi, 1993). Stuttering is a universal reality and is found in almost all people and cultures (Emerick & Haynes, 1986; Van Riper, 1982). Some say the prevalence among different cultural and national groups is nearly comparable (Wingate, 1983), while others suggest greater prevalence among middle and upper-middle socioeconomic class families than those of lower socioeconomic class. Furthermore, while the prevalence of stuttering in Western and other technologically advanced cultures (including Japan) is reported to be approximately 1%, that of other countries reportedly is greater than 1% (the population of Korea; Kawakiutl, Nootka, and Salish Indians of Canada; the Idoma and Ibo tribes of West Africa; and school children in Dakar and the Accra district of the Gold Coast) or less than 1% (the Mundugumar, Arapesh, Tchambuli, Manus, Dobuan, New Hanover, Tabor, and Kamamentira tribes of New Guinea; the Aborigines of Australia; Polar Eskimos; the Bannock and Shoshone tribes of American Indians; and Polynesians) (Silverman, 1996).

Does stuttering result from one's environment?

Environmental factors are of great interest because of their potential impact on causing stuttering and inhibiting its remission. Conversely, environmental factors could prevent stuttering from occurring even in people who have such a predisposition or they could facilitate remission (Andrews et al., 1983). We noted earlier that certain conditions associated with perinatal brain damage (i.e., mental retardation, epilepsy, cerebral palsy, and other syndromes) reveal a higher than expected prevalence of stuttering. Perinatal brain damage appears to be the only environmental event that is causally related to idiopathic or developmental stuttering. Otherwise, Andrews et al. (1983) noted:

> There are no other established facts about the more obvious features in a stutterer's environment that might point to the cause or maintenance of stuttering, be they family structures, race, socio-cultural factors, or parental characteristics. Stutterers appear to come from the same environment as do nonstutterers, with one exception; they come from families with an excess of stuttering relatives. (pp. 228–229)

Nevertheless, the risk of stuttering among first-degree relatives (for the child of a parent who stutters) is three times the general risk. The greatest risk is for male children of females who stutter (which is four times the risk of female children of males who stutter).

A related area of inquiry, twin studies, attempts to distinguish the relative influence of inheritance and that of the environment. Identical twins (monozygotic twins) have identical genes. Fraternal twins (dizygotic twins) are genetically like any other siblings, sharing up to half of their genes. Peters and Guitar (1991) noted that any greater similarity in the traits of identical twins compared to that of fraternal twins generally is attributed to the role of inheritance. Twin studies of stuttering indicate that there is more concordance of stuttering in identical twins than fraternal twins. This means that stuttering occurs more often in both members of identical twin pairs than in both members of fraternal twin pairs, supporting the notion that stuttering is inherited. However, the cases of discordance among identical twins, or when only one member of an identical twin pair stutters, suggest environmental as well as genetic influences. These and other data suggest that predisposition to stutter could be influenced by genetic factors (Ambrose, Yairi, & Cox, 1993; Andrews et al., 1983; Cox, 1988, 1993; Felsenfeld, 1996, 1997; Van Riper, 1982). Kidd (1984) argued that "an inherited neurologic susceptibility underlies most cases of stuttering" (p. 149), yet concurred that stuttering is determined both by nature (inherited factors) and nurture (environmental influences). Nevertheless, stuttering may be precipitated and perpetuated by certain environmental events, particularly the critical, demanding behaviors of significant others (Haynes et al., 1992). Environmental events are of particular interest to clinicians and researchers alike because they can be influenced early in treatment.

What is stuttering like in its developed form?

In advanced stages, stuttering typically has both overt and covert features. Much of the observed escape and avoidance behaviors of advanced stuttering are overt attempts to cope with the emission of speech disfluency. Other than disfluency, stuttering also is characterized by speech and voice abnormalities (e.g., narrow pitch range, vocal tension, lack of vocal expression, muscular lags and asynchronies) that can be detected in nonstuttered speech. These associated observations may be effects of stuttering or may reflect (i.e., to be determined) an impairment in phonation, respiration, neuromotor coordination, or cortical integration (Haynes et al., 1992; Peters & Guitar, 1991; Van Riper, 1982). Taken as a whole, the pieces of stuttering represent a social-psychological event. About this event, Emerick and Haynes (1986) noted the following:

> The acoustic and visual phenomena that occur during the motor act of stuttering are noxious stimuli in a communication context, and listeners tend to react in various explicit and implicit ways. The stutterer tends in turn to react to these listener responses. (p. 191)

Furthermore, stuttering is a personal problem. People who stutter report feelings of fear, frustration, social penalty, dissatisfaction with themselves, lower level of aspiration, and loss of social esteem (Haynes et al., 1992).

Differences Between People Who Stutter and Those Who Do Not

What is known about the intelligence of people who stutter?

Children who stutter score one half of a standard deviation lower on verbal and nonverbal tests of intelligence and lag 6 months behind their peers in school performance (Andrews et al., 1983; Guyette & Baumgartner, 1988; Peters & Guitar, 1991). There is controversy in interpreting these results. Some have argued that the measured deficit might be a result of stuttering rather than a cause of it. This interpretation seems plausible given the emphasis on verbal skills in both traditional intellectual and educational assessment, and the emotional consequence of stuttering on a person who stutters. However, the studies revealing that people who stutter performed more poorly on verbal and motor subtests are interpreted by some as suggesting that stuttering might be related to inadequacy in linguistic and motor domains (Peters & Guitar, 1991). Given this line of argument, it might be predicted that a greater deficit in cerebral functioning (deficient resources underlying both linguistic and motor performance) would predict stuttering. Indeed, it is the case that intelligence is negatively related to stuttering (i.e., as level of intelligence goes down, the prevalence of stuttering goes up; e.g., people with mental retardation demonstrate a 3% prevalence of stuttering) (Andrews et al., 1983; Guyette & Baumgartner, 1988). In other words, lower intelligence does seem to correlate with and predict a greater prevalence of stuttering. However, it is both unfortunate and inaccurate when people assume that stuttering correlates with and predicts a lower level of intelligence. As noted above, there is no difference in the intelligence of people who stutter when compared to those who do not, other than the former group demonstrates a slight gap in early intellectual and educational assessment. This gap is likely a consequence of stuttering rather than a cause of it.

Do people who stutter have a different personality?

There is no difference on measures of neurotic behavior. However, people who stutter show more problems in social adjustment, perhaps a result rather than a cause of stuttering (Guyette & Baumgartner, 1988).

Do children who stutter show a different pattern of speech and language development?

Children who stutter are more likely to have a history of delayed speech or language development, and at least two and one half times the incidence of articulation or phonological disorders as that found in children who do not stutter. It is unclear whether these differences continue into adulthood (Guyette & Baumgartner, 1988; Wingate, 1983). It is also uncertain how speech and language disorders are related to stuttering, if at all. Some suggest that difficulty in speech and language leads to anticipatory struggle and frustration resulting in stuttering (Bloodstein, 1958); others hypothesize that stuttering, language disorders, and articulation errors share a common, genetically predisposed deficit found in the brain structure or function (Peters & Guitar, 1991).

Does the central nervous system of people who stutter work differently?

Though not conclusive, studies of hemispheric dominance indicate that people who stutter are more likely to process meaningful linguistic material in the right hemisphere (i.e., less left hemisphere dominance for speech and language than the general population) (Andrews et al., 1983; Guyette & Baumgartner, 1988). Other studies of central auditory processing have shown that people who stutter are poorer at recognition and recall of competing messages and demon-strate reduced pain thresholds for intense auditory stimulation (Andrews et al., 1983). Likewise, studies of motor speech behavior have indicated that voice onset times, voice initiation times, and speech initiation times are slower in people who stutter. Muscle activity increases and abductor and adductor laryn-geal muscles co-contract during stuttered speech. This co-contraction also occurs during silent periods prior to fluent speech. These data suggest motor speech differences in laryngeal behavior during stuttering but a causal rela-tionship has not been established. The fluent speech of people who stutter also demonstrates lower speed and degree of lip and jaw movement as well as greater movement onset times. Combined, these findings suggest differences between people who do and those who do not stutter in both the fluent and dis-fluent speech (Guyette & Baumgartner, 1988).

Variability and Predictability of Stuttering

What commonalities are there among people who stutter?

There are a number of patterns that are consistent among people who stutter. These include anticipation, consistency, and adaptation; language factors; fluency-inducing conditions; and fluency-inhibiting conditions.

First, people who stutter predict with accuracy the words on which they will stutter (anticipation) and, upon repeated readings of the same passage, tend to stutter on the same words each time (consistency), yet demonstrate a decrease in the overall frequency of stuttering across the passage (adaptation).

Second, there are certain language-related factors that are predictable. Most adults who stutter do so more frequently on consonants; on sounds in word-initial position; in contextual speech (vs. isolated words); on content words including nouns, verbs, adjectives, and adverbs (vs. function words; that is, articles, prepositions, pronouns, and conjunctions); on longer words; on words of greater uncertainty; on words at the beginnings of sentences; and on stressed syllables (Andrews et al., 1983; Peters & Guitar, 1991; Starkweather, 1987).

Third, still defying explanation are the predictable fluency-inducing con-ditions. We find reliably that stuttering is immediately eliminated in choral, lipped, prolonged, or rhythmic speech; and during shadowing, singing, and instructions to slow down. Stuttering is more gradually eliminated by response-contingent stimulation. Immediate reduction of stuttering is observed when the person who stutters speaks alone (when no other person is present) or with rhythmic movement, delayed auditory feedback, masking, change in pitch, or whispering. More gradual reduction of stuttering results from haloperidol, EMG feedback from speech muscles, and adaptation (reduction in baseline stuttering upon repeated reading of the same material) (Andrews et al., 1983). Other conditions that markedly reduce or eliminate stuttering include speaking when relaxed, to an animal or an infant, in a dialect, or while simultaneously writing, swearing, or receiving reinforcement for fluent speech (Bloodstein, 1995; Peters & Guitar, 1991). In general, stuttering is temporarily reduced when speaking in a nonhabitual or novel manner including altering speaking rate, pitch, voice quality, accent, intonation, and vowel duration, and when using conversational interjections, nonverbal movements, and deliberate impersonations (Silverman, 1996).

Finally, a corollary of fluency-inducing conditions is fluency-inhibiting conditions. Such situations in which a temporary increase of stuttering is observed include, with some reported variation, speaking on the telephone, saying one's name, telling jokes, repeating a message that was not understood, waiting to respond, speaking to authority figures, speaking to a relatively large audience, and attempting to conceal stuttering, among others (Silverman, 1996; Van Riper, 1982; Young, 1985). These patterns of variability and predictability are critical in the differential diagnosis of stuttering from other disorders of fluency, which are reviewed in Chapter 4.

Such factors that characterize stuttering also have been used by speech–language pathologists to verify whether a person really has a fluency disorder or is malingering (Bloodstein, 1988; Shirkey, 1987). For example, Shirkey (1987) was asked to verify the stuttering of a 33-year-old man accused of a series of sexual assaults on young girls and one woman. Pivotal testimony in a previous acquittal was that none of the victims reported that the attacker stuttered. Shirkey subsequently analyzed the suspect's communication-related attitudes and speech fluency during conversation and reading and described the adaptation and consistency effects. Exceptional, if not contrary, observations included that the suspect demonstrated appropriate vowels during syllabic repetitions, inability to speak fluently using a rhythmic speaking pattern and external stimulus, and increased frequency of stuttering during prolonged speech and simple linguistic tasks. Shirkey concluded that the suspect's overt and covert features were more consistent than not with adults who stutter, and that this individual demonstrated significant, yet not atypical, variability in his stuttering behavior. Ultimately, the suspect was convicted and sentenced to 101 years in prison.

Similarly, Bloodstein (1988) was asked to verify the stuttering of another suspect in his 30s accused of armed robbery whose defense was that, as a person who stutters, he could not have said fluently, "This is a stickup. Get down on the floor and don't make a move or I'll blow your head off." Bloodstein also analyzed and reported on the suspect's feelings and attitudes in addition to anticipation, adaptation, consistency, and adjacency effects; loci of stuttering; and effect of masking noise and contingent stimuli. Bloodstein also concluded that the suspect's stuttering was legitimate, thus contributing to testimony leading to an anticipated acquittal. Both Shirkey (1987) and Bloodstein (1988) raise important questions regarding our profession's ability to diagnose malingering in stuttering, particularly in light of the heterogeneity among people who stutter and atypical stuttering, and encourage research efforts to improve current methods. Such an endeavor presents an interesting challenge since faking stuttering (pseudostuttering) is a deliberate component of treatment programs (Van Riper, 1973) and has been used by political prisoners during interrogations to allow for processing time in order to prevent contradictions and minimize information given (Lew, 1995).

Treatment

What does the clinical literature tell us about designing effective treatment?

Bloodstein (1995) presented 12 specific criteria for treatment to be considered successful. The treatment must be successful with (a) an ample and representative group of people who stutter when measured (b) objectively (e.g., frequency of stuttering or rate of speech and by judges' ratings of severity at least before, during, and after treatment) and (c) repeatedly (d) across non-clinic situations (e) over a period of no less than 18 months to 2 years (including unexpected, unannounced assessments). (f) Control conditions must be used to demonstrate that reduction in stuttering is indeed the result of treatment. In addition, the speech should sound (g) natural and (h) automatic, (i) abnormal speech attitudes should be normalized, and (j) results should not be invalidated from excessive client attrition or spontaneous remission. Finally, the treatment should continue to be effective (k) when conducted in different clinics by different clinicians and (l) when the treatment is no longer new (pp. 437–445). Using an earlier version of these criteria (Bloodstein, 1981), Andrews et al. (1983) reported that only prolonged speech and precision fluency shaping have been demonstrated to produce significant long-term benefits. Attitude therapy, rhythmic speech, and airflow therapy have been found to be of some benefit, but to a lesser degree. Hours of therapy correlate positively to treatment outcome (Andrews, Guitar, & Howie, 1980; Andrews et al., 1983). Finally, different therapies are found to employ some similar methods (Wingate, 1983).

Summary—Nature of Stuttering

The majority of children who stutter begin stuttering between 2 and 5 years of age, often demonstrating more part-word repetitions and prolongations than children who do not. Prevalence of stuttering is about 1%; incidence is about 5%. The ratio of males who stutter to females who stutter is approximately 3:1 and increases with age, although some cultural variation is reported. Girls appear to recover from stuttering more frequently and quickly than boys. The environment of people who stutter is the same as those who do not, except that those who stutter have more relatives who stutter. These and other observations suggest both environmental and genetic influences on stuttering. Compared to people who do not stutter, those who stutter demonstrate a small measured deficit on verbal and nonverbal tests of intelligence, school performance, social adjustment, speech and language development, sound production skills, discrimination of competing auditory messages, and reaction time. People who stutter demonstrate the effects of anticipation, consistency, and adaptation; specific influences of language on stuttering; and fluency-inducing and fluency-inhibiting conditions. The commonalities among people who stutter have been used for differential diagnosis. Finally, on the basis of criteria reviewed for designing effective treatment, four treatment methods have been found to be beneficial, and time in treatment is one predictor of treatment outcome.

CHAPTER SUMMARY

Because assumptions about stuttering and people who stutter can affect the intervention process, clinicians must be aware explicitly of their assumptions and must possess a basic understanding of the onset, development, and nature of stuttering; etiology and treatment from past and present perspectives; and different fluency disorders. This chapter provided an overview of some developmental and descriptive categories of stuttering. While these categories can be helpful in understanding how stuttering develops, clinicians must remember that each client is unique and should not and cannot be fit into specific categories. Instead, these categories may be used as a basis of comparison to understand the client's individual experiences.

Among the descriptive categories reviewed were those of Bluemel, Froeschels, Van Riper, and Bloodstein. Bluemel described stuttering as consisting of two stages, primary and secondary stuttering. Primary stuttering is characterized by easy, effortless, intermittent repetitions of the first word or syllable in a sentence; secondary stuttering by more obvious physical effort, use of starters and synonyms, attempts to conceal stuttering, and observed fears. Froeschels described a similar progression, but differentiated between easy syllable and sound repetitions (clonic types of stuttering) and more rapid, tense behaviors involving muscle tension, interrupted breathing, and facial tension (tonic types of stuttering).

Van Riper expanded Bluemel's categories by adding two categories. The most frequently occurring pattern of development is Track 1, characterized by gradual, inconsistent development of stuttering between the ages of 2.5 and 4.0 years, with long periods of remission. Typical behaviors include frequent gentle syllable repetitions on initial or function words. In Track 2, rate and frequency of repetitions increase and are accompanied by prolongations and pitch increases. Tension and frustration become evident and word and situation fears develop. In Track 3, stuttering typically appears abruptly after a traumatic experience and develops steadily with few remissions. Tense, prolonged fixations, struggle, and breathing interruptions are common. In Track 4, stuttering also appears suddenly after long periods of fluency. Repetition of whole words on first and content words is typical with little observed fear or frustration. Bloodstein proposed four phases of stuttering reflecting developmental points along a continuum. Phase 1 occurs typically between 2 and 6 years of age under conditions of stress or emotional arousal, and is characterized by whole-word repetitions at the beginning of sentences, clauses, and phrases and on content and function words. Phase 2 typically emerges during the elementary school years, where disfluency notably occurs on content words, becomes chronic, and affects how the child views himself as a communicator. Phase 3 is observed in late childhood or early adolescence, with disfluency typically linked to certain situations, words, or sounds. Circumlocutions and substitutions are observed; however, the person continues to speak freely. Finally, Phase 4 is seen in late adolescence or early adulthood, and involves sound, word, and situation fears. Behaviors may include word substitution and situation avoidance, and fears and embarrassment become evident.

In addition to presenting several patterns of onset and development of stuttering, this chapter summarized the nature of stuttering, including types of disfluency; symptoms, prevalence, and incidence; differences between people who stutter and those who do not; variability and predictability of stuttering; and effective treatment. Frequently occurring questions regarding symptoms, prevalence, and incidence were addressed including:

- What do we know about the speech of young children and particularly the symptoms of stuttering at its onset?

- When does stuttering develop?

- How prevalent is stuttering and what is the likelihood of recovery?

- What about the male:female ratio for stuttering and how widespread is stuttering?

- Does stuttering result from one's environment?

- What does stuttering look like in developed form?

Questions addressed relating to differences between people who stutter and those who do not included:

- What is known about the intelligence of people who stutter?

- Do people who stutter have a different personality?

- Do children who stutter show a different pattern of speech and language development?

- Does the central nervous system of people who stutter work differently?

Variability and predictability of stuttering (i.e., What commonalities are there among people who stutter?) were considered in terms of the anticipation, consistency, and adaptation effects; language factors; fluency-inducing conditions; and fluency-inhibiting conditions. Finally, treatment (i.e., What does the clinical literature tell us about designing effective treatment?) was addressed on the basis of 12 specific criteria.

Chapter 2 Study Questions

1. Throughout this chapter, many questions were raised about the onset, development, and nature of stuttering, as summarized above. How would you address each of the questions raised?

2. An explicit understanding of one's assumptions (i.e., one's personal construct) is essential for effective assessment and treatment with people who stutter. What are your assumptions about the onset, development, and nature of stuttering, and how might these impact your intervention with people who stutter? How have your assumptions about stuttering and people who stutter changed as a result of reading this chapter?

3. Several classification systems were discussed in this chapter. Which do you feel to be most clinically useful and why? What do you feel are the dangers in using developmental categories when assessing and treating a person who stutters? How do your experiences with young children beginning to stutter relate (compare and contrast) to the classification systems discussed?

4. Why do you believe more males than females stutter? What are possible explanations for the more frequent and faster recovery among girls than boys who stutter?

5. While our knowledge of stuttering and people who stutter has grown tremendously in recent years, many inroads are yet to be made. What do we know and what do we need to learn? With all that is known, what might be the reasons for perpetuation of negative attitudes among the general public, allied education and health professionals, and student clinicians and professional speech–language pathologists? How might the confusion about the disorder contribute to the stereotypes, and what can be done about it?

6. Bloodstein presented 12 criteria for effective treatment. Which of these criteria do you believe are most and least important and why? In what ways might these criteria impact your treatment?

7. Johnson (1939) was quoted as saying, "So long as an individual retains and operates on assumptions regarding stuttering and speech, which are characteristics of stutterers, he will not become the sort of individual we refer to as a normal speaker." What are possible implications of this statement for the client, the clinician, and the client–clinician interaction?

Unit I

• • • • • • • • • • • • • • • •

Stuttering in Relief:
A Foundation
for Intervention

Chapter 1
The Nexus of Stuttering: An Introduction

Chapter 2
The Onset, Development, and Nature of Stuttering

Chapter 3
Etiology and Treatment of Stuttering: Past and Present

Chapter 4
Other Fluency Disorders

Chapter 3

Etiology and Treatment of Stuttering: Past and Present

◆ ◆ ◆ ◆ ◆ ◆ ◆ ◆ ◆ ◆ ◆ ◆ ◆ ◆ ◆ ◆ ◆ ◆ ◆

History of Stuttering: The Past   60

"If You Stutter, You're Not Alone"   60

Stuttering in Egyptian Hieroglyphics   61

Stuttering in the Bible   63

Stuttering in Professional Literature   64

Stuttering as an Anatomical Defect   65

Stuttering as a Medical Problem Requiring Surgery   66

Stuttering as a Disorder of Articulation   66

Stuttering as a Disorder of Respiration   67

Stuttering as a Disorder of Neuroanatomy/Motor Speech Dysfunction   67

Stuttering as a Psychoneurosis   68

Stuttering as a Learned Behavior   69

Summary—History of Stuttering   69

Etiology of Stuttering: The Present   70

Etiology Defined: Three Ps   70

Predisposing Factors   70

Precipitating Factors   71

Identification and Interaction of Predisposing and Precipitating Factors   71

Perpetuating Factors   72

Theoretical Explanations   73

Stuttering as a Neurotic Response (i.e., Repressed Need Theory)   73

Stuttering as Communicative Failure and Anticipatory Struggle Behavior   74

The Diagnosogenic Theory   74

The Continuity Hypothesis   75

Preparatory Set (i.e., Primary Stuttering Theory)   76

Stuttering as Learned Behavior   77

Stuttering as an Avoidance Response   77

Conflict Theory of Stuttering and Avoidance Reduction   77

Operant Conditioning and Stuttering   77

Instrumental Avoidance Act Theory   78

Stuttering as an Interaction of Behavioral Phenomena   78

Two-Factor Learning Theory of Stuttering   78

Stuttering as a Physiological Deficit   79

Stuttering as a Function of Incomplete Cerebral Dominance   79

Dysphemia and Biochemical Theory   79

Perseveration Theory   79

Stuttering as a Consequence of Brain Lesion   80

Stuttering as the Result of Disturbed Feedback (i.e., Cybernetic Theory)   80

Demands and Capacities Model   81

Summary and Synthesis—Etiology of Stuttering and Theoretical Explanations   82
What factors render one child more at risk than another for beginning to stutter?   82
Why do people stutter?   84
Why do people continue to stutter?   85

A Personal Postscript on Theory   86

Chapter Summary   91

Chapter 3 Study Questions   93

The longer I work with stuttering the more tolerant I become of any one who has any therapeutic ideas at all concerning it . . . . There is no such thing as the method for treating stuttering, and the fact that so many different methods are more or less successful is of far more than incidental interest. We need not, however, carry our tolerance to the point of uncritical acceptance of every therapeutical approach with the same degree of enthusiasm.

(JOHNSON, 1939, P. 170)

G enerally we need to know where we have been to understand how we arrived at where we are and the rationale for where we are going. Intervention with people who stutter is no exception. To this point, we have addressed a number of seminal concepts and reviewed the onset, development, and nature of stuttering. This chapter highlights the evolution of our thinking throughout recorded history about stuttering and people who stutter. This foundation contributes to our understanding of contemporary theories of etiology and related treatment practices.

HISTORY OF STUTTERING: THE PAST

"If You Stutter, You're Not Alone"

Stuttering and people who stutter are events of historical and contemporary significance. It is of historical interest to know that there have been many prominent and accomplished figures whose stuttering did not hold them back. This information also is of clinical interest and may be used as a positive and motivating influence during assessment and treatment interactions with people who stutter. Famous people who also stutter are receiving increasing attention (Silverman, 1996; Van Riper, 1982; leaflets from the National Stuttering Project and the Stuttering Foundation of America).

Some of these historical figures who attest to stuttering as an old problem include: Moses (prophet), Demosthenes (Greek orator), Virgil (Roman poet), Claudius (Roman emperor), Aesop (Greek storyteller), Isaac Newton (scientist), King Charles I of England, Charles Darwin (naturalist and author), Erasmus Darwin (physician, author, grandfather of Charles), Charles Lamb (British essayist), Moses Mendelssohn (18th century Jewish philosopher), Arnold Bennett (British writer), Clara Barton (founder of the American Red Cross), Cotton Mather (Puritan leader), Lewis Carroll (author of *Alice in Wonderland*), Henry James (American novelist), Marilyn Monroe (actress), Kim Philby (British spy), Aneurin Bevan (British labor leader), Winston Churchill (prime minister), Somerset Maugham (British writer), Henry Luce (magazine founder), Field Marshall Lord Carver (British military leader), Patrick Campbell (British humorist), King George VI of England, Kenneth Tynan (British drama critic), Raymond Massey (actor), Robert Heinlein (writer). Others include Lenin (Russian leader), Theodore Roosevelt (U. S. president), Washington Irving (author),

George Washington (U. S. president), Aristotle (Greek orator, philosopher), Napoleon the First (French emperor), and Michael Ramsey (100th Archbishop of Canterbury).

More contemporary figures who did or continue to stutter include: James Earl Jones (actor), Ben Johnson (runner), Bob Love (basketball star, Chicago Bulls), Ron Harper (basketball star, Chicago Bulls), Neville Shute (novelist), Margaret Drabble (British novelist), Jonathan Miller (British director), Bruce Willis (actor), Greg Luganis (diver), Tommy John (pitcher, Yankees), Dave Taylor (hockey star, L. A. Kings), Lester Hayes (football star, Oakland/L. A. Raiders), Ken Venturi (golfer), Butch Baird (golfer), John Updike (novelist), Annie Glenn (public speaker and wife of John Glenn), Carly Simon (singer), Mel Tillis (singer), Robert Merrill (singer), Richard Condon (novelist), Bruce Oldfield (British fashion designer), Jake Eberts (film producer), Joseph Biden (senator), Frank Wolf (congressman), John Welch (Chairman of General Electric), Austin Pendleton (actor), Henry Rogers (public relations pioneer), Bo Jackson (football and baseball star), John Stossel (reporter), Jimmy Stewart (actor), Anthony Quinn (actor), Chris Zorich (lineman, Chicago Bears), Pat Leahy (kicker, N. Y. Jets), Sam Neill (actor), and Peggy Lipton (actress), among many others.

Interesting accounts are available addressing the impact of stuttering on the lives of some of these people (Attanasio, 1987b; Emerick, 1966; Terry, 1994; Tillis & Wagner, 1984). Stuttering and people who stutter have been present throughout recorded history. The National Stuttering Project (NSP), a large self-help and support network with over 4,000 members including people who stutter and interested others, has published on buttons and posters, "If you stutter, you're not alone." The facts that stuttering is an old affliction and that people who stutter are in good company are both clinically relevant.

Stuttering in Egyptian Hieroglyphics

People have attempted to explain stuttering (or stammering) in various ways for over 4,000 years. From the middle of the ancient Egyptian Empire (2,000 B.C.), Egyptian hieroglyphics were found that included a determinative (i.e., a symbol or icon), represented in Figure 3.1, of a figure pointing with one hand to the mouth and the other to the ground (Clark & Murray, 1965; Curlee, 1993; Manning, 1996). This symbol within the context of the other symbols is said to represent a reduplicated verb root, "njtjt" (L. H. Corcoran, personal communication, May 1, 1997), interpreted by Egyptologists from the graphic form to mean "to talk hesitantly" or "to stutter" (Clark & Murray, 1965, p. 132). Clark and Murray noted the following:

> Its basic sense refers to a retarding movement of the walking mechanism, in a figurative sense it refers to the "gait" of talking with the vehicle of the tongue. What was originally a picture of the reluctant retarded stepping of the legs, was figuratively applied to the stepping (walking) movements of the tongue. (p. 132)

Originally from "The Tale of the Shipwrecked Sailor" (De Buck, 1970, p. 100), the symbols are read from right to left. The verb has the determinative

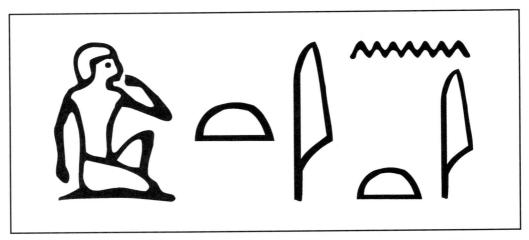

Figure 3.1. Egyptian Hieroglyphics for Stuttering. *Note.* From L. H. Corcoran and A. Webb, personal communication, May 1, 1997. Reprinted with permission.

of "walking legs" and is used in the sense of an impediment of movement. With the substitution of the determinative of the person with the hand to mouth, however, the ancient Egyptians successfully conveyed the concept of an impediment to one's speech (L. H. Corcoran, personal communication, February 6, 1997; W. H. Manning, personal communication, October 16, 1996). The symbols represent the oldest evidence of a speech defect (Clark & Murray, 1965) and may be one of the earliest retrievable references to stuttering (Curlee, 1993; Manning, 1996). This would indicate that the disorder of stuttering has affected speakers for as long as human civilization has been recorded, if not longer.

"The Tale of the Shipwrecked Sailor" is a prose tale set in a narrative frame. The original copy, which is on papyrus, was discovered by W. Golenischeff, is called P. Leningrad 1115, and is preserved currently in Moscow (Clark & Murray, 1965; Lichtheim, 1973). The tale, translated by Lichtheim (1973), tells of a high official returning from a failed expedition who is despondent and fearful about the reception he is about to receive at the royal court. One of his attendants encourages him to take courage, and as an example of how a disaster may turn into success, tells him of an adventure (being shipwrecked) that happened to him many years before. The attendant advised:

> Now listen to me, my lord! I am not exaggerating. Wash yourself, pour water over your fingers. You must answer when questioned. You must speak to the king with presence of mind. You must answer without stammering! A man's mouth can save him. His speech makes one forgive him. (p. 212)

The attendant told of being shipwrecked on an island and encountering a large snake. Interestingly, the snake demonstrates a pattern of phrase and sentence repetition, as follows:

> Then he opened his mouth to me, while I was on my belly before him. He said to me: "Who brought you, who brought you, fellow, who brought you? If you delay telling me who brought you to this island, I shall make you find yourself reduced to ashes, becoming like a thing unseen." (pp. 212–213)

After telling the story of the shipwreck, the sailor was comforted by the snake, "Don't be afraid, don't be afraid, fellow; don't be pale-faced, now that you have come to me. It is god who has let you live and brought you to this island" (p. 213). The snake then foretold the sailor's rescue:

> You shall pass month upon month until you have completed four months in this island. Then a ship will come from home with sailors in it whom you know. You shall go home with them, you shall die in your town. (p. 213)

The snake added words of encouragement: "How happy is he who tells what he has tasted, when the calamity has passed" (p. 213); "If you are brave and control your heart, you shall embrace your children, you shall kiss your wife, you shall see your home" (p. 213). And so it came to be that ultimate joy reined over temporary sorrow.

Stuttering in the Bible

Other early references can be found in the Bible. The book of Exodus, representing 1350–1200 B.C. (May & Metzger, 1962), tells of Israel's emancipation from Egyptian bondage and the establishment of the covenant between God and the people of Israel. Moses was God's agent in delivering Israel from slavery and the mediator of the covenant. There is evidence in this book suggesting that Moses stuttered. When God called Moses to approach Pharaoh and lead the Jews out of Egypt, Moses protested:

> And Moses said unto the Lord: "Oh Lord, I am not a man of words, neither heretofore, nor since Thou hast spoken unto Thy servant; for I am slow of speech, and of a slow tongue." And the Lord said unto him: "Who hath made man's mouth? Or who maketh a man dumb, or deaf, or seeing, or blind? Is it not I the Lord? Now therefore go, and I will be with thy mouth, and teach thee what thou shalt speak." (Exodus, 4:10–12; Jewish Publication Society, 1965, p. 76)

In response to Moses' protests, God instructed Moses to bring Aaron, Moses' brother, as his spokesman.

> Is there not Aaron thy brother the Levite? I know that he can speak well. . . . And thou shalt speak unto him, and put the words in his mouth; and I will be with thy mouth, and with his mouth, and will teach you what ye shall do. And he shall be thy spokesman unto the people; and it shall come to pass, that he shall be to thee a mouth, and thou shalt be to him in God's stead. (Exodus, 4:14–16; Jewish Publication Society, 1965, p. 76)

Then, according to the text, Aaron, not Moses, spoke God's words and performed God's signs. Then Moses and Aaron went to the Pharaoh, and together they presented God's order: "Let My people go . . ." (Exodus, 5:1; Jewish Publication Society, 1965, p. 77). We noted earlier that people who stutter generally become immediately fluent when speaking in unison with another person. Moses and Aaron went repeatedly from God to Pharaoh, conveying the respective messages between the plagues. All the while, Moses gradually became more the spokesman, and Aaron, while present, grew increasingly silent. During the last four plagues, Moses spoke to the people and to Pharaoh, no longer complaining about his speech or seeking Aaron's help. In fact, Moses became an eloquent speaker.

How did Moses first begin to stutter? A midrash (a story from the Talmud told by Rabbis) explained:

> While Moses was still an infant, the Pharaoh was advised to kill him, for one day, it was predicted, Moses would rise up against him. The Pharaoh at first shrugged, then decided to put Moses to the test. He placed two bowls before Moses, one filled with gold, the other, with hot coals. If Moses chose the gold, he would be slain. Of course Moses reached for the gleaming gold, but an angel intervened and struck his hand. So he grabbed a hot coal and put it in his mouth. And thereafter stuttered. (Goldberg, 1989, p. 71)

Siegel (1990) noted that the early Rabbis seemed to hold a physical cause for stuttering and believed that such afflictions came directly from God. Furthermore, Siegel questioned how people can turn to God for strength and understanding if God is the source of the affliction, and concluded that an impediment does not need to disqualify a person from important work, leadership, or vision. Siegel stated the following:

> We don't have to be perfect to lead rich and ennobling lives. All of us have impediments of one sort or another, but for all of us there is a role to play, there are deserts to cross, people who need our help, in our own time and our own domains, in the circles or semicircles that frame our lives. We may not hear God calling to us directly, but we are surrounded by burning bushes and God is pleading with us, even as Moses pleaded with God, to make holy these places where we walk. (p. VII-12)

I believe that Siegel's words have clinical application. In actuality, we will never be certain that Moses stuttered. It is clearer, however, that the disorder was known to Isaiah who, between 742–687 B.C. (May & Metzger, 1962), admonished social injustice and proclaimed that private and public lives should reflect confidence in the omnipotence of God: "The heart also of the rash shall understand knowledge, And the tongue of the stammerers shall be ready to speak plainly" (Isaiah, 32:4; Jewish Publication Society, 1965, p. 573).

Stuttering in Professional Literature

The cause and treatment of stuttering have been foci of speculation for more than 2,500 years. Herodotus (484–424 B.C.), the Greek historian, recorded the treatment of stuttering by a Pythian priestess, who recommended emigration south to Libya. Hippocrates (450–357 B.C.), the Greek physician known as "the Father of Medicine," commented that chronic diarrhea, not of words, was common to people who stutter and recommended its cure by varices, dilating or twisting veins, arteries, or lymph vessels. He viewed the cause to be a disturbance in the mingling of the four "humours" including heat, cold, moisture, and dryness. Aristotle (384–322 B.C.), trained as an orator, attributed stuttering entirely to the tongue. Satyrus, the Greek actor, is said to have cured Demosthenes (383–322 B.C.), who stuttered and demonstrated voice and articulation errors, by having him perform voice exercises with pebbles in his mouth while declaiming and walking uphill. Galen (131–201 A.D.) thought that stuttering was caused by debility of the muscles resulting from diminution of heat and used cauterization as a remedy. Avicenna (980–1037 A.D.), philosopher and physician in Arabia, believed that humidity caused mollification of the tongue and recommended deep inspiration before speaking. Bacon (1560–1626 A.D.) thought stuttering was caused by refrigeration of the tongue resulting in dryness and immobility, for which he recommended drinking wine "because it heateth."

This is only a sample of the diverse thinking across time. In my review of the history of stuttering, I discovered a number of excellent sources (Bloodstein, 1993; Bluemel, 1957; Clark, 1964; Culatta & Goldberg, 1995; Diehl, 1958; Freund, 1966; Hahn & Hahn, 1956; Lewis, 1899; Murray & Edwards, 1980; Shames & Rubin, 1986; Silverman, 1996; Van Riper, 1973, 1982; Wingate, 1976; among many others.) One remarkable article was that of Klingbeil (1939), who described the evolution of etiological concepts and treatments of stuttering from 484 B.C. to 1915 A.D. The following highlights were adapted from these sources. For each contributor, the two dates noted refer to the year of birth and death. When only one date is given, it refers to the approximate time in which the theory was published or became known.

Stuttering as an Anatomical Defect

Throughout history, different anatomical structures have been implicated as the cause of stuttering. The tongue has been mentioned frequently. AEgineta (seventh century), Menjot (1615–1696), Kustner (1716), and Savary (1812) all ascribed stuttering chiefly to malformation of the tongue. Others holding similar views attempted to reduce the size (Chegoin, 1830) or alter position (Wutzner, 1850) of the tongue by mechanical methods. Hagemann (1845) recommended placing an *n* sound before each difficult syllable. Hahn (1694–1745) and Morgagni (1682–1771) both argued that the hyoid bone was responsible. Among those blaming the glottis were Yates (1828), a New York doctor and inventor of "the American Method," who recommended raising the tongue tip to the palate while speaking (this method also has been associated with Mrs. Leigh, whose husband stuttered, who directed an institute using this method, and who was the governess of Yates' daughter); Arnott (1788–1874), a Scottish physician, who recommended continuous phonation of *e* between each word to keep the glottis open; Muller (1801–1858), a German physiologist, who recommended omission of plosive sounds to keep the glottis open; Hoffman (1818–1892), who advocated physical relaxation and elimination of vocal tension; and Graves (1797–1853), an Irish physician, who advised directing the attention of the patient away from speech by having him strike an object simultaneously with speaking, in order to keep time. Santorini (1681–1737), an Italian anatomist, believed that an abnormal size of two holes in the middle region of the palate was the cause of stuttering. Others implicated a combination of structures. Thelwall (1764–1834), an English lawyer, differentiated four types of stuttering on the assumed causal basis of the lips, tongue, pharynx, or bronchi, all of which were treated by rhythm. Harnisch (1832) held that the larynx or posterior part of the tongue was responsible and had speaking rules governing movement of the tongue and lips.

Stuttering as a Medical Problem Requiring Surgery

Surgical intervention for stuttering (notably without the benefit of anesthesia), popular in the early to middle 19th century, varied considerably. AEtiuus (1542), a royal physician to Justinian at Byzantium, implicated the tongue and recommended surgical division of the lingual frenum. De Chauliac (1300–1380), a French surgeon, ascribed stuttering to a defect in the tongue, paralysis, or moisture of the nerves or muscles, and recommended embrocations to desiccate the brain and cauteries for the vertebrae. Dieffenbach (1795–1847), a German surgeon, assumed a connection between defective articulation and strabismus, addressed stuttering by making a horizontal section at the root of the tongue, excising a triangular wedge completely across and nearly through it, in order to interrupt the innervation, thereby modifying the muscular spasm. Velpeau (1795–1867), a French professor of clinical surgery, held that stuttering originated from an unusual depth of the palate, and therefore surgically divided the hyoglossus, geniohyoglossus, and styloglossus muscles. Other French surgeons including Amussat (1796–1856), Baudens (1804–1857), and Bonnet (1841) surgically divided the geniohyoglossus muscle. Froriep (1804–1861), a German surgeon, utilized an electrical form of intervention and also divided the genio-hyoglossus muscle, however, on one side only. Braid (1795–1860), an English surgeon, excised the tonsils or uvula. Parker (1806–1866), an American professor of surgery, introduced surgical intervention for stuttering to the United States, which was subsequently practiced in New York by Mott (1785–1865) and Post (1806–1866). In general, the German school followed the surgical methods of Dieffenbach, the French followed those of Velpeau, and the English those of Braid. Because of the dangers incurred (sometimes death) and the minimal improvement reported (less than 5% receiving permanent benefit), the procedures were abandoned.

Stuttering as a Disorder of Articulation

Colombat de l'Isere (1831) viewed stuttering as a result of spasmodic action of the articulators or rigidity of the laryngeal, pharyngeal, and respiratory muscles. For these conditions, he recommended rhythmic vocal gymnastics, focused practice on opposing movements of articulatory muscles, or mechanical devices including the rhythmic pace-setter, the *muthonome* (metronome). Good (1840) also held that stuttering was the result of defective articulation, and that the will should be strengthened to establish better control of the muscles of articulation. Bishop (1851) proposed that stuttering was the result of attempts to speak without vocal cord vibration, thus indicating disassociation between the articulatory and vocal organs. Others implicating defective articulators included the Hunts (1870) (father and son by the name James Hunt) of England who recommended disciplined exercise; Bristowe (1879) of London, who recommended breathing exercises and precise articulation; and Bates (1884), an American, who used various appliances, including a narrow flattened tube of silver applied to the palatal midline, to facilitate formation of lingua-palatal sounds. Bates also used a hollow biconvex disk with a projecting silver tube placed between the lips to help with labial and dental–labial sounds, and a belt and spring adjusted over the thyroid cartilage to help with velar sounds. Other treatments intending to add articulatory precision were those of Dupuytren (1817), who utilized speech in a singing tone, marking intervals by movement of the foot; Serre d'Alais (1829), who used forcible pronunciation of every syllable aided by synchronous arm gestures; and Comstock (mid-1800s), a Philadelphia physician, who used elocutionary exercises by reading aloud in unison with others.

Stuttering as a Disorder of Respiration

Theories of stuttering as a result of defective articulation often overlapped with those implicating defective breathing. Du Soit (1840) attributed stuttering to spasms of the respiratory system, as did Becquerel (1847) who proposed that the defect was in the respiratory muscles, which permitted air to escape prematurely, and recommended retention and controlled use of breath. Coen (1879) of Vienna viewed stuttering as the result of deficient atmospheric pressure in the lungs or pathological changes in the respiratory system, and recommended elocutionary exercises. Findlay (1885) believed that both the respiratory musculature and the structures of articulation and voice are responsible for stuttering, and that gestures could normalize movement of the diaphragm for fluent speech. Similarly, Rouma (1907) advocated use of arm gestures—however, the rationale was to facilitate overflow of cerebral activity from the arms to the speech centers. Other treatments included those of McCormac (1828), an English doctor, who recommended deep inspirations and forcible expirations, based on the assumption that stuttering resulted from speaking on emptied lungs; and Kingsley (1819–1875), an English orator and writer, whose recommendations from his own experience of stuttering included speaking with an open mouth and full lungs, inhaling at every stop, keeping the tongue down, exercising with weights to help breathing, keeping a piece of cork between the back teeth when speaking, and keeping the upper lip drawn down tightly.

Stuttering as a Disorder of Neuroanatomy/Motor Speech Dysfunction

Both theories of articulation and breathing disorder overlapped with those of neuromotor disorder. Erasmus Darwin (1731–1802), an English physician and naturalist and grandfather of Charles Darwin, held that emotions such as awe and bashfulness interrupted movement of the speech apparatus and recommended softening initial consonants. Itard (1817), a French surgeon, ascribed stuttering to a muscular deficit and used a golden or ivory fork, placed in the cavity of the alveolar arch of the lower jaw, to support the tongue. Rullier (1821) proposed that stuttering results from a disproportion between the rate at which the brain produces thoughts and that at which it transfers them to sites of innervation. He argued that the speech organs are unable to function properly because of the high demand placed upon them when profusion of stimuli must be processed so rapidly by the brain. Rullier's thinking introduced an early version of the Demands and Capacities model presented later in this chapter. Voisin (1821), a French doctor, held similar etiological views to those of Rullier, but added the treatment recommendation of pressing one's thumb against the chin while speaking. Astrie (1824) also located the cause in some modification of brain action, but recommended precise articulation and use of Itard's fork. Deleau (1797–1862) held that stuttering resulted from organic lesions yielding incomplete cerebral action or deficient innervation, and identified three aspects of stuttering including faulty tongue action and spasmodic closure of the lips or glottis. His treatment consisted of maximizing visual feedback for precise articulation. Schulthess (1830) identified stuttering as "phonophobia," a spasm of the glottis extending through nerve associations to the speech organs. Bell (1774–1842), a Scottish anatomist, held that stuttering resulted from inadequate capacity of the nerves to coordinate speech, which causes subsequent respiratory disruption, and emphasized the role of the larynx in articulation. Chervin (1867) concluded that the higher brain was responsible for stuttering, and recommended education to strengthen the will, imitation, and precise articulation. Guillaume (1868) also implicated the central nervous system and stressed the importance of whispering, lip gymnastics, keeping the tongue in contact with the palate during speech, and taking deep inspirations at every sentence.

Others attributing stuttering to motor incoordination resulting from central nervous system involvement included Hall-Marshall (1790–1857), who spoke of the involuntary action of the reflex spinal center and recommended a continuous, flowing manner of speaking; Rosenthal (1861), who blamed the coordinative disorder on an injury received during childhood to the medulla oblongata and recommended rhythmic exercises; Wolff (1861), who held that the nerves or organs themselves were at fault and recommended trying all methods, almost all drugs, and eventually surgical division of the hypoglossal nerve; and Shuldam (1879), who proposed the interaction of nervous weakness and muscular spasm and recommended elocutionary exercises of a rhythmic nature and regulation of respiration.

Stuttering as a Psychoneurosis

Mendelssohn (1729–1786), a philosopher, saw stuttering as the result of collision of too many ideas flowing simultaneously from the brain, and recommended slow reading with systematic disclosure. Others who believed stuttering to be an aspect of psychoneurosis included Lee (1773–1877), an English physician, who recommended surgical treatment and Wyneken (1868), who emphasized building faith in the client regarding the client's ability, speech and breathing exercises, and rhythmic beating of time. Kussmail (1822–1902), a German surgeon, defined stuttering as "lalloneurosis," "disarthria syllabaris," and "intermittent spasmodic neurosis," and recommended strengthening the willpower, breathing and articulatory exercises, and rhythmic speech. Some felt that stuttering was triggered by negative emotions including dread of speaking or excessive eagerness to speak (Sandow, 1898), fear and anxiety (Steckel, 1908), and embarrassment and lack of confidence (Thome, 1867). Thome, however, also held that stuttering is an aspect of motor speech and respiratory breakdown. Klencke (1813–1881), a German physician who emphasized the importance of the scientific method as a foundation for intervention, indicated that stuttering represents the person's need for psychological help, and opened an institution for treatment of people who stutter that placed particular focus on the unique personality disturbance from which stuttering originates. As always, treatments varied, including correcting the overt manifestations of stuttering by drill and exercise (Hudson-Makuen, 1910), rest and relaxation (Sandow, 1898); distraction (Bertrand, 1795–1831); and psychoanalysis (Appelt, 1911; Coriat, 1915; Netskatschen, 1909; Steckel, 1908).

Stuttering as a Learned Behavior

The following theories viewed stuttering as a bad habit or learned behavior. Amman (1667–1724), a Swiss physician, was among the first to state in print that stuttering was a learned behavior and recommended that it be treated by speaking loudly and slowly. Watson (1809), an English instructor, described stuttering as a "vicious habit" and recommended exercise of the speech organs and strengthening the will. Warren (1837) held that stuttering is a habit induced from weakness in and functional irregularity of the nervous system causing nervous agitation and disruption to the processes of articulation and voice. Merkel (1844), a German anatomist, held that stuttering is a deeply-rooted habit learned from an adynamic state of the speech organs and insufficient will, and should be treated by raising the tone of the whole body, lessening the force of the articulatory organs, and strengthening respiratory function. Kingsley, noted earlier for his treatments emphasizing breath control, held that stuttering was the result of conscious or unconscious imitation. Howard (1879), a speech specialist in New York, proposed that stuttering is a habit in which the glottis contracts, thus contracting the throat, because of insufficient pulmonary energy, and should be treated by relaxation of the chest and throat musculature.

In the latter part of the 19th century, others maintained that stuttering was a learned behavior. These included Butterfield (1880), a professor of vocal physiology, who held stuttering to be a habit-induced spasm of the diaphragm that should be treated by speech and respiratory gymnastics; Alexander Melville Bell (1819–1905), a vocal physiologist and grandfather of the inventor of the telephone, who held that stuttering in any stage of its habit formation could be uprooted by reading aloud in a loud whisper and by counting while breathing to improve pulmonary regularity; and Potter (1882) who maintained that the stuttering spasm was a habit induced by defective nerve function that occurred at the stop points on the vocal chain (i.e., lips, tongue, larynx, glottis).

Summary—History of Stuttering

Stuttering has continued to fascinate and intrigue throughout history. There is evidence of stuttering from the Egyptian Empire (2000 B.C.) in Egyptian hieroglyphics and from Biblical times (1350–1200 B.C.) in the Old Testament. Questions about the origin, nature, and treatment of stuttering have been continuous. Explanations for stuttering have included anatomical defects, medical problems requiring surgery, respiratory disorders, neuroanatomical and motor speech dysfunction, phychoneurosis, and learned behavior, among others. The middle of the 1800s saw unsuccessful attempts to link stuttering and strabismus, as well as frequent implications of the tongue as the cause of stuttering. Mechanical devices and surgery were used to raise or lower the tongue position. The physiological approach was more rational and humane than the surgical or medical approach, and sought to correct defective breathing, vocalization, and articulation. Exercises for breathing, articulation, voice, inflection, elocution, rhythm, continuity, and building multisensory feedback were among the remedies.

It is indeed apparent that our present harvest of theoretical explanations and related treatments were sown in seeds of the past. Goldberg (1989) appropriately referred to historic treatments for stuttering as spanning a period "from pebbles to psychoanalysis" (p. 71). Bluemel's (1957) thoughts are no less current or encouraging today:

> Much remains to be done in the field of disordered speech. . . . The research worker in the speech field need not be discouraged by progress which seems at times to be disappointingly slow. The history of poliomyelitis dates back at least 3500 years, and it was not till 1955 that the Salk vaccine became available. Stammering is as old as language; but now the answer to the riddle of the disorder seems close at hand. (p. 134)

ETIOLOGY OF STUTTERING: THE PRESENT

Throughout recorded time to the present day, we continue to ask, "What causes stuttering?" The apparent simplicity of this question is deceptive. The question is asked frequently by people who stutter, their families, and members of the general public. As indicated earlier in this chapter, the professional community, including speech–language pathologists, physicians, surgeons, anatomists, and psychotherapists, among others, has been on this trail for over 40 centuries. Now, we will focus on present or recent thinking. Today, when asked, "What caused your stuttering?" or "What caused (your family member) to stutter?," responses from anecdotal reports suggest that the term *cause* is often assumed to relate to those factors that were immediately present at the time the stuttering was first observed. Let's consider the concept of *cause* more directly.

Etiology Defined: Three Ps

Haynes et al. (1992) indicated, "The notion of cause has different meanings depending on its distance from the problem" (p. 7). Indeed, causality implies an ongoing or developmental concept and therefore assumes a time frame that must be specified. Traditionally, etiology has been defined in terms of *p*redisposing, *p*recipitating, and *p*erpetuating factors (i.e., causes; a helpful pneumonic device is to remember the three Ps).

Predisposing Factors

Predisposing factors are those agents that incline the person to stutter (Nicolosi et al., 1996) and address the question, "What factors cause one person to be at greater risk than another for beginning to stutter?" (Silverman, 1996, p. 100). An example of predisposing factors is the apparent genetic inclination (predisposition) to stutter; stuttering tends to run in families. However, as will be seen, it might be that environmental or developmental (precipitating) factors or the interactions between predisposing and precipitating factors are the reasons that stuttering surfaces. Another way of looking at the significance of predisposing factors is in their potential link with a third agent (Emerick & Haynes, 1986). For example, one frequently observed predisposing factor is the higher incidence of left-handedness among people who stutter. There is little significance in the left-handedness by itself. However, the implication of basic underlying neurological differences is noteworthy and continues to be a current line of research. The clinician and diagnostician must be watchful for factors that occur with regularity in association with the stuttering. Such predisposing factors may be instrumental in revealing information regarding the nature of stuttering and people who stutter (Emerick & Haynes, 1986; Haynes et al., 1992).

Precipitating Factors

Precipitating factors are those agents thought to have made stuttering surface or those that brought it to its present state (Nicolosi et al., 1996; Haynes et al., 1992). Silverman (1996) indicated that these factors address the question, "What actually causes a person to begin to stutter?" (p. 100). Precipitating factors generally are no longer operating, and therefore may or may not be identifiable. Some may debate the value of identifying factors that are not still operating. Haynes et al. (1992) pointed out, however, that each moment, "a new set of precipitating factors is created that, acting as characteristics of the past, perpetuates behaviors of the present" (p. 7). They indicated that communication disorders, namely stuttering, are not static entities developed at a given point in time; rather they are dynamic, ever-changing characteristics that constantly are influenced by internal and external factors. Examples of precipitating factors might include the rapid growth in speech and language skills during the preschool years, competition among siblings for attention and conversational turns in normally busy homes, and the social adjustments necessary when entering preschool and school settings. As will be seen, these factors place increasing demands on children's developing communication skills.

Identification and Interaction of Predisposing and Precipitating Factors

It should be noted that determination of predisposing and precipitating factors in developmental (i.e., idiopathic) stuttering generally is an estimate at best. I am reminded of a young boy with a language impairment with whom I worked many years ago. At the time, he said "I can't know" for "I don't know." This led me to consider the distinction between that which is not knowable and that which is not known. Often, although not always, we cannot know the causal link between predisposing and precipitating factors and the occurrence of stuttering. For example, consider the case of a boy who presented a family history of stuttering (a predisposing factor), and whose stuttering began around the age of 3 years when his speech and language skills were growing rapidly, whose home routine was busy as both parents worked outside, and who was beginning a part-time preschool program (precipitating factors). The predisposing factors cannot be altered. The clinician worked with the family to reduce the potential influence of the precipitating factors (e.g., facilitating fluent conversation though age-appropriate language content and form in a restructured environment that eliminated interruption and perceived communicative pressure), yet the stuttering persisted.

Ultimately, we cannot know if the child's stuttering would have begun and developed in the absence of the factors noted. How do we explain other children who have similar predisposing and precipitating factors and who develop stuttering with early recovery, or those who do not begin to stutter at all? Perhaps the presence, absence, and outcome of stuttering are independent of the factors identified. Maybe a unique interaction of known or unknown factors is explanatory. Communication is a complex process; thus causal factors including social, learning, motivational, psychological, physiological, linguistic, among others, may singly or collectively hold the hidden key. Previously, I warned that correlation (events that occur in temporal proximity to one another) does not infer causality (a direct link of responsibility between two events, one assumed to be a stimulus, the other assumed to be its direct result). I am mindful that attempts to determine predisposing and precipitating factors might appear to be an imprecise science of diagnosis, yet I am encouraged by the potential for these factors to shed some light on the nature of a person's stuttering experience or help to tailor the treatment experience to the uniqueness of the person who stutters.

Therefore, I maintain that pursuing these factors is essential. Less frequently, the precipitating factors are easily identifiable, as is their causal connection to the stuttering behavior. An example might be the infrequent cases of abrupt onset of stuttering surrounding a traumatic event. When observed, such cases are typically viewed as a distinct subtype of the disorder (e.g., "neurotic stuttering," Haynes et al., 1992; psychogenic disfluency, see Chapter 4). Other cases where precipitating factors are clear and causally linked to the communication disorder include instances of cerebral vascular accident (i.e., stroke), vocal abuse, structural anomalies, and certain congenital conditions (Haynes et al., 1992).

Perpetuating Factors

Perpetuating factors are those variables that are continuing or maintaining the stuttering at the present time (Nicolosi et al., 1996) and address the question, "What causes a person to continue to stutter after the disorder has begun?" (Silverman, 1996, p. 100). Haynes et al. (1992) indicated that habit strength is a prime perpetuating factor since the client has made compensations for the stuttering in terms of cognitive and linguistic strategies, motor adjustments, etc. The clinician needs to uncover environmental and physical factors that reinforce, and therefore perpetuate, the disorder. Occasionally, precipitating factors that are still present might serve to perpetuate the stuttering. For example, environmental influences such as criticism of speech, inappropriate linguistic models, unrealistic expectations, and experienced fluency failure exacerbate the problem and maintain the likelihood of its predictability. Unlike frequently observed with predisposing and precipitating factors, perpetuating factors are nearly always "knowable."

Although many clients do not know or recognize the perpetuating factors, they can know them with the assistance of a supportive and knowledgeable clinician. Sometimes the negative feelings and attitudes that result from repeated frustration and embarrassment with stuttering are the most challenging perpetuating factors to alter. Accommodations are made by the person who stutters and others within his communication system (family, friends, classmates, teachers, colleagues, employers, etc.). Thus the dynamics of communication, including how we perceive ourselves and others as communicators, are established that perpetuate or maintain the disorder. The anticipation of fluency failure so often felt by people who stutter in situations perceived to be important (asking someone out for a date, speaking to one's employer, saying one's own name) is understandable given one's history, yet a barrier to fluency facilitation.

The spouse who continues to order for her husband in restaurants during their 40-year marriage is preventing him frustration and embarrassment, yet perpetuating the likelihood that he will be unable to be fluent in that setting. A man of 55 years who reportedly was severely disfluent for his entire life discovered during trial management that he possessed the potential for remarkable fluency. When asked to consider how an improvement in his fluency would affect him as a communicator or his life, he literally was unable to imagine or dream of those possibilities. He indicated, "I have always stuttered. I cannot imagine what it would be like not to stutter. This is all that I've ever known." This is habit strength. This is what happens when stuttering establishes the perimeters of one's self-concept, of one's personal construct. This is a man who saw himself as a "stutterer." Stuttering was at the heart of his very existence. He reported that in his sleep, he saw himself stuttering in his dreams. Stuttering was the anchor around which all of his life revolved—emotionally, interpersonally, socially, professionally. Indeed, it was hard for him even to consider another paradigm—until he experienced systematic and reliable success in treatment. At the sixth week of treatment, he confessed, "You know, I didn't believe in this stuff (i.e., individualized and joint treatment planning, implementation, evaluation, and follow-up) at the beginning. But now, I'm hooked."

Perpetuating factors vary with each individual and may be simple or complex, subtle or obvious, malleable or resistant to change. Nevertheless, we can know and must know these factors in order to facilitate change. The process, as will be seen, is a tender one at times, in that people learn about themselves and others. Learning constitutes change. Change sometimes is difficult to accept. But a sensitive, caring, and knowledgeable clinician cares for, with, and about the person who stutters, and enters into the process as a "comrade in a common struggle."

Theoretical Explanations

The bottom line is that at present we do not, and quite possibly cannot, know the cause of stuttering. While it is tempting to be drawn into the simplicity of unidimensional conceptualizations of etiology, it is most likely that the etiology of stuttering is multidimensional and might vary across people who stutter. What follows is a number of theoretical explanations in response to the vexing questions generated by the three Ps.

Stuttering as a Neurotic Response (i.e., Repressed Need Theory)

More than 50 years ago, psychoanalytic explanations of stuttering held that stuttering satisfies oral or anal erotic needs or represents repressed hostility. Within this framework, stuttering is an attempt to suppress speech and is a symptom of a deep neurotic conflict. Because other neurotic symptoms were not identified and interpersonal relationships, particularly parent–child, were not found to be disturbed, this theory lost general popularity and no longer is considered valid. Stated directly, "Stuttering is not a neurotic disorder" (Andrews et al., 1983, p. 236). Addressing the relationship between children who stutter and their parents, Wingate (1983) provided support (Johnson & Associates, 1959; Parker, 1979; Yairi & Williams, 1971) to state that "parents of stutterers compare quite favorably with parents of nonstutterers" (p. 259).

Stuttering as Communicative Failure and Anticipatory Struggle Behavior

These theories assume that the person who stutters disrupts the way he speaks because he believes that speech is difficult or that he will fail at speaking.

The Diagnosogenic Theory. Johnson's (1958b, 1959, 1961) diagnosogenic or semantic theory states that stuttering is caused by the parents' or care providers' misdiagnosis of and inappropriate reaction to normal disfluencies in a child's speech, followed by the child's attempts to avoid the disfluencies that are mistakenly assumed to render the child's speech as abnormal. Johnson (1942) stated:

> The parents classified their children as stutterers and then proceeded to react to them largely in terms of the implications of the label. These reactions on the part of parents were not confined to inner states of tension and anxiety or chagrin, but usually also involved overt attempts to influence the child's speech behavior and definite communication to the child of the parental evaluations of his speech. (p. 255)

Johnson (1942) also stated that, "There can be little question of the fact that highly similar varieties of speech in young children are thus differently evaluated by different parents, and there can be little question that the way in which they are evaluated plays a determining role in the subsequent speech development of the child" (p. 256). He concluded that, "Stuttering in its serious forms develops after the diagnosis rather than before and is a consequence of the diagnosis" (p. 257).

Bloodstein (1986) discussed the research and other factors giving rise to the diagnosogenic theory and its significant influence on other theories, research, and therapy. Van Riper (1982) classified Johnson's theory as a cognitive learning theory. Johnson's theory was the most widely accepted theory in the 1940s and 1950s. It strongly criticized the environmental events, namely reactions of parents and other listeners, as a direct precipitator of stuttering, and implied that predisposing or constitutional factors were relatively insignificant. Johnson and his associates (1959) observed that children who stutter demonstrated more sound and syllable repetitions, complete blocks, and prolonged sounds than children who do not stutter; the latter group showing more phrase repetitions, pauses, and interjections than children who stutter. Nevertheless, Johnson chose to emphasize the similarity, rather than the differences, across children to stress the significance that stuttering is first in the parent's ear, not in the child's mouth.

Silverman (1988) uncovered a remarkable unpublished study by one of Johnson's graduate students (Tudor, 1939) in which normally fluent children were reported to have been turned into children who stutter. The study was conducted before Johnson proposed the diagnosogenic theory. Those familiar with the study at the University of Iowa reportedly referred to it as "the monster study." Silverman indicated that the study holds tremendous historical significance because it is the only direct test of the diagnosogenic theory and provides clinical implications contraindicating the wisdom of increasing children's awareness of their speech hesitations. Specifically, Tudor selected six children whose chronological ages were 5, 9, 11, 12, 12, and 15 from an orphanage to serve as subjects. All of the children, selected because of their normal communication development, were told flatly that their speech contained symptoms of a child beginning to stutter and that they should stop this pattern immediately, use willpower, and stop talking unless they can get it right. In addition, the teachers and matrons were told that the children showed "definite symptoms of stuttering," should be watched closely for speech errors, and should be corrected when such errors occur. The subjects reportedly experienced negative communicative changes including decrease in verbal output, rate of speech, and length of utterance; heightened self-consciousness; acceptance that there was something defective in their speech; and nonverbal behavior interfering with the message (e.g., gasping and covering the mouth when speaking, avoiding eye contact, laughing awkwardly and showing embarrassment). Tudor attempted to treat the children and continued to do so for several years, but the communicative changes persisted and at least one child continued to stutter (Silverman, 1988).

The results of Tudor's (1939) study were never disseminated widely because the experimenters regretted the experiment and were remorseful about the outcome. Silverman, a former student and research assistant of Johnson, noted that Johnson never published the findings of this study in any of his writings on the diagnosogenic theory although they directly supported it. The results of this study are significant in that they do indicate that evaluative labeling can influence behavior; specifically, that diagnosing normal disfluency as stuttering can cause stuttering. This study has implications for caution to be exercised in the labeling process and that directions for a child to monitor his speech fluency and attempt to be more fluent should be handled with care.

The Continuity Hypothesis. This theory was proposed by Bloodstein (1975, 1984, 1995) and suggests that stuttering develops from normal disfluency that becomes tense and fragmented as the child experiences frustration and failure in attempts to talk. Many types of experiences can lead the child to experience difficulty with speech, including criticism of normal disfluencies, delay in speech or language development, communication disorders, traumatic experience in oral reading, cluttering and reminders to "slow down," and emotionally traumatic events during which the child tries to speak (Bloodstein, 1975, 1984). Peters and Guitar (1991) indicated that other aspects of the internal and external environment may add pressure and lead a child to expect failure. These influences may include a perfectionistic nature or a high need to perform or meet the perceived standards of others. The level of unconditional acceptance and positive regard within the child's communication environment is critical in influencing the child's attitude and expectation toward himself as a communicator.

Bloodstein (1975) interpreted stuttering, heightened tension and fragmentation, as a form of communication failure resulting from anticipatory struggle (i.e., a response to stimuli representative of past speech failure). Bloodstein (1975) indicated that people who stutter "behave as though they have acquired a belief in the difficulty of speech, or of specific speech segments, and appear to struggle against an imagined obstacle in the process of articulation" (p. 4). Tension and fragmentation represent the embodiment of the speaker's doubts about his ability to speak well, heightened by the perception of a critical audience or the memory of past speech failure or pressure. Bloodstein indicated that most children demonstrate speech tension and fragmentation in their speech, but a difference in children who stutter is the degree to which this tension occurs. This observation formed the core of his continuity hypothesis.

On the surface, the diagnosogenic theory and continuity hypothesis sound similar. In both, the child becomes aware of his speech-related tension and fragmentation and desires to avoid it. However, the diagnosogenic theory suggests that the child does so because of negative reactions of listeners to the disfluency (i.e., the child plays more of a passive role in the evolution of stuttering); while the continuity hypothesis emphasizes the child's own awareness of and increasing concern about his own disfluency (i.e., the child is more active).

Taken to an extreme, Bloodstein's (1975) hypothesis implies that no differential diagnosis can be made on the basis of indicators of developmental stuttering because "most young children stutter" (p. 51). Stuttering only becomes a problem when the child evaluates the breaks in fluency as unpleasant and shows fear, avoidance, and struggle reactions. Bloodstein (1975) concluded:

> Any attempt to make such a "diagnosis" is a futile and meaningless exercise. We can describe his tensions and fragmentations, count them, compare them with norms, find out under what conditions they occur, determine how much of a problem they are for the child or anyone else, and make a judgment about whether he should be getting some help from us because of them. But we cannot tell whether he is or is not a "stutterer." (p. 51)

The literal interpretation of Bloodstein's continuity hypothesis and its implications have been challenged by the clinical literature, particularly as clinicians and researchers have become increasingly aware of the importance of differential diagnosis and appropriate early intervention (Gordon & Luper, 1992a, 1992b; Van Riper, 1982).

Preparatory Set (i.e., Primary Stuttering Theory). Van Riper (1972, 1973, 1982) indicated that stuttering emerges gradually from a child's normal hesitations and repetitions. Such disruptions first occur without effort or apparent awareness by the child, and later become chronic when the child begins to anticipate, avoid, and fear speech and related contexts because of reactions by listeners. Stuttering can originate from learning (environmental), constitutional (organic), or neurotic (emotional) sources. Van Riper (1972) described the onset and development of stuttering on the basis of a topographical map. Accordingly, stuttering has three sources. The major one is represented by "Lake Learning," into which the stream from "Constitutional Reservoir" flows. "Neurosis Pond" also is one of the sources of stuttering, but a smaller one. According to Van Riper (1972), stuttering can come from any of these three sources, as follows:

> As the stream leaves Lake Learning, it flows slowly and many a child caught in its current may make it to shore by himself or with a bit of parental or therapeutic help. Some of them are cast up on Precarious Island and become fluent for a time, only to be swept away again by the swift-moving emotional currents from Neurosis Pond. The second stage in the development of stuttering is represented by Surprise Rapids, and the stutterer begins to know that he is in trouble. It isn't hard to rescue him, however, if you know how to do it.

Once he is swept over Frustration Falls, however, he takes a beating from the many rocks that churn the stream. Despite their random struggling, a few make it to shore even at this stage, the third, but they usually need an understanding therapist and cooperative parents to help them. The river flows even faster here, and soon it enters the Gorge of Fear. This is the worst stretch of the whole stream of stuttering, for below it lies the Whirlpool of Self-Reinforcement. Once the child is caught in its constant circling, there is little hope that he will ever make it to shore by himself. Only an able and stout swimmer who knows not only this part, but all of the river of stuttering, can hope to save him. Where does the river end? King Charles the First knows. (p. 277)

Bloodstein (1995) interpreted Van Riper's (1973) use of the preparatory set in treatment to interpret the anticipatory struggle hypothesis. Specifically, the preparatory set, or alteration of the block before it occurs, is used to counteract the tendency of the person who stutters to place himself in a tense, muscular posture in advance of attempting to say a word he fears or believes will be disfluent. This preposturing influences the shape of the disfluency to follow. Van Riper (1982) offered a tentative explanation that stuttering is related to the difficulty some children experience in mastering the synchronized timing of the motor coordinations required for speech.

Stuttering as Learned Behavior

These theories, within the context of the behavioral sciences, define the processes by which stuttering is originally learned and maintained and postulate motivational factors, stimulus variables, and reinforcing conditions (Nicolosi et al., 1996). Andrews et al. (1983) distinguished between learning theories that view stuttering as an avoidance response and those that view stuttering as an interaction of at least two behavioral phenomena.

Stuttering as an Avoidance Response

CONFLICT THEORY OF STUTTERING AND AVOIDANCE REDUCTION. Sheehan (1958, 1975) viewed stuttering as resulting from a double approach–avoidance conflict between speaking and not speaking and between being silent and not being silent. "The avoidance does not come primarily from the fear of stuttering as such but from the competition between the alternative possibilities of speech and silence, with the stuttering a resultant of this conflict" (Sheehan, 1958, p. 126). When the approach drive is more powerful, fluent speech results; when the avoidance drive is more powerful, disfluency or silence results. When both motivational drives for approach and avoidance of speaking are equally dominant, stuttering results. Theoretically, stuttering reduces the fear underlying the avoidance drive, thus enabling the approach motivational drive to regain dominance.

OPERANT CONDITIONING AND STUTTERING. This theory states that speech is a behavior subject to operant control of positive and negative reinforcements and punishments. There is no simple cause of stuttering that is maintained on a complex schedule of reinforcement. Shames (1975) stated:

Operant behavior is that behavior whose frequency is a function of its consequences. On certain occasions, certain responses generate consequences in the environment. If these consequences affect the frequency of the behavior that they follow, we are dealing with operant behavior. (p. 267)

He indicated that stuttering and disfluency decrease with contingent aversive stimulation through negative reinforcement, and that fluency increases through positive reinforcement. Given the reliability of these observations, Shames noted that conditioning processes are probably active in the onset and development of stuttering. The particular form that these conditioning processes may take in the child's natural environment can only be suggested and have not been experimentally verified.

INSTRUMENTAL AVOIDANCE ACT THEORY. This theory states that stuttering is an acquired response reflecting expectancy, anticipation, adaptation, or anxiety and is motivated by the learned drive of apprehension about the normal disfluencies of speech (Nicolosi et al., 1996). Wischner (1950, 1952) applied the concepts of drive-reduction (namely anxiety) to explain the maintenance of stuttering. Wischner adopted Johnson's postulates that the child reacts to the parents' misdiagnosis with tension, anxiety, and avoidance. Wischner emphasized, however, that the child is not trying to avoid the normal disfluencies, but rather the consequences that are associated with the original disfluent behaviors (i.e., feelings of anxiety, hurt, and shame). Certain cues precipitate these anxieties that the person attempts to lessen by avoidance. Because of the anxiety reduction, the avoidance behaviors are reinforced and thereby developed and maintained. For example, avoidance behaviors such as interjection of a sound (e.g., "um") or phrase (e.g., "Let me see") might prevent or stall the moment of disfluency, thus reducing the anxiety reaction that reinforces the avoidance behavior.

Stuttering as an Interaction of Behavioral Phenomena

TWO-FACTOR LEARNING THEORY OF STUTTERING. Two-factor theorists (Brutten, 1975, Brutten & Shoemaker, 1971) differentiate between classical conditioning (stimulus-contingent learning) and instrumental conditioning (response-contingent learning). Classical conditioning generally describes the conditions within which a person (or other organism) learns to be motivationally or emotionally stimulated by previously neutral stimuli. Classical conditioning increases the number of stimuli that motivate, arouse, or drive a person. Instrumental conditioning generally describes conditions within which a person learns coping responses in order to modify "learned or unlearned drive states" associated with a stimulus context. "Classical conditioning leads to the development of relationships between stimuli and motivational states or emotional responses, and instrumental conditioning leads to the development of relationships between stimuli and relatively specific, goal-oriented behaviors" (Brutten & Shoemaker, p. 1055). These authors propose that the core characteristics of stuttering (such as part-word and word repetitions and prolongations) are the involuntary breakdown of speech resulting from negative emotional responses that are classically conditioned. (Stress may produce autonomic reactions that disrupt the speech. The negative emotions aroused become classically conditioned with concurrent stimuli.) Secondary characteristics (such as escape and avoidance) are instrumentally conditioned responses (or learned adjustments) of the individual to unpleasant experiences (Andrews et al., 1983; Nicolosi et al., 1996).

Summarizing the modern concepts of stuttering as learned behavior, Van Riper (1982) indicated that most current thinking about stuttering reflects the influence of learning theory. He stated, "The different varieties of stuttering reactions, the changes that occur as the disorder develops, the role of situational and verbal cues in its precipitation, all these and many other features of the problem testify to the influence of learning" (p. 284). Van Riper indicated that it is generally agreed that learning plays at least a part in determining the patterns of advanced stuttering. There is much disagreement, however, regarding the exact role that learning plays.

Stuttering as a Physiological Deficit

These theories, also referred to as breakdown theories, characterize the moment of stuttering as an indication of failure or breakdown in the complex coordination required for fluent speech. Most breakdown theories assume that a person who stutters has a constitutional predisposition toward stuttering that is precipitated by psychosocial or environmental stress, and a reduced physiological capacity to coordinate speech. The precise nature of the organic predisposing factors and the role of heredity vary across theorists. Such theorists have postulated perceptual, motor, or central deficits (Andrews et al., 1983; Nicolosi et al., 1996).

Stuttering as a Function of Incomplete Cerebral Dominance. This theory suggests that people who stutter do not show the usual pattern for left hemisphere dominance. Orton and Travis (Travis, 1978) observed that many people who stutter were left handed, but were deliberately changed to right handedness by their parents. They hypothesized that ambidexterity or a change in handedness (i.e., incomplete cerebral dominance or laterality) caused a disruption in the regular flow of nerve impulses to the speech musculature. This disruption caused a conflict between the two hemispheres for the control of speech taking the form of neuromotor disorganization and mistiming resulting in stuttering.

Dysphemia and Biochemical Theory. This theory states that stuttering is a manifestation of an internal condition triggered by illness, emotional or environmental stress (i.e., dysphemia), or biochemical imbalance. West (1958) indicated that "stuttering is primarily an epileptic disorder that manifests itself in dyssynergies of the neuromotor mechanism for oral language. Its spasms are precipitated by social anxieties involved in communication by oral language" (1958, p. 197). These anxieties are more likely to be precipitants of stuttering when they take the form of conscious feelings of guilt, particularly related to the topic of the conversation. West, therefore, viewed stuttering as a convulsive disorder involving a relationship between the person who stutters and his conversational partners within a social communicative context.

Perseveration Theory. This theory states that a person who stutters has an organic predisposition to motor and sensory perseveration of which stuttering is an outward manifestation. Eisenson elaborated his interpretation of stuttering as a perseverative phenomenon (1958, 1975), indicating that "stuttering is a transient disturbance in communicative, propositional language usage" (1975, p. 426). Speech becomes implicated because it is the medium for oral language, that which is temporarily disturbed. He indicated that the majority of people who stutter are constitutionally predisposed to a manner of perseverative oral language behavior (i.e., stuttering). While he distinguished between organically predisposed and functional or nonorganic "stutterers," his premise was that both are the products of constitutionally predisposed perseveration.

Stuttering as a Consequence of Brain Lesion. Based on high speed cineradiographic data, Zimmermann (1980a) studied the movements, positions, and timing of lip and jaw structures in the perceptually fluent production of isolated monosyllables by people who stutter. He compared these productions to those of people who do not stutter. The fluent syllables spoken by people who stutter revealed longer duration of movement onset, slower voice onset, longer latency for peak velocity of lip and jaw movements, longer transition times, and greater lip and jaw movement asynchrony. These patterns were evident during perceptually fluent sounds and syllables, and even more evident during stuttered speech. Zimmermann postulated that stuttering involves changes in the interaction of laryngeal, supralaryngeal, and respiratory reflexes. This proposal implicates the brain stem as the site of lesion, and suggests that stuttering is the consequence of disruption of motor organization, timing, and control (Zimmermann, 1980a, 1980b, 1984; Zimmermann, Smith, & Hanley, 1981). Van Riper (1982) projected that if replicated and corroborated, Zimmermann's research could have significant implications for how overt stuttering emerges. (If perceptually fluent speech of people who stutter is consistently burdened by lags and asynchronies, tension and fear can become disruptive communicative stresses.) Furthermore, Van Riper concurred that stuttering appears to implicate the neuromuscular timing pattern, observing "temporal disruption of the simultaneous and successive programming of muscular movements" (p. 415), and concluded that "we find the essence of the disorder in this fracturing and disruption of the motor sequence of the word" (p. 415).

Stuttering as the Result of Disturbed Feedback (i.e., Cybernetic Theory)

This theory is based on the servomechanism feedback model, in which the ear is the sensor, the vocal organs and motor innervations are the effector, and the brain is the controller. People who stutter are assumed to possess a defective monitoring system for speech. To remain error free, ongoing fluent speech movements require feedback and sensory information. When errors occur, the system corrects itself by searching for the appropriate output until it is achieved. Stuttering is seen as a consequence of this corrective process, the absence of a correct standard pattern for production of a syllable or word, or a perceptual error on the input side of sensory information processing. This theory assumes that the automatic motor sequencing of speech occurs within a closed loop system in which feedback, namely auditory feedback, is critical (Fairbanks, 1954). The feedback systems used to monitor speech potentially have many sources of distortion (e.g., asynchrony or delay of auditory feedback, which can interfere with proprioceptive feedback). Too much feedback distortion and output correction can cause fixation in the system. According to this model, such distortion, interference, and overload can cause stuttering.

Demands and Capacities Model

We already reviewed Starkweather's (1984, 1987) definition of speech fluency, a multidimensional variable composed of continuity, rate, and effort. Fluent speech, therefore, is characterized by continuous production, without effort, and at an appropriate rate. Both the child's capacities for fluent speech and the demands for fluent speech imposed on the child by listeners and himself are increasing. When the demands exceed the child's capacities for fluent speech, stuttering occurs. If the demands are reduced or increased slowly or the child's capacities develop sufficiently, stuttering remits. If the demands continue to outpace the child's capacity for fluent speech, stuttering continues. The continuation of stuttering might be self-perpetuating. In other words, if stuttering continues long enough for the child to develop struggle, tension, and avoidance, his whole approach to speaking is influenced by anticipated fluency failure.

Starkweather, Gottwald, and Halfond (1990) elaborated the demands and capacities model, indicating that the capacities for fluency fall into four categories: speech motor control (i.e., rate of syllable production and coordination of movement), language formulation (i.e., word-finding, formulation of grammatical sentences, and knowledge of conversational rules), social–emotional maturity, and cognitive skill (i.e., general intelligence and metalinguistic skill). The demands for fluency are those conditions that impose a pressure perceived by the child to speak at greater rate (i.e., faster) or with greater continuity (i.e., smoothness). The demands, which increase as the child matures, include time pressure, uncertainty, and avoidance.

Time pressure is imposed when parents or others speak too rapidly in the child's presence, thus conveying that speech time is limited and information is expected to flow rapidly. There is evidence that mothers of children who stutter talk more rapidly and interrupt more often than mothers of children who do not (Meyers & Freeman, 1985a, 1985b), and that a positive correlation exists between the extent to which parents decrease their rate of speech (Gottwald & Starkweather, 1984, 1995) or implement structured conversational turn-taking (Winslow & Guitar, 1994) and the extent to which the child's fluency improves. Negative listener reactions (such as interruptions, finishing the child's sentence, behavior interpreted as displeasure or "hurry up") also impose a time pressure. Likewise, language used with the child, including longer and more complex vocabulary and syntax, presents additional time pressure. Such constructions, which the child attempts to match, are motorically more difficult to plan, time, coordinate, and execute, thus consuming neuromotor resources that would otherwise be devoted to maintaining fluency. Additional sources of time pressure are *demand speech* (that which limits the child's conversational spontaneity, including frequent questions or requests to recite something or recount events), a rushed household or other environment, high levels of excitement or emotionality, and rushed and interrupted pattern of conversational turn-taking. Starkweather et al. (1990) indicated that these and other factors are at risk for lowering the child's sense of self-esteem, thus conveying that neither he nor his conversational contribution is valued. As a consequence, the child feels he is not worthy of much talking time.

Uncertainty, or any event that might introduce change or disruption, can challenge the child's sense of security, thus placing additional demands on the child's existing capacities for fluent speech. Starkweather et al. (1990) provided examples including: moving into a new house or neighborhood, first separation from parents, birth of a sibling, illness of a parent, change in daycare setting or childcare arrangement, and a household charged with emotionality or tension. The uncertainty of these and other circumstances might leave the child feeling unsure of the consequences of behavior, thus causing him to become hesitant to do or say anything. This uncertainty may worsen the frequency and severity of disfluency.

Avoidance of stuttering or speaking is another factor imposing a demand on the child. Such avoidance might originate from inadvertent negative reactions from listeners, such as tensing when the child stutters and relaxing when the child regains fluency, looking away, filling in for the child, tapping fingers, wrinkling brows, or other behaviors that communicate to the child that his stuttering is undesirable and unpleasant. In addition to perceiving pressure to speak faster and smoother, some children experience guilt for the discomfort they feel they have caused their parents or other listeners. Starkweather et al. (1990) concluded:

> We believe that fluent speech is rapid and continuous, and that the capacity to speak fluently increases with maturity. At the same time, the environment, both internal and external, is increasingly demanding of fluency. There is increased pressure to generate more complex ideas within a limited period of time. Parents, reacting to disfluency in the child's speech, may speak more quickly and interrupt more often, and these reactions increase the demands of time pressure even further. In addition, changes in the child's life may lead to increased insecurity and uncertainty of the consequences of speaking. Finally, the reactions of parents to the child's disfluency may lead increasingly to an attitude of avoidance of disfluency. The gap between these demands and capacities widens or narrows as changes in the demands proceed more or less quickly than changes in the capacities. The capacities stem from speech motor control—programming, timing, and coordination—and from linguistic and social skills, such as language formulation and pragmatic knowledge. Both speech and language fluency impact on the ease with which a child can produce meaningful speech, as reflected in the rate and continuity of the child's utterances. (pp. 28–29)

Summary and Synthesis—Etiology of Stuttering and Theoretical Explanations

What factors render one child more at risk than another for beginning to stutter?

These constitutional factors have been discussed as predisposing causes of stuttering. The presence of more such factors seems to increase a child's predisposition to stutter, yet to what extent continues to be unknown (Silverman, 1996). Peters and Guitar (1991) indicated that it is unlikely that any of these factors directly causes stuttering; thus these differences appear to be neither necessary nor sufficient to cause stuttering. The connection between these factors and stuttering may be indirect, in that their presence taxes a child's communication development and that the resulting frustration and failure may lead to stuttering. However, it is possible that these factors are unrelated to stuttering. Nevertheless, the following factors seem to present greater risk or predisposition for stuttering:

- *Gender*—Boys are more likely than girls to stutter.

- *Age*—While stuttering can begin at any age, the majority of children who stutter begin to do so between the ages of 2 and 5 years.

- *Family history*—While stuttering can appear in any family, the risk is greater for a child born to a parent who stutters or into a family with a history of stuttering.

- *Socioeconomic status and nationality*—Children from middle and upper-middle class families and certain groups from Canada, Korea, and West Africa show greater risk.

- *Twins*—A child who is a twin, particularly an identical twin, is at greater risk than a child who is not.

- *Brain injury*—A child with a brain injury is at greater risk than one without.

- *Mental retardation*—A child with mental retardation, particularly Down Syndrome, is at greater risk.

- *Bilingualism*—Bilingual children are at greater risk than unilingual children.

Furthermore, children who stutter demonstrate the following group differences when compared to children who do not stutter:

- Greater likelihood to have a history of delayed articulation or language development

- Poorer performance on verbal and motor tests of intelligence

- Poorer performance on measures of school performance

- More problems in social adjustment

- Less left-hemisphere dominance for speech

- Slower reaction times

- Poorer recognition and recall of competing messages

- Slower speech movements even during fluent speech

Theoretical explanations for the patterns demonstrated by some children to show greater predisposition to stutter include atypical patterns for laterality or handedness (cerebral localization theory), disruption in the motor sequence of the spoken utterance resulting from neuromotor mistiming in the patterns needed for perceiving and producing speech (disorder of timing theory), and problems in learning relationships between the desired sounds and the required motor sequences (reduced capacity for internal modeling, or demands and capacities theory).

Why do people stutter?

Various environmental and developmental factors have been discussed as precipitating causes of stuttering. Again, establishing a causal connection between the factors and the literal beginning of stuttering becomes a speculative exercise. Peters and Guitar (1991) metaphorically compared the developing human brain to a computer stating:

> Like a computer, the brain can work on several things at once. Like a computer, the more tasks it does simultaneously, the slower and less efficiently it does each one . . . . The problem of shared resources is more acute, of course, in children, because their immature nervous systems have less processing capacity to share. Some children are especially at risk for strain on their developing resources. They may be delayed in the development of speech or language skills, yet have to compete in a highly verbal environment. Or their language development may surge ahead of their speech development, giving them much to say, but a limited capacity to express themselves articulately. These children may become excessively disfluent as other developmental demands outpace their more limited ability to coordinate the complex movements of rapid, articulate speech. (p. 46)

The developmental factors that are thought to present significantly competing demands on the production of fluent speech include the following:

- *Physical development*—structural, perceptual, fine and gross motor, sensorimotor, neurological

- *Cognitive development*—perceiving, reasoning, imagining, and problem solving

- *Social and emotional development*—forming social relationships, decentration, coping with stress and arousal, forming self-concept

- *Speech and language development*—syntax, semantics, pragmatics, phonology, integrating speech motor skills with linguistic ability

Other demands imposed by the environment include the following:

- Unrealistic speech-related expectations and standards in the home

- Internal or external expectations for greater communicative speed or complexity

- Life events generating uncertainty or insecurity

- Traumatic or otherwise emotionally arousing experiences

Various theories have been reviewed to explain why people begin to stutter. One such theory rarely claiming support today is that stuttering is a symptom of an unsatisfied repressed emotional need for oral gratification (stuttering as a neurotic response, repressed need theory). Other theories explain the beginning of stuttering as communicative failure and anticipatory struggle. These included that stuttering is precipitated by the parents' misdiagnosis of and inappropriate reaction to normal disfluency (diagnosogenic theory), by the child's awareness of and increasing concern about his own disfluency (continuity hypothesis), or by the child's normal disfluencies that become avoided and feared resulting from negative listener reaction and to which tense prepostures are developed (preparatory set or primary stuttering theory).

Other theories propose that stuttering is a learned avoidance behavior resulting from an attempt to alleviate the double approach–avoidance conflict between speaking and not speaking and between being silent and not silent (conflict theory of stuttering and avoidance reduction), from principles of positive and negative reinforcements and punishments (operant conditioning), or from attempts to prevent the emotionally painful consequences that are associated with the original disfluent behaviors (instrumental avoidance act theory). Other learning theories stress the interaction of at least two behavioral phenomena (two-factor learning theories) including classical conditioning (stimulus-contingent learning) and instrumental conditioning (response-contingent learning).

Still other theories explaining the beginning of stuttering emphasize physiological deficits, also referred to as breakdown theories. Some of these also have been used to explain the predisposition to stuttering, including that cerebral dominance for speech production is not present to a sufficient degree (incomplete cerebral dominance); that a disruptive internal condition is triggered by stress or biochemical imbalance (dysphemia or biochemical imbalance); that the person has an internal transient disturbance in language use (perseveration theory); or that stuttering is the consequence of disruption of motor organization, timing, and control (stuttering as a consequence of brain lesion or a disorder of timing). Other theories view stuttering as a consequence of a defective monitoring system for speech (cybernetic theory of stuttering), or of excessive internal and external demands on the child's capacity for fluent speech production (demands and capacities model). Other hypotheses for the beginning of stuttering do not fit neatly into any of those already noted. Silverman (1996) noted other factors that can precipitate a breakdown in one's speech fluency including stress and anxiety, shocks and fright, illness, imitation, and emotional and/or communicative conflicts.

Why do people continue to stutter?

Identifying the perpetuating causes of stuttering tends to be more promising than identifying the predisposing or precipitating factors. Once the predisposing foundation is in place and stuttering has been precipitated, what keeps people stuttering? Several factors have been considered, all of which resist change:

- Habituated cognitive, linguistic, and motor adjustments

- Maladaptive environmental conditions

- Interpersonal dynamics within communication systems

- Personal construct of a "stutterer"

Theoretical explanations for why people continue to stutter have included that any of the following conditions that predisposed or precipitated stuttering continue to be present: unsatisfied emotional need for oral gratification (repressed need theory); anticipation and fear of stuttering and subsequent struggle to avoid it (communicative failure and anticipatory struggle); learned avoidance behavior to reduce speaking-related conflicts, to respond to environmental reinforcements and punishments, or to prevent painful emotional consequences (stuttering as an avoidance response); learned adjustment to unpleasant experiences (stuttering as an interaction of behavioral phenomena); physiological deficits (breakdowns); disturbed feedback (cybernetic theory); disrupted motor organization, timing, and control (stuttering as a consequence of brain lesion or a disorder of timing); defective monitoring system for speech (cybernetic theory of stuttering); or excessive internal and external demands on the child's capacity for fluent speech production (demands and capacities model); environmental factors including stress, fear, illness, or conflicts.

A PERSONAL POSTSCRIPT ON THEORY

Before throwing my personal hat into the ring, I am reminded of Bloodstein's (1986) admonition: "Anyone who advances a supposedly new idea about stuttering must be put on notice that someone has probably said it before and that someone else will probably disprove it" (p. 130). I am reminded also of *The Fiddler on the Roof,* and particularly the wisdom of Reb Tevya, a scholarly and introspective Rabbi who always weighed all of the evidence before taking a stand or making a judgment. Listening to an argument between two townspeople, Reb Tevya listened carefully to each of two opposing yet equally convincing perspectives. After each one and with sufficient deliberation, Tevya furrowed his brow, pushed his fingers of one hand through his remaining hair, and thoughtfully pulled upon his long gray beard with his other, before saying, "You know, you're right." An astute bystander queried Tevya, "Rabbi, if he is right (pointing to the presenter of the first perspective), then how can he be right (pointing to the second presenter); but if he is right, then how can he be right?" Giving at least equal merit to the perspective just presented in the parceled question, Tevya again furrowed his brow, ran a hand over his scalp, and thoughtfully pulled at his beard searching for sufficient wisdom, then replied, "You know, you are right too."

Sitting here as I am, weighing the merits of the descriptive and explanatory notions of what predisposes, precipitates, and perpetuates the "riddle" (Bluemel, 1957), the "enigma" (Wingate, 1988), the "tangled tongue" (Carlisle, 1985), the "age-old human anguish" (Bloodstein, 1993), I realize the importance of articulating my own assumptions about stuttering. To that end, I hold that stuttering is a multidimensional neuromotor disruption resulting in asynchronous timing of the simultaneous and successive motor movements necessary for relatively effortless, continuous, and rapid speech. This statement recognizes both the observable and acoustic elements of mistiming and the underlying physiological processes of excessive muscular tension and effort. In addition, it does not minimize the significant emotional and cognitive impact that such an experience can have on a person who stutters and his conversational partners. The process of neuromotor control, and thereby maintenance of speech fluency, is influenced by many other multidimensional factors or capacities including speech and language competence, oral and speech motor coordination (and other fine and gross motor control), cognitive and learning potential, and social and emotional maturity. My thinking here is particularly influenced by Peters and Guitar (1991), Starkweather et al. (1990), and Van Riper (1982), among others.

Peters and Guitar (1991) suggested that constitutional factors predispose a child to stutter, and that developmental and environmental factors precipitate the stuttering. As tempting as this proposal is, the authors cautioned that, "In some cases, environmental factors may trigger stuttering in children who have this predisposition. In other cases, the predisposition may be there, but the environment may nurture fluency. These children may never develop stuttering" (p. 24). Therefore, identifying and attributing the role of predisposing and precipitating factors is within "a domain of educated guesses and tentative conclusions" (p. 45). Constitutional factors in stuttering were proposed on the basis of what is known about the role of heredity and group differences between people who stutter and those who do not. After reviewing, as we have already done, the role of heredity (e.g., relatives—particularly first relatives—of people who stutter are at greater risk for stuttering, females seem more resistant, if not resilient, to stuttering than males, etc.), Peters and Guitar (1991) indicated that some unknown predisposing factor or factors appear to be inherited that might act singly or together. Furthermore, after reviewing the group differences (e.g., poorer performance on IQ tests and school achievement, delay in language development, greater likelihood of articulation errors, etc.), Peters and Guitar indicated that as a group, people who stutter differ from those who do not on cognitive, linguistic, and motor tasks. However, studies also show that many people who stutter do not show these differences, and that many who do not stutter perform as deviantly as those who do. Taken together, these differences might or might not be causally related to stuttering. Establishing a causal connection between constitutional factors and stuttering is speculative.

Peters and Guitar (1991) proposed relevant developmental (physical, cognitive, social and emotional, and speech and language) and environmental (parents, speech and language environment, and life events) influences that might precipitate stuttering. The influence of developmental factors is supported by the observation that stuttering frequently begins when children are growing rapidly both mentally and physically in the preschool years. Similarly, the influence of environmental factors comes from reports of stresses often associated with the beginning of stuttering, and remission of stuttering when these stresses are reduced. Nevertheless, Peters and Guitar acknowledged the ordinariness of the environment when stuttering first appears, pointing out that "the conditions at the onset of stuttering are typically not dramatic. The child is usually not under great stress, nor has he just experienced some traumatic event" (pp. 43, 45). Van Riper (1982) expressed a similar observation:

> In the great majority of the children we have carefully studied soon after onset, we were unable to state with any certainty (or even with some feeling of probability) what precipitated the stuttering. In most instances, there simply were no apparent conflicts, no illnesses, no opportunity to imitate, no shocks or frightening experiences. Stuttering seemed to begin under quite normal conditions of living and communicating. We cannot, of course, be sure of this. Who can look within the inner world of a child? All we can say is that usually we could not account for the onset of stuttering in terms of the conditions surrounding it. In only a fraction of our cases do we feel we identified the circumstances that might have been precipitating. (p. 81)

This apparent contradiction between the intuitive (presumed) and actual influence of environmental factors at the time of onset suggests that constitutional predisposition often plays a part in the first appearance of stuttering, which is gradual, and supports the concept of multiple and yet undetermined origins of stuttering.

Reviewing the influence that developmental factors might have on speech fluency, Peters and Guitar (1991) concluded that the brain must share its resources to cope with many demands. They described the child as a system with finite resources, as follows:

> Rapid acquisition of language competes with available resources for the task of speech production. However, as more language is acquired and utterances become longer, speech rate usually increases. But in a system with finite resources, there must be a speed-accuracy trade-off; that is, if speed increases, accuracy decreases. Thus, if the child, already burdened with increasing complexity of language, succumbs to producing his utterances more quickly, before his available resources can meet that demand, he may become less accurate in his productions. Depending on the child, this inaccuracy may manifest itself as stuttering, decreased intelligibility, or some combination thereof. (p. 51)

Peters and Guitar (1991) described the rapid growth between 1 and 6 years of age as a "two-edged sword" for children predisposed to fluency problems:

> Neurological maturation may provide more "functional cerebral space," which supports fluency. But neurological maturation may also spur the development of other motor tasks, which compete with fluency for available neuronal resources. An example of such competition is the common observation that children learn to walk first or talk first, but not both at the same time. (p. 46)

The point is that such new and major tasks as talking or walking consume the available resources. For example, children who are learning a new motor skill often are observed to become temporarily disfluent. Peters and Guitar (1991) described the conflict between the demands imposed by developmental processes on the available resources as creating "noise in their neural circuitry for speech" (p. 50), particularly for children who may be neurophysiologically vulnerable or predisposed to stuttering. Similar concepts, particularly the effect of demands including time pressure, uncertainty, and avoidance on the available capacities were elaborated by Starkweather and colleagues (1990), already reviewed.

Within this postscript, I have highlighted the following assumptions about stuttering:

- Stuttering is a multidimensional neuromotor disruption in the timing and control of speech-related motor movements.
- Stuttering is caused by the interaction of individually determined, yet unknown, predisposing (constitutional) factors with precipitating (developmental and environmental) factors.
- Stuttering is maintained by perpetuating factors that can and must be identified and systematically eliminated in the treatment process.

• The phenomenology of stuttering can best be explained and conceptualized from the delicate and dynamic balance of demands and capacities.

I hold that stuttering is triggered by a multisensory-induced cognitive or affective overload. My own notion of the demands that potentially interact with each individual's capacity for fluent speech production is distinct in at least two respects. First, the demands need to be interpreted from a multisensory and multidimensional perspective including, but not exclusive to, pressures of time, uncertainty, and avoidance. We have become increasingly aware of the risks of presenting any of the following to children: speech models characterized by rapid speech or complex language, negative or impatient listener reaction, demand speech, excessive or busy scheduling, high levels of emotionality, limited turn-taking, dramatic change that challenges the child's sense of security, or other experiences that lead the child to avoid stuttering or the experience of communication in general. One additional item not generally addressed is the impact of multisensory overload—that is, of overburdening the existing avenues of sensory input, particularly the auditory and visual channels. We have reviewed already that, as a group, people who stutter tend to demonstrate less proficiency in recognition, discrimination, and recall of competing auditory messages and slower reaction times when vocal or nonvocal responses are required. My own observations indicate that some children tend to be more prone to disruption of speech fluency in conditions of auditory and visual bombardment. These have included homes where the television or stereo play constantly, presenting both auditory and visual noise during all opportunities for conversational interaction. Other common household interferences include noise from the dishwasher, laundry machines, microwave, exhaust fans, oven timers, and phones (both incoming and outgoing calls). In today's world where technology seems to change by the minute, the same could be said about the potential interference of devices such as computers, fax machines, beepers, and portable and car phones, among others.

Interferences and interrupters certainly are not limited to the home setting. We know that children who stutter demonstrate poorer performance on measurements of intelligence and school performance, whether a cause or result of stuttering. I have often wondered if the deficit in school performance is exacerbated by auditory or visual overload. I am not aware of literature addressing the differential learning strategies of children and adults who stutter. However, in light of the identified differences among the population of people who stutter, the potential benefits of modified teaching methods are yet to be determined. These methods might include reducing the rate at which verbal instructions are given, allowing for processing time between verbal instructions, establishing rules for conversational turn-taking to eliminate interruptions, etc.

The environment beyond home and school is rich with potential sources of sensory overload. Consider the following illustration. Recently, I visited with a 3-year-old boy and his family at night in a local tourist town known for its constant and timeless activities. We walked past the shops and arcades, all overly crowded, booming with different music, and nearly blinding with bright and colored lights. I observed this young boy's distraction, which took the form of kinetic attention to the auditory and visual stimuli. At the same time, his fluency disintegrated gradually to frequent part-word repetitions, though without any visible tension. These disfluencies were managed successfully by providing models of slow, gentle, normal-sounding speech. When we walked by a "haunted house," a commercial dungeon intended to elicit fear, a masked and costumed man shouted "boo" at us. At this, the boy startled and immediately repeated an initial *w* four times, equally spaced, without pitch rise but this time with oral and facial tension ("Wuh–wuh–wuh–wuh–why did he do that?"). His speech continued to be speckled with repetitions of similar form for the next 10 minutes until he was removed from the noise and lights and provided models of normalized speech with more deliberate transitions. Some might argue that it was the fright or the late hour that contributed to the boy's fluency breakdown. Perhaps the fright precipitated the repetitions with oral and facial struggle noted. But previous to that, when bombarded with auditory and visual stimuli, the boy's fluency became increasingly disfluent with repetitions but without any evidence of tension or struggle. This example, while experienced directly, is just an illustration. I am convinced that we all are prone to sensory overload, particularly children who are constitutionally predisposed to stuttering.

A second distinction is that these demands appear to be cumulative rather than episodic. In other words, the conditions of multisensory overload can be reversed or removed, and the child who is at risk for stuttering may regain fluent speech. However, with repeated exposure to such environments, whether at home, school, daycare, camp, or other settings, the child is less able to regain fluency, and the process of reversing the effects of such overload takes an increasingly longer time and has results that are more temporary. Perhaps some children within these environments develop buffering mechanisms that shield them from the potentially damaging effects of sensory overstimulation. This concept is not a new one. The literature addressing wartime activity and imprisonment is replete with examples of how sensory bombardment through auditory, visual, and other channels of input has been used to create cognitive and affective overload. Perhaps children who are prone to stutter are more likely to experience behavioral, affective, and cognitive disorganization from sensory overload. Those who do stutter have been less successful in developing or using strategies to buffer themselves from such overload, thus experiencing the effects of ultimate disintegration of previously organized behaviors, feelings, and thoughts related to communication, specifically speech fluency. An important message here is that controlling for multisensory stimulation and preventing systemic overload are critical in facilitating fluency in both the prevention and intervention processes.

What does all of this mean? It seems likely that there are unique and undetermined predisposing and precipitating factors for each person who stutters. We are aware of neither what these factors are nor what combinations of such factors (and their interactions) would be necessary and sufficient to result in stuttering. Also, we remain unaware of how knowledge of such factors would impact our efforts directed toward prevention and intervention. It seems more than just chance that renders such factors active (necessary and sufficient) for some, yet dormant (neither necessary nor sufficient) for others. In fact, current research has not yet developed a methodology to determine which combinations of factors are necessary and sufficient. There seems to be an orderliness in both the constitutional and developmental/environmental factor proposal, and in the demands and capacities model. However, we still cannot predict to any satisfactory degree who will stutter and who will not. At this point, some will throw up their hands in utter frustration; others will seize the challenge and opportunity to make a meaningful contribution to understanding stuttering and people who stutter. By virtue of you reading these leaves, I know that we share a commitment as comrades to work and learn with and for people who stutter.

CHAPTER SUMMARY

Chapter 3 highlighted the evolution of our thinking throughout recorded history about stuttering and people who stutter as a foundation to understanding contemporary theories of etiology and related treatment practices. Famous people from times past and present, all of whom stutter, were presented to illustrate that stuttering is an old affliction. Indeed, stuttering was traced through Egyptian hieroglyphics (2,000 B.C.), the Bible (1,350–687 B.C.), and professional literature from 484 B.C. to the present day. Theoretical constructions of etiology and treatment have included anatomical defects, medical problems, articulation disorders, respiratory disorders, neuroanatomical or motor speech dysfunctions, psychoneurosis, and learned behavior.

Contemporary interpretations of etiology were defined as the interaction of *predisposing factors* (agents that incline a person to stutter or put one at greater risk for stuttering), *precipitating factors* (agents thought to have triggered the stuttering or brought it to the surface), and *perpetuating factors* (variables that are continuing or maintaining the stuttering at the present time). Six major theoretical explanations for stuttering were reviewed, as follows:

1. Viewed as a neurotic response, stuttering is a consequence of deep *repressed needs*.

2. As a result of communicative failure and anticipatory struggle, stuttering is explained by the *diagnosogenic* or *semantic theory* (stuttering is caused by the parents' or care providers' misdiagnosis of and inappropriate reaction to normal disfluencies in a child's speech, followed by the child's attempts to avoid the disfluencies that are mistakenly assumed to be abnormal), the *continuity hypothesis* (stuttering develops from normal disfluency that becomes tense and fragmented as the child experiences frustration and failure in attempts to talk); and *preparatory set* or *primary stuttering theory* (stuttering emerges gradually from a child's normal hesitations and repetitions and later becomes chronic when the child begins to anticipate, avoid, and fear speech and related contexts because of reactions by listeners).

3. As a learned behavior, stuttering is explained as an avoidance response or as an interaction of behavioral phenomena. Avoidance response explanations include the *conflict theory of stuttering and avoidance reduction* (stuttering is the result of a double approach-avoidance conflict between speaking and not speaking and between being silent and not being silent); *operant conditioning* (speech is a behavior subject to operant control of positive and negative reinforcements and punishments); and *instrumental avoidance act theory* (stuttering is an acquired response reflecting expectancy, anticipation, adaptation, or anxiety and is motivated by the learned drive of apprehension about the normal disfluencies of speech). As an interaction of behavioral phenomena, stuttering is explained by the *two-factor learning theory*

(which differentiates between *classical conditioning,* or stimulus-contingent learning, and *instrumental conditioning,* or response-contingent learning) and states that the core characteristics of stuttering are the involuntary breakdowns of speech resulting from negative emotional responses that are classically conditioned, while the secondary characteristics are instrumentally conditioned responses of the individual to unpleasant experiences).

4. As a physiological deficit, stuttering is explained by the *incomplete cerebral dominance theory* (a result of not showing the usual pattern for left hemisphere dominance), the *dysphemia and biochemical theory* (a manifestation of an internal condition triggered by illness, emotional or environmental stress, or biochemical imbalance), the *perseveration theory* (an organic predisposition to motor and sensory perseveration of which stuttering is an outward manifestation), and as a *consequence of a brain lesion* (damage causing changes in the interaction of laryngeal, supralaryngeal, and respiratory reflexes, thereby disrupting motor organization, timing, and control).

5. As a result of disturbed feedback (*the cybernetic theory*), stuttering results from distortion, interference, or overload of the internal feedback mechanisms to messages received or produced or too much output correction to the internalized distortion.

6. Finally, the *demands and capacities model* views stuttering as the mismatch between the internally or externally imposed demands placed on the child and his finite capacity for fluent speech.

Finally, upon the theoretical and research foundation presented, stuttering was characterized as: a multidimensional neuromotor disruption in the timing and control of speech-related motor movements, an interaction of individually determined yet unknown predisposing (constitutional) factors with precipitating (developmental and environmental) factors, a communication disorder that is maintained by perpetuating factors that can and must be identified and systematically eliminated in the treatment process, and a phenomenology that can be best explained and conceptualized from the delicate and dynamic balance of demands and capacities. These statements recognize both the observable and acoustic elements of mistiming and the underlying physiological processes of excessive muscular tension and effort, and do not minimize the significant emotional and cognitive impact that such an experience can have on a person who stutters and his conversational partners. The potential precipitating and perpetuating effects of multisensory overload were discussed last.

Chapter 3 Study Questions

1. Many people throughout recorded history have stuttered. What relevance is there in this observation to understanding stuttering people who stutter, as well as to the processes of assessment and treatment?

2. Written records attest to an awareness of and beliefs about stuttering over at least the past 4,000 years. Also, the professional literature over the last 2,500 years has addressed the etiology and treatment of stuttering. How have previous notions contributed to our present level of understanding? What are the historical underpinnings of our present understanding about stuttering and people who stutter? How has our thinking developed and changed over time? How do you project our thinking will continue to develop into the future? What inroads are yet to be made?

3. Etiology was conceptualized as three Ps. What are the three Ps, and why is a consideration of all three essential for assessing and understanding stuttering and for designing effective intervention?

4. An understanding of the theoretical explanations is essential for developing your own theory, which is a foundation for designing effective intervention. How would you explain the development of our theoretical understanding as a field about stuttering? Given your understanding of the theories and the importance of the three Ps, what is *your* theoretical explanation for why people stutter? How might your theory impact your design of assessment and treatment?

5. Real or perceived reactions of listeners play a significant role in the development of stuttering. Thinking about your own experiences, how have you reacted to the differences of others (including but not limited to stuttering), and how have others reacted to your differences?

6. Go out into the community with one of your classmates so that each of you can take a turn as a person who stutters. At no time should you reveal that you really speak normally. After the experience, consider your physical, cognitive, and affective reactions, those of your classmate, and those you perceive were experienced by your conversational partner. What insights did you gain from this experience about communication, stuttering, people who stutter, and yourself?

7. We have summarized why some people are at greater risk for stuttering (predisposing factors), why people stutter (precipitating factors), and why people continue to stutter (perpetuating factors). How would you explain each of the factors reviewed? For example, why is greater risk experienced by boys, twins, people from middle and upper-middle socioeconomic families, those from certain countries, and so on?

Unit I

* *

Stuttering in Relief:
A Foundation
for Intervention

Chapter 1
The Nexus of Stuttering: An Introduction

Chapter 2
The Onset, Development, and Nature of Stuttering

Chapter 3
Etiology and Treatment of Stuttering: Past and Present

Chapter 4
Other Fluency Disorders

Chapter 4

Other Fluency Disorders

◆ ◆ ◆ ◆ ◆ ◆ ◆ ◆ ◆ ◆ ◆ ◆ ◆ ◆ ◆ ◆ ◆ ◆ ◆

Cluttering   97

Neurogenic Disfluency   99

    Stroke   104

    Head Trauma   104

    Extrapyramidal Diseases   105

    Dementia and Tumors   106

    Drug Usage   106

    AIDS   106

    Other   107

Psychogenic Disfluency   108

Malingering   109

Adductor Spasmodic (i.e., Spastic) Dysphonia   110

Acquired Disfluency Following Laryngectomy   110

Tourette Syndrome   111

Linguistic Disfluency   113

Normal Developmental Disfluency   114

Other Forms of Disfluency   115

    Disfluency in Manual Communication   115

    Disfluency During the Playing of a Wind Instrument   115

Chapter Summary   116

Chapter 4 Study Questions   116

The generic use of the term stuttering can obscure important differences, despite shared symptoms. Not all headaches are the result of brain tumors; not all neoplasms are carcinogenic; and not all disfluencies are stuttering.

(CULATTA & GOLDBERG, 1995, P. 23)

In previous chapters, we considered the behavioral, affective, and cognitive characteristics of people who stutter and those who do not. We emphasized particularly the speech characteristics of idiopathic (developmental) stuttering and those of normal fluency and disfluency. An all too common misconception is that all abnormal disfluency is stuttering behavior. This chapter distinguishes stuttering from other fluency disorders. Those that will be addressed include cluttering, neurogenic disfluency, psychogenic disfluency, malingering, adductor spasmodic (spastic) dysphonia, acquired disfluency following laryngectomy, Tourette Syndrome, linguistic disfluency, and normal developmental disfluency, among others (those observed in manual forms of communication and others reported during the playing of a wind instrument). Familiarity with different fluency disorders is essential and helps clinicians realize that not all disfluency is stuttering.

CLUTTERING

Cluttering, also referred to as *tachyphemia* or *tachylalia* (a Greek term meaning *fast speech*), is a fluency syndrome disorder that begins during early childhood, frequently occurring with stuttering, and is thought to have a genetic basis (Dalton & Hardcastle, 1989; Daly, 1986, 1993; Silverman, 1996). Referred to as the "orphan" in the family of speech–language pathology because of relative neglect (Weiss, 1964), cluttering has received more attention in the European literature than the American literature. Physicians (Arnold, 1965; Froeschels, 1955; Weiss, 1964) and speech–language pathologists (Daly, 1986, 1993; Diedrich, 1984; St. Louis, 1996; St. Louis & Hinzman, 1986; St. Louis, Hinzman, & Hull, 1985; St. Louis & Myers, 1997; Tiger, Irvine, & Reis, 1980) continue to be intrigued by this multidimensional disorder. As with stuttering, cluttering is difficult to define. Some have defined cluttering as a verbal manifestation of a central language disorder, others as a speech defect, while still others as a combined speech–language disturbance. Daly (1993) defined cluttering as "a disorder of both speech and language processing which manifests itself as rapid, dysrhythmic, sporadic, unorganized, and frequently inarticulate speech by a person who is largely unaware or unconcerned with his difficulty" (p. 181). Others have asserted that cluttering negatively affects all channels of communication and related behavior including grammar, reading, writing, handwriting, rhythm, musicality, coordination, and self-monitoring (Diedrich, 1984; Perkins, 1978; Weiss, 1964). Weiss (1964) is often cited for his iceberg representation (see Figure 4.1) of cluttering as one prominent symptom among multiple deficiencies (delayed speech, dyslalias, reading and writing disorders,

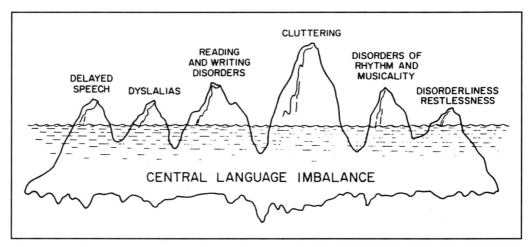

Figure 4.1. Cluttering as One Symptom of a Central Language Imbalance. *Note.* From *Cluttering* (p. 7), by D. A. Weiss, 1964, Englewood Cliffs, NJ: Prentice-Hall. Reprinted with permission.

disorders of rhythm and musicality, and disorderliness and restlessness), all sharing the common pathological basis of central language imbalance. The constellation of symptoms defines cluttering as a clinical syndrome that is related to, but often independent of, stuttering.

Daly (1993) presented eight quantitative and seven qualitative features of cluttering. Quantitative symptoms included:

1. acceleration of speech rate between and within multisyllabic words

2. short attention span and poor concentration

3. vowel stops, or pauses, before vowel-initial words without fear or muscular tension

4. six to eight units of repetition of single syllables, short words, and phrases, without apparent concern

5. articulation errors including /r/ and /l/ phonemes, reduction of consonant clusters, or signs of oral apraxia

6. vocal monotony (lack of speech melody or intonation)

7. reading errors including skipping small words, revising text, or poor concentration

8. writing errors including poor integration of ideas and motor incoordination

Qualitative symptoms included:

1. disorganized speech including abrupt topic shifts, incomplete phrases, and deficient word retrieval skills

2. verbal transpositions without awareness

3. physical immaturity, clumsiness, incoordination, often appearing inattentive, restless, or hyperactive

4. deficits in musical ability and rhythm, often unable to imitate a simple rhythmic pattern

5. familial pattern of cluttering

6. personality characteristics variously described as impulsive, hasty, restless, hyperactive, careless, impatient, and short-tempered

7. unawareness that the speech deviates from normal

Daly (1993) concluded that "cerebral dysfunction and/or heredity may play an even more prominent role in cluttering than in stuttering" (p. 185), that "future research will verify that cluttering and LD [learning disabilities] are frequently interrelated" (p. 186) (cf. Tiger et al., 1980), and that "pure" cluttering is rare. Thus, cluttering and stuttering often occur simultaneously. Daly (1996) presented a useful checklist, represented in Figure 4.2, for assessing and diagnosing cluttering. The checklist, "Daly's Checklist for Possible Cluttering," contains 33 items that are indicative of cluttering, each of which is rated between *0* and *3* depending on the truth of the statement or presence of the symptoms. With a possible total of *99* points, Daly (1993) suggested that a score of *60* or above usually is sufficient to support a diagnosis of cluttering. Scores between *30* and *60* may be indicative of a "clutterer-stutterer" (p. 187). He has found that certain items are more critical for diagnosing cluttering (Item Numbers 2, 3, 7, 9, 10, 12, 14, 20, 25, and 33), and indicated that the checklist is useful for structuring an interview, gathering information, and making decisions about cluttering.

To organize the information from the checklist for treatment planning, Daly (1996) presented a planning profile ("Daly's Cluttering Treatment Planning Profile," represented in Figure 4.3). The 33 items from the checklist are categorized on the profile, which also designates the extent of deviancy from "normal" for each item. The consecutive marks (i.e., designations) are connected by a line, thereby structuring relevant data into a framework for identifying strengths and weaknesses by displaying observable behaviors into four categories. The four categories include *speech and motor coordination* (general and suprasegmental features), *language and cognition* (auditory comprehension, verbal expression, written expression, reading comprehension, attention and concentration, awareness, thought organization, and reasoning/problem solving), *behavioral/pragmatic,* and *developmental observations.* An individual's strengths and weaknesses in these areas are analyzed to design overall treatment goals. Daly noted that whether the client is diagnosed as a *clutterer, clutterer/stutterer,* or *stutterer,* treatment objectives should address speaking rate and level of awareness in addition to other areas as appropriate.

NEUROGENIC DISFLUENCY

Culatta and Goldberg (1995) defined neurogenic disfluency as that which is "the result of an identifiable neuropathology in a speaker with no history of fluency problems prior to occurrence of the pathology" (p. 34), and reported that such disfluency appears at the onset or soon after neurological trauma or progressive disease. Similarly, Helm-Estabrooks (1993) offered the following

Checklist for Possible Cluttering

Client _____ Date _____ Age _____

Respond to each descriptive statement below. Your answer should reflect how well you believe the statement describes you.

	not at all	just a little	pretty much	very much
1. repeats syllables, words, or phrases	0	1	2	3
2. started talking late, onset of words and sentences delayed	0	1	2	3
3. fluency disruptions started early, no remissions, never very fluent	0	1	2	3
4. speech very disorganized, confused wording	0	1	2	3
5. silent gaps or hesitations common, interjections, many "filler" words	0	1	2	3
6. stops before saying initial vowel, no tension, no drawn-out vowels	0	1	2	3
7. rapid rate (speaks too fast), tachylalia, speaks in spurts	0	1	2	3
8. extrovert, high verbal output, compulsive talker	0	1	2	3
9. jerky breathing pattern, respiratory dysrhythmia	0	1	2	3
10. slurred articulation (omits sounds or unstressed syllables)	0	1	2	3
11. mispronunciation of /r/, /l/, and sibilants	0	1	2	3
12. speech better under pressure (during periods of heightened attention)	0	1	2	3
13. difficulty following directions, impatient/disinterested listener	0	1	2	3
14. distractible, attention span problems, poor concentration	0	1	2	3
15. storytelling difficulty (trouble sequencing events)	0	1	2	3
16. demonstrates word-finding difficulties resembling anomia	0	1	2	3
17. inappropriate reference by pronouns is common	0	1	2	3
18. improper language structure, poor grammar and syntax	0	1	2	3
19. clumsy and uncoordinated, motor activities accelerated or hasty	0	1	2	3
20. reading disorder is a prominent disability	0	1	2	3
21. disintegrated and fractionated writing; poor motor control	0	1	2	3
22. writing shows transposition of letters and words (omits letters and syllables)	0	1	2	3
23. left-right confusion, delayed hand preference	0	1	2	3
24. initial loud voice, trails off to a murmur, mumbles	0	1	2	3
25. seems to think faster than s/he can talk or write	0	1	2	3
26. above average in mathematical and abstract reasoning abilities	0	1	2	3
27. poor rhythm, timing, or musical ability (may dislike singing)	0	1	2	3
28. improper stress patterns of speech, poor melodic accenting of syllables	0	1	2	3
29. appears younger than age, small and/or immature	0	1	2	3
30. other family member with similar problem	0	1	2	3
31. untidy, careless, hasty, impulsive, or forgetful	0	1	2	3
32. impatient, superficial, and/or short-tempered	0	1	2	3
33. lack of self-awareness, unconcerned attitude over inappropriateness of many behaviors and responses	0	1	2	3

Total Score _____   Diagnosis _____

Other relevant information determined by interviewer:
- identified in school as learning disabled ❑ yes ❑ no ❑ recommended for testing ❑ don't know
- currently receiving speech-language therapy ❑ yes ❑ no ❑ recommended for testing ❑ don't know
- comments _____

Figure 4.2. Daly's Checklist for Possible Cluttering. *Note.* From *The Source for Stuttering and Cluttering,* by D. A. Daly, 1996, Moline, IL: LinguiSystems. Copyright 1996 by David A. Daly. Reprinted with permission.

Cluttering Treatment Planning Profile

Client _____ Date _____ Age _____

	undesirably different from normal			normal		desirably different from normal	
	-3	-2	-1	0	+1	+2	+3

A. Speech and Motor Coordination

General
- (1) repeats syllables, words, phrases _____
- (5) silent gaps, hesitations, many "filler" words _____
- (6) stops before initial vowels _____
- (9) jerky breathing pattern, respiratory dysrhythmia _____
- (10) slurred articulation (omits sounds/unstressed syllables) _____
- (11) mispronunciation of /r/, /l/, and/or sibilants _____
- (19) clumsy and uncoordinated, hasty motor activities _____
- (21) poor motor control, disintegrated writing _____
- (27) poor rhythm, timing, or musical ability _____

Suprasegmental Features
- (7) rapid rate (tachylalia), speaks in spurts _____
- (24) initial loud voice, trails off to murmur; mumbles _____
- (28) improper stress pattern_____

B. Language and Cognition

Auditory Comprehension
- (13) difficulty following directions, impatient listener _____

Verbal Expression
- (16) word-finding difficulty, resembles anomia_____
- (17) inappropriate pronoun reference_____
- (18) poor grammar and syntax, improper language structure _____

Written Expression
- (22) transposition/omission of letters and/or syllables_____

Reading Comprehension
- (20) reading disorder is prominent disability_____

Attention and Concentration
- (12) speech better under pressure for short periods _____
- (14) distractible, attention span problems_____

Awareness
- (8) extrovert, high verbal output, compulsive talker _____
- (33) lack of self awareness, inappropriate behaviors _____

Thought Organization
- (4) disorganized speech and language, confused wording _____
- (15) storytelling difficulty (trouble sequencing events) _____
- (25) thinks faster than can speak/write_____

Reasoning/Problem Solving
- (26) above average math/abstract reasoning skills _____

C. Behavioral — Pragmatic

- (31) untidy, careless, hasty, impulsive, or forgetful _____
- (32) impatient, superficial, short-tempered_____

D. Developmental

- (2) started talking late, onset of sentences delayed _____
- (3) early fluency disruptions with no remissions, never very fluent_____
- (23) left-right confusion, delayed hand preference _____
- (29) immature, appears young for age _____
- (30) family member with same/similar problem _____

Figure 4.3. Daly's Cluttering Treatment Planning Profile. *Note.* From *The Source for Stuttering and Cluttering,* by D. A. Daly, 1996, Moline, IL: LinguiSystems. Copyright 1996 by David A. Daly. Reprinted with permission.

distinction, borrowing from and building upon the definition of stuttering by the World Health Organization (1977):

> Stuttering refers to disorders in the rhythm of speech in which the individual knows precisely what he or she wishes to say but at the same time is unable to say it because of an involuntary repetition, prolongation, or cessation of a sound. When the behavior first occurs, notably worsens, or recurs in the presence of acquired neurological problems, it is diagnosed as stuttering associated with acquired neurological disorders (SAAND). (p. 207)

A significant point in these and other definitions of neurogenic disfluency is that it must occur subsequent to nervous system damage and not be accountable for in any other way (Rosenbek, 1984). Other terms for disfluencies associated with acquired neurological involvement have included cortical stuttering (Rosenbek, Messert, Collins, & Wertz, 1978) and neurogenic or acquired stuttering (Helm-Estabrooks, 1986; Rosenbek, 1984). Frequent discomfort is expressed, however, over application of the term stuttering, a diagnostic label that identifies idiopathic or developmental disfluency, to the disfluent speech of adults whose adventitious onset following neurological damage is only one symptom of an underlying and identifiable dysfunction (Kent, 1983). Indeed, Rosenbek (1984) identified as a major problem that "too many kinds of disfluency have been called by one name: stuttering" (p. 36). Culatta and Goldberg (1995) concurred that terms such as neurogenic stuttering are misleading because they imply that treatment should parallel that provided to people who stutter, and are inaccurate because they confuse a neurologically based communication disorder (neurogenic disfluency) with one of unknown origin (stuttering). For the purposes of this book, disfluency of known origin, including cerebral damage or disease and psychological trauma, will be so indicated by a descriptive label; the word *stuttering* will be reserved for disfluency of unknown origin as defined and described in the first 3 chapters.

Although interest in neurogenic disfluency has been long-standing, only two published accounts were available in 1978; approximately 50 more by 1991 (Helm-Estabrooks, 1993). The similarities and differences between stuttering and neurogenic disfluency have maintained and heightened interest of clinicians and researchers alike. The uniqueness of an individual's neurogenic disfluency is determined by the site and degree of lesion. Unlike other speech–language deficits, disfluency by itself is of limited utility in differentially diagnosing the site of lesion (Culatta & Goldberg, 1995; Rosenbek, 1984). This becomes particularly apparent in light of the evidence that disfluent speech results from damage to most areas of the nervous system. Rosenbek (1984) observed:

> Various kinds of speech and language deficits can be used to help localize where damage has occurred to the nervous system. Neurogenic stuttering, however, may not be one such deficit. It has occurred following damage to the low and high brainstem, to the basal ganglia, cerebellum, left and right cortical hemispheres, and to the white matter (tracts) of the frontal lobes of both the right and left hemispheres. . . . Stuttering has also been reported after frontal, parietal, and temporal lobe lesions within the left hemisphere. About the only sites within the nervous system which have not been associated with

stuttering are the occipital lobes of the brain, which are devoted primarily to vision and the cranial nerves once they leave the brainstem. (pp. 42-43)

Furthermore, disfluency has originated from diverse neurological events such as cerebral vascular accidents (CVA, or strokes), head trauma, extrapyramidal diseases, tumors, dementia, drug abuse, anoxia, and surgery (Helm-Estabrooks, 1986). Canter (1971) developed a specific list of characteristics of "neurogenic stuttering" including:

1. Repetitions and prolongations occur on final as well as initial and medial syllables.

2. Phonemic foci of disfluency may differ from developmental stuttering.

3. Disfluency is not related to grammatical function (function and content words may be equally troublesome).

4. There may not be a direct relationship between propositionality (linguistic complexity) and disfluency (self-formulated speech may be easier than automatic speech).

5. The adaptation effect is not observed (fluency does not improve with repeated readings of a passage).

6. The speaker may be annoyed but does not appear anxious.

7. Secondary features (facial tension, eye blinking, fist clenching) are not observed.

Others have taken issue with these observations (Rosenbek, 1984; Rosenbek et al., 1978) resulting in a greater appreciation of individual variation based upon degree and site of lesion (Silverman, 1996). Rosenbek (1984) concluded, "Canter may be correct for some neurogenic stutterers, but not for the population as a whole" (p. 33). However, Helm-Estabrooks (1993) recommended Canter's (1971) defining characteristics for diagnosing "stuttering associated with acquired neurological disorders (SAAND)" (p. 207).

There are other differences between neurogenic disfluency and stuttering. People with aphasia or apraxia tend to repeat incorrect sounds and words, but these repetitions stop once the phonemically correct target or close approximation is achieved. In comparison, people who stutter repeat sounds that are correctly articulated except for their frequency of occurrence (Culatta & Goldberg, 1995; Rosenbek, 1984). People with aphasia who experience dysnomia or people with dementia may demonstrate disfluencies in the form of interjections, pauses, and circumlocutions while searching for the correct word. Again, these disfluencies cease once the target word is accessed. In contrast, people who stutter demonstrate disfluencies that may appear similar, but they report being keenly aware of the word they are trying to say before, during, and after the word is spoken (Culatta & Goldberg, 1995). Whereas the onset of neurogenic disfluency usually is abrupt (however, gradual onset, disappearance, reappearance, and worsening of disfluency with subsequent interruption of neurological function have been reported; Helm-Estabrooks, 1993), the onset of stuttering typically is gradual. Neurogenic disfluency also differs in its immunity to behavioral manipulation and lack of developmental history, which often relates to a client's self-image. About such distinctions and relating to a client's self-image, Rosenbek (1984) stated, "Disfluencies beginning after a long period of normal speech–language use may well be different from the disfluencies beginning in childhood, if for no other reason than that the adult may react differently to their appearance" (p. 46). A perplexing problem is that neurogenic disfluency often appears behaviorally similar to stuttering. Such similarities might include prolongation of correct sounds and syllables and revision of syllables to include the *schwa* vowel (Rosenbek, 1984), repetitions and dysrhythmic phonations (Silverman, 1996), and development of secondary characteristics such as facial grimaces (Culatta & Goldberg, 1995). An understanding of these distinctions is essential to prevent misdiagnosis (Culatta & Leeper, 1987, 1988, 1989–1990; Helm-Estabrooks, 1986), which has been responsible for too many people with neurological impairments unnecessarily experiencing emotional trauma, frustration, guilt, and failure when attempting to modify their speech with inappropriate stuttering therapy techniques (Culatta & Goldberg, 1995). Because the known origin is one of the distinguishers of neurogenic disfluency, familiarity with these origins and "typical" fluency-related outcomes, as follows, is important.

Stroke

Strokes result from thrombosis (occlusion of a blood vessel by fatty substances and blood platelets), embolus (occlusion of a blood vessel by detached tissue from a thrombosis), or hemorrhage (rupture of a blood vessel). Disfluency has been reported in people experiencing stroke without aphasia, and within the context of amnestic aphasia, Broca's aphasia, apraxia of speech, conduction aphasia, and Wernicke's aphasia (Helm-Estabrooks, 1986). People who experience a stroke frequently show fluency disruption of abrupt onset on initial phonemes and content words, particularly within conversation. Other contexts are often affected to a lesser extent, including medial phonemes, function words, repetition, automatized sequences, rote paragraphs, singing, and tapped speech. The adaptation effect generally is absent. Concomitant findings sometimes include aphasia and buccofacial apraxia, and rarely subsequent seizure disorders and secondary motor involvement. Performance often is reduced in carrying a tune, tapping rhythms, block designs from a model, stick designs from memory, sequential hand positions, and three dimensional drawing (Helm-Estabrooks, 1986, 1993). Helm-Estabrooks (1986) indicated that the disfluency may be of little relative concern to people with severe aphasia, yet may be a source of frustration inhibiting verbal expression in people with milder aphasia. Therefore, fluency management will be influenced by the nature and extent of the language problem.

Head Trauma

A common brain trauma is closed head injury acquired from car accidents. Focal damage is due to compression of the skull, skull fractures, and hemorrhages. Other more diffuse microscopic damage is possible, resulting in coma or seizure disorders. Closed head injury often results in change or deficit in memory, personality, and cognitive capacity, particularly in abstract thinking. These effects and others from an acquired language disorder might inhibit the treatment process. Helm-Estabrooks (1986, 1993) reported that in such cases, onset of disfluency might be gradual, and typically is observed on initial phonemes in conversation. Disfluencies usually are heard on automatic sequences and rote paragraphs, tapped speech, and singing. Medial phonemes and content and function words are affected less. The adaptation effect rarely is observed. Occasionally, aphasia, seizure disorder, and secondary motor involvement co-occur. Performance may be reduced in carrying a tune, tapping rhythms, block designs from a model, stick designs from memory, sequential hand positions, and three dimensional drawing. A person experiencing a head trauma, compared to one experiencing a stroke, will demonstrate more gradual onset of disfluency, less likelihood to acquire aphasia, more likelihood to experience a seizure disorder, show an adaptation effect, and have secondary motor involvement.

While the patterns described above are observed more commonly, brain injury resulting from head trauma or other circumstances may have communication-related consequences that cannot be predicted. In one such case described by Helm-Estabrooks, Yeo, Geschwind, Freedman, and Weinstein (1986), an ambidextrous 21-year-old man who had stuttered since he was 8 years old fell and struck his head, causing right hemiparesis. Following a period of unconsciousness for 10 days, the injury resulted in disappearance of stuttering; however his speech became slower and dysarthric with slight hypernasality and articulatory imprecision. In another case described by Helm-Estabrooks et al. (1986), a man who stuttered as a child achieved spontaneous fluency by the time he was 8 years old. At 61 years of age, he incurred a stroke with right hemiparesis, resulting in the reappearance of his stuttering. Helm-Estabrooks et al. (1986) noted that these and other such cases indicate how little we know about the brain and its organization related to communication and its disorders, specifically stuttering.

Extrapyramidal Diseases

Dysarthric-type disfluency often is seen in patients with Parkinson's disease. Faulty motor execution is thought to give rise to the characteristic slurred speech and sound prolongations, repetitions, and blocks related to articulatory immobility. These disfluencies, which usually are gradual in onset and progressive in nature, generally are observed on initial phonemes and content words in conversation, and often on medial phonemes and function words. Occasionally, errors of verbal perseveration and reduced verbal output are observed (Downes, Sharp, Costall, Sagar, & Howe, 1993). The adaptation effect may be present. Secondary motor involvement, aphasia, and buccofacial apraxia generally do not co-occur. Performance generally is reduced in carrying a tune, tapping rhythms, and sequential hand positions (Helm-Estabrooks, 1986, 1993). Compared with disfluency in other neurogenic conditions, that resulting from extrapyramidal diseases generally is gradual in onset, without aphasia or buccofacial apraxia, and more likely to show the adaptation effect and stuttering on self-formulated speech and content words.

Dementia and Tumors

Dementia is another progressive disease that has been linked to the onset of disfluency in adults. Several cases were reported of dialysis dementia, in which after prolonged dialysis for kidney disease, disfluent speech was the first symptom preceding intermittent mutism, eventual mutism, and death (cf. Rosenbek, McNeil, Lemme, Prescott, & Alfrey, 1975). Similarly, a 62-year-old business man experienced recurrence of childhood stuttering 7 months before other symptoms of Alzheimer's-type dementia including mild aphasia, cognitive loss, and death within 18 months of the observed disfluency (cf. Quinn & Andrews, 1977). Tumors have been related to speech disfluency as well. Helm, Butler, and Canter (1980) reported on a woman of 54 years who had a metastatic brain tumor. Three weeks after symptoms of ataxic gait and right hyperreflexia, she became disfluent on initial phonemes of content and function words with no evidence of the adaptation effect. Her condition worsened, leading to mutism and eventual death. Helm-Estabrooks (1993) reported on a man with sudden onset of mildly disfluent speech who was found by the attending physician to have no positive neurological signs for the speech disruption. One week later, the speech–language pathologist detected a slight right facial weakness. Several months later, the man died of a brain tumor. Helm-Estabrooks (1986) stressed that "onset of stuttering in a well-adjusted adult should be regarded as a possible symptom of neurological disease" (p. 201). The early identification and appropriate referral for neurophysiological evaluation "may be the major contribution made by the speech pathologist in cases of progressive dementia" (p. 202).

Drug Usage

Anecdotal accounts document co-occurrence of disfluency with introduction of different pharmacological agents, and elimination of disfluency with removal of the agent. Such reports suggesting a chemical reaction have implicated amitriptyline, a tricyclic antidepressant (Quader, 1977) and theophylline, a broncho dialator used for asthma with a 4-year-old boy (McCarthy, 1981). Another drug, phenothiazine, has been used to control both psychosis and stuttering in people with schizophrenia (Nurnberg & Greenwald, 1981). However, the effects seemed to be mutually exclusive (i.e., low dosage left patients fluent but psychotic; higher dosage controlled the psychosis but not the stuttering). Most label warnings do not include information about the effects that medications have on speech fluency. Some have urged speech–language pathologists to inquire about a client's medication, especially if the disfluency reported is of recent onset (Culatta & Goldberg, 1995; Culatta & Leeper, 1989–1990).

AIDS

The human acquired immunodeficiency syndrome (AIDS) virus causes a variety of neurological symptoms reflective of progressive neuropathology. One symptom unreported until recently was speech disfluency. Fantry (1990) described one of her male patients who, at 27 years old, tested positive for the

AIDS virus antibody and developed "stuttering" for the first time. This symptom was concomitant with other more predictable symptoms including weight loss, fever, fatigue, diarrhea, difficulty with memory, and "haziness of mind." Fantry reported, "During the clinic visit, the patient was observed stuttering on three separate occasions with no impairment of language function" (p. 38). Another physician (Vinnard, 1990a) labeled the disfluency reported by Fantry as "AIDS-related acquired stuttering" (p. 6). It is unfortunate, however, that Fantry reported neither the speech-related nor psychoemotional characteristics of the patient. Fantry indicated that the disfluency "decreased" after 2 weeks of zidovudine (AZT) treatment and "completely resolved" after an additional 4 weeks of treatment. Furthermore, she suggested that "certain sites in the brain may have structural or vascular abnormalities that lead to stuttering" (p. 6), and concluded that "it is entirely possible that zidovudine therapy could account for the cessation of stuttering, just as removal of focal central nervous system lesions has relieved acquired stuttering in other patients" (p. 6).

More recently, Lopez et al. (1994) analyzed and described the "speech motor control disorder" (SMCD) characteristics of six patients infected with the AIDS virus. These characteristics, which are progressive in nature, included irregular articulatory breakdowns in consonants and vowels (in terms of range, rate, and direction of movement), prolongation of phonemes and the intervals between them, dysrhythmia of speech and syllable repetition, greater difficulty initiating than completing single word production, harsh voice, and monopitch and monoloudness (occasionally interrupted by patterns of excessive loudness variation), respiratory and vocal arrest, and slow and effortful cognitive processing associated with motor speed and attentional tasks. The authors concluded that the deficits were the consequence of cerebellar dysfunction, possibly accompanied by basal ganglia deficits. No intervention was used to alter the observed speech–motor characteristics, however.

Other

Helm-Estabrooks (1986) reported several cases of adults who acquired disfluent speech associated with other neuropathologies. One 48-year-old man became disfluent and developed memory loss following brain anoxia during open heart surgery. Another man, with adolescent onset of seizures, developed transient disfluency following an overdose of dilantin. A 16-year-old male developed severe disfluency and dysarthria following surgery to the right thalamus. Earlier treatment to the right thalamus did not affect speech fluency. Another man (a 30-year-old electrician) experienced transient disfluency (about 6 weeks in duration) following inhalation of toxic fumes. Byrne, Byrne, and Zibin (1993) described a man who, at 25 years of age, acquired speech disfluency ("transient neurogenic stuttering") as a result of impairment of brain function secondary to chronic starvation. Statements of symptoms included "dysfluency . . . finishing sentences," "repetitions of syllables," "difficulty with both functors and substantives," "difficulties when pronouncing small words," and "repetition did not improve his performance in these areas" (p. 512). After receiving a well balanced diet during 2 weeks of hospitalization, all symptoms of speech disfluency disappeared.

A familiarity with neurogenic disfluency is essential, lest we assume erroneously that all disfluency is stuttering. It is beyond the scope of our purposes here to review the assessment and treatment methods for such disfluency. Suffice it to say that it is important to distinguish the motor–speech aspects of the disfluency from the aphasia-related word retrieval or formulation deficits. This distinction is made on the basis of standardized tests (for aphasia, buccofacial apraxia, and nonverbal motor and cognitive skills), repeated readings of phonetically balanced (standard) speech passages, automatized recitations, singing familiar songs, and conversational analysis. Both differential diagnosis and differential treatment are critical. Neurogenic disfluency may be transient or persistent. Treatments for persistent disfluency have included pacing techniques, delayed auditory feedback and masking noise, transcutaneous nerve stimulation, biofeedback and relaxation, pharmacological agents, surgery, and thalamic stimulation, among others (Helm-Estabrooks, 1986, 1993).

PSYCHOGENIC DISFLUENCY

The literature contains a number of reports of disfluency that began in adulthood in association with psychological disturbance or reaction to emotionally traumatic events (Arnold, 1965; Attanasio, 1987a; Deal, 1982; Deal & Doro, 1987). In each of these cases, the client had neither a history of childhood stuttering nor any positive indication of neuropathology. The onset of the disfluency usually was sudden, but occasionally gradual, progressive, and episodic. For example, clients have experienced onset of psychogenic disfluency following combat fatigue during World War II (Peacher & Harris, 1946), a direct missile attack to a ship during the Korean conflict (Dempsey & Granich, 1978), anxiety attacks (Culatta & Goldberg, 1995; Wallen, 1961), each of two suicide attempts (Deal, 1982), a traumatic business experience (Weiner, 1981), and other emotionally disturbing events such as recalling memories of sexual abuse (Mahr & Leith, 1992) and separating from a failing and ultimately terminated marriage (Attanasio, 1987a). In some cases, the presence of psychopathology was determined (Cox, 1986). Emotionally based disfluency has been referred to as hysterical stuttering (Arnold, 1965; Bluemel, 1935; Deal & Doro, 1987; Silverman, 1996), psychogenic acquired stuttering (Silverman, 1996), neurotic stuttering (Haynes et al., 1992), and other such terms. In fact, Freund (1966) documented historical use of such terms as expectancy neurosis, compulsive neurosis, anxiety hysteria, lalophobia, phonophobia, paralalia syllabaris, pregenital conversion neurosis, and socio-affective dysphasia, among others.

Deal (1982) described the following characteristics that may reflect disfluency subsequent to psychological trauma:

1. Onset is sudden.

2. Onset is temporally related to a significant event that could reflect extreme psychological stress.

3. Disfluency is primarily repetition of initial or stressed syllables.

4. Disfluency pattern is affected little by choral reading, white noise, delayed auditory feedback, singing, and different communication situations.

5. There may be no conditions in which fluency is observed.

6. Attitude toward stuttering is indifference (also referred to as "la belle indifference" in the psychiatric literature; cf. Roth, Aronson, & Davis, 1989).

7. Secondary symptoms (sound, word, and situation avoidance, or other attempts to inhibit the disfluency) are not observed.

8. No change in the disfluency is observed during mimed reading aloud.

Others researching psychogenic disfluency have added that normal eye contact is observed (Freund, 1966; Deal & Doro, 1987); cited criteria using psychiatric terminology for conversion disorders (Roth et al., 1989); and combined speech–language pathology (Deal, 1982) and psychiatric (Roth et al., 1989) criteria to propose defining and associated symptoms for stuttering as a conversion symptom (Mahr & Leith, 1992). Silverman (1996) summarized psychogenic disfluency as follows:

> Hence, a typical patient who has this disorder is an adult, with no previous history of stuttering, who suddenly begins to stutter after (or while) experiencing a great deal of psychological stress and who has no neurological condition that could account for the behavior. Furthermore, the patient's disfluency may not vary on a situational basis and he or she may not exhibit any behavior that indicates a desire to avoid it. (p. 224)

MALINGERING

Silverman (1996) indicated that, "Whenever a person being evaluated has something to gain by being labeled a stutterer, the possibility should be considered that he or she is malingering" (p. 229). Likewise, Culatta and Goldberg (1995) noted that, "Not only is a conscious volitional component of the disorder needed for diagnosis, but also a recognizable gain from the behavior needs to be obvious before the disfluency could be labeled malingering in nature" (p. 39). Recall from Chapter 2 how what is known about the nature, variability, and predictability of stuttering and people who stutter was used to verify whether two different people really had a fluency disorder or whether they were malingering (Bloodstein, 1988; Shirkey, 1987).

Lew (1995) reported that he was a political prisoner in China during 1989 because of anti-government activity at Tiananmen Square in Beijing. Self-described as a "stutterer," he deliberately planned to worsen his stuttering in order to reduce on himself the impact of the police interrogation. Under pressure, however, Lew found that his stuttering naturally disintegrated. This experience, he reported, helped convince the police that because of his stuttering, he would not have been sponsored as a spokesperson by an "anti-revolutionary organization," thus leading to his ultimate release from captivity. The point is that Lew prepared to malinger his speech to effect a more severe stuttering pattern. He recalled, "My stuttering helped me to be released. It not only helped me. It saved me . . . My stuttering saved my life" (p. 5).

Culatta and Goldberg (1995) reported on a 20-year-old man who admittedly malingered stuttering to maintain his deferment from military service, thus preventing himself from being drafted to Vietnam. He reportedly intended to maintain this behavior until "after the war is over or until I am too old to go" (p. 40). As noted earlier, Bloodstein (1988) and Shirkey (1987) identified as insufficient our current methods for verifying stuttering in a suspected malinger and recommended that future research address this area. Making such a distinction indeed requires a knowledgeable observer who can quantify and qualify fluent and disfluent behaviors, and relate these to what we know about communication, stuttering, and people who stutter.

ADDUCTOR SPASMODIC (I.E., SPASTIC) DYSPHONIA

Spastic dysphonia is characterized by spasms of the adductor laryngeal muscles resulting in sounds that intermittently are strained and strangled. This voice condition has been referred to as "stammering of the vocal cords" and "laryngeal stuttering" (Aronson, 1973, 1990; Nicolosi et al., 1996). In some ways, the symptomatology of spastic dysphonia and stuttering is similar. Both are intermittent disruptions in the control of the speech (particularly laryngeal) musculature, the severity of which depends on similar situational factors, including the perception held by the speaker toward the listener and the significance of the communicative act. People with spastic dysphonia speak normally when reading in chorus; singing; repeating a memorized verse; speaking to children, animals, and when alone; and demonstrate an adaptation effect (the number of strained, strangled syllables decreases upon repeated readings of the same passage). There also is a debate over whether the causes of spastic dysphonia are neurological or psychological. Proponents of the former argue that it is the result of a degenerative process in the central nervous system, supporting this notion by observing that some speakers demonstrate neuropathology; proponents of the latter state that it is related to psychological trauma, supporting their argument by observing that speakers with this condition can speak normally at times. The age of onset and frequency of occurrence of spastic dysphonia and stuttering are different, however. While in most cases, stuttering begins during early childhood, spastic dysphonia begins in middle age. And while stuttering is more frequently seen in males than females, this is not the case with spastic dysphonia (Silverman, 1996).

ACQUIRED DISFLUENCY FOLLOWING LARYNGECTOMY

Silverman (1996) summarized the literature related to stuttering following laryngectomy and indicated that (a) some people who stutter continue to do so after relearning to speak using esophageal speech or an electrolarynx, (b) it is not unusual for laryngectomized patients to be highly disfluent at the early stages of relearning speech, and (c) there is some evidence that stuttering may be acquired following laryngectomy. The few case reports available in the professional literature imply that acquired disfluency of a lasting nature following laryngectomy is a relatively rare phenomenon.

TOURETTE SYNDROME

Tourette Syndrome is a neurological disorder that was first described in the medical literature in 1825 by Gilles de la Tourette, a French neurologist after whom the disorder is named. The syndrome is characterized by chronic tics (repetitive, rapid, sudden, involuntary movements or utterances) and thought to be caused by abnormal metabolism of dopamine, a neurotransmitter. The prevalence in adolescent males is 2.9% (Comings, 1995), with an overall male to female ratio of 3:1 (Colligan, 1989; Tapia, 1969). Over 100,000 people in the United States alone have this disorder, which demonstrates genetic predisposition (Colligan, 1989). It has been estimated that nearly one third of patients with Tourette also stutter (Comings, 1995; Vinnard, 1990b). Characteristics of this disorder have been described recently (Bruun & Bruun, 1994; Colligan, 1989; Comings, 1995; Lohr & Wisniewski, 1987; Scahill, Lynch, & Ort, 1995; Wand, Matazow, Shady, Furer, & Staley, 1993) and include the following:

- Both multiple motor and one or more vocal tics are present at some time during the illness (not necessarily concurrently).

- The tics occur nearly daily, usually in bouts, persisting for at least 1 year with no tic-free period of more than 3 months.

- The tics can be voluntarily suppressed for periods of minutes to hours.

- The anatomic location, number, frequency, complexity, and severity of the tics vary over time.

- Onset is before 18 years.

- Occurrence is not limited to periods of drug abuse or central nervous system disease.

Colligan (1989) presented a particularly useful guide—Teacher's Checklist on Tourette Syndrome: Range of Symptoms—that is represented in Figure 4.4. In it, she distinguished between motor and phonic symptoms. Motor symptoms were classified either as *simple motor tics,* which are fast, darting, and meaningless (such as eye blinking; grimacing; kicking; finger moving; nose twitching; and rapid jerking or tensing of the arm, head, or any other part of the body), or *complex motor tics,* which are slower or more purposeful (such as hopping; clapping; touching; arranging; gyrating or bending; biting, hurting, or picking at oneself or others; making odd expressions; and perseverating behaviors such as writing the same word or letter over and over or tearing paper or books). Phonic symptoms were classified either as *simple phonic tics,* which are fast, meaningless sounds (such as whistling, coughing, spitting, screeching, barking, grunting, hissing, and sucking), or *complex phonic tics* consisting of

Instructions: Mark an X on the symptoms you have observed. This is not a diagnosis. This is simply an observation of symptoms for referral purposes.

Motor Symptoms			
Simple Motor Tics: fast, darting, meaningless		17. Kissing	
		18. Pinching	
1. Eye blinking		19. Writing, over and over, same word or letter	
2. Grimacing		20. Pulling back on pencil while writing	
3. Nose twitching		21. Tearing paper or books	
4. Lip pouting		**Phonic Symptoms**	
5. Shoulder shrugs			
6. Arm jerks		**Simple Phonic Tics: fast, meaningless sounds**	
7. Head jerks			
8. Abdominal tensing		1. Whistling	
9. Kicks		2. Coughing	
10. Finger movements		3. Sniffling	
11. Jaw snaps		4. Spitting	
12. Tooth clicking		5. Screeching	
13. Frowning		6. Barking	
14. Tensing parts of body		7. Grunting	
15. Rapid jerking of any part of body		8. Gurgling	
Complex Motor Tics: slower, purposeful		9. Clacking	
		10. Hawking	
1. Hopping		11. Hissing	
2. Clapping		12. Sucking	
3. Touching objects (or others, or self)		13. Uh-uh, eee, ah-uh, and other sounds	
4. Throwing		**Complex Phonic Tics: words, phrases, statements**	
5. Arranging			
6. Gyrating and bending		Shut up, stop that! Oh, I've got it! Right! How about it? (others)	
7. "Dystonic postures"			
8. Biting mouth, lip, arm (circle which)		Rituals: counting, repeating a phrase until it is "just right"	
9. Headbanging			
10. Thrusting arms		Coprolalia: obscene and aggressive words and statements (these may be obscured to sound like the letters *fff* or *sss*)	
11. Striking out			
12. Picking scabs			
13. Writhing movements		Palilalia: repeating one's own words	
14. Rolling eyes to ceiling		Echolalia: repeating words of others	
15. Holding funny expressions			
16. Sticking out the tongue			

Problems with hyperactivity? ____ Short attention span?____ On medication for hyperactivity? ____

_____ _____ _____
Date Student's Name Nurse's/Teacher's Signature

*A signature provides more accountability in providing the list of symptoms observed.

Figure 4.4. Teacher's Checklist on Tourette Syndrome: Range of Symptoms. *Note.* From "Recognizing Tourette Syndrome in the Classroom," by N. Colligan, 1989, *School Nurse,* p. 3. Copyright 1989 by Tourette Syndrome Association. Reprinted with permission.

words, phrases, or statements (commands such as Shut up!, Stop that!, Right!; rituals such as counting, repeating a phrase until it is just right; coprolalia, or involuntary obscene and aggressive words and statements; papilalia, or repeating one's own words; and echolalia, or repeating words of others).

Various associated problems may be associated with Tourette Syndrome, including attention deficit disorder (poor attention and concentration, distractibility, impulsivity), hyperactivity (fidgety, ceaseless movement), emotional disorder, obsessive–compulsive disorder (often indistinguishable from complex motor tics), and conduct disorder (short temper, rage attacks over nothing, opposition, lying, stealing, starting fires). Other coexisting problems may include learning disabilities, dyslexia, depression, mania, sleep disorders, and stuttering (Bruun & Bruun, 1994; Colligan, 1989; Comings, 1995; Pauls, Leckman, & Cohen, 1993). While there is no cure for Tourette, intervention has most often been neuropharmacological. Agents used have included haloperidol, clonidine, pimozide, fluphenazine, and clonazepam (Bruun & Bruun, 1994; Colligan, 1989). Of continuing research interest are the differential effects of haloperidol (Haldol) on Tourette and stuttering (Brady, 1991; Ludlow & Braun, 1993; Quinn & Peachey, 1973; Tapia, 1969; Wells & Malcolm, 1971; Vinnard, 1990b). Other treatments have included relaxation techniques, biofeedback, psychotherapy, and behavior modification (Bruun & Bruun, 1994; Colligan, 1989; Tolchard, 1995). Excellent personal accounts are available about well-known people who have a history of Tourette Syndrome, such as Mahmoud Abdul-Rauf, formerly Chris Jackson, Denver Nuggets basketball guard; Jim Eisenreich, Philadelphia Phillies baseball outfielder; Samuel Johnson, English author and lexicographer, known for *A Dictionary of the English Language* published in 1755; among others. Numerous informative pamphlets are available from the Tourette Syndrome Association (42-40 Bell Boulevard, Bayside, NY 11361; phone: 718-224-2999).

LINGUISTIC DISFLUENCY

The existence of a relationship between language delay or disorder and stuttering is documented, yet not clearly understood (Culatta & Leeper, 1989–1990; Wall & Myers, 1995). Various accounts have noted the increase in disfluency with the initiation of language treatment and emerging language skills, and the decrease in disfluency with the development of linguistic sophistication (Colburn & Mysak, 1982a, 1982b; Hall, 1977; Hall, Wray, & Conti, 1986; Wexler, 1982). This is not terribly dissimilar to the observed co-occurrence between phonological errors and those in other aspects of language (lexical, syntactic, semantic, and pragmatic). Fey (1986) reported that improvements from language intervention often effect positive changes in phonology, and improvements in phonological intervention often effect positive changes in language. These overlaps between different aspects of communication should not be surprising, since their distinction is in the mind of the observer; the child's communication skills represent a multidimensional outcome of an integrated system. The form of disfluency reflective of linguistic emergence is somewhat different than that of stuttering. The former demonstrates primarily part-word repetitions, prolongations, and dysrhythmic phonation (Hall, 1977;

Hall et al., 1986). Why disfluency increases with the child's attempt to use new linguistic processes is uncertain. This could be explained from the Demands and Capacities model discussed earlier. As always, there are many other possible explanations.

Karniol (1992) presented a striking case report of a bilingual child who began to stutter in both languages at age 25 months, the point of transition into grammatical sentence construction. When the stuttering became severe, the parents responded to the child's request to drop the nondominant language (English), whereupon the child became a nonstuttering monolingual (Hebrew) speaker. When the nondominant language was reintroduced at 39 months, no stuttering returned. Karniol proposed stuttering as a function of syntactic overload. Others have offered explanations that syntax is a determinant of stuttering (Colburn & Mysak, 1982a, 1982b; Ratner & Benitez, 1985). Essential points are that the individual's communication competence must be understood in light of strengths and both primary and secondary exceptionalities, and that clinicians must not assume that all disfluency is stuttering. Hall et al. (1986) indicated that initial increase in disfluency among children with language delay who enter treatment is not reflective of stuttering, but the result of challenge to the child's communication system imposed by new linguistic rules. Culatta and Goldberg (1995) proposed that the method of identifying the disfluencies of children with language impairments has a major impact on treatment.

I maintain that as clinicians, we must recognize the child's communication system as uniquely organized and integrated, and be mindful that gains in one area of communication ultimately affect gains in others. This observation provides a challenge for insightful differential diagnosis and an opportunity for systematic planning of individualized communication intervention, both of which are addressed in greater detail in Unit III (Chapters 8, 9, and 10).

NORMAL DEVELOPMENTAL DISFLUENCY

Often mistaken as abnormal, disfluency is a normal occurrence reflecting developmental stages of language learning and communication development. Children who are developing communication skills normally will be their most disfluent typically between the ages of 2.5 and 4 years. These disfluencies are characterized by effortless and rhythmic repetition of whole words and phrases, the most gentle sound prolongations, and occasional sound interjections. Parents and other care providers, as well as people within the child's communication system, need to be informed that such disfluencies reflect a temporary and developmental stage, necessary for the establishment of communication proficiency (Ainsworth & Fraser, 1989; Gordon & Luper, 1992a, 1992b; Pindzola & White, 1986; Van Riper, 1982; Walle, 1976). Distinguishing between disfluencies that are normal and a necessary part of communication and those that represent the danger of incipient stuttering is a critical skill for speech–language pathologists. This will be addressed further in Chapter 8.

OTHER FORMS OF DISFLUENCY

Disfluency in Manual Communication

Some people present a communication disorder so severe that their speech is not of functional utility. Many such people use manual communication (finger spelling or sign language) in combination with their speech (as an augmentative communication system) or as a replacement for their speech (as an alternative communication system). Simultaneously using speech and manual communication is referred to as "total" communication. As noted earlier in Chapter 2, there are relatively few publications (e.g., Liles, Lerman, Christensen, & St. Ledger, 1992; Montgomery & Fitch, 1988; Silverman & Silverman, 1971) that document disfluencies in manual communication including repetitions or hesitations of signs and initial letters in finger spelling, in addition to involuntary interjections and extraneous hand and finger movements. When manual communication was used to augment speech, the manual disfluencies including part-word repetitions, word repetitions, and prolongations sometimes were accompanied by speech disfluencies and at other times were not.

Disfluency in manual communication that might be compared to stuttering during oral speech appears to be a relatively rare phenomenon. Silverman and Silverman (1971) reported that of the 78 responses received from teachers of deaf children at residential schools, 13 reported "stutter-like behavior in manual communication of the deaf" (p. 45). Even more indicative of its infrequency, Montgomery and Fitch (1988) identified only 12 cases in the 9,930 students with hearing impairments whom they surveyed. These findings have been interpreted variously. Van Riper (1982) indicated that "perhaps, in their manual communication, some deaf individuals show behaviors equivalent to stuttering" (p. 47). Silverman (1996) hypothesized that "certainly, conditions that result in neurogenic-acquired stuttering and psychogenic acquired stuttering could as easily affect the musculature of the upper extremities as that of the mouth" (p. 228). Silverman also suggested that theoretical explanations for stuttering, such as anticipatory-struggle behavior or demands exceeding capacities, could as well explain disfluency in manual communication.

Disfluency During the Playing of a Wind Instrument

There are very few published accounts of disfluent-like behavior occurring during the playing of a wind instrument. Those reported involved the trumpet (Van Riper, 1973), the flute (Silverman & Bohlman, 1988), and the French horn (Meltzer, 1992). Meltzer (1992) provided the following description:

> a blocking of the flow of sound as a result of closure and tightening in the throat and a breakdown in coordination of tonguing movements. The frequency of occurrence varied, increasing under conditions of fatigue, stress, anticipation, speed, and the need to maintain a high standard of performance. (p. 260)

Each of the three people on whom the reports focused also stuttered. Silverman (1996) hypothesized that because playing a wind instrument requires use of the same muscle groups as does connected speech (respiratory, laryngeal, and oropharyngeal), the cause or causes of stuttering could also interfere with playing a wind instrument. While disfluency during playing a wind instrument would seem to be relatively rare by virtue of the few published accounts, Silverman (1996) reminded that both the prevalence of such a disorder and the likelihood that a person who does not stutter can develop one, remain uncertain.

CHAPTER SUMMARY

This chapter conveyed that not all disfluency is stuttering. Clinicians must be able to distinguish between stuttering and other fluency disorders. Those reviewed here include cluttering, neurogenic disfluency (associated with stroke, head trauma, extrapyramidal disease, dementia and tumor, drug usage, AIDS, and other neuropathologies), psychogenic disfluency, malingering, adductor spastic dysphonia, acquired stuttering following laryngectomy, Tourette Syndrome, linguistic disfluency, and normal developmental disfluency, among others (including disfluency in manual communication and disfluency during playing a wind instrument). Making differential diagnostic distinctions presents a unique opportunity to understand how each client's communication system is uniquely organized and integrated, and how such an understanding relates to individualized and effective communication intervention.

Chapter 4 Study Questions

1. This chapter addressed fluency disorders other than stuttering. Why is it important to differentiate between stuttering and other fluency disorders? What are the similarities and differences between the disorders in terms of behavioral, cognitive, and affective considerations?

2. What differences might be observed in verbal and nonverbal behaviors and expressed attitudes when comparing people who stutter and those who are malingering? Why might a person malinger, and how would you distinguish between stuttering and malingering?

Unit II

• •

Central and Guiding Intervention Assumptions

Chapter 5
Personal Constructs and Family Systems: Intrafamily Considerations

Chapter 6
Interdisciplinary Teaming and Multicultural Awareness: Extrafamily Considerations

Chapter 7
Stuttering Modification and Fluency Shaping: Psychotherapeutic Considerations

Chapter 5

Personal Constructs and Family Systems: Intrafamily Considerations

◆ ◆ ◆ ◆ ◆ ◆ ◆ ◆ ◆ ◆ ◆ ◆ ◆ ◆ ◆ ◆ ◆ ◆

Personal Construct Theory 120

    Personal Constructs Defined 120

    Personal Constructs Applied to Intervention 120

    Case Example 123

    Summary and Extension—Personal Construct Theory 124

Family Systems Theory 125

    A Paradigm Shift 125

        Shifting from Monocular to Polyocular Perspectives 125

        Shifting from Labeling to Understanding 126

        Shifting from Behaviors to Systems 127

    Family Based Treatment—Families and Professionals as Partners 127

    Family Based Treatment—Modeling Characteristics of Optimal Families 128

    Family Based Treatment—Modeling Characteristics of Successful Families 129

    Family Based Treatment and Heightened Effectiveness 130

    Family Based Treatment and Fluency Disorders 132

    Family Diversity 134

    Family Characteristics 134

        Characteristics of the Exceptionality 135

        Characteristics of the Family 135

        Personal Characteristics 136

        Special Challenges 137

    Family Interactions 138

        Family Cohesion 139

        Family Adaptability 140

        Family Patterns and Change 140

    Family Functions 142

    Family Life Cycle 145

        Family Roles Affect Fluency Treatment 145

        Family Stress Affects Fluency Treatment 146

        Families as Portraits of Development and Change 147

    Summary—Family Based Treatment 149

Chapter Summary 150

Chapter 5 Study Questions 151

Man creates his own ways of seeing the world in which he lives; the world does not create them for him. . . . Each individual man formulates in his own way constructs through which he views the world of events. As a scientist, man seeks to predict, and thus control, the course of events. It follows, then, that the constructs which he formulates are intended to aid him in his predictive efforts.

(KELLY, 1955A, P. 12)

dentifying and describing the concepts that form the core of our working assumptions in clinical intervention is more than an academic exercise. Doing so explains, if not justifies, what we do with people who stutter. Why do we need to explain or justify what we do? Because all of us, by virtue of making a professional commitment to understanding stuttering and people who stutter, have sworn an oath to do our utmost to facilitate positive change in someone's communication world (ASHA, 1994a, 1996b). This commitment requires that we understand what we are doing and the rationale for why we believe our methods will result in positive change. What we do in clinical intervention is not arbitrary. Our methods are based on systematic application of knowledge to the clinical process within an explicit and coherent theoretic context (Johnston, 1983). No less critical is our sincere belief in our clients and their potential for communication growth and change, and in ourselves as professional facilitators of this change process (Daly, 1988). Too often, I have heard clinicians justify what they are doing clinically by saying, "That's how I was trained." Such thinking falls short of our ethical, legal, and social obligation to people who stutter (Messick, 1980). Furthermore, it fails to reflect the excitement within the challenge and privilege facing us in communicating with and coming to understand the world of another person.

In the first three chapters of Unit I, we established that how we approach intervention and what we do within the process reflect in part our understanding of stuttering including its onset, development, nature, and etiology and treatment from past and present perspectives. In Chapter 4, we also established that not all disfluency is stuttering, thus the importance of being able to distinguish stuttering from other fluency disorders. In the present unit, we now will begin to identify and address the central and guiding assumptions that are at the very core of our assessment and treatment experience with people who stutter. These assumptions address intrafamily considerations (Chapter 5), extrafamily considerations (Chapter 6), and psychotherapeutic considerations (Chapter 7). In this chapter, we will establish the following:

- Stuttering is a personal construct. Stuttering-related thoughts, feelings, and behavior reflect in part the consequence of active and alternative choices.

- Stuttering and other communication disorders exist, and therefore must be addressed, within a family context. The experiences of and changes in a person who stutters trigger compensatory changes in family members and significant others.

PERSONAL CONSTRUCT THEORY

Personal Constructs Defined

That all people, including people who stutter, have alternative choices is a basic postulate to effective treatment and healthy living. This premise is central to personal construct theory (Kelly, 1955a, 1955b). The philosophical assumption to personal contruct theory is "constructive alternativism," expressed as follows:

> We assume that all of our present interpretations of the universe are subject to revision or replacement. . . . We take the stand that there are always some alternative constructions available to choose among in dealing with the world. No one needs to paint himself into a corner; no one needs to be completely hemmed in by circumstances; no one needs to be the victim of his biography. (Kelly, 1955a, p. 15)

This highly optimistic view assumes that we have the ability to change every aspect of our feelings, thoughts, and behavior. We are highly adaptable because we have individually created an interwoven network of personal constructs, viewpoints of reality based upon past experience in life situations. Because life experiences are varied, typically we bring many personal constructs to bear on our interpretation of the world in which we live.

Defining constructs, Kelly (1955a) noted, "Man looks at his world through transparent patterns or templets which he creates and then attempts to fit over the realities of which the world is composed" (pp. 8–9). The primary purpose of constructs is prediction of the future. According to this theory, we actively try to anticipate what may happen in the future and develop plans to cope effectively given a variety of different outcomes. A central point is that people are not passive participants in the unveiling of the future. Rather, we plan long-term goals and prepare in advance for the challenges that inevitably arise in pursuit of these goals. Personal construct systems should always be evolving, ever changing in light of new information and experiences.

Personal Constructs Applied to Intervention

Personal construct theory relates directly to our clinical interactions with people who stutter. In this theory, the client's personal experience and understanding of the social world, particularly the clinician–client relationship, are critical to the change process. Botterill and Cook (1987) stated:

> PCT [Personal Construct Theory] holds that if therapists are to play a significant part in the exploration of another person's construct system there must be trust, empathic understanding and genuine respect between client and clinician. Effective help only occurs when the therapist is able to see events through the eyes of her client. This understanding will in turn lead to changes in the way the client construes his therapist. We feel that this level of mutual understanding is a prerequisite for effective therapy. (p. 149)

Personal construct theory is based on the fundamental postulate of constructive alternativism that "a person's processes are psychologically channelized by the ways in which he anticipates events" (Kelly, 1955b, p. 561). As stated earlier, constructs serve to anticipate and ultimately cope with events based on past, and thus predictable, experience. This fundamental postulate was elaborated into 11 corollaries (Kelly, 1955b, pp. 561–562), several of which are noted below with an application to the clinical process with people who stutter, for illustration.

• *"Construction Corollary: A person anticipates events by construing their replications."* This means that we anticipate our future on the basis of our past. A 55-year-old client cannot envision what it might be like to talk fluently because stuttering is all he has ever known. People who stutter anticipate the words on which and situations within which they will stutter. Clients' motivation in treatment will continue only if they have experienced, and thereby can anticipate, success. A clinician's attitude toward stuttering therapy and the likelihood of a client's success will be affected by the relative success of treatment with previous clients.

• *"Dichotomy Corollary: A person's construction system is composed of a finite number of dichotomous constructs."* In other words, people view the world in terms of opposites. The common conceptualization of people as "stutterers" or "fluent speakers" embodies a dichotomous construct that obscures the reality that fluency is a continuous variable and that people who stutter (and their clinicians) are a heterogeneous population.

• *"Choice Corollary: A person chooses for himself that alternative in a dichotomized construct through which he anticipates the greater possibility for extension and definition of his system."* This means that all people have and make choices, either implicitly or explicitly. Both stuttered and fluent speech are the consequences of what someone does, feels, and thinks. Once provided ownership of stuttered and fluent speech as realistic options, the person who stutters may choose, with guidance, accordingly.

• *"Experience Corollary: A person's construction system varies as he successively construes the replications of events."* Building on the construction corollary, this means that both our anticipation of events and our view of the world evolve on the basis of past and particularly repeated experiences. This is how stuttering gains habit strength. "I have always stuttered. I stutter. Therefore, I will stutter." However, this same corollary can be used by clinicians to break the habit strength of stuttering by creating an opportunity for the client to build a foundation of successful fluency experiences, upon which he begins to anticipate future fluency success. In other words, by creating opportunities for success (a primary objective in effective treatment), success begets success.

• *"Individuality Corollary: Persons differ from each other in their constructions of events."* This means that people are likely to hold vastly different interpretations of the very same observed event. Because all people who stutter are different in how they construe and predict the world, treatment must be tailored to fit each individual. Also, this corollary may explain why clinicians may hold different treatment recommendations for the same client.

• *"Commonality Corollary: To the extent that one person employs a construction of experience which is similar to that employed by another, his psychological processes are similar to those of the other person."* This argues for the client and clinician to create and use opportunities to shift perspective so as to consider other points of view—that is, for the client to see through the eyes of (experience the construct systems of) fluent speakers, and the clinician to see through the eyes of the client.

• *"Sociality Corollary: To the extent that one person construes the construction processes of another he may play a role in a social process involving the other person."* This is an extension of the commonality corollary. People often do share common perceptions of the same experience. Examples might include the camaraderie noted at conventions held by self-help and support groups for people who stutter, or the sense of inclusion experienced by members sharing a cultural identity. Others, however, at least temporarily can come to see as others do by shifting perspective. To the extent that we can share the perspective of another person, we can begin to understand and participate within his or her reality. Such shifting of perspective is difficult yet essential for effective change (such as learning, growth, transfer, and maintenance) and, as I will note later, perhaps is the essence of shared respect for individuals and groups representing all people, the heart of multicultural sensitivity.

The point is that all people, including people who stutter and clinicians, come to view their world and themselves on the basis of unique systems of personal constructs that develop from previous experience. These systems help us anticipate and respond to, if not shape, future events. When explicitly aware of our clients' personal constructs, we can use this awareness to effect positive and proactive change in his communication skills and the way he views himself as a communicator. When aware of our own personal constructs regarding our role as a clinician and as a facilitator of change, we can plan for and effect growth in our own professional development. When only implicitly aware or relatively unaware of our constructs, we inevitably maintain the status quo and inadvertently dilute any effort to effect change. We do not have to stick with the past. If we become aware that our interpretation of past events, and thereby anticipation of future events, was incorrect or undesirable, we may revise our construct system to achieve outcomes that were not or did not seem possible previously (such as speaking with greater fluency, using self-corrections more often, and using fluency facilitating controls in outside settings).

Personal construct theory indicates that people have choices—an active, deliberate, and conscious process—and that "all of our present interpretations of the universe are subject to revision and replacement" (Kelly, 1955a, p. 15). The ways we view and interpret the world, the words we use to discuss our personal constructs, and the areas within which we envision change are idiosyncratic and, perhaps, the very essence of constructive alternativism. The clinician, therefore, must gain an appreciation of the client's system of personal constructs in order to understand the client's conception of himself as a person and as a communicator within a social world, vision for targeted change, and portrait of presenting abilities and problems. Furthermore, the clinician must determine the relative coherence among these three components. In other words, the clinician must shift perspective so as to see the client's world as the client sees it (Klein & Moses, 1994; Moses & Shapiro, 1992, 1996; Shapiro, 1987, 1994a, 1994b, in press; Shapiro & Moses, 1989), and must assess whether the client's personal constructs can accommodate (i.e., will facilitate) or will inadvertently hinder the desired change. Fransella (1972) noted that people who stutter ultimately choose to stutter because this role is the most familiar and predictable based on acquired experience. Making the transition from disfluency to fluency presents a difficult challenge of internal adjustments to one's system of personal constructs, a far greater challenge than simply bringing overt disfluent behaviors under control. This distinction provides an explanation for why the long-term transfer and maintenance of feelings, thoughts, and behaviors that are characteristic of fluency prove to be so difficult. In Fransella's (1972) words, "The road from stuttering to fluency is paved by reconstructions" (p. 70).

Case Example

Consider the following example. Some 11 years ago, I conducted the diagnostic evaluation of a 32-year-old woman who described herself as a "stutterer," and who reported feelings of insecurity and embarrassment related to her stuttering and particular concern regarding the listener's first impression of her as a communicator. After a thorough evaluation, I was left utterly unable to detect any overt behavior that might resemble stuttering. In fact, she was both skillful at communication and eloquent as a communicator. Nevertheless, the woman was visibly anxious that she might stutter and appeared shamed at the slightest twinge of normal disfluency. To me, she was an excellent illustration of an "interiorized stutterer" (Douglass & Quarrington, 1952), and a good reminder that even though the clinician might perceive an individual's stuttering as mild or nonexistent, that perception is not necessarily shared. Recall that the very same event, disfluency in this case, might generate vastly different interpretations (seeming normal to one person but communicatively handicapping to another). Bloodstein (1993) noted that "some of the most severe problems are presented by people who seem to talk with perfectly normal fluency" (p. 4).

In this particular case, it became clear that the woman's personal construct of herself as a communicator was inhibiting her recognition of her own communicative and interpersonal strengths, thus confining her perceived potential in other areas. For example, she had completed an associate's degree from a 2-year college and was working as a clerical assistant in a dentist's office. While she longed to pursue her education, she felt unable and that ultimately she would be unsuccessful. Her communication treatment involved providing an opportunity for her to identify and better understand her own system of personal constructs and to determine whether these were appropriate for her based upon past, and thereby projected future experience. She was regularly involved in recording and analyzing audio- and videotapes and comparing her assessment with conversational partners' assessment of her communication skills. In short order, the mismatch between her perception and that of her listeners became evident to her. This procedure was successful in helping her to identify and shift her own perspective about herself as a communicator on the basis of concrete data and a steadily growing foundation of communication success. I have followed this woman's progress for 10 years post treatment. Several years ago, I learned that she completed dental school and was successful in her practice of dentistry.

Summary and Extension—Personal Construct Theory

Kelly's (1955a, 1955b) personal construct theory indicates that all people, on the basis of past experience, construct systems to help anticipate and cope with life events. This is particularly true when coping with personal difficulties, including stuttering. This theory has direct application to personal change and reconstruction, which are core elements of effective treatment. One key concept is that the client is actively involved in all aspects of the treatment process including identifying, reassessing, and revising (as appropriate) his own system of personal constructs. Another key concept is that the client has choices to make among alternatives and is responsible for his own actions. Within limits, fluency and disfluency are alternative choices representing bipolar components within a personal construct. Both fluency and disfluency represent the composite outcome of feelings, thoughts, and behaviors of a person who stutters.

Botterill and Cook (1987) discussed three treatment stages of problem solving leading to the clients' ability to see alternatives in situations (circumspection), arrive at a choice of action from among these alternatives (pre-emption), and ultimately bring a situation under control (control). They emphasized that the relative success of the chosen strategy is less important than the resulting refinement of the individual's construct system. The point is the importance of client-initiated change, both in terms of its construction and its action. The clinician serves as a facilitator, all the while transferring responsibility for treatment design, implementation, evaluation, and follow-up to the client. As will be seen later, I maintain that the process of transferring fluency skills to extraclinical settings is begun from the beginning, not the end, of treatment and is supported by all aspects throughout the treatment process. Botterill and Cook (1987) offered an insightful conclusion:

> It is our role as therapists to help clients explore their construct systems and appreciate how construct systems provide both the basis of current functioning and the vehicle for future change. . . . For many clients the chance to reconstrue themselves and their communication difficulties can at the very least make the problem more acceptable. For others such basic reconstruction is the prelude to more comprehensive change in many areas of social functioning including speech fluency. We do not suggest that all there is to the treatment of stuttering is a period of personal reconstruction; but equally we are convinced that it takes more than motor speech training to achieve lasting change in the treatment dysfluency. (p. 165)

To this point in the present chapter, we have examined personal construct theory and its relevance to working with people who stutter. We looked within the individual and determined that stuttering-related thoughts, feelings, and behavior reflect, to some degree, alternative choices, whether they are made implicitly or explicitly. We now will move from the individual to the family. We will see that experiences and changes in a person who stutters trigger compensatory changes in family members and significant others. Therefore, stuttering and other communication disorders exist and must be addressed within a family context.

FAMILY SYSTEMS THEORY

Among the central tenets of family systems theory is that the family, with few exceptions, is the most powerful emotional unit to which we ever belong that continues to affect the course and outcome of our lives (Carter & Orfanidis, 1976). Furthermore, members of the family unit or communication system are interdependent; thus, experiences or changes of one member trigger compensatory changes in other members. This primary impact makes the family unit our greatest potential resource for clinical intervention (Bowen, 1976; Whitaker, 1976). One part of the family cannot be understood in isolation from the other members of the system (Epstein & Bishop, 1981). Luterman (1996) said this aptly:

> When there is a communication disorder in a family, everyone is affected by it, and it therefore becomes the responsibility of the speech pathologist and the audiologist to work with the needs of all members of the family. A communication disorder always exists within a "family" context. It cannot be confined to a single individual because the disorder manifests itself only within the milieu of a relationship. For us to be effective, to be clinicians, we must examine and deal with the whole relationship. . . . Failure to deal with family needs almost invariably limits therapeutic effectiveness. (pp. xxiv–xxv)

A Paradigm Shift

While clinicians traditionally have tried to involve family members in the intervention process, such attempts have been based on a linear treatment model, in which an individual is the center of the treatment process (Andrews & Andrews, 1990). Mothers, and occasionally other family members, are directed by the speech–language pathologist to engage in treatment-related activity in settings outside of the treatment room. Under this arrangement, the most significant changes are viewed as occurring in the treatment session that might be enhanced by family cooperation and understanding. Nevertheless, the individual with the communication disorder is the unit of treatment, and family participation is secondary to the role of the professional. Changing this conception of treatment, which is so deeply rooted in behavioral tradition, would require (and currently is exacting) a paradigm shift, adopting a new construct or way of looking at the clinical world. That is, we must move from a linear assumption already described to one of a more systemic nature requiring several critical shifts of perspective described by Andrews and Andrews (1990).

Shifting from Monocular to Polyocular Perspectives

The first shift is from a monocular to polyocular perspective, where different interpretations of the same event are not only accepted, but are invited and nurtured. Such a perspective is consistent with the importance of being able to shift perspective, distinguishing an event from its multiple potential interpretations, and the notion of personal construct theory where we actively choose a perspective from multiple alternatives. Andrews and Andrews (1990) provided the following example:

> One of the language delayed children that we treated was seen as stubborn by his mother, mechanically gifted by his father, cute by his grandfather, autistic by a school psychologist, retarded by his teacher, and language impaired by a speech–language pathologist. Each of these views, though different, was correct from the perspective of the person expressing a "truth." Many factors, of course, influenced each view including the professional, personal, and family relationship of each person to the child. The clinician must honestly view all these perspectives as accurate when considered from the point of view of the person expressing the opinion. (pp. 7–8)

A corollary to adopting a polyocular view is accepting different interpretations of an event as potentially equally correct. For example, parents with different parenting styles (such as orderly and structured versus playful, relaxed, and spontaneous) will need to recognize and use the benefits of both as a broad exposure for childrearing, lest the difference become a source of tension. Likewise, clinicians must see the significance in differing perspectives on a clinical matter, even though such perspectives often are not in agreement with our own. The importance of being able to shift perspective cannot be overstated.

Shifting from Labeling to Understanding

A second shift is moving from labeling behaviors to identifying interactive patterns and understanding the relevance of a problem within a meaningful communicative context. A corollary related to identifying communicative relevance is moving from a focus on problems to one of finding solutions. For example, rather than focusing initially on disfluent behavior, as most people who stutter have come to expect, I find it highly motivating and far more solution-focused first to identify the nature of one's fluency and then to create opportunities for more frequent demonstration of such fluency. In other words, I provide guidance for the person who stutters to do more of what he is already doing that is conducive to fluency. Identifying what the person who stutters is doing (and to a lesser extent initially, feeling and thinking) that facilitates fluency, as well as helping him to do more of this, is significantly different than initially identifying what he is doing wrong and assisting him in doing this less often. The former shows a person who stutters that he is capable of fluency, is an active and vital member of the change process, and already possesses target behaviors that need to be demonstrated more frequently; the latter conveys the contrary, that he is to rebuild his speech pattern under the control of the clinician who is the primary member of the treatment team. Simply put, how many of us would continue to be motivated when what we are doing wrong, the problem (i.e., disfluent speech behavior) receives primary focus? This process "gets old" in a hurry, and we wonder why clients' cooperation and attendance slack off. I find that focusing on what the client is already doing "right" and providing guidance in how to do more of what he is already doing right (including thoughts, feelings, and behaviors) "hooks" people who stutter and their families into a positive process that is motivating, rewarding, and surely solution-focused.

Shifting from Behaviors to Systems

A third shift is moving from a cause–effect consideration to one that focuses on transformations within an integrated communication system. We already have discussed improvements in language functioning effecting changes in phonology, or changes in fluency effecting changes in self-concept, personal hygiene, academic performance, professional aspirations, and so on. Too often, labels applied to behavior fall short of conveying an understanding of the nature of one's communication strengths and weaknesses within meaningful contexts. Too often, behaviors are identified with an emphasis on communication DIS-order rather than on disORDER. Therefore, we are surprised by such related yet unplanned improvements beyond the target behaviors. Such surprise reveals that the clinician's intervention posture typically is reactive. Rather, I stress that we need to be more proactive, understanding communication-related changes that occur within a communication system, and thus not only prepared to handle and nurture them but to plan systematically for them (becoming aware for the first time of new choices—personal outlooks on oneself, relationships, personal and professional options, etc.; feelings of confusion and insecurity by other family members needing role clarification and support, such as spouses, parents, significant others, and teachers). The point is that we must plan for cause–effect changes and system transformations, only some of which can be predicted. Nevertheless, while facilitating the processes of change, self-actualization, and growth, we can expect the unexpected, learn from previous and present experience, and recognize the uniqueness of each person who stutters within a family system.

Family Based Treatment—Families and Professionals as Partners

In treating a person who stutters, within the context of a family system the entire family is involved in all aspects of assessment and treatment. Such involvement requires understanding by the clinician of the nature and dynamics of the individual family. Indeed, Turnbull and Turnbull (1990) discussed the "special partnership" between families, people with exceptionalities, and professionals as follows:

> We address the family in all its diversity: size, cultural background, geographic location, values, interaction styles, met and unmet needs, and the changing characteristics of a given family over time. By addressing the family as a system, we are not bounded by a focus on one family member, typically the person with an exceptionality. Indeed, we seek to show the complex interrelatedness of all members in a family and the importance of adopting a comprehensive view of professional interventions. We stress that each family must maintain its own critical balance, its unique center of gravity in order to allow any professional intervention to be beneficial to a family member or to the entire family. We encourage professional support of families. (pp. viii–ix)

We noted already that within family based intervention, the family, rather than the individual, is the unit of treatment. Family members become equal partners with the professional members of the treatment team. Counseling is the medium for discussing aspects of family interactive patterns that facilitate or inhibit the targeted changes that are jointly determined. Throughout the literature on family therapy, different principles guide the practice of intervention within a systems perspective. Andrews and Andrews (1990, pp. 16–21) adapted the following overlapping principles from family therapy (Epstein & Bishop, 1981) and applied them to family based treatment in communication disorders:

• *"One part of the family cannot be understood in isolation from the rest of the system."* The behavior of each family member is understood more completely when interpreted within the context of family beliefs, patterns, and customs. This is surely the case when observing, assessing, and treating the behavior of a person who stutters, within the environment of the family rather than in isolation.

• *"The parts of a family are interrelated; change in one part influences change in other parts of the system."* When one member of a family stutters, all other members are affected by it and the treatment process.

• *"Transactional patterns of the family shape the behavior of family members."* A fluency disorder frequently is embedded in the pattern of family interaction.

• *"A family's structure, organization, and developmental stage are important factors in determining the behavior of family members."* Every family develops and adopts certain roles over time, an understanding of which is critical to involving the family meaningfully in treatment-related activities.

An obvious question at this point might be, "Why should a family systems approach be taken seriously by clinicians working with people who stutter?" Or by implication, "Isn't working exclusively with the person who stutters a more direct and time-efficient approach?" In response, I want to share a few observations illustrating that in a family systems approach, clinicians have an opportunity to participate actively in and model the very behaviors we hope to nurture in the families of our clients who stutter. Then, I want to provide some representative data that support such methods.

Family Based Treatment—Modeling Characteristics of Optimal Families

Luterman (1996) noted that when clinicians approach intervention from a family therapy perspective, we become united with the family. He stated:

> Our job as professionals in working with persons with communicative disorders is to help the family become optimal, or as close to it as possible. We can teach parents, mainly by modeling, how to manage conflict, how to communicate openly and honestly with their children, and how to display their affection and

caring for their children. In effect, what we must do is parent the parents and create for them in our relationship an optimal family. The parents then can take from our optimal clinical family the information and skills necessary for their own home situation. (p. 161)

Indicating that we are to demonstrate what we intend for our clients and their families, Luterman (1996) summarized characteristics of optimal (pp. 159–161) families. He noted that optimal families produce well-functioning individuals, both with and without exceptionality. About optimal families, Luterman indicated the following:

• *"Communication among all family members is clear and direct."* Communication is explicit, contains content and feeling, and is balanced by empathy and humor.

• *"Roles and responsibilities are clearly delineated, overlapping, and flexible."* Boundaries within and across family subsystems (e.g., parent–parent, parent–child, child–child; reviewed later in the section titled "Family Interactions") are clear, allowing for parental authority balanced with open communication. Roles and responsibilities change and are renegotiated to maintain a well-functioning unit.

• *"The family members accept limits for the resolution of conflict."* Conflict is viewed as normal and healthy, resulting in growth and change. Resolution of conflict is fair, taking individual needs into account, allowing everyone to "win" in part of the solution. Luterman noted that clinicians' modeling conflict resolution for families is essential.

• *"Intimacy is prevalent and is a function of frequent, equal-powered transactions."* Caring and affection, in observable or more subtle ways, are communicated and received while respecting the need for space and distance. "Optimal families are cohesive without being enmeshed." (These concepts are reviewed later in the section titled "Family Interactions.")

• *"A healthy balance exists between change and the maintenance of stability."* Some change is predictable (i.e., see later section titled "Family Life Cycle") and some is not (e.g., who will stutter, cf. Yairi, 1993). The balance between accommodating change and maintaining stability (i.e., homeostasis) is accomplished by open, clear communication and role flexibility so others can help when demands increase on family time, mutual caring, and effective conflict resolution.

Family Based Treatment—Modeling Characteristics of Successful Families

Families that are successful in coping with the changes and challenges required when a member has an exceptionality demonstrate other related characteristics. Luterman (1996) reviewed a number of such characteristics (pp. 161–165), which again should be nurtured and modeled by the clinician. These include the following:

- *"A successful family is one that feels empowered."* People who stutter and their families need to feel that they own (have participated in the development of) the intervention strategy, and that what they can do will make a positive difference. I am greatly concerned with professionals who present a bleak picture, taking away the spark of hope. For this reason, I recommend focusing initially on what the person who stutters can, rather than cannot, do and helping him to do more of what he is already doing that is conducive to fluency and feelings associated with fluency control. When experiencing success, one is motivated and wants to do more. Ownership and success are empowering.

- *"In successful families the self-esteem, especially of the mother, is high."* Related to empowerment, parents, spouses, and other family members need to be and feel needed, involved, and successful. These experiences replace the need for denial as a coping strategy.

- *"In successful families there is a feeling that the burden is shared."* Members of the family and occasionally friends share tasks and/or emotional support related to the intervention process. Luterman indicated that to prevent parents from becoming overwhelmed with feelings of total responsibility, he tells them:

> This business is really in thirds—one third is your responsibility, one third is mine as a professional, and one third is the child's. You just be sure that you do your third, I'll do my third, and both of us will see that the child does his third. (p. 163)

- *"Successful families need to make philosophical sense of the situation."* When bad or challenging things happen, many people ask, "Why me?" Successful families have an answer, whatever it might be (such as biological, theological, or philosophical). Not having an answer breeds unproductive bitterness, negativity, and anger. Successful families come to see that growth results from challenge and stress. Luterman (1996) conveyed his personal thoughts from sharing his wife's struggle with multiple sclerosis and professional thoughts from working with families of people with hearing impairments:

> For me there has always been growth in stress. I am pushed by the stress to develop more capacity in order to reduce the stress. We generally give to life what life demands. When life demands more, I am forced to expand. That increased capacity is my growth. I see this happening in all the families I have worked with, and although I can empathize and perhaps sympathize with the pain involved, I know that if they can just hang in, they will learn and grow. They have a powerful teacher in the disorder; and we as professionals must allow the process of growth to take place. We can facilitate the growth by not overhelping; by at all times respecting the dignity and the capacity of our clients to grow. Very often we have to let go of our preconceived notions. (pp. 164–165)

Family Based Treatment and Heightened Effectiveness

Another support for a family systems approach to intervention is the growing body of supportive efficacy data. The amount of attention being given to family oriented approaches to intervention in the published literature is increasing.

My reading of this literature across disciplines indicates that positive treatment outcome for an individual with an exceptionality, defined in different terms and variables that are unique to that exceptionality, is related to the emotional and communicative health of the family members and their respective involvement in and commitment to the treatment process. This has been shown over and over. Luterman (1996) stated:

> I have found in my professional life by working intimately with parents of deaf children, if you take good care of the parents, the children will do well. This admonition applies equally well to the chronically ill; if you take good care of the spouse and other family members, the identified patient also will do well. Failure to deal with family needs almost invariably limits therapeutic effectiveness. (pp. xxix–xxv)

Turnbull et al. (1993) compiled first person accounts by families that have experienced a member's developmental disability across the life span. Their collective voices powerfully convey the varied resources of family strength that were used for cognitive coping—for constructively approaching challenging situations in ways that enhanced self-esteem, feelings of control, and a sense of meaning. Such methods enabled families to interpret the experience of having a member with a disability as an opportunity rather than a tragedy, to find positive benefit from the experience, and to enhance family well-being.

Rivara et al. (1993) studied changes in children's functioning in the year following traumatic brain injury and reported the following:

> A strong overall preinjury family functioning score, a high level of family cohesion, positive family relationships, and a low level of control (family hierarchy and rules that are rigid) are predictive of good child adaptive functioning, social competence and global functioning 1 year following TBI. (p. 1052)

Within this context, Rivara et al. (1993) reviewed studies of childhood chronic illness indicating that level of family functioning and extent of illness significantly predicted (was directly, positively correlated with) subsequent physiological, psychological, and social wellness of children with disorders of psychological adjustment, childhood diabetes, severe juvenile rheumatoid arthritis, and congenital or acquired limb deficiencies.

Similarly, Luterman (1996) summarized studies indicating that level of family empathy and positive treatment involvement contributed to (again, directly, positively correlated with): (a) the recovery rate of people who have incurred a stroke, (b) gains in academic achievement with children who have learning disabilities, (c) the success of young children using augmentative and alternative communications programs, and (d) the outcome of children with cystic fibrosis.

Zarski, DePompei, and Zook (1988) supported the importance of understanding family functioning when assessing a family's adaptation to a major stressor—in particular, a head injury to a family member. Zarski et al. (1988) noted that:

> Families that adjust successfully to the trauma reorganize by changing their power structure, role relationships, and relationship rules in response to the situational stress. In addition, emotional bonding, boundaries, coalitions, and

decision-making factors are utilized in ways that focus on the head-injured member's normalcy rather than the symptomatology. In contrast, as families struggle to cope with the many social, physical, cognitive, linguistic, and emotional changes that accompany head injury, some families respond to the theme of loss by focusing on the limitations of the head-injured member, thereby organizing around the dysfunction. . . . These families are unprepared to deal with these changes and use denial as a major block to family reintegration. . . . The more severe the denial, the higher the risk the family will enter a severe crisis stage, further jeopardizing the recovery process. (pp. 38–39)

Several of Zarski et al.'s (1988) themes noted here, such as the positive relationship between cohesion and adaptability and a family's adjustment, and between the focus on ability rather than disability and the overall treatment and recovery outcome, are themes that will be revisited in Unit III, in which we design intervention procedures for people who stutter.

Taken together, these and other studies argue for the importance of assessing and understanding the family's strengths, needs, and level of functioning as factors in the intervention process. Furthermore, problems experienced by families when a member has an illness or exceptionality often are more related to their own resources, coping styles, and organization than to the member's limitations.

Family Based Treatment and Fluency Disorders

The literature directly related to a family systems approach when working with people who stutter is limited at best. The empirical basis appears to be borrowed from allied disciplines as noted in the absence of efficacy studies comparing family systems approaches to other methods of intervention with people who stutter. In fact, Rollin (1987) stated, "Although a comprehensive search of the literature in family systems theory and therapy has failed to reveal any discussion or documentation of stuttering, we believe it is useful to explore the role that family environment may play in its development" (p. 122). One decade later, his words are no less true. Rollin (1987) reviewed basic tenets of family systems theory and then indicated that, "We contend that stuttering in a child may be a behavioral manifestation produced by family tensions, particularly between parents, that have not been resolved through other means" (pp. 121–122). Departing from clinical research and studies of families of people who stutter, Rollin postulated:

Stuttering families can be differentiated from nonstuttering families on the basis of unique family systems processes irrespective of psychopathology per se. That is, our stuttering families constitute a special and often unique combination of circumstances, reactions, conditions, behaviors, and personalities from which stuttering itself has evolved. In some cases, stuttering occurs as a primary instigator for effecting changes in family dynamics, whereas in others, stuttering manifests itself as one possible response to family conflict. (p. 124)

He offered general guidelines, albeit without inclusion or exclusion criteria or supportive empirical or clinical data, for using a family systems approach for fluency intervention. These included the following:

(1) evidence of continued family dysfunction; (2) mild to moderate degree of secondary stuttering characteristics; (3) evidence of parental pressure on the child; (4) motivation—the desire by all family members to participate in the family therapy process; and (5) no evidence of severe psychopathology in the child or other family members. (p. 130)

The guidelines were followed by a general recommendation for treatment methodology. Rollin admitted, "Although the choice of family therapy method may be difficult to decide, because of the many approaches described in the literature, we have selected a general approach that would be most appropriate for the 'stuttering family' " (p. 130).

Rustin (1987) presented a program to treat disfluency in young children through active parental involvement. Making the point that stuttering is highly context-sensitive, Rustin noted that the most significant context for the child is the family, and that the school setting is nearly as critical. Emphasizing that clinicians focus on the family and social contexts of early stuttering, Rustin stated:

> If the problem of speech dysfluency is the result of an interaction between child and environment then intervention must be targeted at both; too often we 'treat' the problem from only one perspective. To include any contextual intervention it is vital to involve the family. . . . The family is seen as the main focus for early intervention with the young dysfluent child. At the simplest level family participation involves parental training in the techniques of improving motor speech fluency. At the social level it means studying family dynamics with a view to promoting changes in the family systems which are likely to lead to further fluency development. (pp. 167–168)

Rustin and Purser (1991) reported preliminary findings from a survey of parents addressing the developmental history and family circumstances of children who stutter. Among many interesting findings on the 209 sampled (163 boys and 46 girls—mean chronological age, 8.4 years; mean age at onset, 3 years, 6 months), they reported that 52% of the boys and 36% of the girls were prone to "inconsolable temper tantrums" (p. 11); that there was a relationship between birth order in the family and stuttering—of the children sampled, all of whom stutter, (a) most were the youngest (34% boys, 36% girls) or oldest (40% boys, 32% girls), (b) fewer were only children (16% boys, 25% girls), and (c) fewest were middle children (10% boys, 7% girls); and that only 42% of the parents of the boys and 50% of the parents of the girls who stutter reported their marital relationship as "good," with the remainder characterizing it as "not completely satisfactory, with the atmosphere at home often being uncertain and volatile" (p. 14) or offered responses that could not be classified. Rustin and Purser concluded:

> It seems to us that even these broad findings do illustrate the need for a careful and systematic appraisal of the family dynamics as well as focusing on problems that child experiences in conjunction with disfluency. . . . Understanding the contexts in which fluency problems arise, both in terms of the individual child and the family system in which that child is developing, offers considerable scope for more effective intervention. (p. 16)

Many treatment programs incorporate parents and other family members into the treatment process; however, the rationale is more practical (to facilitate development and maintenance of fluency) than conceptual (based in family systems principles) in nature. For example, parents have been incorporated by reducing fluency disrupters and creating conditions that facilitate fluency (Van Riper, 1973); supervising the child's use of fluency initiating gestures (FIGs) (Cooper, 1976, 1987b, 1990b; Cooper & Cooper, 1985b, 1993); participating in group counseling sessions, instructing in fluency techniques, and reinforcing correct use of these techniques (Gregory, 1984, 1986a, 1986b); and observing and recording stuttering and fluent speech behaviors (Shine, 1980, 1984). These and many other programs are reviewed more thoroughly elsewhere (Bloodstein, 1993, 1995; Culatta & Goldberg, 1995; Shames & Rubin, 1986; Silverman, 1996; Van Riper, 1973). The importance of approaching stuttering intervention from a family systems perspective cannot be overstated. Empirical support for this perspective has come more from allied disciplines than from communication disorders.

In order to understand more fully the manner in which a family affects and is affected by a member who stutters, we need to understand the nature of that family from a systems framework. Because families are becoming increasingly diverse, as will be noted, each family must be treated as unique, thus our approach to working with families must be individualized. To build this understanding, we focus next on the nature and dynamics of the family unit.

Family Diversity

Turnbull and Turnbull (1990) studied the diversity among American families and addressed the variables that impact how a member's exceptionality affects the family. They indicated that traditional, somewhat nostalgic associations with the word *family* (father as breadwinner, mother at home, two or three children, all under the same roof) are not only outdated; it is unlikely that such a reality of the American family ever existed. Attempts to characterize families in general terms are futile because they are so diverse. In actuality, many people today are delaying marriage or living alone. The vast majority of married women between 18–34 years of age with or without children are employed outside the home. The divorce rate has topped 55%, and 20% of families with children under 18 are headed by a single parent. Beyond demographics, families differ in religion, ethnicity, education, socioeconomic status, location, values, beliefs, family and social structure, among other ways. The point is that each family is unique. Turnbull and Turnbull (1990) conceptualized family systems as dynamic composites of family characteristics, interactions, and functions that develop and change over the life span. We will look briefly at some of their ideas to help us understand the reciprocal interactions between people who stutter and their families.

Family Characteristics

Turnbull and Turnbull (1990) looked at four variables that influence the impact of an exceptionality on the family. These included: (a) characteristics of the exceptionality, (b) characteristics of the family, (c) personal characteristics, and (d) special challenges.

Characteristics of the Exceptionality

First, the characteristics of the exceptionality itself affect the family's reactions. "Exceptionality includes non-normative conditions of a person's senses (hearing and sight), health (heart, lungs, or other internal organs), body (limbs), mind (mental capacity or learning disability), affect (emotional disorder), and language (speech)" (p. 22). For our purposes, we will address only their last category, speech, specifically stuttering. Nevertheless, the nature of each exceptionality presents its unique challenges, special needs, and positive contributions. Likewise, the nature and severity of the exceptionality create unique demands on the family. It cannot be assumed, however, that the greater severity, particularly with stuttering, presents greater demands. Recall the discussion of interiorized stuttering where adults who stuttered as children suppressed their overt, outward symptoms, but not their more covert or inner experience of stuttering (Bloodstein, 1993; Douglass & Quarrington, 1952). Also, the degree of severity of stuttering behavior was not a factor that influenced parental behavior reported by children in the sixth and seventh grade (Yairi & Williams, 1971).

Characteristics of the Family

Second, the characteristics of the family affect its reactions to an exceptionality. These characteristics include the family's size and form, cultural background, socioeconomic status, and geographic locations. The clinician must become aware of the presence, nature, and number of children, parents, stepparents, extended family, among others. Turnbull and Turnbull (1990) reported on a literature indicating that larger families and those with two parents tend to adapt more positively to a member with an exceptionality (than smaller families and those with one parent present). The authors indicated also that it is likely that clinicians will encounter families of more than two parents because one or both parents from the original family has remarried. The resulting "blended family" presents an array of family variations and emotional situations. They warned against prejudgment and stereotyping and offered the following advice:

> In your work with families, remember that no family should be considered "broken" whether it is a nuclear, remarried, adoptive, or foster family. The home atmosphere, the quality of the family's interactions, and the family's perception of itself affect the quality of the family life. (Turnbull & Turnbull, 1990, p. 32)

The individual family's cultural background often influences its rituals, traditions, and foods, in addition to its perspectives and values, which influence the members' attitudes and reactions to an exceptionality. More will be said later in this chapter about the importance of understanding cultural differences. Another factor potentially influencing a family's reactions is socioeconomic status (SES), including income, level of education, occupations, and implied social status. While higher socioeconomic status often translates to greater access to and knowledge about available services, these resources do not necessarily imply better coping skills. Families of lower socioeconomic status might have large families and broad social support networks that can be valuable resources. Related to socioeconomic status are values that impact a family's attitude toward exceptionality. For example, Turnbull and Turnbull reported that higher socioeconomic status often relates to more achievement orientation and control of one's environment, both of which might result in greater disappointment by parents toward their aspirations for a child with an exceptionality. On the other hand, families of lower socioeconomic status might regard family solidarity and happiness as more important than achievement and control, perhaps resulting in greater acceptance and nurturing. Turnbull and Turnbull (1990) summarized aptly:

> On the one hand, therefore, higher SES families may be more stressed by an event, such as an exceptionality, that contradicts their belief that they are in control of their lives. Lower SES families, on the other hand, may have difficulty considering future options for their child and might be caught unprepared. . . Furthermore, a belief that it is useless to try to control a situation or to plan ahead may make lower SES families less active participants in educational decision making. (pp. 38–39)

Again, prejudgments must not be made. Every family is unique. I remember very clearly a 3-year-old girl who stuttered with whom I worked for nearly a year before the father was transferred by his work to a city over 200 miles away. This family of few financial means did everything imaginable to be actively involved in all aspects of the intervention process, in addition to traveling the distance in an unreliable vehicle, arranging for housing with relatives, and caring for other pressing concerns. At one point the family moved locally in order to receive services, which resulted in either temporary separation from or extensive commutes for the father. While I was utterly moved by this family's commitment to one another and to its continuing and abiding faith (never once did I hear a complaint or unkind word), I was uncomfortable nevertheless with being responsible for the family being apart and incurring additional burden. This arrangement was alleviated when we investigated together similar and affordable intervention services in the city, supplemented by ongoing indirect and less frequent direct intervention from me. This anecdote also conveys another factor—geographic location—that influences availability and affordability of services, either of which can influence a family's attitude toward the exceptionality. The point is that all people within families present both needs and positive contributions. We must work with each family individually and learn with and from them.

Personal Characteristics

Third, personal characteristics including tolerance to stress, coping styles, and intellectual capacity, among others, affect a family's and its members' reactions to stuttering. These characteristics might be strengths or limitations for the individual family and will affect the clinician's approach to the family. Many factors influence one's tolerance to stress, including coping styles. Turnbull and Turnbull (1990) discussed various methods for coping, or reducing feelings of stress, including passive appraisal (ignoring a problem), reframing (changing one's perspective about a problem to help solve it or view it as less stressful), spiritual support (gaining comfort and direction from spiritual beliefs), social support (receiving assistance from friends and family), and professional support (receiving help from human service professionals).

Turnbull and colleagues (1993) presented a series of moving essays conveying how individuals and families cope with exceptional circumstances. In one of these essays, Schulz (1993) defined cognitive coping as "the process of restructuring stressful events in positive ways" (p. 31), and indicated that her family openly discusses stressful issues and uses coping strategies including family support, previous successful experience with coping, and humor. Schulz raised important questions that might be considered by service providers including whether cognitive coping strategies can be taught to families and people with exceptionalites to help them solve their own problems. Nevertheless, clinicians must be aware of the coping strategies being used so that intervention and recommendations are appropriate to the individual family. Another personal variable is the intellectual capacity of the family members including the person who stutters. In other words, the extent to which people understand and can be helped to understand what is happening will affect their attitudes toward stuttering and the intervention process, and will affect how they are included as active participants.

I remember a boy of 4 years with whom I worked because of his stuttering. Recognizing the young mother's significant cognitive limitations, I included her in the intervention process but to a different extent than I would other parents who were more cognitively able. Specifically, she was taught how to take conversational turns with her son. This was the only expectation placed upon her. Working with her was a good reminder of what we will discuss in Unit III about how to prepare parents and others to participate meaningfully in the intervention process. Such preparation, or teaching, involves no less than three distinct steps: telling, showing, and then directly coaching the person in doing what you expect. Unfortunately, this mother's limitations were neither recognized nor accounted for by other service providers. When her son became absent from treatment for an extended time, I investigated and learned that the boy was hospitalized. This was why. He first became ill when the mother bathed him in a partially frozen creek. The boy's illness prolonged, whereupon the case workers urged the mother to bring the boy for medical attention. Following directions as she interpreted them, she filled the boy's prescription and fed him the entire bottle at one sitting. Although the instructions were printed plainly on the bottle, she was unable to read them. The point is that all persons can and should be involved in the intervention process. However, the nature of involvement must take into account a variety of personal strengths and limitations without prejudgment. This requires that clinicians come to know their clients and their families.

Special Challenges

Finally, some families find themselves facing special challenges that not only might affect reactions toward the exceptionality, but the family's apparent willingness to participate in and contribute to intervention programs. Such situations include families who live in poverty, in rural areas, in homes where abuse occurs, or where one or more members are ill or disabled. Too often, professionals assume that parents who do not participate in the intervention process care less about their children than those who do. Another interpretation, often verified if given the opportunity, is that for some people, more basic needs of their children including food, shelter, and health take precedence, thus leaving few available resources in terms of time, money, and physical and emotional energy to address the child's communication needs.

I remember interviewing a mother who referred to me her 9-year-old son because of stuttering. The mother was 34 years old, African American, and took the day off work to travel 120 miles for the evaluation. At first, her manner was at best "guarded" and her communication style was passive. She responded briefly to questions asked of her, offered little elaboration, and did not initiate topics for discussion when invited to do so or when provided silence. What I most recall was that when we were seated, she demonstrated no direct eye contact, focusing instead downward, a forward slouching posture, and constantly fidgeting hands. This woman was tense. The evaluation proceeded, after which I conferenced with her again to describe my observations and evaluation. As usual, I began by highlighting the aspects of the interaction I observed between the woman and her son that were particularly facilitative of fluency and gentle, uninterrupted conversational turn-taking. I also expressed my sincere appreciation to her for doing all she had to in order to be present for the evaluation. As the summary continued, I noticed that she began to participate more in the conversation, asking questions, seeking clarification, and initiating topics. Her posture became more inviting, and when she offered me her eye contact, I noticed that her eyes were reddening. What followed would best be described as a conversationally and emotionally cathartic experience for this woman. The following statement was taken from among the many significant feelings and observations she shared:

> You are the first professional who has made me feel that I am worth a damn. Most of the others think that because I am on Welfare that I am not a good mother. I love my boy. He's all I got. I would do anything for him. But I got to work. All the others tell me what I do wrong, tell what I should do. They don't know me. They don't want to know me. They judge me. I know it. You tell me I do something right. That is everything.

Families who live in rural areas often report feelings of loneliness and social isolation, particularly with respect to having others with whom to discuss feelings and experiences related to stuttering. Also, those in rural areas might incur geographic, in addition to financial, limitations in accessing services. Unique challenges are experienced by families in which abusive situations exist and when other members, including parents, are ill or disabled. These and other such situations already described are reminders of the importance of individualizing treatment with families, and working from a team approach, a topic to be explored later in this chapter.

Family Interactions

In addition to being keenly aware of family characteristics, clinicians must become knowledgeable of the unique patterns of interaction within each family.

Turnbull and Turnbull (1990) indicated that "the family is a unit consisting of many interactions—an interactional system. Events affecting any one member can have an impact upon all family members" (p. 53). Schulz (1993), referring to family members as "heroes in disguise," added that "in family system theory, we frequently state that what happens to a person with a disability happens to the entire family. What we fail to mention is that what happens to the family also happens to the person with a disability" (p. 31). Turnbull and Turnbull (1990) discussed four family subsystems that must be recognized and understood. These are the *marital subsystem* (husband and wife interactions), *parental subsystem* (parent and child interactions), *sibling subsystem* (child and child interactions), and *extended family subsystem* (interactions of the family and its individual members with extended family, friends, neighbors, and professionals). Within each of these subsystems, the impact of a family member with an exceptionality is experienced in many different ways. Thoughts, feelings, and behaviors all are affected. Such an experience can have a positive, bonding impact within the interactions, or can have a negative, interpersonally destructive impact within the family. Again, without prejudgment, the clinician must assess the impact of the exceptionality, namely stuttering, and tailor the intervention and the respective participation of the family members accordingly. Before discussing the interaction between family patterns and the change process, I will introduce the concepts of family cohesion and adaptability as aspects of family interaction.

Family Cohesion

Elements of interaction including cohesion and adaptability have been used to help understand the ways people within a family interact. *Family cohesion* has been described as "the close emotional bonding that members have toward each other and the level of independence individuals feel within the family system" (Turnbull & Turnbull, 1990, p. 69). Cohesion within interpersonal relationships has been characterized as falling along a continuum from high *enmeshment* on one end and high *disengagement* on the other (Luterman, 1996; Minuchin, 1974; Minuchin & Fishman, 1981; Turnbull & Turnbull, 1990). Both enmeshment and disengagement define the relative degree to which boundaries are open versus closed for relationships within and across the interpersonal subsystems described. High enmeshment means that boundaries between family subsystems are not well defined; thus relationships often are characterized by overinvolvement, overprotection, and insulation from demands requiring independence or risk taking. Most decisions and activities are family focused, allowing little privacy for individual family members. In such families, one often finds the stuttering to be the center of the family's existence around which most activity and interactions are based, thus isolating the family from contact with others.

In contrast to highly enmeshed families are those described as disengaged. Highly disengaged families maintain strict boundaries between family subsystems. The family may deny the existence of the stuttering, thus withdrawing emotional support and friendship toward the member who stutters and who may experience loneliness. Such families are characterized by little involvement among its members, few shared interests, extensive privacy, more time apart than together, and independent rather than joint decision making. Most healthy families experience a balance between enmeshment and disengagement, clearly understanding family limits and boundaries, thus inviting close bonding and nurturing independence and autonomy. As noted earlier, clinicians need to be aware of the level of cohesion within and between family subsystems in order to tailor intervention and recommendations that are sensitive and responsive to each family, thus best helping the individual who stutters.

Family Adaptability

Another variable for clinicians to consider is *family adaptability,* the ability to change or adjust in response to stresses. Just as individuals need to have an awareness of, so as to use, their personal constructs, families need to understand their view of a problem to accommodate change when appropriate. Families that are unwilling or unable to change are considered rigid; those always changing without a sense of structure or plan are considered chaotic. Just as healthy families have struck a balance between enmeshment and disengagement, they too fall between the extremes of *rigidity* and *chaos.* Families that are rigid experience high control and structure, strict rules and role definitions, and little sharing or negotiation. The intervention process from a systems perspective requires that family members actively participate and support the person who stutters. This expectation will prove problematic with rigid families. While structure varies with each individual family, as noted, there are still some in which the mother is expected to meet the child's ever changing academic, social, extracurricular, and developmental needs. In such families where roles are firmly and inflexibly established, the mother may feel overly burdened and stressed by addressing alone the added accommodations required when a child stutters. Without shared family ownership of the challenges presented by a person who stutters and the resulting intervention plan (i.e., when only the mother is expected to participate in intervention), the potential effectiveness of intervention is significantly reduced. Furthermore, the reality of stuttering and the intervention may be denied, if not rejected, by the other family members, thus causing further conflict.

In contrast to rigid families are those described as chaotic. Chaotic families are relatively unstructured and their interactions are guided by few rules, which are rarely enforced and frequently change. People outside of the family can no more count on commitments made by the family than the members can among themselves. Often there is no family leadership, which results in little control, endless discussion and negotiation, unclear family role distinctions, and little concern for future planning. All families experience temporary periods of rigidity and chaos during particularly stressful life events. Most families fall somewhere between the two polar opposites. Only when such extremes become a family's mode of operation does a problem arise for working with its members in a program of fluency intervention. In any case, intervention and related recommendations must reflect an awareness of and account for the uniqueness of each family system and its members.

Family Patterns and Change

Family interactions tend to be highly reciprocal, patterned, and repetitive (Carter & Orfanidis, 1976). We already noted that a systems perspective assumes the interactions are indeed systemic (circular) rather than linear (Andrews & Andrews, 1990). In other words, it is of limited utility for family members (or a clinician) to look exclusively for direct cause and effect relationships. For example, while it might be tempting to find someone to blame for a family member's worsening stuttering, doing so falls short of identifying interactive and perpetuating patterns and tracing their flow. Carter and Orfanidis (1976) noted that all family patterns, once established, are perpetuated by everyone involved in them. Nevertheless, when stress inevitably enters into any of the two person subsystems discussed (parent–parent, parent–child, child–child), a pattern of scapegoating, or *triangulation*, frequently is observed. This means that the two people experiencing a problem come to focus on a third person (or thing, or external issue) in order to divert anxiety in the relationship. This pattern is dysfunctional in that it offers stabilization by diversion, thus perpetuating the problem, rather than working toward resolution or change. Luterman (1996) noted that often a child is triangulated into a marital conflict and that the child's symptoms, whatever they might be, serve to distract the parents from their other problems. The cost to the child, however, is significant. If the child's symptoms are removed or alleviated, the family's homeostasis, or conditions operating to promote status quo functioning, would be threatened. Therefore, family members experience conflict— they alleviate the child's symptoms (gain) at the expense of the parent's shared focus (cost), or maintain the child's symptoms (cost) to promote apparent harmony among the parents (gain). In any case, this zero sum conflict (if one gains, then the other loses) exacts a mighty toll on the child who already is experiencing significant demands and therefore is likely to be functioning under reduced capacity.

Hartman and Laird (1983) described the potential benefits and drawbacks of change within a family as creating a paradox, as follows:

> Change can be frightening. In some families, any change is perceived as an enemy which must be warded off—a threat to coherence, stability, or even continued existence. . . . Families over a period of time propagate rules and patterns of behavior which gain certain coherence and which serve to preserve the family. "Symptoms" or problematic behaviors are often an essential, indeed key part, of the family's effort to maintain itself. . . . The symptom should be understood, then, not as a problem but rather as a solution to another more grievous or threatening problem, one which might expose a feared secret, threaten the family with dissolution, or otherwise shake its very foundations. Such a family is in a paradoxical situation in the sense that they want the disturbing symptom to change but they do not want, or rather are afraid for, the family itself to change. Yet one cannot happen without the other. (pp. 326–327)

Others have documented marital partners in conflict who triangulated a family member, frequently a child, with exceptionalities including psychiatric disturbance (Satir, 1967), psychosomatic illnesses (e.g., asthma, anorexia, diabetes), dependence, depression, academic failure, sexual promiscuity (Hartman & Laird, 1983), and stuttering (Rollin, 1987). All recommended that intervention occur at the level of the family rather than the individual. Hartman and Laird (1983) noted that the family unit is both a resource and target for change that must be understood within the context of its own unique ecological environment (the complex interrelationships among physical, social, psychological, and cultural forces). Luterman (1996) reminded that many of the families with whom we work are stressed because they include a person with a communication disorder and are not necessarily dysfunctional. Clinicians must be aware of and sensitive to issues and concepts related to family interaction including the subsystems and relative cohesion and adaptability of the members.

Turnbull and Turnbull (1990) indicated that family interactions are influenced by available resources, characteristics of the exceptionality, values, and ethnic background. The nature of the subsystems and the respective interactions change as a family moves through the life cycle. Clinicians are reminded that intervention with people who stutter should not be approached in isolation, or from what has been referred to as a linear perspective. My own observations, however, unfortunately suggest that this is often the case. Rather, people who stutter, like all other people, interact within a system of interpersonal and interdependent relationships. Thus, changes in one member of the communication system affect all other members. Luterman (1996) concluded as follows:

> The family is a system in which all of the components are interdependent. Every family member affects every other component of the family. For the family therapist, there is no such thing as individual therapy; any time a change occurs in one member of the family, everybody in the family is impacted. Working in individual therapy with an identified patient in a dysfunctional family burdens the individual to become a change agent for the family. This is often too difficult a task for the patient, especially if it is a child. Family therapists find it much more efficacious to work at the systems level; in fact many family therapists refuse to work with individuals. (p. 133)

Family Functions

Sometimes in our interactions with people who stutter and their families, we clinicians inadvertently assume that their sole function is to participate within our intervention plan. As a consequence, we experience a measure of discouragement in what appears to be our clients' failure to recognize the source and degree of inspiration from which the plan was derived. I am not making light of the fact that a high level of sincere motivation and commitment from both the client and clinician is essential to the clinical process. However, I do want to underscore that clinicians' expectations must be tempered by an explicit understanding of the different, and at times conflicting, functions of our clients and their families that might occasionally interfere with participation in intervention. Family functions are interdependent and pose occasionally conflicting demands. These functions have been distinguished into seven broad categories: economic, daily care, recreation, socialization, self-definition, affection, and educational/vocational (Turnbull & Turnbull, 1990). While these and other functions are distinct, any one dimension of family functioning often impacts other dimensions.

For example, it is easy to see how economic needs can limit resources and outlets for recreation, socialization, education, and other dimensions. Furthermore, family tension can be increased by financial pressure, thus negatively impacting the affection offered to others, particularly those, because of stuttering or another exceptionality, who might pose an additional financial burden. Turnbull and Turnbull (1990) pointed out that "the presence of a family member with an exceptionality can create special economic needs by increasing the family's consumptive demands and decreasing its productive capacity" (p. 83). Furthermore, "Just as the presence of a family member with an exceptionality can negatively affect the amount of money the family has to spend on other needs, so it can negatively affect the amount of money a family can produce" (p. 84).

I am reminded of a man in his 50s who, with absolute support and participation of his family, demonstrated a model commitment to the treatment process. During one of our many conversations, he discussed the actual cost incurred by his family for the treatment process. The direct cost of treatment was only the beginning. The time he took off from work to attend treatment had a significant financial impact because he was paid on an hourly basis. When it was possible for him to make up the hours, he was paid at the regular, rather than the overtime, rate. His wife, an active and regular participant in the treatment process, also needed to adjust her work schedule which required administrative approval although presented no additional financial burden. He pointed out that the long drive necessitated additional car repairs, which to him seemed minor in the long run. While the man's tone was positive and did not present even the shadow of a complaint, this discussion was a good reminder for me of the commitment offered by this man and his family. One day during treatment, the man indicated that he would be absent for one session the following month. He explained that he and his family had planned an important social and recreational activity that would be fairly expensive, and when combined with treatment would create a financial hardship for that month. How easy it would have been for me or any other clinician to misinterpret this honest expression as an indication of the client's waning commitment for treatment. Rather, I chose to express appreciation for his candor, particularly in light of his resolute participation in the treatment process, and to share the importance of the social event to him and his family.

I have said that we must value people who stutter as members of a family system, all of whose functions including, but not limited to, fluency intervention must be acknowledged and respected. In this case, I arranged to waive the fee for treatment during that particular week so that the client could engage in both important activities. While the suggestion of this arrangement startled the client and caused visible reactions of embarrassment, conducting the session as planned and at no cost sent a powerful message regarding the degree to which he and his family were valued as people and active participants in family functioning including the treatment process. My intention here is not to recommend my decision for other clinicians, to discuss the implications of fees for service, or to debate the sincerity of the client's candor. Rather my point is that we clinicians, when designing and implementing treatment, must value people who stutter as functioning in capacities beyond those that we directly observe. That value must be appreciated implicitly and acknowledged explicitly.

Another reminder is that for all of us, including people who stutter, there are just so many hours in a day. Yet it is true and often said that work expands to fill the time. Nevertheless, clinicians need to be mindful of the many and often conflicting demands upon our clients as participants in different family functions. I will be emphasizing several points later, including that transfer activities, which generalize fluency skills to outside settings, begin at the outset of treatment if not before, and that valuable treatment activities must occur regularly between scheduled treatment sessions. The point here is that such activities must be planned with, rather than for, our clients with an appreciation of the many demands upon them. Believe me, I am not reluctant to hold people who stutter to their treatment obligations, albeit within a positive framework. However, a client's occasional lack of follow-through might have alternative interpretations.

Another client who stuttered comes to mind. This one was 35 years old and in a failing marriage. While he was in fluency treatment, his marriage dissolved and he gained sole custody of his two sons, then aged 7 and 9 years. To make ends meet, this man worked three jobs and was a full time college student pursuing a career in computer programming. While his parents helped occasionally with child care, the demands of daily living combined with economic hardship were keen. This man, in my estimation, was responsible to a fault. Assignments were always jointly designed and completed satisfactorily. Independently, he initiated and designed a personalized evaluation system to critique his extraclinical speech-related activities, which were recorded frequently each day in a pocket journal. Treatment was canceled frequently, however, due to the demands related to his family obligations including children's illness, teacher conferences, doctor appointments, among others. One time, he called to explain that he had just pulled out of his garage on the way to treatment when his old truck caught fire. The firemen were extinguishing the blaze as we spoke. Surely, these frequent interruptions reduced treatment progress. We discussed this and other issues of treatment continuity and transfer and compensated as much as possible through tailored home assignments. Some clinicians would have terminated his enrollment because of breach of attendance. I chose not to. I believed that he demonstrated absolute commitment and responsibility to all of his obligations and family functions, including fluency intervention. As he progressed through treatment, which was protracted and adjusted frequently to meet his unique needs, he gained control of his fluency and other aspects of his life. He is a successful father, college graduate, computer programmer, respected citizen, and yes, fluent speaker. I admire his dedication and his personal constructs, which helped him maintain strength and perseverance through adversity. He recently shared with me his excitement over having met a wonderful woman. My classes have been inspired and moved to tears on more than one occasion when he and his sons have shared their experiences and their appreciation for the support and understanding they feel they received during the treatment process.

Once again, we need to remind ourselves that we all, clients and clinicians, are members of family systems and experience interdependent functions and occasionally conflicting demands. When we work with people who stutter, we are challenged not to become narrowly focused in our efforts or judgmental in our interpretations. The mother of a 15-year-old boy who stutters, actively participating in the treatment process, realized that she, not the clinician, had become too narrowly focused on problems that commanded her immediate attention. The mother's words might remind clinicians of the importance of viewing people who stutter as able members of a family and communication systems and of incorporating that view into the treatment process. Her words, taken from a letter to the clinician, follow:

> Observing you with my son helped me understand the "magic" of your success with him. You are so interested in who he is and who he is becoming, in his goals, in what is important to him. You are excited by his interests. Your genuine acceptance and approval of him is very inspiring to him. You honor the adolescent struggle of forging a separate identity. Listening to you rekindled that awareness in me. You reminded me to celebrate this "rite of passage." I am ashamed that I allow the urgent, daily life to overshadow these more important things. Thank you for helping me to refocus on this awesome developmental process.

Family Life Cycle

Describing the family life cycle, McGoldrick and Carter (1982) referred to "the family as a system moving through time" (p. 168). It is within this cycle that the family is viewed as the major context for the development of its members. Each family frames and approaches challenges within the contexts of past and present experiences in addressing challenges and problems, and the future toward which the family is moving. The experience of stuttering and its influence on members of the family system can be viewed as one such challenge. McGoldrick and Carter indicated that distinct phases in the developmental cycle can be identified and predicted. An understanding of the family life cycle is essential to dealing with people who stutter, all of whom are members of, influence, and are influenced by respective family units. Consideration of the potential influence of and on a family should not be restricted to the members of a particular household. McGoldrick and Carter viewed family as comprising the entire emotional system of at least three generations, as follows:

> It has rarely been taken adequately into account that the family life cycle is a complex process involving at least three and now more often four generations moving among together in time. The tremendous impact of one generation on those following is hard to overestimate. For one thing, the three or four different generations must accommodate to life cycle transitions simultaneously. While one generation is moving toward older age, the next is contending with the empty nest, the third with young adulthood and the forming of couples, and the fourth with the process of becoming the newest members of the system. Naturally, there is an intermingling of the generations, and events at one level have a powerful effect on relationships at each other level. (pp. 168–169)

Family Roles Affect Fluency Treatment

Some may ask why an understanding of a family life cycle is important to working with people who stutter. We already underscored the point that anything happening to one person affects and is affected by other members of the family system. For this reason alone, it is foolhardy to direct our clinical efforts to the person who stutters without consideration of the others with whom this person communicates regularly. The needs of all involved must be taken into account for treatment to be effective and generalizable.

For example, when adjusting the clinical activities for home programming with a man who stutters and his wife, both of whom are in their 50s, I deliberately asked how the fluency changes were being addressed by the couple. The man said things were fine. The woman expressed uncertainty as to the limits of her responsibility. He was to talk with her as part of his assignments to report fluent words and experiences of self-correction, and she was to feel comfortable providing positive feedback when she heard him use his fluency controls. She was not expected, however, to correct him in respect to the nature of their relationship as husband and wife, and not to assume that she was the clinician in absentia. Furthermore, we had discussed that he needed to handle increasing amounts of responsibility for fluency independence, and guard against building dependence on the clinician, his wife, or anyone else. Although the respective involvement of each was a topic of weekly discussion, followed by modeling and feedback, both had come to assume that she was to correct him when he failed to use his fluency controls. Both expressed feelings that she was letting him down when she did not correct him, or keep him to task. The subsequent discussion was essential to restate and redemonstrate the roles of each, and particularly to provide her with an opportunity to continue to feel needed and appreciated in ways other than as his spokesperson. Without such regular discussion and attention to the needs of both, her involvement would likely have become an irritant and an inhibitor rather than a facilitator of treatment.

Family Stress Affects Fluency Treatment

Another reason that we need to understand the family life cycle is to recognize stressful experiences for what they are and how they may affect a person's fluency and the treatment process. Stress experienced within a family often occurs around transition points in the life cycle, frequently disrupting the cycle or producing symptoms of dysfunction (McGoldrick & Carter, 1982). Stuttering can be one such symptom of stress or disruption (Rollin, 1987). We already noted that stress increases the demand on a person, which can limit one's capacity for fluency and other aspects of coping. For these reasons, we need to know what stages a family might be experiencing to better understand the effect of the stressful events. Furthermore, one's readiness for treatment must in part consider the stage within the life cycle being experienced by the person who stutters and the family.

For example, the parents of a preschool child who is beginning to stutter will need to adjust the demanding family functions to accommodate the requirements of treatment (such as time for participating in treatment, home activities, financial cost, and rescheduling of other activities). Likewise, if one of the parents requests fluency intervention for himself or herself, a realistic question will involve the extent to which the family can accommodate the requirements of treatment. I have worked with a number of young parents who have demonstrated to themselves the ability to speak fluently, but because of other conflicting demands (i.e., newly born infant, recovery of mother, work demands, and others) were unable to put themselves and their speech fluency as a priority. The relative priority of the fluency treatment within the existing demands on the person and the family will impact a clinician's decision regarding the appropriateness of the timing for intervention and the viability of the person as a candidate for intervention. Perkins (1983, 1984) spoke of clients' opting disfluency over fluency because the constant cost, measured in the effort expended to maintain fluency, proved too high.

Families as Portraits of Development and Change

We already reviewed that every family's experience is unique. Nevertheless, there are distinct developmental stages during which each member is engaged in fairly regular tasks related to his or her period in life. Such tasks are influenced by factors already discussed, including family characteristics (size, membership, ethnicity, values, and special challenges, among others), interactions within and between family subsystems, and diverse and at times conflicting family functions and individual commitments. Turnbull and Turnbull (1990) pointed out that all life-cycle interpretations are culturally and historically specific, generalized representations of family change, and therefore unique to each family. Common family changes are experienced, for example, as its members are born, grow up, leave home, develop long-term relationships, retire, and die. Consequently, the characteristics and functions of the family and its members also change developmentally with such transitions and idiosyncratic variation.

Different authors have presented varying representations of the family life cycle. When becoming familiar with and thinking about such models, clinicians should consider the reciprocal interaction between the family's stage and its experiences related to the person who stutters. McGoldrick and Carter (1982) presented what they considered to be the normal (i.e., statistically predictable) family life cycle in middle-class America in the last quarter of the 20th century, and noted that such realities are changing. These changes are being precipitated by lower birth rates, longer life expectancy, and increasing divorce and remarriage rates. While childrearing once occupied adults for their entire active life span, it now consumes less than half the time span prior to old age. Conceptualizations of family, therefore, are changing because they are no longer organized primarily around this activity and because both men and women are considering more varied personal and professional options. McGoldrick and Carter described the family life cycle as a sequence of six stages, with particular emphasis on the emotional network and transitions within the family as follows:

- The unattached young adult, who is between family systems, is in the process of separating from parents, which requires differentiating self from family, developing peer relationships, and establishing oneself in work.

- The newly married couple, which has joined families through marriage, is establishing a commitment to a new system. This requires formation of a marital family system and realignment of relationships with extended families and friends to include the spouse.

- The family with young children, which is in the process of accepting new members into the system, must adjust the marital system to make room for the child or children, take on new parenting roles, and realign relationships with extended family to include parenting and grandparenting roles.

- The family with adolescents, which increases flexibility of family boundaries to accommodate children's independence, must adjust the parent–child relationship, refocus on midlife marital and career issues, and begin to focus on concerns of older generation.

- The family that is launching children and moving on must accept a multitude of exits from and entries into the family system. At the same time, the partners must renegotiate the marital system as a dyad, nurture adult relationships with grown children, realign relationships to include in-laws and grandchildren, and deal with failing health of parents (i.e., grandparents).

- The family in later life must accept the shifting of generational roles. This requires maintaining one's own and the couple's functioning and interests during physiological decline, exploring new family and social role options, supporting the more central role for the middle generation, making room in the system for the needs and wisdom of the older generation, preparing for and dealing with loss of spouse, siblings, and peers, and preparing for one's own death. This is the period of life review and integration.

McGoldrick and Carter (1982) noted that many events result in variations in the family life cycle. Such variations include divorce and remarriage, child custody issues, experiences of people who are in a socioeconomically lower or poverty status, and cultural (i.e., ethnicity and religion) factors. Issues related to multicultural awareness and human diversity will be explored further in Chapter 6.

Turnbull and Turnbull (1990) identified four life-cycle stages of family development while emphasizing the potential impact that an exceptionality of one member may have on the family unit. A summary of their thoughts follows:

- *Birth and Early Childhood (ages 0–5 years):* The parents have had some experience integrating their own values and responding to each other's needs and now are challenged to nurture the child's needs without forgetting their own. Also, this stage is often when the exceptionality is identified, when families are in first contact with educational and allied health professionals, and when expectations are established or revised for the children. The authors emphasized that providers of early intervention should "establish and capitalize upon the child's positive contributions" (p. 115). These experiences and the need for a positive outlook are particularly relevant to developmental stuttering.

- *School Age (ages 6–12 years):* Children, upon entry into school, broaden social horizons and establish friendships. Parents begin a long process of letting go, turning over responsibility for their child to others. Children with exceptionalities often move from noncategorical to categorical intervention where clinical labels are applied. They are apt to encounter their first experience of social stigma for being different. The authors stressed the importance of friendships to all people including those with exceptionalities, and reminded service providers that "concentrating on the strengths of the family will improve the members' confidence in dealing with the exceptionality as well as facilitate a family/professional partnership" (p. 118).

- *Adolescence (ages 12–21 years):* This stage is characterized by stressful changes, both physical and psychological. Coinciding with puberty is a variety of challenging tasks including development of self-identity, development of positive body image, adjustment to sexual maturation, emotional independence from parents, and development of mature social relationships. Parents often find this period stressful as well because their authority is challenged by their child's growing independence and because they begin to face issues of mid-life; for example, their own perceived attractiveness and youthfulness begin to decline at the very time their children are becoming attractive adults. Adolescents who stutter must balance the implications of social stigma with the development of self-advocacy skills.

• *Adulthood (ages 21+ years):* There are many cultural variations for when and how adulthood is attained. Generally, however, this means the acquisition of greater independence and responsibility. In the last quarter of this century for middle class America, this has meant finding employment and moving away from the parents' home. Other cultures do not separate emotionally or geographically.

Summary—Family Based Treatment

Many models exist to represent the family life cycle. They attempt to represent the ongoing and developmental process of change within families. At each developmental stage and particularly at points of transition, changes occur within families' interactions and approach to life. I have made the point that clinicians working with people who stutter must address their needs from a family systems perspective. One member of a family (i.e., a person who stutters) cannot be understood in isolation from the rest of the system. A family's structure, organization, and interactional patterns are among the factors that determine the behavior of the person who stutters and that of the other members. Therefore, changes in the behavior of one member of a family affect and are affected by the other members of the family. For these and other reasons, clinicians must be aware of such factors when approaching the challenges of fluency intervention. Turnbull and Turnbull (1990) pointed out that under the best of circumstances, life transitions within families are difficult. This difficulty is compounded when a family member has an exceptionality. They summarized valuable implications for clinicians working from a family systems perspective with a person who has an exceptionality:

1. Every family brings a different set of characteristics, values, and styles to their experience with exceptionality; thus, you will need to individualize your approach to working with families.

2. Families have an interactional style that dictates the way the members fall into subsystems as well as their preferred levels of closeness and flexibility. To be effective, you will find it helpful to encourage balance and to adapt interventions according to family needs and preferences.

3. Families have a variety of coping skills that enable them to meet their tangible and intangible needs. Respect each family's priorities and encourage the family to attend to the different needs of all its members.

4. Families change over time; therefore, families will need you to help them meet the needs of different developmental stages and also to ease the stress of transition from one stage to another. (p. 141)

CHAPTER SUMMARY

This chapter reviewed central and guiding intervention assumptions from intrafamily perspectives. Specifically, we addressed personal constructs and family systems.

An understanding of personal construct theory and its relevance to intervention reveals that stuttering-related thoughts, feelings, and behavior reflect in part the consequence of active and alternative choices. All people, including those who stutter and their clinicians, develop a perspective about the world and themselves based on previous experiences. These systems of personal constructs help us anticipate and respond to, if not shape, future events. When we are aware explicitly of our clients' personal constructs, we can use this awareness to effect positive and proactive changes in his communication skills and how he views himself as a communicator. When we are aware explicitly of our own personal constructs regarding our role as a clinician and as a facilitator of change, we can make necessary adjustments to meet our clients' objectives while planning for and effecting growth in our own professional development. Personal construct theory tells us that we do not need to stick with the past or maintain the status quo. By becoming aware of our assumptions, and thereby our interpretation of past events, clients and clinicians may evaluate the appropriateness of the constructs that have formed. If the constructs are found to be incorrect, inappropriate, or undesirable, then we may consciously revise them to achieve the outcomes that were not or did not seem possible previously (such as speaking with greater fluency, using self-corrections more often, or considering the client's point of view). Personal construct theory conveys that all people have choices (i.e., active, deliberate, conscious decisions) and that "all of our present interpretations of the universe are subject to revision and replacement" (Kelly, 1955a, p. 15). This constructive freedom combined with personal responsibility is at the heart of "constructive alternativism." Clinicians, therefore, must shift perspective so as to see and understand the client's world as the client sees it.

Family systems theory emphasizes that the changes in or experiences of one member trigger compensatory changes in other members. Furthermore, one part of the family cannot be understood in isolation from the other members of the system. This makes it incumbent upon clinicians to understand and work with the families of their clients who stutter. Doing so requires that clinicians shift from a monocular to a polyocular perspective (from holding one perspective as correct to viewing different interpretations of the same event as potentially equally correct), from labeling to understanding (moving from labeling behaviors to identifying interactive patterns and finding solutions), and from behaviors to systems (moving from a focus on cause–effects to transformations within an integrated communication system). Family based treatment requires that families and professionals interact as partners, and that clinicians understand, model, and nurture the characteristics of optimal and successful families. Various studies were reviewed that empirically support the efficacy of family based treatment. In order to understand the manner in which a family affects and is affected by a member who stutters, the nature and dynamics of the family unit were addressed including family diversity, characteristics, interaction, functions, and life cycle.

Chapter 5 Study Questions

1. Understanding our own and our client's personal constructs is essential for providing effective intervention. How might a client's and/or clinician's personal constructs impact the assessment and treatment processes? What can be done to maximize a positive treatment outcome?

2. Constructive alternativism invites constructive freedom combined with personal responsibility. What is the relevance of constructive alternativism to assessing and treating people who stutter, predicting treatment outcome, and working with families? What is the relevance to engaging in professional preparation (the academic, clinical, and supervisory processes), maintaining professional growth, and engaging in lifelong learning?

3. A family systems approach to intervention emphasizes the importance of working with families, rather than just with individuals who stutter. Indeed, clinicians' interpersonal (i.e., counseling) skills are critical for effective intervention. How will you as a clinician remain within the limits of your professional training and competence? What challenges do you feel are within the boundaries of your training? Which exceed the limits of your training? How will you recognize the difference and what will you do should you find yourself expected to perform outside these limits? What other challenges do you feel you will encounter from a family systems perspective? What are the similarities/differences and advantages/disadvantages when considering a family systems approach and more traditional forms of intervention? In what ways might working from a family systems approach facilitate interdisciplinary forms of intervention?

4. We have emphasized the importance of understanding the nature and dynamics of families. How does an understanding of the family life cycle affect you personally and professionally? How has your understanding developed over time? How will your understanding continue to develop? In what ways might this understanding impact your work with clients who stutter and their families?

5. Intervention is affected by many different variables. One such variable is setting. How might different treatment settings (school, university, private clinic, hospital, or daycare, among others) influence your potential application of personal construct theory and family systems theory? What about the impact of other variables (status, power, degree, professional training, gender, age, cultural differences, and others)?

Unit II

* * * * * * * * * * * * * * * * * * *

Central and Guiding Intervention Assumptions

Chapter 5
Personal Constructs and Family Systems: Intrafamily Considerations

Chapter 6
Interdisciplinary Teaming and Multicultural Awareness: Extrafamily Considerations

Chapter 7
Stuttering Modification and Fluency Shaping: Psychotherapeutic Considerations

Chapter 6

Interdisciplinary Teaming and Multicultural Awareness: Extrafamily Considerations

◆　◆　◆　◆　◆　◆　◆　◆　◆　◆　◆　◆　◆　◆　◆　◆　◆　◆

Interdisciplinary Practice   155

Interdisciplinary Practice Defined   156

Case Example   157

Background and Justification for Interdisciplinary Teaming   158

Models of Team Practice   159

Conceptual Foundation and Necessary Competencies for Interdisciplinary Practice   160

Conceptual Foundation   160

Necessary Competencies   161

Summary—Interdisciplinary Practice   163

Multicultural Awareness   163

A Context for Multicultural Appreciation   163

Background Related to Multicultural Awareness   166

Multicultural Considerations in Research on Stuttering   168

Multicultural Considerations in Intervention   169

Cultural Sensitivity and the Clinical Process   172

Summary—Multicultural Awareness   175

Chapter Summary   175

Chapter 6 Study Questions   177

Can anything more than profound confusion be indicated by this admixture of diverse fields and concerns?

(KUHN, 1970, P. 9)

In the previous chapter, we underscored the importance of intrafamily considerations in approaching and planning for the intervention process with people who stutter. First, we addressed how a client's system of personal constructs impacts his view of himself as a communicator and his potential for change. Secondly, we emphasized that stuttering must be addressed within a family context because experiences of and changes to a person who stutters effect compensatory changes in family members and significant others. Both of these considerations focus within the family unit, specifically on the thoughts, feelings, and dynamics within the individual and the family itself.

The present chapter addresses two other sets of considerations, this time focusing more outside, yet still influencing and influenced by, the family unit. These extrafamily considerations are interdisciplinary teaming and multicultural awareness, both of which also are critical to effective and responsive intervention with people who stutter. Within this chapter, we will make and elaborate the following two points:

- Interdisciplinary practice provides for collaborative opportunities to work with and learn from people who stutter, family members, and allied professionals while ensuring the highest quality of service delivery.

- Multicultural education invites clinicians to appreciate human diversity in all of its forms and to resolve to approach each person, including those who stutter and their family members, as individuals who are blessed with similarities and differences.

INTERDISCIPLINARY PRACTICE

The concept of interdisciplinary practice or collective collaboration among allied professionals is not a new idea. Our enthusiasm for this process, our expectation for people with exceptionalities and their families to participate actively in this process, and our concern over the paucity of efficacy data to validate the process, however, are relatively recent events. Interdiscipliniary team intervention has been described as both "family-centered" and "community-based" (Rokusek, 1995, p. 1), concepts that naturally stem from several others reviewed earlier. These include viewing people who stutter as able individuals who are responsible for actively interpreting and making decisions about their communication world based on their unique systems of personal constructs, and as interactive members within family systems. In other words, interdisciplinary teams evoke the idea of a "partnership [that] requires a shift from valuing the individual to valuing the individual within the family within the community" (Sokoly & Dokecki, 1992, p. 24). This partnership entailing people who stutter, their families, allied professionals, paraprofessionals, and community resources, among others, assumes a balance of shared responsibility for individually tailored and effective intervention. In support of the partnership, Rubin (1995) indicated the following:

> While it is quite reasonable to isolate any aspect of knowledge for detailed scientific study or investigation, it becomes necessary to combine areas of knowledge to appreciate the understanding of its application. In truth, one cannot exist without the other. The enhancement of knowledge and understanding must focus on specific, well-delineated concepts, while the application of that knowledge and understanding requires a broader perspective and conceptual framework that almost invariably incorporates knowledge and understanding from a variety of disciplines. (p. viii)

Interdisciplinary Practice Defined

As with most other concepts within the human service professions, there are at least as many definitions for interdisciplinary practice as there are practitioners. One of the most succinct is "involving, or joining, two or more disciplines" (Thyer & Kropf, 1995, p. i). Others have elaborated this seminal structure. Rokusek (1995) indicated that interdisciplinary process involves "individuals coming together to identify the course of action that is most effective and reasonable for the challenge(s) presented. It means equal input and respect from all persons to reach a goal—or scores of goals" (p. 1). Rokusek also indicated the following:

> Interdisciplinary practice is the ability to practice one's own profession while linking into the work of others. Interdisciplinary practice requires knowledge and skill that differentiates one's work from that of others within a single frame of reference. Consumers/patients gain from the numerous advantages of interdependent practice in that various (and often numerous) needs are met, continuity of service is likely, and professionals/practitioners are open to several approaches and options. (p. 4)

Ogletree, Saddler, and Bowers (1995) defined interdisciplinary practice as "collaborative goal-setting from a 'whole-person' perspective . . . [that] depends on the integrated efforts of numerous team members, each of whom brings unique contributions to the assessment and treatment of persons with disabilities" (p. 220). Others have defined one key element of interdisciplinary practice: *collaboration,* such as, "the shared effort of allied professionals and families to bring diverse perspectives, expertise, and emotional support to the planning and implementation of intervention goals and procedures" (Klein & Moses, 1994, p. 249) and "direct interaction between at least two coequal parties voluntarily engaged in shared decision making as they work toward a common goal" (Friend & Cook, 1996, p. 6). While terms used to refer to interdisciplinary practice vary, most capture the concepts of collaboration of diverse members, each of whom shares valuable expertise, thus ensuring that multiple perspectives are considered during the assessment and intervention processes. The participants necessarily include the person who stutters, family or significant others, and professional and paraprofessional practitioners. Klein and Moses (1994) advised that while sharing insights about observed behaviors, practitioners should retain rather than abandon their professional identity as experts in their respective area of specialized knowledge. For example, the speech–language pathologist will be viewed as the expert in communication disorders who is receptive to related or contrasting views about communication from others outside of the discipline, just as the classroom teacher is the expert in academic design who is open to feedback or suggestions about curricular planning. Such a depiction is one of colleagueship, where each participant is viewed as a valued contributor who flexibly gives and receives, always with the communicative interests of the person who stutters and the family in mind.

Case Example

Consider the following case example. Ginny was a junior in high school when she came to my attention. She presented a composite of learning disabilities including receptive and expressive language deficits, in addition to noticeable stuttering. Her academic performance had plateaued and was presently falling. She expressed frustration with the school experience, particularly feeling unable to understand and master the curriculum (which was increasingly challenging conceptually), unable to communicate in classroom and social settings because of her stuttering and subsequent embarrassment, and discouraged by her inactive social life. Because of her home situation, Ginny worked in the afternoon and evening to contribute money to her family. For these and other reasons, she expressed that she was considering dropping out of school.

The interdisciplinary team meetings included Ginny and her mother, several classroom teachers, the learning disabilities specialist, the guidance counselor, and me (i.e., speech–language pathologist). The team realized the urgency of and need for effective and integrated intervention if Ginny was to succeed and stay in school. Each member shared insights reflecting respective expertise. The communication intervention plan involved identifying areas in which Ginny felt and experienced academic success, using them within a communication context with particular emphasis on conceptual processing, problem solving, and transfer and maintenance of speech fluency skills. From this positive foundation, and with the full support and understanding of all team members, I served as a resource providing additional curricular support in challenging academic content areas, with the foci noted above. The positive, successful context in which Ginny and I designed opportunities for her to experience and acknowledge her own success, combined with an integrated approach in which communication skills were viewed as pivotal to all other areas of learning, resulted in dramatic changes in Ginny's performance and her expressed attitudes about herself as a person and as a communicator. Some of the activities included teaching her to reauditorize verbal instructions and to take telegraphic notes so as to retain information for subsequent recall and processing; improving money changing, check writing, and financial balancing skills; relating content of one class to that of others; and finding daily application for apparently unrelated class content, among others.

Significant and continuing improvements were observed during the ensuing year and a half in classroom participation, performance on examinations, standardized testing of language-related conceptual processing, and most noticeably, in conversational speech fluency. Ginny now expressed feelings of success and pride. Secondary improvements were observed in her personal hygiene and grooming, posture, and positive and inviting manner of interpersonal communication. Ginny graduated high school and completed a degree at a technical college. Indeed, this story illustrates the importance of interdisciplinary teaming, and the impact of success across a person's communication and life skills.

Background and Justification for Interdisciplinary Teaming

Rokusek (1995) reviewed the history of interdisciplinary teams under various labels in medicine, education, and social service from 1920 to the present date. The term "interdisciplinary teams" and an understanding of them did not receive focus until World War II when many rehabilitation centers representing different disciplines were established across this country. Readers who are interested in this history will want to refer to Rokusek (1995).

Klein and Moses (1994) highlighted three events that stimulated emergence of collaborative models of service delivery including interdisciplinary teams. These included, first, the passage of P.L. 94-142 (Education of All Handicapped Children Act) in 1975 and subsequent amendments in P.L. 99-457 in 1986, which stipulated that the individualized educational plan (IEP) is a legal document and must be developed in collaboration with the child's parents or legal guardians. The parents, who ultimately had the power to approve or reject the IEP, became recognized as legal partners in the design of goals and procedures. Secondly, collaborative models of service delivery emerged from the field of early intervention which, during the 1980s, addressed "transdisciplinary" service programs. More will be said about such programs shortly. Suffice it now to say that the term *transdisciplinary* signifies actual crossover in roles assumed by allied professionals and family members. In this way, the different team members participate in one another's goals and procedures and learn treatment techniques from one another. Thirdly, collaborative models of assessment and intervention emerged from the recent interest in "whole language." This concept assumes a linguistic foundation underlying the development of oral language and literacy, both of which are predicated on the individual's active construction of meaning. Klein and Moses (1994) indicated that interest in *whole language theory* resulted in naturalistic techniques to facilitate language development and literacy. These included using manipulable materials in the classroom, engaging children in conversations about a variety of subjects, and using storytelling and group problem solving techniques, among others. Other catalysts for interdisciplinary practice included paradigm shifts in how and where people with disabilities should be served (i.e., addressing functional needs in naturalistic settings), demographic shifts toward increasingly older populations, and trends toward movement of people with special needs into community-based programs (Rokusek, 1995).

While retaining professional identity and being valued for unique areas of expertise, as noted, individual professionals and service providers no longer are viewed as possessing all of the knowledge and skills necessary for intervention planning (Klein & Moses, 1994) or for meeting the diverse needs of people with exceptionalities living integrated, independent, productive lives within communities (Rokusek, 1995). In addition to the team members noted previously, some argue that team size and make-up should be dictated by the needs and desires of the person being served, opening potential membership to such diverse persons as community planners, clergy, architects, engineers, attorneys, chamber of commerce representatives, business managers, fundraisers, police officers, hospital aides, multi-skilled technicians, human resource leaders, and city housing, labor, and transportation representatives (Rokusek, 1995). The point is that intervention from an interdisciplinary perspective has helped bring the strengths and needs of people with exceptionalities into focus. People who stutter and their families stand to benefit from these advances.

Models of Team Practice

When designing intervention with people who stutter, it is important for clinicians to be aware of different treatment models. Recently, Ogletree and Daniels (1995) presented a concise discussion of four different models (*unidisciplinary, multidisciplinary, interdisciplinary,* and *transdisciplinary*), as follows:

> The unidisciplinary model is best characterized by independent service provision. Although popular, unidisciplinary services are limited by a lack of interprofessional collaboration (i.e., interaction). As a result, treatments may not be "cutting edge" and are often poorly coordinated. . . . Unlike unidisciplinary services, the remaining models allow for some degree of collaboration. In a multidisciplinary model, professionals provide services independently, yet have a formal means of collaboration (e.g., staffings). An interdisciplinary model, while allowing independent functioning, emphasizes a greater degree of interaction between professionals, typically resulting in joint decision making regarding treatment goals and strategies. Finally, a transdisciplinary model incorporates the concept of professional role release where disciplines share roles and responsibilities. (p. 231)

Rokusek (1995) elaborated these models and indicated that discipline professionals need to feel comfortable in a unidisciplinary, also called an intradisciplinary, setting before they are comfortable in more collaborative environments. A multidisciplinary model, from a traditional medical setting, identifies a team leader or chair who ultimately is responsible for the direction and final decision making of the group. The focus is on providing input to the team leader who assimilates and directs the outcome or recommendations. Interdisciplinary teaming, also called interprofessional teaming, assumes that each member is an equal in all decision making and consensus building, where the work relationship is interdependent. Transdisciplinary teaming, derived from interdisciplinary practice, addresses collectively a specific need and brings in other team members as necessary. This final setting again assumes equal team membership and a high level of discipline comfort, but also emphasizes cross-discipline understanding permitting the role release referred to earlier. Various authors have elaborated these and other concepts related to models of treatment or team practice (Friend & Cook, 1996; McGonigel & Garland, 1988; Sokoly & Dokecki, 1992; Stoneman & Malone, 1995; Wilcox, 1989). Ogletree and Daniels (1995) acknowledged that a variety of factors impacts decisions regarding appropriate treatment models, including family needs and the availability and attitudes of professionals. While collaborative models appear more consistent with the public legislation noted earlier, they may not be preferred by families, or they may not be possible because of unavailability of practitioners in certain regions or inflexibility of some professionals to adjust their style of service delivery.

Conceptual Foundation and Necessary Competencies for Interdisciplinary Practice

Rokusek (1995) and Stoneman and Malone (1995) addressed the reasons why practitioners should take interdisciplinary practice seriously and defined the necessary competencies for such collaboration. In my estimation, both of these foci have significant import for clinicians who design intervention with people who stutter.

Conceptual Foundation

The foundation for interdisciplinary practice is first and foremost a commitment to the welfare of a person with an exceptionality. The foundation also reflects a commitment to one's own individual discipline and to the value of related human service disciplines. Similarly, Rokusek (1995) indicated that the conceptual foundation of interdisciplinary practice primarily is "a commitment to one's individual discipline or experiential background, to recognizing the value of others' disciplines and backgrounds, and to integrating the work of others with one's own" (p. 6). She indicated that this premise leads to at least four significant conceptual derivatives:

- "an ability to look at the 'whole' in the delivery of services that focus on a consumer in holistic fashion while operating in numerous personal and professional environments"

- "recognition of the interdependency of disciplinary practice and other environmental input from paraprofessionals, families and consumers"

- "respect for the expertise of all disciplinary professionals, paraprofessionals, families and consumers"

- "recognition of the ultimate benefit to consumers and their families through increased knowledge and skills and cross-disciplined assessment, problem-solving, intervention, prevention, and short- and long-term planning" (p. 6)

Similarly, Stoneman and Malone (1995) indicated that current changes in the design and delivery of services for people with disabilities reflect a "conceptual revolution" (p. 236). Indeed, "Professionals who work with individuals with disabilities have been challenged to set aside their belief that determining the best interests of their constituents is solely within their jurisdiction" (p. 234). Stoneman and Malone reported that adopting and implementing interdisciplinary considerations reflect a number of conceptual underpinnings including the following:

- *Shift to a support paradigm.* This means focusing on community partnerships including the community member with an exceptionality (i.e., interdependence), and moving from interdisciplinary teams that are professionally dominated to those that include family, friends, and community members.

• *Self-advocacy.* People with exceptionalities are demonstrating that through organized political action, they can effect changes in laws, regulations, and practices that affect their lives (The Stuttering Foundation of America, National Stuttering Project, and other organizations advocate for and among people who stutter by fostering interpersonal and international understanding and acceptance, eliminating discrimination, expanding opportunities, and working toward other transition goals—see Appendix B).

• *Person-centered approaches.* The person with an exceptionality explores what he wants for his life (i.e., whole-life planning), and the clinician and other team members engage in joint problem solving to help realize these dreams (e.g., to be able say what is on one's mind without fear of ridicule).

• *Natural and informal supports.* People who care about the person with an exceptionality are identified (friends, family members, neighbors, and community members) and engaged in intervention. For example, a best friend might assist a child with transference of fluency to the classroom, or a spouse might offer praise when the person who stutters demonstrates gentle contacts when ordering in the restaurant.

• *Family-focused, family-driven supports.* The family is viewed as central in the lives of all people. Viewed as advocates for the person with an exceptionality, families need to be involved in all aspects of the intervention process, leading to feelings of shared ownership of the process and its outcome, thereby leading to empowerment.

• *Full community inclusion and inclusive education.* This means that the person with an exceptionality will participate in all aspects of community life, and will be educated in regular education classrooms with peers who do not have exceptionalities. Although the primary focus of legislation (P.L. 94-142 and P.L. 99-457, noted earlier; Part H of P.L. 102-119, the Individuals with Disabilities Education Act, formerly P.L. 99-457; and P.L. 101-336, the Americans with Disabilities Act of 1990), these concepts continue to stimulate heated debate (Villa & Thousand's *Creating an Inclusive School,* 1995; Kauffman & Hallahan's *The Illusion of Full Inclusion,* 1995).

• *Blurring of professional roles and turf.* Focus shifts from professional domains to the multifaceted needs of the person being served.

• *Cost containment.* Interdisciplinary teams are potentially expensive. Stoneman and Malone (1995) stated that "human need is increasing, but fiscal resources to support that need are finite" (p. 239). They argued that use of interdisciplinary teams within a support model will decrease the cost for most people but will increase the cost for some. The need for efficacy data is critical.

• *Accountability.* Stoneman and Malone (1995) stated that "theoretically, and intuitively, interdisciplinary teams provide a relatively good fit with holistic models of human development" (p. 239). However, "Few, if any, published studies exist which document that interdisciplinary teams are better than other modes of service delivery" (p. 239). Again, the need for efficacy data is critical.

Necessary Competencies

Rokusek (1995) indicated that dominance, control, superiority, and extreme individualism are not compatible with interdisciplinary practice. Rather, she noted that all members of interdisciplinary teams must share the ability to:

- "understand a common professional language"

- "decrease control of all work boundaries"

- "understand the delivery system(s) available and remain open to all available resources"

- "communicate openly and effectively to peers and others in and outside of the professional work environment"

- "integrate their professional abilities and unique personal qualities into the team, and recognize the specialized culture, values, traditions, knowledge, training, personal emotions, and experiences that the other members bring to the team"

- "work well in teams and contribute towards consensus building" (pp. 5–6)

To these vital requirements, I would add that clinicians must have an understanding of and sensitivity toward the people and interpersonal dynamics within the family system as described in the previous chapter.

Similarly, Stoneman and Malone (1995) addressed the necessary competencies to be an effective team member. In doing so, they recalled Garner, Uhl, and Cox's (1992) "10 Cs," which might be viewed as individual members' skills or team characteristics, as follows: communication, cooperation, collaboration, confronting problems, compromise, consensus decision-making, coordination, consistency, caring, and commitment. Stoneman and Malone (1995) noted that additional competencies for interdisciplinary team practice include:

- *Relinquishing professional power.* The person with the exceptionality is a key member of the team, thus negotiating, rather than imposing our professional will, is essential. "Respecting the family's right to self-determination, while acknowledging that families do not always make the best choices for the family member with a disability, requires a difficult blend of compromise and advocacy" (p. 241).

- *Shared dreaming.* The ability to dream with and to facilitate in another person things that he may never have imagined possible indeed is a professional competency. Stoneman and Malone warned that "the gift of dreaming has been extinguished in all too many professionals" (p. 241). Rather than engaging in dreams of fantasy, dreams or visions should be reality-based. Recall Daly's (1988) reminder of the importance of the clinician truly believing in the client's potential. This cannot be overstated.

- *Holistic thinking.* The ability to think holistically enables a clinician to shift from "fixing" the person who stutters (addressing disfluent speech only) to accentuating, better understanding, and facilitating the fluency already demonstrated by that person. As noted earlier, the person who stutters is viewed as one with many abilities rather than as a "stutterer." Fluency is viewed as the root of disFLUENCY.

- *Community-building skills.* In order to interface the person who stutters with opportunities within the community, clinicians must be comfortable with advocacy and leadership skills, coalition-building, conflict resolution, resource management, and negotiation strategies.

- *Building systems of natural and informal supports.* The concept of natural supports was reviewed earlier as part of the conceptual foundation to interdisciplinary teaming. Here, building such supports is viewed as a necessary competency for collaborative clinicians. Those skills noted with community-building skills above are relevant here as well.

• *Providing supports to people where they are.* Both assessment and treatment with people who stutter must reflect ecological contexts (i.e., settings that directly resemble where they need to use, and therefore improve, their speech fluency skills). This means that intervention must not be limited to clinical settings and must facilitate transfer to optimally meaningful communication contexts from the earliest contact.

• *Taking responsibility for finding solutions.* Clinicians have a responsibility to see to it that, after getting to know, listening to, gaining trust from, dreaming with, and thereby building a meaningful relationship with a person who stutters, intervention plans are carried out to the point of solution. Too often in a traditional diagnostic model, clinicians design plans for someone else to carry out, and never know if the plans were implemented.

• *Creativity in problem solving.* As people who stutter actively design and achieve their own communication life goals, new challenges are encountered. Many years ago, a wise couple told me that meaningful challenges take a long time to accomplish, and those that are seemingly impossible take a bit longer. So it is for people who stutter. Valuable problem-solving skills include listening, facilitating, identifying and administering supports and resources, and achieving solutions (Moses & Shapiro, 1996; Shapiro & Moses, 1989; for a discussion of a constructivist foundation and related strategies for creative problem solving). An important point made earlier is that our intervention, problem solving, and solutions are conducted with, rather than for, people who stutter.

Summary—Interdisciplinary Practice

Interdisciplinary team practice was variously defined as a process of collective collaboration. Being both family centered and community based, interdisciplinary practice was presented as an outgrowth of concepts presented earlier, specifically that people who stutter are viewed as able individuals who actively interpret and make decisions about their communication and the world based on their personal constructs and as interactive members within family systems. Thus, interdisciplinary teams are partnerships entailing people who stutter, their families, allied professionals, paraprofessionals, and community resources in shared responsibility for designing and implementing individually tailored and effective intervention. Interdisciplinary practice was defined and justified as an appropriate mechanism for clinical intervention with people who stutter. Models of interdisciplinary practice were presented, as were the conceptual underpinnings and necessary competencies for such intervention.

MULTICULTURAL AWARENESS

A Context for Multicultural Appreciation

Over the last several chapters, we have considered diversity in its many forms, such as the nature of disfluency, personal constructs, family systems, and interdisciplinary team considerations. One thing is for sure. Human beings have a remarkable capacity for richness and variation in communication behavior, interpersonal dynamics, and conceptual interpretation. It is little wonder that understanding communication and its disorders, particularly intervention with people who stutter, is no small undertaking. We have made the point that each person, including those who stutter, usually experiences a sense of belonging to a family. Families may identify with some larger group within society, and that larger group with a still larger group. Ethnicity and religion often influence our daily lives including the foods we eat, our rituals, our traditions, and other aspects (Turnbull & Turnbull, 1990). Such aspects that contribute to our cultural heritage shape our values and perspectives on the world, including our attitudes toward communication, its disorders, and specifically stuttering. Battle (1993) clarified that race, ethnicity, and culture are not synonymous terms. She stated:

> Race is a statement about biological and anatomical attributes and functions such as skin color, facial features, and hair texture. Ethnicity is about race, origin, characteristics, and institutions. Culture is about the behavior, beliefs, and values of a group of people who are brought together by their commonality. Ethnography refers to a fully developed sense of meaning of a culture and the complicated manner in which one comes to understand the intricacies of the culture. An ethnographical understanding of a culture implies a fully developed sense of the complex web of meanings, perceptions, actions, symbols, and adaptations that make a people who they are. Ethnography is the lens through which individuals view the world as they maneuver through life. (p. xvii)

Battle illustrated that two people may be of the same biological race, but may differ vastly in their cultural identity, personal history, and view of the world. Indeed, race is an entirely physical phenomenon determined by heredity. Ethnicity is determined by heritage and refers to belonging to groups that share unique social and cultural traditions often passed from one generation to the next. Ethnic heritage is often identified by and associated with patterns of family life, language, recreation, and religion, among other patterns (Johnson & Mata-Pistokache, 1996). Battle (1993) indicated that culture can be distinguished by explicit and implicit behaviors. Explicit cultural behaviors are those that are visible and thus identify members as a group to observers. Such behaviors include dress, language and speaking patterns, eating habits, customs, and lifestyles. Implicit cultural behaviors are less visible, but no less significant in contributing to the essence of the person with whom we communicate within and outside the clinical process. More implicit behaviors are associated with age, gender, family, roles within the family, childrearing practices, socioeconomic status, education, religion and spiritual beliefs, fears, attitudes, values, perception of what is considered handicapping, and exposure to and adoption of other cultural ways. Battle provided the following meaningful advice to all practitioners in speech–language pathology and audiology:

> Speech, language, and communication are embedded in culture. Therefore, one cannot understand communication by a group of persons without a thorough understanding of the ethnographic and cultural factors that are related to communication by the group. These factors are embedded in the historical, geographical, social, and political history that binds the group and gives it commonality. (Battle, 1993, p. xviii)

Battle's point is that we cannot study or understand communication and its disorders without reference to cultural, historical, and societal bases of communication by members of the culture. For example, the conversational partners one chooses, what they talk about, when and where they talk, and even what constitutes meaningful communication and what represents a communication disorder must be interpreted and understood within a cultural context. "One must understand the salient cultural values, perceptions, attitudes, and history of a group in order to draw conclusions about the communication competence of a particular person within a group" (Battle, 1993, pp. xix–xx). The speech–language pathologist, when assessing a client's speech fluency, must be mindful that cultural factors may impact the client's willingness to initiate conversation, to discuss feelings, to have or maintain eye contact, or even to speak with a particular partner. Clinicians must be knowledgeable about and sensitive to the cultural heritage of those with whom we interact, and must realize that culture influences how each of us views the world.

If heightened multicultural knowledge, awareness, and sensitivities are positive attributes of clinicians working with people who stutter, there is also a significant, yet implicit, caution. In our sincere efforts to better understand, accept, and accommodate, we must be careful not to assume that all members of a particular cultural group share the same values and beliefs held by the group as a whole (Turnbull & Turnbull, 1990). In fact, working with families of diverse cultural backgrounds has taught me that different members of the same family may hold differing values and beliefs. I am reminded of a young woman from a traditional Greek Orthodox family who, as part of her fluency treatment, discussed the challenges she experienced in having parents who are immigrants and whose expectations of her are different than those she holds for herself. Some of the differences involved career ambition (she wished not to stay at home, but practice medicine), dress (she wished not to wear traditional black garb, but more contemporary clothing), and social etiquette (her parents were horrified that she would call a man to initiate a social engagement).

Many of our students at this university are among the first generation in their family to pursue a college degree. This is not an uncommon experience for the adult children of families from mountainous regions in rural Appalachia. These students bring with them all of the experiences, needs, and fears of those who have broken the traditional family mold. Many years ago, a television advertisement pictured a man with Native American features eating a rye bread sandwich. After visibly enjoying the sandwich, the caption boasted, "You don't have to be Jewish to love Levi's (Jewish Rye bread)." The point is that people differ. Learning about cultural tendencies runs the real risk of inadvertently promoting cultural stereotypes, the antithesis of multicultural awareness and sensitivity. We have reviewed that people who stutter are often negatively stereotyped by diverse groups including parents, school personnel, and students and professionals in speech–language pathology, among others. Cooper and Cooper (1993) cautioned, "Vigilance will be required if we are to avoid creating new stereotypes as we strive to identify culture-dependent influences on the assessment and treatment of stuttering" (p. 190). Similarly, Cole (1989) cautioned:

> There is a delicate balance between recognition of cultural orientations and stereotyping. Care must be taken to avoid over generalizing or over emphasizing

such differences to the point that they interfere with effective service delivery. Nevertheless, service providers must be cognizant of cultural tendencies that could pose possible barriers to effective service delivery. (p. 68)

Multicultural education leads clinicians to appreciate human diversity in all of its forms, and to resolve to approach each person, including those who stutter and their families, as individuals who are blessed with similarities and differences. This notion is consistent with and grows out of the concepts reviewed previously addressing variation in disfluencies, personal constructs, family systems, and interdisciplinary approaches.

Background Related to Multicultural Awareness

Johnson's (1944) early claim—which was later challenged (Van Riper, 1982; Zimmermann, Liljeblad, Frank, & Cleeland, 1983)—stating that the Hopi people in the American Southwest did not demonstrate stuttering behavior because they did not so label it, was frequently cited in the literature of our professions' early stages. Recalling Johnson's article, Taylor and Clarke (1994) stated that the importance of cultural considerations undergirding our understanding of communication and its disorders is not a new idea. Nevertheless, Taylor (1986) stated that "prior to 1968, little interest was shown within the professions of speech pathology and audiology in addressing the unique clinical needs of individuals with communication disorders from culturally and linguistically diverse populations (p. 3). Taylor (1986) recalled a debate (as have others—Battle, 1993; Cole, 1989; Wiggins, 1994) between himself and John Michel at the Annual Convention of the American Speech and Hearing Association (ASHA) in 1968 in Denver, Colorado as significant in bringing ASHA's attention to issues of cultural relevance and to a number of related professional developments. These included formation of the ASHA Black Caucus, which expressed concern that speech pathologists were viewing the language differences among African Americans from a pathology model, and urged ASHA to require coursework in sociolinguistics and Black history and to stimulate training and research opportunities in these areas. Taylor reviewed the history of ASHA's and the professions' positive responses and related legal, legislative, research, and training developments. Interested readers are referred to this informative source.

Since that time, others have documented historical and more recent developments in the assessment of speech and language disorders in culturally diverse populations and related management and educational issues (Adler, 1993; Screen & Anderson, 1994). Throughout, ASHA has maintained and enforced its policies opposing discrimination and promoting affirmative action and cultural diversity (ASHA, 1991, 1992a; Cole, 1992). These policies have determined acceptable locations for national meetings, defined ethical conduct and clinical practice, influenced appointments to committees and boards, determined topics and faculty for educational programming, and motivated an assortment of official position statements, guidelines, and definitions regarding multicultural issues. These and other activities reflective of ASHA's ongoing commitment to minority concerns and heightened understanding and acceptance among the general membership culminated in 1991 with a published plan, "Multicultural Action Agenda 2000" (ASHA, 1991). This plan specified objectives to be completed by 2000 that addressed increasing the proportion of people who identify with federally designated racial and ethnic minority groups in ASHA's general membership, leadership roles, and national office staff and managerial positions. ASHA advised its members that it is their responsibility to upgrade their own knowledge and skills to better understand and serve multicultural populations. Within this context, ASHA seeks to ensure that its programs related to cultural diversity are maintained and become prominent, that educational opportunities are available and sponsored, that multicultural understanding and commitment are interwoven with certification and accreditation requirements, and that its governmental, legislative, and public relation efforts are consistent with its policies.

To understand the significance of ASHA's and its members' commitment to the "Multicultural Action Agenda 2000," particularly the commitment to multicultural diversity in clinical education, practice, and research, clinicians need to appreciate the demographic changes of increasing cultural diversity that are taking place in the United States. Various authors (Battle, 1993; Johnson & Mata-Pistokache, 1996; Taylor, 1993) have cited the 1990 U.S. census (U.S. Bureau of the Census, 1990) in order to characterize the evolving and continuous changes. This census indicated that over 60 million people (at least 25% of the American population) were of an ethnic or racial minority group. Taylor (1993) indicated that this census undercounted such minorities, thus, the actual count would be significantly greater. According to the census, 11.48% were African American, 8.56% Hispanic (Cuban, Mexican, Puerto Rican, other), 2.78% Asian/Pacific Islander, and 0.75% Native American and Eskimo. The remaining 76.43% were Caucasian. The rate of population growth was 110% for Asian/Pacific Americans, 55% for Hispanics, 38% for Native Americans and Eskimos, and 15% for African Americans, compared to 3% for Caucasians. Taylor (1993), reflecting on this pattern, stated, "If current trends continue, demographers assert that by the year 2010, one-third of the population of New America will be people of color and by the middle of the twenty-first century, whites will be a minority" (p. xii).

Our country is becoming increasingly diverse, both culturally and linguistically. Speech–language pathologists are being called upon, more than ever before, to work with people from a variety of cultures having different cultural behaviors, learning and interpersonal styles, social beliefs, and world views. Nevertheless, there is a significant shortage in the number of professionals who are qualified to work with people who identify themselves with ethnic or racial minority groups. Taylor (1993) reported the results of a recent study conducted at Howard University that revealed that approximately 75% of the speech–language pathologists certified by ASHA stated that they did not have sufficient knowledge to feel competent to provide clinical services to bilingual or nonstandard English-speaking clients. Furthermore, Johnson and Mata-Pistokache (1996) cited studies indicating that in 1985, 91% of the certified speech–language pathologists reported having received no training in minority-language populations in preprofessional or graduate training (Campbell, 1985) and that in 1986, only 8% of the applicants for the Certificate of Clinical Competence had elected to take a course in multicultural communication (ASHA, 1987). What this means is that all speech–language pathologists and audiologists must take seriously ASHA's "Multicultural Action Agenda 2000" and commit to participating in and developing ongoing educational opportunities for achieving improved cultural literacy, thereby becoming competent to serve people whose culture is different from their own.

Multicultural Considerations in Research on Stuttering

Although it is indisputable that stuttering is a universal phenomenon (Bloodstein, 1995; Van Riper, 1982), there are few data related to the influence of cultural factors on the nature of stuttering. Cooper and Cooper (1993) demonstrated that this dearth of knowledge is the unfortunate result of conscientious researchers who have successfully isolated independent variables by keeping their research population homogeneous. As a consequence of excluding minority group members from research, we know little about fluency-related characteristics of minority groups and culturally divergent populations. Another obstacle in our knowledge on cultural variations in fluency disorders is the historical and continuing lack of universally accepted or standard definitions for key terms (such as fluency, disfluency, stuttering, and stammering), particularly in studies from other than White English-speaking Western cultures. This problem with definitions, reviewed more thoroughly in Chapter 1, significantly limits the potential for comparison and generalizability of the results from studies to other studies and to clinical application. More recently, however, studies have used solid empirical design and techniques to address fluency disorders in minority populations and in cross-cultural investigations.

Acknowledging the comparative limitations noted above, various reviews (Bloodstein, 1995; Culatta & Goldberg, 1995; Leith, 1986) have summarized what is known about the prevalence (occurrence at a specific time) and incidence (occurrence over the lifetime) of stuttering in different cultural populations. For example, Cooper and Cooper (1993) reviewed the occurrence of stuttering in the mainstream United States population compared with that of African American, African, West Indies, Hispanic, and Asian populations. Results suggest that prevalence of fluency disorders varies among the different cultures, and that stuttering tends to be higher among Black populations than White or Asian populations. Speculations abound about why the prevalence of stuttering varies across cultures. Some have argued provocatively that the inherent relative stress within a culture affects the prevalence of stuttering. For example, Leith (1986) stated that:

> The sociocultural variables we consider when appraising cultural influences would be the cultural value placed on such attributes as competitiveness and achievement, child-rearing practices as related to the amount of pressure put on the child, attitudes toward language and expressive behaviors, and the treatment of defective or handicapped individuals in the culture. Cultures that have all or most of these characteristics have a higher incidence of stuttering, since they are "stress cultures" or "tough" cultures. Cultures that have few if any of these characteristics have a lower incidence of stuttering, since they are not "stress cultures"; they are "easy" cultures. (p. 13)

Similarly, presenting data depicting occurrence of stuttering in various ethnic cultures (i.e., in increasing frequency of occurrence; Bantu, South Dakota

Indians, England, United States), Culatta and Goldberg (1995) stated that "the percentage of occurrence is lower for aboriginal cultures than industrialized societies, which may be the result of a less stressful or demanding life style or other microcultural values that have not been identified" (p. 117). Cooper and Cooper (1993) challenged such interpretations stating, "As fetchingly simplistic and patently plausible as these recurrent speculations might appear, neither the prevalence data nor any significant body of data pertaining to the etiology of stuttering support them" (p. 197). Furthermore, they questioned the usefulness of conceptualizing the world into two types of societies, cautioned those who might allow preconceived notions about stuttering to limit their interpretations of what they observe ("the danger of being hung by our frameworks," p. 192), and concluded that "the frequency of fluency disorders does vary from one culture to another, but the universality of the problem tells us that fluency disorders are not simply the result of cultural considerations" (p. 197).

Multicultural Considerations in Intervention

When striving to understand the cultural influences on people who stutter, clinicians must be mindful to approach each person and his family as an individual entity unto itself, without preconceived notions or stereotypical assumptions about the family's general cultural group. Leith (1986) advised clinicians to become aware of a variety of factors that might have precipitated or might be perpetuating the stuttering. These include the family's child-rearing practices, reactions to stuttering, and other special cultural factors that might interfere with fluency facilitation. These will be addressed separately.

First, while different families demonstrate different child-rearing practices and interpersonal styles with their children, concern arises when a child stutters and the family is oriented more toward adult needs and values than toward those of the child. In such families, "children are to be seen and not heard" (i.e., the child is expected to be silent unless spoken to). Potentially, this puts significant pressure on the child who wishes to or needs to speak with an adult. The child feels that he is intruding in an adult world and anticipates scolding for such interference, regardless of the importance of what is to be said. Leith (1986) indicated that the content and function of such infrequent interactions are noteworthy as well, typically taking the form of commands, instructions, or reprimands from the adult to the child, and the briefest responses from the child to the adult only when directed or invited to do so. Likewise, the family's performance expectations for the child in different domains including speech can pressure and penalize the child, and thus may contribute to the development or maintenance of stuttering. In any case, the absence of easy dialogue or presence of high expectations for the child's performance may contribute to stuttering and may interfere with treatment progress.

Secondly, Leith (1986) pointed out that the reactions received toward one's stuttering also may reflect cultural beliefs. For example, if the cultural group believes that stuttering is due to religious or superstitious factors such as the child being "possessed" or under a spell of the "evil eye" (recall that in the first half of the twentieth century in this country, many children who were left handed were forcibly changed to right handedness), the child would be penalized by negative reactions and would be made aware of his being possessed or under a spell. He and the family might experience shame and might explore cultural treatments such as ritualistic dances, prayers, and folk remedies. Other cultures might either respond with ridicule, assuming the child who stutters is being foolish, or react with anger, assuming volitional stuttering. Leith highlighted that people who stutter experience a double jeopardy—a fairly predictable reaction from their own cultural group, and a more unpredictable reaction from the general American culture. Furthermore, the familial lineage, whether traced through patriarchal or matriarchal lines, will influence attitudes toward stuttering. In a patriarchal society, where the male is the dominant figure, stuttering in a boy is considered grievous, because of its projected influence on his role in society. Stuttering in a girl is less serious, but noteworthy, in its impact on marriageability. In a matriarchal society, however, stuttering in a girl is more serious because it not only will impact marriageability, but her later role in society as well.

Thirdly, there are special cultural influences including the role that verbal communication plays in a particular culture, the diverse roles that different members fill in that culture, among others. Leith (1986) presented an enlightening assortment of scenarios from his clinical experiences that clearly indicate that an interaction within the clinical context may be interpreted very differently, and misinterpreted, from different cultural orientations. We discussed earlier the importance of distinguishing between an event and its multiple interpretations (Shapiro & Moses, 1989). Acknowledging and interpreting an event from multiple perspectives is critical when working with people who stutter, particularly in order to understand the participants and to nuture the clinical process. The events Leith described, each of which caused the client discomfort, address a variety of cultural factors. The events are summarized here, followed by the clinician's interpretation (or that of the mainstream United States) and then a unique cultural interpretation:

• *Family arrived late for their scheduled appointment and was admonished by the clinician.* Family is irresponsible and unmotivated versus family's culture is not time oriented. *Recommendation:* Clinician might schedule this family earlier to allow for late arrival.

• *Clinician who is feeling time pressure began an interview by asking parents questions about the child's development.* Clinician used clinical time efficiently versus clinician rudely discussed business before social interaction. *Recommendation*: Value people and build interpersonal rapport first.

• *Clinician directed questions to the mother who did not respond and who deferred to the father who was present.* Mother was conversationally passive and uninvolved versus in this patriarchal family, the father speaks for the family and the wife does not speak when the husband is present. *Recommendation*: Address both parents and allow them to decide who will respond; address each parent in separate settings.

• *Clinician determined that the father speaks for the family and directed questions to him. The father seemed awkward and responded tentatively.* Father became upset at questions versus father was not accustomed to a female (i.e., clinician) being in authority and questioning his responses. *Recommendation*: Share purposes and accept tentative responses.

- *Clinician interviewed the parents about communication-related family matters.* Parents became silent and agitated versus family matters are private and not to be shared with strangers. *Recommendation*: Plan treatment based on general information.

- *Clinician repeatedly praised child and child's behavior to the parent.* Mother was uncomfortable hearing compliments versus mother believed clinician would abduct the child or cast the evil eye (a powerful spell) on the child. *Recommendation*: Be positive but not to excess.

- *Family refused to allow a male clinician to escort a female child away from her parents to the clinical room.* Family had trouble with separation versus culture does not allow a female child to be alone with a male stranger (i.e., male not related to her family). *Recommendation*: Allow parent to accompany child, or assign a female clinician.

- *Clinician patted child on head.* Clinician offered nonverbal form of reward versus clinician broke a religious rule that the hair is sacred and not to be touched by a stranger and thereby insulted the family. *Recommendation*: Know the family before using touch as a nonverbal form of reward or affection.

- *Client did not stutter openly as directed by the treatment program and clinician.* Client was not committed to treatment process versus culture highly regards speech, thus disfluency invites ridicule by others within that culture. *Recommendation*: Use a more fluency-oriented program.

- *Client refused to maintain eye contact with the clinician as prompted by clinician.* Client did not follow instructions versus client's culture views direct eye contact as a sign of hostile or sexually aggressive behavior and lowering the eyes is a sign of respect. *Recommendation*: Interpret apparent resistance from multiple perspectives.

- *Clinician offered a gesture (forming a circle with tip of thumb touching index finger) after which client fell silent.* Clinician's gesture was a form of nonverbal praise versus the gesture is interpreted as an obscenity in the client's culture. *Recommendation*: Use verbal forms of feedback.

- *Client did not observe or perform deliberate repetition of a disfluency on a word containing "th."* Client was noncompliant versus client was reluctant to expose the tongue, which is considered impolite. *Recommendation*: Modify behavior so that tongue is barely visible between the teeth.

- *Child did not perform transfer activities at home.* Client was noncompliant versus client's home is not child-oriented, thus speech initiation by child is penalized. *Recommendation*: Interpret apparent resistance from multiple perspectives.

- *Child refused to dialogue with clinician.* Child was conversationally passive versus child was taught not to speak with strangers (this cultural lesson might also interfere with extra-clinical transfer activities). *Recommendation*: Interpret resistance from multiple perspectives.

- *Child did not complete assignments or maintain fluency.* Child was uncooperative versus child is punished at the home for using new speech (i.e., Parents believe that stuttering is punishment for sin, and that stuttering will disappear when they atone. Reducing stuttering by treatment interferes with their belief and reduces their punishment, thus parents maintain stuttering in accordance with their religious beliefs). *Recommendation*: Invite and understand client's and family's causal assumptions about stuttering and expectations for treatment.

It is both impossible and undesirable to anticipate all of the potential exchanges we might have with our clients who stutter and their families, particularly those whose cultural framework is different than that of the clinician. As always, clinicians need to be both sensitive to and accepting of differences that exist within such an increasingly pluralistic society. Every interaction is an opportunity to learn about others and ourselves. That is the message here. To increase the likelihood of constructive interactions and effective communication, clinicians are advised to remember the importance of considering all exchanges from multiple perspectives, particularly those contrasting with our own, and to remain flexible. Differences provide a source of richness and an opportunity to appreciate human diversity. Differences are not to be tolerated, but rather invited and nurtured (Shapiro, 1987, 1994a, 1994b). Cole (1989) pointed out that "E Pluribus Unum" ("From Many, One") describes the homogenization of the U.S. population since the day the Declaration of Independence was signed, and stated:

> Although this motto may still represent our common belief in democratic ideals, it has a less noble meaning when considering the diversity of the people who inhabit this land. The dramatic demographic shift that is jolting this nation makes E PLURIBUS PLURIBUS (From Many, Many) a more accurate motto. (p. 65)

Cultural Sensitivity and the Clinical Process

We have emphasized that every person and every family is unique. Any objective and positive attempt to characterize patterns or trends that represent members of a cultural group aims to sensitize clinicians to the infinite diversity among human beings. A serious risk, however, is run by considering such information because doing so tends to establish or reinforce stereotypes. In this way, an aspect of multicultural education presents a potential paradox. Specifically, an awareness of cultural patterns heightens sensitivity toward and appreciation of differences among all people. Yet we must remain mindful to guard against generalizations, which form the core of stereotypes. Cooper and Cooper (1993) cautioned as follows:

> Generalizations concerning the feelings, attitudes, and behaviors of a culture are seldom, if ever, helpful to the practicing clinician. Such lists are helpful only to the extent that they sensitize us to the infinite and joyous heterogeneity of the human condition. (p. 202)

Similar cautions and inviting lists of cultural trends that clinicians might find relevant when working with people who stutter and their families have been provided (Cooper & Cooper, 1993; Cole, 1989; Culatta & Goldberg, 1995; Johnson & Mata-Pistokache, 1996; Nellum-Davis, 1993; Turnbull & Turnbull, 1990), as have discussions addressing the challenges in providing valid and reliable assessment and treatment with people who have culturally or linguistically diverse backgrounds (Adler, 1993; Bess, Clark, & Mitchell, 1986; Hamayan & Damico, 1991; Keys & Ruder, 1992; Paul, 1995; Screen & Anderson, 1994; Westby, 1994). Our purpose now, however, is to provide a number of recommendations, some specific, some general, that might be useful when working with people from different cultures who stutter. The recommendations are intended neither to be all inclusive nor necessarily applicable to all people with diverse backgrounds. Rather, they are intended to help us remember to guard against preconceptions; to address all people, including members of the same family, as individuals; and to invite and nurture our understanding and acceptance of different behaviors and beliefs as opportunities to learn about ourselves, our clients, and our world.

Leith (1986) recommended that clinicians remember that there is no standard cultural group. Any group is made of subcultures, depending on degree of assimilation, socioeconomic level, geographic location, educational level, and other factors. Cultural variation often exists across members of the same family. An awareness of this variation should help prevent cultural stereotyping. Similarly, Culatta and Goldberg (1995) advised clinicians to determine the client's macroculture and microculture. Macroculture consists of the values that bind a population together as a whole and on which most political and social institutions of a country are based. For example, the macroculture of the United States values occupation, education, and financial worth; work and achievement; access to comforts of living; cleanliness; self-governance, humanitarianism, and so forth. Microculture represents the individual's interpretation of values, speech and linguistic patterns, learning styles, and behavioral patterns based on such variables as ethnic or national origin, religion, sex, age, exceptionality, geographic region, and class. Culatta and Goldberg (1995) indicated that for most people in the United States, cultural identification involves a blending of different microcultures.

Leith (1986) advised clinicians to determine the cultural group's and the client's own beliefs about and assumptions regarding a number of factors that might influence the assessment and treatment processes. The factors include:

• *Privacy about family and personal lives.* Families will demonstrate different degrees of willingness and comfort to discuss such matters.

• *Protectiveness toward the children.* Parents and children will demonstrate different levels of comfort for the children to communicate with adults outside of the family.

• *Appropriate level of speaking loudness.* Some clients may appear shy, but in actuality are reluctant to speak or be spoken to in a loud (impolite) voice.

• *Attitudes toward stuttering and people who stutter.* Such attitudes will influence receptivity toward treatment programs and should be a factor in treatment design.

• *Roles of male and female children and adults.* These roles might impact who provides information for the family, reticence of males to acknowledge fear, and reactions toward female clinicians and others in the helping or authority capacity. Also, if a family is not child-oriented, efforts to seek parental cooperation in home programming may fail.

- *Communication with people from other cultures.* In some cultures, females do not interact with people from other cultures, which would result in difficulty for the clinician in conducting home visits and establishing home programming.

- *Interpretation of eye contact, touch, and gestures.* Such requests and behaviors may be misunderstood by clients holding different cultural interpretations than the clinician.

- *Reluctance to sign forms.* In some cultures, families may be reluctant to sign documents, because doing so brings embarrassment or shame to the family.

- *Status accrued for oral ability.* If oral ability is accorded high status, a person who stutters may feel a keen social stigma, and common treatment procedures such as voluntary stuttering or discussion of feelings may be both stressful and distasteful.

- *Views about etiology.* If a family views stuttering as a curse or a God-given condition, treatment will need to account for such beliefs. Otherwise, clinicians inadvertently could challenge clients to decide between clinician's advice and personal beliefs.

- *Stuttering in native language.* Stuttering in a child's native language may contraindicate teaching English as a second language until stuttering is resolved. Communicative stress is a factor in the development and maintenance of stuttering.

Battle (1993) offered a number of related suggestions for working with people from different cultures than our own. These suggestions included:

- *Use the name of that culture as assigned by its members.* This will reduce cultural conflicts and help us know how to refer correctly to a group (Black or African American, Latino or Hispanic, Asian or Oriental, American Indian or Native American, White or Caucasian).

- *Use accurate and appropriately descriptive terms to refer to one's race or ethnicity.* For example, use African American, not minority; Hispanic, not bilingual; and nonwhite, not culturally diverse or multicultural.

- *Beware the inaccurate, albeit common, assumption that most or all members of a racial or ethnic group are the same.* We must acknowledge intragroup variation, even intrafamily variation as noted earlier, based on gender, age, socioeconomic status, and education, among other factors.

- *Avoid pejorative terms that assume European Americans are the standard (such as culturally deprived, at-risk, minority, culturally disadvantaged) and qualifiers that reinforce racial or ethnic stereotypes (such as Indian giver, black sheep, articulate Black student).*

- *Beware nonverbal (spacial distance, appropriate topics for conversation, social rituals) and verbal (beginning the professional agenda immediately vs. establishing social and interpersonal rapport) sources of cultural conflict and miscommunication.*

Summary—Multicultural Awareness

Multicultural education invites clinicians to appreciate human diversity in all of its forms and to resolve to approach all people, including those who stutter and their family members, as individuals. Aspects of diversity addressed previously include the nature of disfluency, personal constructs, family systems, and interdisciplinary team considerations. Race, ethnicity, and culture were defined and distinguished. As clinicians, we need to be knowledgeable about and sensitive to the cultural heritage of those with whom we interact and realize the influence that culture has on how each of us views and reacts within our own communicative worlds. At the same time, however, we must not assume that all members of any particular group share the same values and beliefs held by the group as a whole. In other words, in our sincere efforts to better understand, accept, and accommodate our clients and their families, we must be mindful to prevent cultural stereotyping. This section reviewed the background to our professions' appreciation of multiculturalism and multicultural literacy, and discussed multicultural considerations that influence research on stuttering and the clinical process with people who stutter and their families. Related recommendations for clinicians were offered as a reminder and facilitator to invite and nurture our understanding and acceptance of different behaviors and beliefs as opportunities to learn about ourselves, our clients, and our world.

CHAPTER SUMMARY

This chapter explored extrafamily considerations that must be taken into account when developing intervention plans with people who stutter. These considerations included interdisciplinary teaming and multicultural awareness.

Interdisciplinary teaming provides for collaborative opportunities to work with and learn from people who stutter, family members, and allied professions while ensuring the highest quality of service delivery. Such collaboration requires objective consideration of multiple and diverse perspectives regarding all aspects of case management. Three significant events were catalysts to emergence of collaborative models of service delivery. These events included passage of legislation (such as P.L. 94-142 in 1975, P.L. 99-457 in 1986), which stipulated that the individualized educational plan is a legal document and must be developed in collaboration with the child's parents or legal guardians, emergence of early intervention transdisciplinary programs in the 1980s, and recent interest in the concept of whole language intervention.

Models of treatment (i.e., unidisciplinary, multidisciplinary, interdisciplinary, and transdisciplinary) were reviewed. The foundation of interdisciplinary practice is a commitment to the welfare of the person and family being served (ASHA, 1994a) and to one's own discipline and related disciplines. The conceptual underpinnings necessary for adopting and implementing interdisciplinary practice include shifting to a support paradigm, self-advocacy, person-centered approaches, natural and informal supports, family-focused and family-driven supports, full community inclusion and inclusive education, blurring of professional roles and turf, cost containment, and accountability. Members of interdisciplinary teams must share the ability to understand a common professional language; decrease control of work boundaries; understand the delivery systems and remain open to available resources; communicate openly and effectively to peers and others; integrate their professional abilities and unique personal qualities into the team and recognize the specialized culture, values, traditions, knowledge, training, personal emotions, and experiences that the other members bring to the team; and work well in teams and contribute toward consensus building. Other related competencies were reviewed.

Multicultural awareness invites clinicians to appreciate human diversity in all of its forms and to resolve to approach each person, including those who stutter and their family members, as individuals with similarities and differences. While clinicians must be aware of differences in race, ethnicity, and culture, they must be careful not to allow this awareness to lead inadvertently to stereotypes about racial, ethnic, or cultural groups. Despite the continuing growth of minority groups and increasing cultural and linguistic diversity in the United States, few professionals are qualified to work with people who identify themselves with ethnic or racial minority groups. Prevalence and incidence of stuttering appear to differ among different cultural populations, suggesting that cultural factors may precipitate or perpetuate stuttering. Such factors include child-rearing practices, reactions to stuttering, and the role that communication plays and family members fill in the culture.

Cultural factors that may influence the assessment and treatment processes include privacy about family and personal lives; protectiveness toward the children; appropriate level of speaking loudness; attitudes toward stuttering and people who stutter; roles of male and female children and adults; communication with people from other cultures; interpretation of eye contact, touch, gestures, and other nonverbal behaviors; reluctance to sign forms; status accrued for oral ability; views about etiology; and stuttering in native language. Battle (1993) suggested that professionals working with people whose culture is different than their own should use the name of the culture as assigned by its members, use accurate and appropriately descriptive terms to refer to one's race or ethnicity, beware the inaccurate assumption that most or all members of a racial or ethnic group are the same, avoid pejorative terms that assume that European Americans are the standard and qualifiers that reinforce racial or ethnic stereotypes, and beware nonverbal and verbal sources of cultural conflict and miscommunication.

Chapter 6 Study Questions

1. Rokusek (1995) stated that professionals need to feel comfortable in a unidisciplinary setting before they can function effectively in more collaborative environments. What implications does this statement hold for professional preparation?

2. Some models of interdisciplinary practice advocate role release among professionals, while others suggest that professionals retain their identity as experts in their respective area of specialized knowledge. How does each philosophy impact the effectiveness of the assessment and treatment processes? As a clinician, which do you feel more comfortable with and why? What factors would indicate one intervention approach over another?

3. Interdisciplinary practice implies sharing and exchanging information and skills for the sake of providing clinical services of the highest quality. How could such an arrangement impact and be impacted by confidentiality? What should be shared and what should not? What should you do if the information that the client or family provided to you confidentially could be of use to other professionals serving the same people? What is confidentiality and what are its limits?

4. Clinicians must be sensitive to cultural differences that might influence assessment and treatment. However, might a clinician's professional values or judgment be compromised when accommodating a client's cultural differences? For example, if a client's culture does not allow a female child to be alone with a male who is not a family member, is it appropriate to assign a female clinician when a male clinician is qualified to provide the treatment? In a university training setting, when might the missions of service delivery and clinical instruction be in conflict?

5. We have reviewed intrafamily (personal constructs and family systems) and extrafamily (interdisciplinary teaming and multicultural awareness) intervention considerations. How does the concept of diversity relate to both intrafamily and extrafamily considerations? How do these areas of diversity relate to assessment and treatment with people who stutter and their families?

6. This chapter began with a quotation by Thomas Kuhn, author of *The Structure of Scientific Revolutions*. He asked, "Can anything more than profound confusion be indicated by this admixture of diverse fields and concerns?" Given your understanding of intrafamily and extrafamily considerations and the relevance of both of these to the intervention process, how would you respond to his question?

Unit II

* * * * * * * * * * * * * * * * * * *

Central and Guiding Intervention Assumptions

Chapter 5
Personal Constructs and Family Systems:
Intrafamily Considerations

Chapter 6
Interdisciplinary Teaming and Multicultural Awareness:
Extrafamily Considerations

Chapter 7
Stuttering Modification and Fluency Shaping:
Psychotherapeutic Considerations

Chapter 7

Stuttering Modification and Fluency Shaping: Psychotherapeutic Considerations

◆ ◆ ◆ ◆ ◆ ◆ ◆ ◆ ◆ ◆ ◆ ◆ ◆ ◆ ◆ ◆ ◆ ◆ ◆

General Definitions 182

Stuttering Modification   182

Fluency Shaping   183

Significant Differences   184

Premise   184

Behavioral Treatment Goals 184

Spontaneous Fluency   184

Controlled Fluency   185

Acceptable Stuttering   186

Stuttering Modification and Fluency Shaping   186

Affective Treatment Goals   186

Stuttering Modification   186

Fluency Shaping   187

Treatment Procedures   187

Stuttering Modification   187

Fluency Shaping   188

Treatment Structure   188

Stuttering Modification   188

Fluency Shaping   188

Advantages and Disadvantages   188

Stuttering Modification   188

Fluency Shaping   189

Differential Diagnostic Indicators for Treatment Design   189

Stuttering Modification   190

Fluency Shaping   191

Combined Stuttering Modification and Fluency Shaping Approaches   192

Exemplar Treatments   192

Stuttering Modification   193

Diagnosis   194

Motivation   195

Identification   196

Desensitization   197

Variation/Modification   199
Approximation/Modification   200
Stabilization   201

Fluency Shaping   203
Stuttering Interview (SI)   203
Counting, Charting, Timing   205
Criterion Test   205
Establishment   205
GILCU   205
DAF   206
Transfer   207
Maintenance   208
Postscript   208

Chapter Summary   209

Chapter 7 Study Questions   211

Many clinicians believe they need to decide to use one approach or the other [i.e., stuttering modification or fluency shaping] in working with their clients. They believe that either they need to modify their clients' moments of stuttering or they need to target their overall speaking patterns. The two approaches appear to them to be incompatible. To many clinicians, this can be a difficult and confusing choice. Fortunately, however, the two approaches are not necessarily antagonistic. On the contrary, techniques based on one approach can be helpful to the clinician employing the other approach.

(PETERS & GUITAR, 1991, P. 116)

In the previous two chapters, we addressed both intra- and extrafamily considerations that are critical to intervention with people who stutter. Intrafamily considerations underscored that stuttering and fluency represent different personal constructs, and that changes in a person who stutters trigger compensatory changes in family members and significant others. Extrafamily considerations emphasized and illustrated the importance of approaching intervention from a collaborative, interdisciplinary perspective in which all participants value human diversity in all of its forms. This chapter, the last in Unit II, provides a third set of considerations. Specifically, stuttering modification and fluency shaping are presented as bipolar endpoints of a psychotherapeutic continuum. Understanding these two elements and the continuum that lies between them is useful for distinguishing the many treatments available and currently being used with people who stutter. The primary purpose of presenting the continuum, however, is to provide a theoretical framework for tailoring the design of treatment for each individual who stutters. We will underscore the point that the design of effective treatment is not arbitrary; rather, it is systematic and based on coherent, psychotherapeutic decision rules. Following this chapter, we will begin Unit III, which focuses on assessment and treatment with people who stutter, while applying intrafamily (personal constructs and family systems), extrafamily (interdisciplinary teaming and multicultural awareness), and psychotherapeutic (stuttering modification and fluency shaping) considerations.

GENERAL DEFINITIONS

Stuttering Modification

Stuttering modification therapy (Guitar & Peters, 1980; Peters & Guitar, 1991) refers to a category of intervention approaches used *with* people who stutter. These approaches assume that stuttering results from avoiding or struggling with disfluency, avoiding feared words, and avoiding feared situations. The intervention process seeks to reduce speech-related avoidance behaviors, fears, and negative attitudes, while modifying the form of stuttering. Guitar and Peters (1980) explained that this can be accomplished by different methods, including reducing the struggle behavior, smoothing out the form of stuttering, and reducing the tension and rate of stuttering by stuttering in a more relaxed and deliberate way. Such techniques are used to help a person who demonstrates advanced stuttering to stutter in a more fluent manner. Gregory (1979) grouped these techniques into a category he described as "stutter more fluently" (p. 2). Similarly, Curlee and Perkins (1984) characterized these techniques as "those that manage stuttering" (p. iii). Taken together, stuttering modification approaches help the person who stutters to stutter more fluently (i.e., with less effort, struggle, and abnormality). Gregory (1979) emphasized that the person who stutters must make his speech behavior the object of study, become familiar with it, and gradually modify his stuttering by thinking about, identifying, and practicing methods of stuttering more easily. By allowing the stuttering to occur so as to study and modify the behavior, the person who stutters changes his speech-related behavior, feelings, and attitudes, thus reducing his avoidance behavior.

One of the best known exemplars of stuttering modification therapy is Van Riper's (1973) treatment for the "confirmed stutterer" (p. 203) referred to as MIDVAS (*M*otivation, *I*dentification, *D*esensitization, *V*ariation, *A*pproximation, *S*tabilization) (Van Riper, 1972, 1973). Other approaches that are reflective of stuttering modification include, but are not limited to, those of Bloodstein (1975), Conture (1990b), Dell (1979), Luper and Mulder (1964), Sheehan (1970), and Williams (1957, 1971, 1979).

Fluency Shaping

On the other end of the continuum is fluency shaping therapy (Guitar & Peters, 1980; Peters & Guitar, 1991). This category refers to intervention approaches used *for* people who stutter, and assumes that stuttering is learned. Therefore, intervention is based on principles of behavior modification (i.e., operant conditioning and programming). Unlike stuttering modification where the goal of treatment is to modify stuttering into an easier, gentler form, fluency shaping first seeks to establish fluent speech by eliminating stuttering in a controlled stimulus environment. The fluent response is reinforced (positively and/or negatively) and stuttering behavior is punished. Through successive approximation, fluency gradually is modified to approximate normal sounding conversational speech in a controlled clinical setting. Then, efforts are directed to generalize the fluent speech into the person's natural speaking environments. Gregory (1979) characterized such treatments as those that direct the person who stutters to "speak more fluently" (p. 5). Likewise, Curlee and Perkins (1984) categorized these treatments as "those that manage fluency" (p. iii). Taken together, fluency shaping techniques increase the length and complexity of the fluent responses of a person who stutters, first in the treatment setting and then in extraclinical settings, ultimately so as to replace the stuttering behavior.

Programmed Conditioning for Fluency (Ryan & Van Kirk, 1971) and *Programmed Therapy for Stuttering in Children and Adults* (Ryan, 1974) represent a well-known example of fluency shaping therapy. In this form of treatment, fluency is established in one of four programs. One program is referred to as GILCU (*G*radual *I*ncrease in *L*ength and *C*omplexity of *U*tterance) whereby the client is directed to talk slowly and to generate a fluent (not stuttered, by definition in this case) single-word response. The response gradually is increased to two, three, and so on to six words before a sentence becomes the target response. Another establishment program is known as DAF (*D*elayed *A*uditory *F*eedback). In this, the client uses headphones to hear his speech in 50 millisecond decrements of delay from 250 to 0 milliseconds. This delayed auditory feedback helps the person who stutters to speak in a slow, prolonged, nonstuttered manner. The third establishment program (Programmed Traditional) shapes a fluent response first by identifying stuttered words and then by using cancellations, pull-outs, and preparatory sets (terms borrowed from Van Riper, 1973, which will be discussed later in this chapter). The last establishment program (Punishment) reduces the frequency of stuttering by presenting aversive events. Other proponents of fluency shaping treatments include, but are not limited to, Boberg (1981, 1984), Boberg and Kully (1985), Costello (1980, 1983), Goldiamond (1965), Perkins (1973a, 1973b), Perkins, Rudas, Johnson, Michael, and Curlee (1974), Shames and Florance (1980), Shine (1980, 1984), Webster (1979), and Wingate (1969, 1976).

SIGNIFICANT DIFFERENCES

Before discussing advantages and disadvantages of stuttering modification and fluency shaping, differential diagnostic indicators, and an exemplar of each form of treatment, stuttering modification and fluency shaping will be distinguished further on the bases of treatment premise, behavioral treatment goals, affective treatment goals, procedures, and structure (Guitar & Peters, 1980). These distinctions follow and are represented in Table 7.1.

Premise

We noted earlier that stuttering modification assumes that stuttering results from avoiding or struggling with disfluency, feared words, feared situations, and negative attitudes. Fluency shaping, on the other hand, assumes that stuttering is learned like any other behavior through conditioning principles.

Behavioral Treatment Goals

Three different behavioral treatment goals for people who stutter have been outlined (Guitar & Peters, 1980; Peters & Guitar, 1991). They will be discussed individually.

Spontaneous Fluency

The most desirous goal is spontaneous speech fluency, which is characteristic of the "normal" speaker. Neither tension nor struggle behaviors are observed, thus revealing ongoing smoothness of speech. Repetitions and prolongations

Table 7.1. Distinctions Between Stuttering Modification (SM) and Fluency Shaping (FS)

Premise

SM: Stuttering results from avoiding or struggling with disfluencies, fears, and negative attitudes.

FS: Stuttering is learned.

Behavioral Treatment Goals

SM: In decreasing order of desirability, goals include spontaneous fluency, controlled fluency, or acceptable stuttering.

FS: Only spontaneous or controlled fluency are acceptable goals. Any evidence of noticeable stuttering is regarded as a program failure.

Affective Treatment Goals

SM: Fears and avoidances related to stuttering are reduced by identifying, studying, and understanding thoughts, feelings, and attitudes about communication and oneself as a communicator. Positive social and vocational adjustments are targeted directly.

FS: No attempt is made to reduce communication-related fears and avoidances or impact the attitudes of the person who stutters. As a result of improved fluency, however, fears often reduce and positive social and vocational adjustments occur indirectly.

Procedures

SM: Much attention is given to reducing speech fears and avoidance behaviors. The client is taught to be more fluent by various techniques to modify stuttering. Fluency is maintained by reduction of fears and avoidance behaviors.

FS: Little attention is given to reduction of speech fears and avoidance behaviors. The client is "programmed" for stutter-free speech via specific contingencies. Fluency is maintained by modifying the manner of speaking and, if necessary, reinstatement of fluency by recycling through the original program.

Structure

SM: A less structured format (such as a teaching or counseling interaction) is used.

FS: In contrast, the format is highly structured (which is typical of behavioral conditioning and programming).

Note. From *Stuttering: An Integration of Contemporary Therapies* (pp. 13–23), by B. Guitar and T. J. Peters, 1980, Memphis, TN: Stuttering Foundation of America. Adapted with permission.

are easy, nearly effortless, and occur only occasionally. The rate and rhythm are even, regular, and without notice. The relative effort is minor; thus the speaker attends to the thoughts and ideas being conveyed and exchanged rather than to his speech itself.

Controlled Fluency

The smoothness (continuity) of speech in controlled fluency is similar to that of spontaneous fluency. However, in order to maintain controlled fluency, the person who stutters must monitor and adjust his speech to maintain natural, or normal, sounding speech. Peters and Guitar (1991) indicated that this might be achieved in various ways including making a fluency adjustment before (preparatory set) or during (pull-out) a disfluent word is being spoken, reducing rate of speech, softening articulatory contacts, prolonging syllables, responding to auditory and proprioceptive feedback, among other methods. These adjustments might be slightly noticeable to an astute listener. By attending to and adjusting speech rate and rhythm, a person who achieves controlled fluency expends greater effort in order to achieve near normal sounding speech smoothness. Distinguishing spontaneous from controlled fluency, Guitar and Peters (1980) indicated that the former "is the fluency of the normal speaker" (p. 15), while in the latter "the speaker exhibits normal sounding speech by paying attention to how he is talking" (p. 15).

Acceptable Stuttering

The third and least preferred goal is acceptable stuttering in which the speaker demonstrates noticeable disfluency that is of relatively low severity. Furthermore, the speaker demonstrates and reports feeling relative comfort in his role as a communicator despite his stuttering. As with controlled fluency, the person who demonstrates acceptable stuttering monitors his speech and makes adjustments to maintain a reduced or acceptable level of stuttering. However, with acceptable stuttering, all dimensions of fluency (rate, rhythm, continuity, and effort) are affected and potentially noticeable to conversational partners.

Stuttering Modification and Fluency Shaping

Both stuttering modification and fluency shaping clinicians work toward the ultimate goal of spontaneous fluency. Clinical research indicates that this objective becomes increasingly challenged as stuttering advances through the life span. If spontaneous fluency proves unattainable as a realistic objective, then clinicians of both theoretical orientations would treat controlled fluency as the next best objective. If both spontaneous fluency and controlled fluency prove unattainable, the stuttering modification clinician then would turn to acceptable stuttering as the most appropriate treatment goal. For a fluency shaping clinician, however, any form of noticeable stuttering is regarded as evidence of a program failure. Therefore, acceptable stuttering typically is not a viable treatment objective for fluency shaping clinicians.

Affective Treatment Goals

Another way that stuttering modification and fluency shaping differ is on the basis of the affective treatment goals—the extent to which and how the communication-related feelings and attitudes of the person who stutters are addressed.

Stuttering Modification

Stuttering modification emphasizes the importance of identifying, studying, and understanding such feelings and attitudes, thereby reducing the fears and avoidances related to stuttering. People who stutter are encouraged to seek out and systematically master speaking situations that were formerly avoided.

Through desensitization and strategically designed successes, the person who stutters develops communication competence and confidence, thereby achieving a more positive attitude toward his speech, the process of communication, and himself as a communicator. Furthermore, stuttering modification attempts to impact the overall adjustment of the person who stutters, thus facilitating development of his social and vocational skills.

Fluency Shaping

Fluency shaping, on the other hand, does not attempt to reduce the communication-related fears and avoidances or otherwise impact the attitudes of the person who stutters. As a consequence of fluency success from programmed treatment, however, often fears are reduced and attitudes are improved, albeit indirectly. Likewise, while fluency shaping does not attempt to impact the social or vocational adjustment of the person who stutters, such changes may occur as a by-product of programmed treatment.

Treatment Procedures

Both stuttering modification and fluency shaping attempt to help the person who stutters achieve an initial measure of fluency by using deliberate and controlled techniques. These might include speaking in slow, gentle speech (speech with prolonged, gradual onset) with or without use of a delayed auditory feedback device, engaging in choral reading, or shadowing the speech of the clinician. After initial fluency is established, however, stuttering modification and fluency shaping methods differ with respect to how later objectives (such as spontaneous or controlled fluency) are achieved.

Stuttering Modification

As noted earlier, stuttering modification seeks to facilitate fluency by reducing communication-related fears, avoidances, and negative attitudes, and looks for adjustments in such internal dimensions as a consequence of improved fluency. Once fluency is established, people who stutter are encouraged to combat the natural tendency to avoid feared words and situations. They are guided in how to approach such feared contexts by using techniques for controlling and canceling instances of stuttering. Furthermore, since the morale and self-esteem of people who stutter are considered to be critical factors in the maintenance of fluency, stuttering modification seeks to monitor and enhance, if appropriate, the social and emotional adjustment of such persons. Peters and Guitar (1991) indicated that relapse into periods of uncontrolled stuttering is a significant issue, particularly for people whose stuttering has advanced. To reduce the likelihood of such occurrences, the authors indicated that stuttering modification clinicians urge clients to combat the tendency to avoid words or situations, keep speech fears at a minimum level, master stuttering modification skills, and become their own clinician and thereby assume responsibility for their own therapy. Other strategies to facilitate transfer of fluency skills and to minimize the likelihood of relapse that I will address include beginning transfer activities from the very first contact with the client, identifying and modifying as necessary one's personal construct, working within family systems and interdisciplinary contexts, and preparing for relapse so as to minimize its negative effects, among others. Stuttering modification, therefore, tends to consider the person who stutters in dynamic totality.

Fluency Shaping

Fluency shaping addresses directly observable speech behavior to the exclusion of fears, avoidances, and negative emotions. This is consistent with the assumption reviewed earlier that stuttering is acquired through conditioning principles. Therefore, fluency (stutter-free speech) is established in a controlled stimulus environment and maintained by the use of techniques such as slowing speech rate and monitoring the ease of speech onset. Often such techniques are found in behaviorally (operantly) designed programs that seek to instate or reinstate fluency through sequenced steps in which the response expectation is prescribed and increased systematically. Should relapse occur, the client is recycled through the earlier steps in the program, which enabled him to achieve his fluency prior to relapse. Guitar and Peters (1980) indicated that within fluency shaping, "It is the manner of speaking rather than the moment of stuttering that is modified" (p. 16).

Treatment Structure

Stuttering Modification

Stuttering modification treatment typically is conducted within a teaching or counseling context in which dialogue between the clinician and client is the medium of exchange. The interaction, while systematically planned, is relatively unstructured, with the clinician and client interacting as equal participants, each with dynamic roles and contributions to the treatment process.

Fluency Shaping

Fluency shaping treatment typically is a highly structured approach in which stimuli, responses, and subsequent events are preprogrammed. Regarding fluency shaping, Peters and Guitar (1991) noted that "specific responses are called for from the stutterer with specific reactions to these responses required from the clinician" (p. 124).

ADVANTAGES AND DISADVANTAGES

Stuttering Modification

Stuttering modification techniques directly address the communication-related feelings and attitudes of people who stutter in addition to their speech behaviors. Furthermore, as noted, the person who stutters is an active participant in all aspects of the treatment process, requiring particular interpersonal, problem solving, and professional skills on the part of the clinician. Some may interpret as a disadvantage that the actual change in speech behavior takes relatively longer in stuttering modification (when compared to fluency shaping) because of the nature and context of the change. However, this observation is compensated by the advantage that change occurs not only to speech behavior, but to feelings and attitudes as well, thus facilitating the maintenance and transfer of fluency over time and communicative settings. In other words, stuttering modification tends to result in slower observable fluency change, but is more effective in reducing speech fears and reversing negative attitudes while strengthening generalization of the speech behaviors. Guitar and Peters (1980) pointed out that stuttering modification is a dynamic process in which the person who stutters is not directed to speak in an abnormal pattern (as in fluency shaping), but is expected and supported to confront his communication-related fears and avoidances (unlike fluency shaping). While clinicians find stuttering modification to be less structured and often more conversationally inviting than fluency shaping, such a dynamic, interactive clinical context requires more advanced professional skills of the clinician. These abilities include providing emotional support, clinical problem solving, and responding to clients' individual differences, some of which prove troublesome for beginning clinicians. These and other clinician competencies will be addressed in the chapters to follow, particularly in Chapter 11.

Fluency Shaping

Fluency shaping techniques, on the other hand, target speech behaviors only. The person who stutters is more passively involved in a relatively highly structured program designed and directed by the clinician. Observed behavior change occurs relatively rapidly. Balancing this potential advantage, however, is the observation that maintenance and transfer of the fluency skills usually are not as promising as in stuttering modification. In other words, fluency shaping produces more rapid fluency improvement, the duration of which is more challenged than with stuttering modification. Guitar and Peters (1980) indicated that fluency shaping procedures tend to engage the client in an abnormal or artificial pattern of speaking in order to achieve stutter-free speech. Highly prescribed, the procedures tend to be less motivating, if not boring. Many commercially available fluency shaping programs direct both the clinician and client through a clinical script, indicating what to do and when to do it. Clients do not directly confront speaking-related fears or avoidances. Thus, the delivery of services requires less advanced professional skills, less clinical insight, and less clinical sensitivity on the part of the clinician.

DIFFERENTIAL DIAGNOSTIC INDICATORS FOR TREATMENT DESIGN

As noted earlier, the purpose of reviewing stuttering modification and fluency shaping is to establish a theoretical framework for individualizing treatment for people who stutter. The most effective treatment for an individual typically falls somewhere between the anchor points of stuttering modification and fluency shaping. It is incumbent, therefore, for clinicians to know how to combine the stuttering modification and fluency shaping considerations already presented, while designing treatment for each individual who stutters. Both schools of thought have merit when applied judiciously. Neither is appropriate for all people who stutter.

Guitar and Peters (1980) reported that stuttering modification and fluency shaping treatments are most distinct when designed for adults who stutter (those of or beyond the high school years), less distinct for children in elementary school (particularly among the lower age range), and least distinct for preschool children. They commented that, "the stuttering modification approach and the fluency shaping approach begin to become more similar at the elementary school age level; this is particularly true for the lower age range of the group" (p. 53). One reason for this distinction is that the factors guiding the design of treatment, such as a person's history and emotional reaction to stuttering, are more pronounced as he accumulates experience with stuttering. For reasons of illustration, this discussion focuses on the differential diagnostic indicators for the design of treatment for adults who stutter.

We will discuss later (in Chapters 8 and 9) how treatment is modified for individuals who have less experience stuttering and who may be experiencing less penalty. Guitar and Peters (1980) noted that as a person continues to stutter, overt speech behavior often becomes more severe and related feelings and attitudes become more handicapping. With respect to planning treatment, they commented, "In reality the six or seven year old is often more like the preschool stutterer. The twelve year old stutterer, on the other hand, can be more like the high school stutterer" (p. 53). Therefore, the factors guiding the design of treatment extend beyond one's chronological age and severity of overt symptomatology. Specifically, one of the most deciding factors in the design of treatment is the extent to which a person tends to conceal stuttering or avoid communicative situations that incline him to stutter. These factors are discussed now and relate to how the person who stutters confronts his feelings about himself as a person and as a communicator.

Stuttering Modification

Guitar and Peters (1980) noted that a stuttering modification approach is neither indicated nor contraindicated by the severity of stuttering. They noted the following:

> This approach works as well with mild as with severe stutterers. The important thing to consider is how much the stutterer avoids or hides his stuttering. If he spends considerable energy disguising his stuttering, he is more likely to profit from stuttering modification therapy. (p. 34)

Furthermore, stuttering modification is indicated when a person experiences a personal penalty for stuttering. Such penalties may take the form of feeling poorly about oneself as a communicator, feeling that others are not accepting of oneself because of the stuttering, or feeling that stuttering interferes with one's life dreams or future ambitions. As will be seen, the extent to which a person may perceive a personal penalty can be determined from the diagnostic process, from trial management within and subsequent to the diagnostic interview, and from informal, unstructured (conversationally based) and more standardized (attitude questionnaires) assessment of feelings and attitudes. Another indication for stuttering modification is when the person demonstrates a more positive response to trial management taking the form of stuttering modification than to that of fluency shaping. This means that the person responds positively to opportunities to discuss the nature of observed fluency and disfluency, practice ways of stuttering more easily, and address feelings and attitudes about himself as a communicator. Furthermore, this person may express discomfort when using the fluency shaping techniques that seem to be communicatively artificial or imposed. In other words, an intervention approach more in the direction of stuttering modification is indicated when the person who stutters demonstrates the following:

- hides or disguises his stuttering

- avoids speaking

- perceives personal penalty as a consequence of stuttering

- feels poorly about himself as a communicator

- demonstrates a more positive response to stuttering modification trial management

Fluency Shaping

On the other hand, Guitar and Peters (1980) noted that a candidate for fluency shaping is more likely to demonstrate a positive self-image as a communicator. This person's stuttering does not seem to be maintained by negative emotions. Thus, the person is talkative whether or not he stutters severely. Although the stuttering may be represented as an annoyance and even as an impediment to his life, this person nevertheless remains positive, does not feel that the stuttering is a significant handicap, and feels accepted by family, friends, and associates despite his stuttering. Furthermore, a person for whom fluency shaping is indicated does not attempt to conceal his stuttering or avoid speaking situations. His stuttering, therefore, is easily observable. A positive response to fluency shaping trial management is observed and the candidate expresses acceptance of the prolonged speech pattern often characteristic of fluency shaping. In fact, he may express relief to have gained increased conversational fluency by use of such methods. In summary, indications for intervention of a fluency shaping nature include an individual who:

- stutters openly,

- does not avoid speaking,

- perceives annoyance or interference but no personal penalty from stuttering,

- feels positive about himself as a communicator, and

- demonstrates a positive response to fluency shaping trial management.

Combined Stuttering Modification and Fluency Shaping Approaches

In reality, most people who stutter present indications both from those presented for stuttering modification and for fluency shaping. Most forms of intervention, therefore, are combined. Again, a challenge facing clinicians is knowing how to combine the approaches most effectively for each person who stutters. Guitar and Peters (1980) noted:

> In our experience, most clients will benefit from a combination of stuttering modification and fluency shaping approaches at some stage of their treatment. We believe this for the following reasons. We think that fluency shaping therapy is more efficient than stuttering modification therapy for changing speech patterns. We also think, however, that stuttering modification therapy is more effective in reducing speech fears and improving speech attitudes for those clients who need it. (p. 36)

Furthermore, candidates for a combined approach typically have some fear of stuttering, but not to the extent of internalizing deep hurt, rejection, and penalty. Variation in the frequency and severity of stuttering may be present. Similarly, evidence of occasional avoidance including circumlocutions and stalling tactics may be observed. Usually candidates for a combined approach have a somewhat positive response to both fluency shaping and stuttering modification trial management. In other words, the reduction in disfluency resulting from fluency shaping is as motivating to candidates for a combined approach as is the opportunity to discuss and better understand the nature of one's own fluency and disfluency, as well as related feelings. Therefore, an approach combining stuttering modification and fluency shaping is indicated for a person who:

- stutters openly, but may demonstrate some avoidance,
- perceives some sense of personal penalty and negative feelings from stuttering, but not to an extreme or handicapping degree,
- feels relatively positive about himself as a communicator, but wishes for personal change, and
- demonstrates a positive response both to stuttering modification and fluency shaping trial management.

EXEMPLAR TREATMENTS

We are nearly ready to address intervention that integrates stuttering modification and fluency shaping in addition to the intrafamily and extrafamily considerations reviewed earlier in Chapters 5 and 6. Before doing so, it is helpful to be familiar with treatments that represent the anchor points of stuttering modification and fluency shaping. In this way, clinicians better understand the nature of how treatments can be combined, particularly when they see the origins of different aspects of the combined treatment. To this end, we will look more closely at two different treatments referred to earlier. Specifically, Charles

Van Riper's treatment (MIDVAS; 1972, 1973) will be discussed as a form of stuttering modification; Bruce Ryan's treatment (*Programmed Conditioning for Fluency,* Ryan & Van Kirk, 1971; *Programmed Therapy for Stuttering in Children and Adults,* Ryan, 1974) as a form of fluency shaping therapy. Many other treatments referred to earlier could be discussed as well. We will not do so, however, with space limitations in mind. Interested clinicians are encouraged to investigate these treatments and to read any of a number of excellent sources that review different treatments (Culatta & Goldberg, 1995; Ham, 1986, 1990; Peters & Guitar, 1991; Shames & Rubin, 1986; Van Riper, 1973; Wall & Myers, 1995). For purposes of illustration, the treatments summarized will address intervention with young adults who demonstrate confirmed or advanced characteristics of stuttering.

Stuttering Modification

Van Riper (1972) indicated that two facts are important cornerstones in his form of treatment. Specifically, stuttering is intermittent, and the occurrence, frequency, and severity of stuttering vary systematically with the strength of certain specific, observable, and therefore manipulable factors. In other words, Van Riper stated:

> If we can focus our therapy on these factors so that those which make stuttering worse are weakened sufficiently and those which make for less stuttering are strengthened, the frequency and severity of stuttering will decrease, and ultimately stuttering will disappear. (1972, p. 283)

Van Riper underscored that like all other human behavior, stuttering obeys certain predictable patterns or laws. For example, conditions that tend to worsen stuttering include the following: penalty, frustration, anxiety, guilt, and hostility; situation fears based on memory of past stuttering unpleasantness in similar situations; word and phonetic fears based on memory of past stuttering unpleasantness on similar words and sounds; and greater real or perceived communication importance or meaningfulness of what is being said. Such predictability and individuality of the stuttering experience result in three principles that ground the intervention process: learning theory, servotheory, and psychotherapy (Van Riper, 1973).

With respect to learning theory, the person who stutters is guided to unlearn old maladaptive responses to the fear and experience of fluency disruption and to learn new more adaptive ones. Secondly, servotheory indicates that speech is automatically controlled by feedback and suggests that stuttering is a consequence of failure in the auditory processing system. Therefore, Van Riper's treatment emphasizes monitoring speech by proprioception, essentially bypassing or reducing the reliance upon the auditory feedback system. Finally, Van Riper acknowledged that adolescents and adults who stutter often "come to us with intense fears, frustrations, and other emotional reactions due to their disrupted speech and feelings of deviance" (1973, p. 204). For this reason, the treatment is designed so that psychotherapy for secondary or expectancy type neurosis is interwoven within all interactions. When a more primary or central neurosis exists, a referral is made to an appropriate practitioner.

Diagnosis

Before entertaining treatment, Van Riper advised that the diagnostic evaluation must begin to appraise the person and the presenting problem, a process of assessment that in reality continues throughout treatment. Factors being assessed include overt (stuttering severity, nature of fluency) and covert (motivation, frustration, anxiety, guilt, shame, hostility, fears, ego strength) manifestations of communication. Conducted within an interview format, Van Riper (1973) recommended the following general procedures:

- Discuss with the client an outline of the diagnostic process.

- Invite the client to describe the presenting problem, and verbalize the client's likely feelings.

- Engage the client in conversation and reading. Discuss with the client the observed stuttering behavior (e.g., comparison to client's usual speech, hierarchic sequences, strategic function).

- Analyze core behaviors (e.g., speed, regularity, coarticulation of syllabic repetitions), noting the simultaneous and successive motor movements; how and where tremors begin and end; timing of respiration, phonation, and articulation; and other factors. Also analyze avoidance and release behaviors, noting variability and consistency.

- Analyze the client's fluent speech (e.g., rate, pitch, intensity, quality).

- Determine the client's prediction of stuttering, from which to discover phonemic or situation cues.

- Explore the onset and development of stuttering, penalties and rejections, possible profits and secondary gains, and emotionality.

- Explore attitudes and perceptions through formal and informal assessment.

- Determine the impact of communication stress (e.g., listener loss, interruptions, time pressure, phone calling, speaking to a small group).

- Conduct trial therapy and summarize impressions. The diagnostic session should end by assigning the client to prepare a thorough autobiography addressing significant experiences that shaped him and the people who influenced him.

The clinician must interpret the strength, frequency, and duration of the client's habits of avoidance and struggle, and differentially diagnose possible organicity and other types of disfluency. Van Riper cautioned that "we cannot rely solely on frequency counts of stutterings. The disorder is too variable, too influenced by too many external and internal stimuli. We cannot treat the stuttering alone. We must treat the stutterer" (p. 219). It generally is not possible in the initial evaluation to explore fully and in depth all of the client's communication strengths and limitations. Therefore, following establishment of initial impressions, the clinician must continue to question and learn about the client as a person and as a communicator throughout the treatment process.

Van Riper's treatment contains four sequential phases. The *identification phase* is intended for the person who stutters to explore, analyze, and classify overt behaviors and covert experiences characteristic of his stuttering. Second, the *desensitization phase* decreases speech anxieties and other related negative emotions, and "toughens" the person who stutters to the threat and experience of fluency failure. Third, the *modification phase* is intended first to vary and then to unlearn the habitual avoidance and struggle responses, and then to learn to use counterconditioning in a new, more fluent, and less abnormal way of stuttering. Finally, the *stabilization phase* is to help the person who stutters make the less abnormal, more fluent way of stuttering more automatic, and to develop proprioceptive monitoring of his speech. Van Riper noted that his methods must not been seen as a static template to be applied to all people who stutter. Rather, he emphasized the importance of tailoring treatment to each client's special strengths and needs.

Within these four phases, there are a number of main steps of overlapping subphases referred to by the acronym MIDVAS (Van Riper, 1972, 1973). As noted earlier, the letters each stand for a phase of treatment in sequence. In other words, treatment begins with *M*otivation, followed by *I*dentification, *D*esensitization, *V*ariation, *A*pproximation, and *S*tabilization. The treatment is cumulative and overlapping, so that each phase has a special emphasis based on all previous goals. The phases will be summarized briefly.

Motivation

According to Van Riper, no other phase in treatment is more important to its success or failure than the assessment, understanding, and management of one's motivation. In this phase, the clinician conveys her role as a companion and guide, one who is willing to share the burden of stuttering and is both positive and optimistic about its management. Van Riper noted that "out of the therapist's faith can come the stutterer's hope" (1973, p. 230). The clinician demonstrates her genuine interest in the person who stutters as a person. Verbally recognizing and identifying the components of the client's speech and the client's related feelings with complete acceptance, the clinician thus conveys support, permissiveness, and understanding. The clinician may replicate the stuttering in her own mouth. Doing so helps to initiate a close relationship and to extinguish, at least partially, the evil effects and hurt experienced from previous stuttering. Encouraging the client to express feelings about stuttering and himself as a communicator, the clinician verbalizes the client's feelings tentatively and invites correction.

From the clinician's patience, understanding, and acceptance, the client learns that he can share anxiety, guilt, and hostility, thus reducing through sharing the fears associated with stuttering. The client is helped to realize that his present speech possesses a certain degree of fluency and fluent, non-struggled stuttering. Furthermore, the clinician might adjust tentatively through modeling a characteristic or two of the client's stuttering. This builds an understanding that the client can speak more fluently and possesses certain abilities and choices (concepts that will be pivotal to the intervention methods presented in later chapters). He comes to see that the problem is his inefficient, learned coping reactions to the fear associated with stuttering. By learning to stutter more fluently and with less abnormality, both the severity and frequency of stuttering will decrease. The clinician provides a brief overview of treatment, and discusses the importance of the client accepting responsibility as an active participant in all aspects including setting goals and making and completing assignments. The client must understand and accept the "cost" of treatment (time, energy, and discipline) for its anticipated outcome (more fluent speech, less abnormal stuttering, more efficient coping reactions). Likewise, the clinician must appreciate that clients will not work with continued motivation and commitment without the demonstration of "payoff."

Van Riper indicated that people who stutter severely tend to have more positive prognosis than those with milder stuttering because the former know that they have far to go and expect to work harder. Their expectations regarding the costs of treatment are more realistic and their expected payoff is greater. It also is true, however, that those who stutter more severely may demonstrate decreased motivation prematurely when they feel that they have progressed enough to communicate effectively. Waning motivation often is observed in the terminal stages of treatment in which the person who stutters is enjoying his fluency that seems so far removed from the original stuttering. Van Riper noted that management of motivation is a continual challenge because it wanes and waxes daily. This challenge is met by understanding and relating to the client's unique motives, establishing realistic objectives with the client, responding to the client's fears to reenter situations in which he may have been grievously wounded, respecting the cost:profit ratio, and by providing undaunted support and commitment to the client. Reflecting the essence of motivation and its management with people who stutter, Van Riper (1973) noted:

> Somehow we blow the trumpet that sends the stutterer forward into the battle for his freedom and somehow we get him to blow it himself. Faith is said to move mountains but it is the therapist's dedicated care and concern, if not love, that moves stutterers. (p. 243)

Identification

The basic goal in this phase is to engage the person who stutters in identifying and evaluating the unique factors that comprise his stuttering. Typically, this person is only globally aware of what he does when he speaks. Describing and dialoguing about what he does with respect to what he thinks he does within a context of clinician's interest and freedom from punishment creates an opportunity for "unlearning, relearning, and new learning" (Van Riper, 1973, p. 245). Van Riper highlighted that within this phase, the valuable process of desensitization begins. He noted, "For once, the experience that he has always avoided is sought and desired. The untouchable can be touched" (p. 247). The major premise being addressed in this phase is that any learned habits are easier to change once they are made conscious. Habits persist when they are automatic and subconscious. Four critical functions being addressed include the following: combating denial, discriminating behaviors and feelings so as to identify what is and what needs to be changed, desensitizing through examining stuttering behaviors with the clinician, and providing the client a role and responsibility in treatment (establishing the client as an active participant in the treatment process). These goals and objectives are accomplished through a variety of procedures, all of which facilitate identification. Overt behaviors are identified including fluently spoken words, easy stutterings, and ultimately hard stuttering and avoidance behaviors.

Van Riper noted that at first, the person who stutters is not expected to modify his stuttering. Rather, "His role is that of a collector and cataloguer, not corrector or extinguisher. We want to know and we want him to know what he does when he says he stutters. We are defining and learning the problem" (1973, p. 249). Also defined are the precipitants of stuttering including verbal, situational, and emotional cues; core behaviors; loci of tension; recoil behaviors; post-stuttering reactions, feelings of frustration, shame, hostility, and other factors. A critical emphasis of this phase is on self-therapy. The person who stutters is encouraged to complete assignments, which are increasingly designed by him. These are specific to ensure success and evoke reporting of experiences and feelings, both of which are rewarded. An important observation is that the person who stutters comes to seek speaking experiences rather than avoid them. The identification experience often leads to sharing and exploring the client's feelings about himself. Van Riper (1973) noted:

> As hostility begins to pour forth, the therapist must expect to become the target of some of this long repressed aggression especially in those stutterers who have turned their hatred inward upon themselves because they couldn't project it outwardly for fear of being clobbered some more. We are not appalled when this happens. The therapist's receptacle should be large enough to receive such evil. Better to have it come out than to keep it within. Better to have it expressed in words rather than in stuttering behavior. Good therapists are self-flushing anyway. (pp. 264–265)

He noted also that the identification phase is one of exploration, which by itself often produces nearly immediate decreases in the amount and severity of stuttering, fear, and avoidance. Such reductions are temporary at best and not yet a direct objective of treatment. As with motivation, identification will continue throughout treatment.

Desensitization

Desensitization implies stress. Unless reduced, stress maintains the avoidance and escape behaviors, which are noticeable characteristics in stuttering. This phase aims to reduce the speech-related anxieties and negative emotions held by the person who stutters so that he can learn new ways of coping with and responding to stuttering. The methods used are more direct than those in motivation and identification. Van Riper (1973) again emphasized the role of the clinician who creates in the treatment room a "zone of safety and security, where basically the stuttering is felt with little frustration and where the listener is not punitive" (p. 268). At the same time, the clinician is to "toughen" the client to the factors that formerly resulted in disintegration and stuttering. A concomitant reduction in avoidance is important in order to begin to approach stuttering with the intention of modifying it (i.e., we cannot modify that which we avoid). As avoidances are reduced, the client's feelings of anger, fear, and hostility often surface and may be shared with, if not directed at, the clinician. Furthermore, the client's stuttering may become more severe, albeit temporarily. The clinician needs to verbalize her understanding and acceptance of the client's emotions and explain that the heightened disfluency reflects greater awareness of what needs to be changed.

Both of these patterns (emotionality and greater disfluency) expressed in a benign, nurturing environment enable the person who stutters to prepare for the change process. Using different procedures and assignments, the clinician determines the client's stress tolerance, regulates the amount of stress, and again verbally acknowledges the amount of stress the client is feeling. One assignment is for the client and clinician to build a communicative situational stress hierarchy. Speaking contexts (involving situations, listeners, and others) that later become clinical tasks and assignments are progressively ordered from least to most challenging. The client will move up the hierarchy in the smallest possible steps to ensure success. The clinician often will model the task several times before the client attempts it. For example, the clinician might enter a store with the client and pseudostutter (i.e., fake stuttering) to a clerk. From this experience, the clinician will convey that she is not upset and recall and discuss with the client what the clerk did and how the clinician and client honestly felt. That another person would be willing and able to undergo such an experience and remain integrated conveys a powerful message of support to the client. Activities such as these provide opportunities for the client to unlearn old reactions and learn new ones, all the while confronting stuttering (seeing, hearing, feeling, and identifying core behaviors, listener reactions, and one's own related thoughts and feelings). Desensitization involves counter-conditioning, or linking old stimuli with new reactions, involving assertive training (seeking out stuttering so that it can be modified) and disinhibition (reversing habituated tendency to be on guard, always scanning speech for feared sounds or words, thus speaking tentatively as though expecting trauma). Desensitization also involves the following:

• *Relaxation*—clinician-induced visualization promoting cognitive restructuring (i.e., Van Riper reported poor transfer of this technique to actual stuttering).

• *Pseudostuttering*—volitional, intentional stuttering.

• *Adaptation*—collecting, logging, analyzing stuttering (flooding the client with heightened awareness of stuttering so as to strengthen the approach gradient and decrease the avoidance gradient).

• *Nonreinforcement*—repeating certain words on which the client stutters over and over until he says each of them fluently and then continuing to say that word with increasing loudness.

• *Negative suggestion and flooding*—presenting the internalized fears of the client as a probability (e.g., "I bet you will stutter miserably on this next phone call.").

• *Response prevention*—the client deliberately stutters on nonfeared sounds of nonfeared words until the clinician signals to release.

• *Adaptation with negative suggestion*—verbalizing for the client feelings that he has reported during real fixations (e.g., "Oh no, I'm stuck again. I'm helpless!"), first during pseudostuttering and eventually during real stuttering.

• *Adaptation to stress*—flooding the client with communicatively stressful situations in which he must speak fluently so that in comparison his daily speaking challenges seem less onerous.

• *Eliminating other sources of anxiety*—helping the client resolve other conflicts (such as finding a job, passing a course, and other sources of stress) so that stuttering-related fears will reduce. Van Riper noted the following about his life and the lives of other people who stutter:

We who stutter must learn to live better lives than normal speakers if only so that we can keep from amplifying our stuttering fears. Even after we have learned to speak and stutter fluently, we cannot afford to let other sources of guilt, hostility, or anxiety convert themselves into precipitants of stuttering. Sad as the prospect may seem, we must deny ourselves the human privilege of wallowing in the muck of sin and folly. If we do, then we pay the price in fear and in stuttering. If there is any injustice involved in having to be a stutterer and to be fluent in spite of stuttering, it is in this denial of the right to live foolishly. This author has always resented this constraint. (1973, p. 298)

• *Reassurance*—providing realistic, undaunted positive support for the client's potential as a communicator. Van Riper (1973) noted about clients that "they know that they are no longer alone and this special kind of reassurance is one of the most potent attenuators of negative emotion ever invented" (p. 299).

• *Anxiety reduction by modifying stuttering*—reducing client's fears and negative emotions by helping him learn a new way of stuttering that will not evoke penalties and frustration.

Summarizing the significance of desensitization, Van Riper stated about the client that:

He comes to us full of anxiety and shame, unable to confront his problem, disguising it, avoiding contact with it. Through a preliminary period of desensitization we calm him and gentle him enough so that he can do this new learning. And as he realizes he is coming to grips with his problem and making progress, his morale goes up and his fears go down. And so does his stuttering. (1973, p. 299)

Variation/Modification

In this phase, the person who stutters learns that it is possible to stutter and be more fluent (i.e., stutter more fluently). The purpose is to break up the stereotype of the client's old responses and to attach new responses to old cues. Much of the strength of the habitual compulsive reactions lies in their stereotype or consistency of their pattern. Varying these patterns weakens them. The variation phase typically is short in duration because it passes naturally into the next one (i.e., approximation). Having already collected and identified many instances of easy, unforced stuttering, the client in this phase is encouraged to experiment with change, to realize that he has a range of responses from which he can choose. Van Riper proposed a wide range of behaviors for the client to vary. He cautioned, however, that the assignments by themselves have little value. "Only when shared with the therapist and when feelings are expressed and when rewards are appropriately timed, do the experiences they evoke have potency in modifying the attitudes and outward behavior of the stutterer" (1972, p. 327). The assignments and procedures address the following:

• *Exploration of self*—recognizing the way a person characteristically behaves and identifying the idiosyncratic patterns of thinking, feeling, and acting, which comprise one's way of living (such as patterns of sitting, walking, talking, eating, and reading: also dress, appearance, manner, and routines).

• *"Rut breakers"*—deliberately varying the habitual patterns that were identified.

• *Role playing*—deliberately assuming a different role or the role of another person to facilitate variation of behavior.

• *Attitudinal change*—deliberately shifting from one mood of feeling to another (e.g., recognizing the influence of previous negative autosuggestion, a client first might express such thoughts aloud and then formulate alternative thoughts and memories).

• *Varying the stuttering behaviors*—deliberately changing the form of the anticipatory behaviors (i.e., postponement and avoidance reactions). For example, if the client prolongs "ah" or repeatedly interjects "well" before attempting a fluency modification, he might shorten or break up the "ah" into units, or interject a different word or words.

• *Varying the escape behaviors*—adjusting the behaviors that closely reflect feelings of blockage (such as sudden eye closings, abnormal mouth positions, jaw jerks, breathing abnormalities). Van Riper noted that these behaviors are the most resistant to change. He suggested a modeling approach in which the clinician assumes the client's abnormal mouth postures and revises them before finishing the word, or stutters in unison, adopting the first part of the abnormality but then introducing a variation and asking the client to follow the model presented. Through such modification, clients increase the repertoire of responses available to them.

Approximation/Modification

Once the client can vary his reactions to the factors that typically make stuttering worse, the objective of approximation is to learn new responses that gradually will diminish stuttering. The aim now is to modify the form of stuttering so that fluency is reinforced and that the appropriate motor sequence of the word is being approximated. The easy, more fluent form of stuttering, which has already been discovered occasionally and analyzed, will serve as the template. Van Riper emphasized the importance of clarifying the sequence of the motor model and heightening proprioceptive awareness through masking, delayed auditory feedback, and pantomiming, among other methods. Specific methods for approximating properly sequenced, more fluent speech include the following:

• *Stuttering in unison*—The clinician stutters with the client, first duplicating the behavior, then easing out of the tremors, ceasing the struggle, and smoothly finishing the word. The clinician shares the client's initial behavior and then diverges. Modifications are made in small steps (e.g., first stutter with eyes open rather than closed, then with relaxed rather than tense lips) and with a manageable and deliberate degree of stress. Expression of feelings is encouraged. The mutual sharing, faith, and acceptance creates a favorable context for change and growth.

• *Cancellation*—This is a vehicle for learning new responses to stimuli that trigger stuttering responses. The client stops immediately after a stuttered word is completely uttered. After a deliberate pause for reposturing, he then says the word with the modification he just learned. In other words, the modification is used after the word containing the disfluency has been spoken. Communication stops once he stutters, and continues only after he has used a more appropriate stuttering response. This procedure shifts the reinforcement to become the word finally spoken fluently, thus removing the reinforcement value of the old struggle behaviors.

• *Pull-outs*—Once the modifications have been practiced in unison with the clinician and in cancellation, the client incorporates them within the moment of stuttering (while the disfluency is occurring without any pauses). Therefore, the modification is moved forward in time, from the period just following the stuttering into the moment of stuttering itself.

• *Preparatory sets*—The modification now is moved into the period of anticipation of stuttering. Typically, people who stutter covertly rehearse before an anticipated instance of disfluency. Having used the modification after and during the actual stuttering, the client now is challenged to implement the modification before the stuttering occurs, during the stage of anticipatory rehearsal.

The stuttering modification techniques just reviewed—cancellation, pull-out, and preparatory set—are illustrated in Figure 7.1. Van Riper (1972) noted that as clients master the different techniques, both the severity and frequency of stuttering tend to decrease. Fears of words and then situations decrease as well. Self-confidence grows, as does tolerance of communicative stress.

Stabilization

At this point, the client is using reliable fluency. He no longer responds to fluency challenge with helplessness, and feels good about communication and himself as a communicator. Van Riper (1973) indicated that often treatment is terminated prematurely at this point. This phase is to help the client consolidate his gains, make his new form of more fluent speech and stuttering more automatic, heighten proprioceptive monitoring of his fluent speech, and adjust his self-concept and pragmatic skills to that of a fluent speaker. At this point, individual treatment decreases in favor of group treatment. Self-treatment is encouraged in which the client is responsible for charting, logging, and analyzing behaviors, thoughts, and feelings. Specific procedures include the following:

• *Fluency practice*—To remove any remaining gaps in the speech where disfluency used to occur and to heighten the feeling of fluency, the client is encouraged to shadow (use echo speech) or pantomime the speech of a fluent speaker on television or radio, repeat whole sentences in which he or another speaker demonstrated a disfluency, and to self-talk when alone.

• *Faking*—To heighten control, the client is directed to fake easy, repetitive or prolonged stuttering within fluent speech casually in certain daily situations. Also, the client fakes an occasional disfluency in the original form and follows it with a cancellation or pull-out. Although these procedures strengthen the fluency controls, most clients resist this phase of stabilization.

• *Assessment*—The client must inventory his fluency-related behaviors, thoughts, and feelings on an ongoing and daily basis.

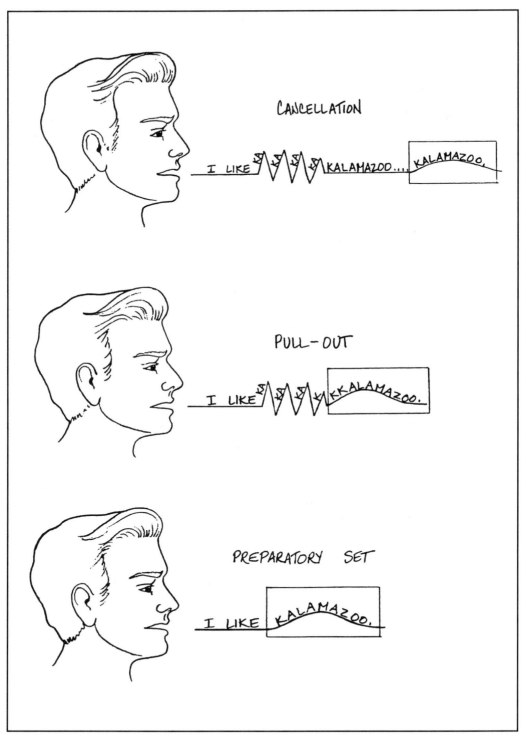

Figure 7.1. Stuttering Modification Techniques. *Note.* From *Stuttering: An Integrated Approach to its Nature and Treatment* (p. 196), by T. J. Peters and B. Guitar, 1991, Baltimore, MD: Williams & Wilkins. Copyright 1991 by Williams & Wilkins. Reprinted with permission.

- *Resistance therapy*—To maintain the methods of fluent stuttering and fluent speaking within the context of varied communicative stresses, conditions are created in which pressures to stutter in the old way are strong and the client must do his utmost to resist them. By seeking out and entering situations that were feared in the past, the client strengthens the new behavioral responses to the old cues (i.e., to the old stimuli that resulted in abnormal responses of avoidance and struggle). Other forms of negative practice that again foster resistance to old habits include teasing, interruption, and suggestion (i.e., during fluent speech in unison, the clinician stutters and the client is expected to remain fluent).

- *Terminating treatment*—Dismissal follows achievement of all objectives and reflects communication independence. Van Riper suggests that cases be followed for 2 years post treatment.

Fluency Shaping

Programmed Therapy for Stuttering in Children and Adults (Ryan, 1974), also referred to as *Programmed Conditioning for Fluency* (Ryan & Van Kirk, 1971), is based on the principles of fluency shaping. Ryan (1974) articulated the premise of fluency intervention as follows:

> Stuttering is viewed as learned behavior. The approach to therapy can be best characterized as behavior modification or contingency management or operant conditioning or programmed instruction. All of these systems draw from the same basic source of learning principles. (p. v)

Further, he indicated that "the new behavioral technology suggests that one should limit himself to behaviors which he can systematically observe, count and manipulate. . . . The major goal in this system is normal fluent speech" (p. v). Ryan and Van Kirk (1971) indicated that the treatment is intended for children and adults who stutter, focuses on slow speech, and can be expected to require between 10 and 20 hours of total treatment time. A summary of the treatment program follows and is outlined in Figure 7.2.

Stuttering Interview (SI)

The prospective client first is given the stuttering interview, which determines whether or not he is a candidate for the fluency program. There are two interview forms (Form A, for young children; Form B, for upper elementary, junior high school, and senior high school students and adults). Requiring about 30 minutes to administer, the interview forms provide a sample of talking in different speech categories including the following: automatic (counting, saying alphabet, singing, reciting poem), echoic (imitating words and sentences), reading, picture naming, speaking alone (clinician leaves room), monologue, speaking with puppet, command speech (client directs clinician), talking with gestures, talking with time pressure, talking with drawing, phonemic difficulty (imitating complex words), responding to and asking questions, speaking on telephone, conversational speech, and observation in natural setting. A stuttering

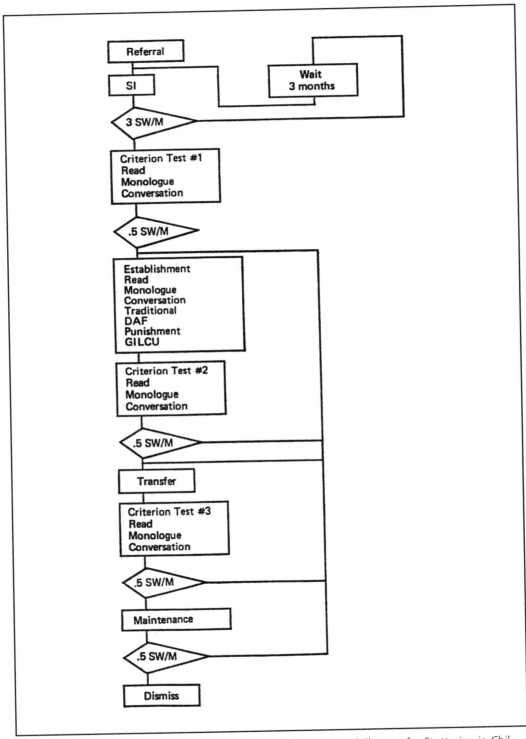

Figure 7.2. Outline of Fluency Training. *Note.* From *Programmed Therapy for Stuttering in Children and Adults* (p. 67), by B. P. Ryan, 1974, Springfield, IL: Charles C. Thomas. Copyright 1974 by Charles C. Thomas. Reprinted with permission.

rate (stuttered words/minute, SW/M) is computed (see "Counting, Charting, Timing" section below). A rate of 3.0 SW/M or more indicates the person is a candidate for fluency training; a rate of less, with few exceptions, indicates the person is not a candidate pending the results of a reevaluation scheduled in 3 months. The stuttering interview is tape-recorded for later analysis.

Counting, Charting, Timing

The program uses two different measurements. First, the stuttering rate (stuttered words/minute, SW/M) is figured by counting only the number of words that demonstrate whole-word repetition, part-word repetition, prolongation, or struggle. Each stuttered word is counted only once, and only according to these four categories. The number of stuttered words is divided by the talk time (e.g., 15 stuttered words/5 minutes = 3 SW/M). Only the client's talking is timed. Secondly, the talking rate (total words read or spoken) is computed in the same way, but only done in the SI and Criterion Tests. Both the stuttering rate (SW/M) and talking rate (total words spoken/minute, WS/M; total words read/minute, WR/M) are charted for visual demonstration and evaluation of treatment.

Criterion Test

If the person is selected for treatment, he is given a criterion test consisting of 5 minutes each of reading, monologue, and conversation. The first criterion test provides his baseline or pretreatment rate of stuttering. If his stuttering rate is more than .5 SW/M in any of the three modes (reading, monologue, or conversation), he is put through an establishment of fluency program in that mode or modes. The criterion test is a measure of stuttering rate (stuttered word output) and talking rate (total word output) before and after each of the three phases of therapy: Establishment, Transfer, and Maintenance. The criterion test is the same each time it is given. Withholding reinforcement, the clinician directs the client to read, monologue, and converse for 5 minutes each. A stuttering rate of more than .5 SW/M indicates that the client needs training or recycling of training; less than .5 SW/M indicates that the client can advance to the next phase.

Establishment

Clinicians can select from among four different establishment programs. Ryan and Van Kirk (1971) originally presented the Gradual Increase in Length and Complexity of Utterance (GILCU) and the Delayed Auditory Feedback (DAF) establishment programs. The more recent work (Ryan, 1974) retained these two but added two others (Programmed Traditional and Punishment). For illustration purposes, only the GILCU and DAF establishment programs will be summarized here. The authors indicated that they are all effective. The client is to complete each mode in the establishment phase, provided he demonstrates a stuttering rate of more than .5 SW/M and is capable of the requisite tasks (reading, monologue, and conversation). Reading is omitted for nonreaders.

GILCU. This program has 54 steps and starts with reading a single word and works up to 5 minutes of fluent conversation in the clinic room. The minimum run time for this program is 90 minutes (Ryan, 1974) and requires no special equipment other than a stopwatch. The client is instructed to read slowly (i.e., verbal stimulus) and is reinstructed to slow down contingent on each stuttered word. The target responses progress from reading fluently one word, to two words, three words and so on to six words; reading fluently one sentence, two sentences, to four sentences; reading fluently for 30 seconds to 5 minutes with 30-second increments; and ultimately advancing to the next mode (i.e., monologue or conversation). In each subsequent mode, the same stimulus and response structure is followed (verbal instruction to engage in monologue or conversation, starting with fluent single words and working up to 5 fluent minutes in that mode). The client receives reinforcement (verbal, social, or redeemable tokens) for each novel fluent response. If the client persists on the same step for either 60 minutes (Ryan & Van Kirk, 1971; or 40 minutes, Ryan, 1974) of training or three sessions, whichever comes first, the client is put on a branching program designed for the clinician to model the correct response. If the client cannot produce correct responses, the clinician models them and gradually reduces the modeling through the branch steps until the client can produce the desired response without the model. Once the model is faded, the client returns to the establishment program. If the client cannot produce the response independently, branch index step #245 is exercised in which the clinician is directed to do the following:

> Anything that seems reasonable to help the person pass that step. Try to respond to the type of error. If he is having trouble on particular words or sounds, do special practice on them. Try different response changes such as whispering, singing, prolonging, loose contacts, sliding, talking softly, etc. May also have to break down response unit into sound or syllable. If all else is unsuccessful, consider using DAF program. (Ryan & Van Kirk, 1971, p. 17)

If the client fails the post-establishment program criterion test (demonstrates a stuttering rate of more than .5 SW/M), he is recycled through the program in that mode or modes with a reduced criterion of performance. Ryan (1974) presented several modifications of the GILCU establishment program.

DAF. This establishment program requires a delayed auditory feedback device with at least six settings (i.e., 250, 200, 150, 100, 50, and 0 milliseconds of delay of auditory feedback [DAF]) and requires a minimum of 111 minutes for completion (Ryan, 1974). The clinician provides brief verbal instructions to speak slowly (i.e., stimulus), appropriate to each of the 27 steps within this program. The client's target response is "super-fluent prolonged speech" (Ryan, 1974, p. 79) within the clinic room. This means that the client speaks slowly, prolonging each sound and word, thus eliminating juncture and significantly reducing inflection. Ryan (1974) provided the following example: "Mmmmmmyyyyyy-nnnnnnaaaaaammmmmmiiiiiissssssssMmmmmmaaaaaarrrrrryyyyyy (My name is Mary)" (p. 75). The client first identifies stuttered words during reading, after which he is instructed to read slowly to accommodate the maximum DAF setting (250 millisecond delay). Within each mode, the rate of prolonged speech (i.e., response) gradually increases by decreasing the amount of delay in five steps by 50 millisecond units (i.e., stimulus; 250, 200, 150, 100, 50, 0 millisecond or no delay). After fading the use of headphones, the client is taken off the DAF machine. This same structure is used in the subsequent modes of monologue and conversation. The client should approximate a "normal" rate of speech, "arbitrarily" defined as 120 words read per minute (i.e., 120 WR/M) and

100 words spoken per minute (i.e., 100 WS/M) in monologue and conversation. If the client persists on the same step for either 60 minutes (Ryan & Van Kirk, 1971; or 40 minutes, Ryan, 1974) of training or three sessions, whichever comes first, the client goes through a branching program similar to that described for GILCU. Essentially, the branching program takes the client back to a previous step with more reinforcement. When the client passes the branch steps, he returns to the regular program step. If he fails the branch steps, a special branch index (i.e., #245) similar to that described for GILCU is available. In it, the client is reinstructed and provided models for a smooth, prolonged speaking pattern. If even it proves to be unsuccessful, the clinician is advised to consider the DAF program. If the client fails Criterion Test #2 (failing to achieve a stuttering rate of less than .5 SW/M), he is recycled through the program using every other step in that mode or modes, after which he again is given Criterion Test #2. A rate control program is available, if necessary, to speed up the rate to "normal." About the DAF establishment program, Ryan (1974) commented:

> The client comes out of this program being able to prolong, count stuttered words, articulate more precisely, and be generally fluent although the client may feel dependent upon the machine. The clinician can help the client avoid addiction to or dependency on the machine by adhering to the rules of the program and getting the client through the steps as quickly as possible. . . . We view the DAF Program as one of the most powerful establishment programs available to us in operant stuttering therapy. Its effect is dramatic and quite consistent across clients. For best results, however, it should be used in a systematic, programmed manner. Simply exposing a client to brief, random periods on the DAF machine may not produce positive changes. (pp. 80, 82)

Transfer

Once fluent speech has been established in the treatment room, the goal of the transfer phase is to use this speech in a wide variety of settings and with many different people. This phase requires between 10 and 15 hours of treatment time (Ryan, 1974). Typically, transfer takes less time if the older children and adults have been engaged in regular home practice during the establishment phase. Most of the transfer steps target the response of fluent conversation, although some target fluent speech in large group settings. As in the establishment program, the clinician instructs the client to speak slowly and fluently. A criterion of between 5 and 10 minutes of fluent speech (0 SW/M) is set for each step. Only social reinforcement is offered during the transfer phase, which contains between 22 and 50 steps, depending on the client's age. The contexts targeted for transfer of fluent speech (Ryan & Van Kirk, 1971) include the following:

- *Physical settings.* Increasing distance from the treatment room with the clinician present.

- *Audiences.* Increasing the size of the audience and distance from the treatment room (e.g., transitioning in small steps from interacting with one other person in the clinic room to giving a speech to 15 people).

- *Classroom.* Increasing the size of the interactive group and the level of communicative demand with and then without the clinician present (e.g., moving from small to large group activity to giving a speech to the class).

- *Home.* Increasing the size of the family audience at home, first with and then without the clinician present.

- *Telephone.* Making phone calls first to the clinician, then with and ultimately without the clinician present to family, friends, relatives, and eventually strangers.

- *Strangers.* Conversing with strangers in settings of increasing distance from the clinic.

- *Work.* Conversing at work with the clinician, friends, co-workers, and people in increasing authority, in small and eventually large groups.

- *Residual.* Addressing any remaining situations in which the client reports continuing difficulty.

- *All day.* Extending gradually the number of hours spent targeting fluent speech, based on a 16-hour day.

These transfer contexts are adjusted to accommodate the individual (e.g., older adults do not interact in the classroom, children do not interact with strangers). Ryan (1974) recommended branching steps if a client fails to achieve 0 SW/M on the transfer phase for three sessions or 40 minutes on one step. Criterion Test #3 is given after completion of the transfer phase. Greater than .5 SW/M requires recycling through the transfer phase. Less than .5 SW/M allows for advancement to the maintenance phase.

Maintenance

Similar to the transfer phase, the goal of the maintenance phase is fluent speech in a wide variety of settings and with many different people. However, the maintenance phase emphasizes the test of time (continuing to use fluent speech over years). Basically, this is done by fading the number of treatment activities until the client can direct the treatment or until he no longer needs it. The client engages in counting the number of stuttered words each day, home practice, and clinic contact for measurement and reinstruction. This phase provides for clinic rechecks, which are faded out over a 2-year period. Three-minute samples of reading, monologue, and conversation are collected at each recheck to evaluate fluency maintenance. A rate above .5 SW/M indicates the need for more training. The clinician inquires about fluency in other environments and additional training in reported difficult situations such as telephone calling or giving speeches may be instituted. Maintenance rechecks are held one time each week for the first month, then held again in 1 month, 3 months, 6 months, and finally in 12 months. When the client can maintain less than .5 SW/M in each mode during the last scheduled rechecks, he is dismissed.

Postscript

At the conclusion of Ryan's (1974) presentation, he reiterated the goal of fluency intervention based upon operant learning theory: "The emphasis is and should be on fluency. All of the data presented in this book make one point; normal fluency is a reasonable goal for people who stutter" (p. 159). Ryan then used the premise that "normal fluency is a realistic, achievable goal" (p. 159) to reflect on the implications for clinicians who stutter. He indicated that such clinicians should be able to carry out most of the procedures, except for those requiring fluent modeling or a fluent conversational partner. He raised the following point:

> It does seem reasonable, however, that a clinician running a successful operant speech fluency program which is helping many clients achieve normal fluency would also want to achieve such fluency. The important point is that the clinician who stutters has the opportunity now, through operant speech fluency programs, to become fluent. The clinician may also choose to continue to stutter. (p. 159)

Two important points in this postscript are Ryan's insistence that we focus on our clients' fluency, and that people who stutter, including clinicians, might do so in part as a consequence of having made a choice. These two points will be visited again as we address my suggestions for intervention methods that integrate stuttering modification and fluency shaping principles. I do not agree, however, that "normal fluency" is necessarily "a realistic, achievable goal." In fact, for some people who stutter, it is not.

CHAPTER SUMMARY

This chapter examined psychotherapeutic considerations, the third and final set of central and guiding intervention assumptions addressed in Unit II. Stuttering modification and fluency shaping approaches were presented as endpoints of a psychotherapeutic continuum. A thorough understanding of these types of treatment, combined with consideration of intrafamily (personal constructs and family systems) and extrafamily (interdisciplinary teaming and multicultural awareness) factors, is necessary for designing effective intervention.

Stuttering modification approaches assume that stuttering results from avoiding or struggling with disfluency and avoiding feared words or situations. These approaches emphasize reduction of fears, negative attitudes, and avoidance behaviors while seeking to modify the form of stuttering. The client is directed in how to study his own communication behaviors, thus becoming familiar with and learning to modify his behavior, feelings, and attitudes. While spontaneous fluency is the ultimate behavioral treatment goal, controlled fluency and acceptable stuttering are considered appropriate goals if higher levels of fluency remain unattainable. Affective treatment goals include reducing the client's stuttering-related fears and avoidances, thereby helping him form a more positive view of himself as a communicator. The clinician offers guidance in how to approach feared words and situations and teaches the client techniques for controlling or canceling instances of stuttering. Treatment sessions are relatively unstructured wherein the clinician and client interact as equal partners in the treatment process. Because stuttering modification techniques address behaviors, feelings, and attitudes, observed changes in speech behavior tend to take longer, but are transferred and maintained more readily. Stuttering modification intervention typically is indicated for persons who avoid speaking, hide or disguise their stuttering, feel poorly about themselves as communicators, perceive a personal penalty as a consequence of stuttering, and demonstrate a more positive response to stuttering modification trial management. Van Riper's program was discussed as an exemplar of stuttering modification. He recommended a thorough diagnosis of the fluency disorder and four sequential phases of treatment: identification, desensitization, modification, and stabilization. Within these four phases, a number of overlapping steps are represented by the acronym MIDVAS: motivation, identification, desensitization, variation/modification, approximation/modification, and stabilization.

Fluency shaping approaches assume that stuttering is learned and apply the principles of behavior modification to fluency treatment. Stuttering first is eliminated in a controlled stimulus environment through operant procedures and then generalized to more natural environments. Spontaneous fluency is the ultimate goal of fluency shaping approaches, although controlled fluency is considered acceptable if higher levels of fluency prove unattainable. Any form of noticeable stuttering, however, is considered to be evidence of program failure. While not addressing directly the feelings and attitudes of the individual client, improvement in these areas may be a by-product of improved fluency. Treatment sessions typically are highly structured and use programmed techniques to improve speech fluency. Behavioral change is relatively rapid; however, transfer and maintenance tend to be more difficult than in stuttering modification techniques. Fluency shaping treatment is indicated typically for persons who stutter openly, do not avoid speaking, perceive annoyance or interference but no personal penalty from stuttering, feel positive about themselves as communicators, and demonstrate a positive response to fluency shaping trial management. Ryan's *Programmed Therapy for Stuttering in Children and Adults* is based upon the principles of fluency shaping and consists of the following: stuttering interview; counting, charting, timing; criterion test; establishment; transfer; and maintenance.

In reality, most intervention is designed by combining stuttering modification and fluency shaping principles, depending on the unique strengths and needs of each client. Combined stuttering modification and fluency shaping treatment typically is indicated for persons who stutter openly but may demonstrate some avoidance; perceive some sense of personal penalty and negative feelings from stuttering, but not to an extreme or handicapping degree; feel relatively positive about themselves as communicators, but wish for personal change; and demonstrate a positive response both to stuttering modification and fluency shaping trial management.

Chapter 7 Study Questions

1. This chapter reviewed psychotherapeutic considerations related to stuttering modification and fluency shaping. How do psychotherapeutic considerations relate to intrafamily considerations (personal constructs and family systems) reviewed in Chapter 5 and to extrafamily considerations (interdisciplinary teaming and multicultural awareness) reviewed in Chapter 6?

2. This chapter familiarized you with the similarities and differences between and implications of stuttering modification and fluency shaping. How do the premises and principles of stuttering modification relate to those of fluency shaping? How would you determine which type of treatment or combined treatment is "right" for a particular client? How might the client's needs vary such that one type of program may be appropriate at one time, and either another type or different type of combined program may be appropriate at another?

3. Van Riper stated that people with more severe stuttering have a more positive prognosis than those with milder stuttering. The reasoning is that those who have more severe symptoms know they have further to go and more to gain; therefore, they are willing to work harder because they expect greater improvement. In other words, those whose stuttering is more severe typically experience greater or more pronounced need. How might this information be useful clinically and how might it impact the clinical process?

4. Motivation is the first of Van Riper's phases in treatment. What does this imply about Van Riper's philosophy of treatment? How does such a philosophy compare and contrast to that of Ryan and to your own philosophy? What avenues are available for a clinician whose client or family is lacking in motivation? Why might a client be lacking in motivation? Does that mean that the client will not or cannot succeed? What is the clinician to do?

5. Stuttering modification treatment approaches require more advanced clinical skills than do fluency shaping approaches, including the ability to provide emotional support, clinical problem solving, and responding to individual client differences. How might this observation be related to the structure or style of intervention designed and provided by clinicians? Considering avenues of professional preparation and lifelong learning, what are some ways in which clinicians might improve their skills in order to provide clients the most effective intervention possible?

6. Stuttering modification approaches address communication-related behaviors, thoughts, feelings, and attitudes directly. Fluency shaping approaches directly address behaviors only, and interpret changes in the affective domain as a by-product of programmed treatment. Why might thoughts, feelings, and attitudes vary among people who stutter and others within their communication system? In working with these people, how would you ensure that your methods for addressing thoughts, feelings, and attitudes are within the domain of your training and ASHA's Scope of Practice? How would you know if you were beginning to function outside of these boundaries? What would you do in that event?

7. We noted that for some people who stutter, spontaneous or controlled fluency is not a realistic or achievable goal. How should a clinician determine whether or not such a goal is realistic for a particular client? How do timing and each individual client's life circumstances impact his potential for fluency improvement? How can we explain clients who failed to make significant improvement during over 50 years of intermittent treatment and then achieve spontaneous or controlled fluency in treatment during their later or senior years?

Unit III

Assessment and Treatment Strategies with People Who Stutter: A Life Span Perspective

Chapter 8
Preschool Children: Assessment and Treatment

Chapter 9
School-Age Children Who Stutter: Assessment and Treatment

Chapter 10
Adolescents, Adults, and Senior Adults Who Stutter: Assessment and Treatment

Chapter 8

Preschool Children: Assessment and Treatment

◆ ◆ ◆ ◆ ◆ ◆ ◆ ◆ ◆ ◆ ◆ ◆ ◆ ◆ ◆ ◆ ◆

General Precepts About Preschool Children   217

Preassessment Procedures   218
    Case History Form   218
    Audio- or Videotape Recording   218
    A Preliminary Phone Call   223

Assessment Procedures   223
    General Considerations   223
    Parent Interview   224
      Preparation   224
      Social Greeting   225
      Questions and Dialogue   225
    Parent–Child Interaction   227
    Child–Clinician Interaction   229
      Speech–Language Sample Without Communicative Pressure   229
      Structured Activities Without Communicative Pressure   233
      Speech–Language Sample and Structured Activities with Communicative Pressure   234
    Trial Management   235
      Fluency Shaping   235
      Stuttering Modification   235

Post-Assessment Procedures   236
    Normal Disfluency and Incipient Stuttering   236
    Speech Analysis   239
      Frequency of Speech Disfluency (i.e., Disfluency Frequency Index)   239
      Type of Speech Disfluency (i.e., Disfluency Type Index)   246
      Molecular Description of Disfluency   247
      Rate of Speech   248
      Secondary Characteristics   250
      Severity Rating   250
      Adaptation and Consistency   251
      Other   256
    Diagnosis   257
    Prognosis and Recommendations   258
    Post-Assessment Parent Interview   259

Treatment   262

> Parent Intervention   263
>
> > Behaviors   264
> >
> > > The parents' aim should be to react to and interact with the child without drawing attention to the disfluency   264
> > >
> > > Encourage the parents to be good listeners   264
> > >
> > > Simplify, soften, and slow the daily speech model to which the child is exposed; Reduce other forms of stimulus bombardment (visual, auditory, emotional) to the extent possible within the communicative environment   264
> > >
> > > Give the child as much fluent talking experience as possible; Try to minimize the amount of experience the child has of talking disfluently   266
> > >
> > > Keep the child from becoming aware of his stuttering   267
> > >
> > > Reduce the pace of activities and overall tension as much as possible   267
> > >
> > > Identify and reduce or eliminate all fluency disrupters   268
> >
> > Thoughts and Feelings   270
>
> Direct Intervention   272
>
> > Goals   273
> >
> > Objectives   273
> >
> > Rationale   273
> >
> > Procedures   274
> >
> > > Establish and transfer fluent speech   274
> > >
> > > Develop resistance to the potential effects of fluency disrupters   277
> > >
> > > Encourage expressions of feeling about communication and oneself as a communicator, as appropriate   278
> > >
> > > Maintain the fluency-inducing effects of treatment   279

Clinical Portrait: Amy Stiles   280

> Selected Background Information   280
>
> Abbreviated Speech–Language Analysis   280
>
> Recommendations   281
>
> Follow-Up   281
>
> Treatment Snapshot   281
>
> Follow-Up and Epilogue   283
>
> Central and Guiding Intervention Assumptions   284
>
> > Intrafamily Considerations   284
> >
> > Extrafamily Considerations   284
> >
> > Psychotherapeutic Considerations   285

Chapter Summary   285

Chapter 8 Study Questions   287

Over the years one of the questions that has haunted most respon-sible clinicians is "How do I tell if a person is 'really' stuttering or if he or she just has a great many normal disfluencies?" It's easy to become enmeshed in this trap. The trap is there only if clinicians turn their attention solely to the speaking behavior of the child and on the basis of it attempt to make a decision. . . . There is no person alive today who can describe exactly the point on the continuum of disfluency at which a child would fall from the category of "speak-ing normally" into that of "stuttering."

(WILLIAMS, 1978, PP. 285–286)

I dentifying and distinguishing between normal disfluencies and incipient stuttering is one of the most vexing challenges facing parents, teachers, and clinicians alike. We will see that making such a distinction involves both quantitative and qualitative considerations, the essence of which requires both careful description and subsequent evaluation. Equally challenging is planning intervention for preschool children who are at risk for stuttering or who are beginning to stutter. Williams (1978) noted that "stuttering" is an evaluative word, not a descriptive one. Description requires observation, analysis, and reporting in molecular form. Because most children demonstrate disfluencies of repetition and prolongation and because children are remarkably heteroge-neous (i.e., highly variable), clinicians often are asked questions about a child's speech such as "Is he normal?" or "Is he stuttering?" and questions about a child's disfluency such as "Is he doing too much of it?" Williams (1978) noted that " 'Too much' is a floating cork on the continuum of disfluency" (p. 285).

In the first unit, we underscored that planning and conducting interven-tion with people who stutter require a broad understanding of stuttering including its onset, development, nature, and etiology and treatment from past and present perspectives. We also established the importance of being able to distinguish stuttering from other fluency disorders. In the second unit, we dis-cussed a variety of central and guiding assumptions (intrafamily, extrafamily, and psychotherapeutic considerations) that are essential for designing and implementing effective intervention. In the present unit, we now will apply the material presented so far and present specific assessment and treatment strategies from a life span perspective with people who stutter. Each chapter concludes with a clinical portrait that spotlights an individual communicator and emphasizes the importance of the central and guiding assumptions. Using this format, we will address preschool children (Chapter 8), school-age children (Chapter 9), and adolescents, adults, and senior adults (Chapter 10). This order was selected partly because "stuttering is constantly developing in complexity the longer the child lives and copes with the problem" (Williams, 1978, p. 285). These groupings, however, were chosen for instructional purposes as well. We will see that in reality, the procedures for a person in one group frequently over-lap with those of another.

In this chapter, we will discuss how to structure the communication assessment of a preschool child and the family, what to look for, and how to design different methods for intervention with the child and significant others. In doing so, we will emphasize the following major points:

- There is a fine and invisible line between normal disfluency and incipient stuttering. Identifying this line and making such a distinction requires analysis of the child's behaviors, thoughts, and feelings, and a professional judgment on the part of the clinician.

- Intervention with preschool children and their families requires understanding of the communication environment, full support and involvement of all members within the communication system, and identification and elimination of potential precipitating and/or perpetuating factors.

GENERAL PRECEPTS ABOUT PRESCHOOL CHILDREN

All people are different and present unique opportunities and challenges. Taking a bird's eye perspective initially creates a general view of a territory. Moving in for a closer look brings uniqueness and individuality into focus. We will do this now with preschool children and subsequently with the other populations noted. The process of moving from a molar to more molecular perspective will prepare us for the assessment and treatment decisions that lie ahead.

The following represent general considerations of preschool children as a group. As always, individual members often demonstrate different or contrasting patterns. Hence, preschool children, as do all groups of people, represent a heterogeneous category within which individual differences are valued and nurtured.

- *The preschool period is a time of intense development, both quantitatively and qualitatively.* Speech fluency and disfluency vary within and across children as do their relative awareness of and observed frustration over such fluctuation. Maintaining the child's positive attitude toward communication is a critical factor in the prevention of stuttering.

- *Play and fun represent the language of childhood.* Too often, clinicians emphasize the medium of questions and questioning to the near exclusion of play, thus turning a potentially fun, interactive opportunity into an interrogation. More will be said later about stages of play. When in doubt, ask less and play and observe more.

- *Children vary in their apprehension of the clinical setting.* Haynes et al. (1992) noted that such fear results from one or more of the following: inadequate preparation for the assessment or treatment appointment; uncertainty over what will be done to or with the child by the clinician; traumatic memories of visits to dentists, physicians, and other professionals; contagious anxieties of parents; stress and conflicts recalled from past listener reactions to speech impairments. Clinicians must be mindful of children's fears, thus giving them a responsible role and engaging them in the play interaction.

- *While vulnerable in their tendency to do whatever they are told, children are affectively insightful.* Occasionally, children will mirror the clinician's (or other adult's) emotions before either is keenly aware of them. This means that clinicians should be sincerely positive about working with young children (children rapidly perceive disinterest or lack of confidence), use absolute honesty in all interactions (always keep your promise for activities, rewards, and punishments), maintain appropriate complexity of language presented to children; and provide but limit choices offered to children (limit choices for which the alternatives conflict with the clinical goals). With respect to choices presented, for example, do not ask if the child would like to go with you, do this activity, or other such questions. Children invariably will say, "No." The questions imply that a promise will be kept. When the child's refusal, which was invited, is not accepted, the implied promise is broken. It is more effective to provide choices for which the alternatives are acceptable. The clinician might ask, "Do you want to play here *or* here?" or "Which do you want to do first, activity X *or* Y?"

• *People of all ages have a story to tell* (Shapiro, in press). Preschool children are no exception. While children may lack the relative cognitive insight to analyze a problem objectively (Haynes et al., 1992), children's and adults' stories differ more on the basis of subject matter than in the depth of feeling or inherent quality (Johnson, Sickels, & Sayers, 1970). Clinicians have the responsibility to create opportunities for children to tell their story and thereby the privilege to learn from them and to see again only as children do.

PREASSESSMENT PROCEDURES

Case History Form

When a preschool child is referred for a communication evaluation, a case history form, similar to that represented in Figure 8.1, is sent to the primary care provider (parents, relative, guardian) in advance of the scheduled appointment. (As implied here and discussed in Chapter 5, the person or persons serving as the child's primary care provider may vary across families. While remaining sensitive to individual families, I use the term "parents" generically to refer to any person serving in this responsible role.) The information provided informs the clinician about the child's developmental and medical history; family structure; communication strengths and limitations; and onset, development, and current perceptions regarding the presenting communication problem. This information also gives the clinician an indication of questions that need to be asked during the parent interview and previous service providers that may need to be contacted for related information.

Audio- or Videotape Recording

When possible, it is helpful to receive a tape recording (audio or video) of the child interacting with his family or other members of the household. This tape serves a variety of functions. First, it reflects the communication and interpersonal dynamics of the members of the child's family. Furthermore, it reveals the nature of the communication concern at the time it was expressed. This is particularly important when there is a lapse between the initial referral and the time of the evaluation. We noted previously that speech fluency of preschool

(*text continues on p. 223*)

Please complete this form as completely as possible. Feel free to add information on the back or on additional sheets.

Person completing this form: _____ Date: _____

Identifying Information

Child's name: _____ Date of birth: _____

Social Security #: _____Insurance/Medicaid #: _____

Address: _____

Telephone #: _____ Gender: _____ Race: _____

Child's physician: _____

Address/Phone: _____

In case of emergency, contact: _____

Address/Phone: _____

Family Information

Mother's name: _____ Age: _____

Occupation/Employer: _____ Education: _____

Father's name: _____ Age: _____

Occupation/Employer: _____ Education: _____

If address of either parent is different from that of the child, please indicate: _____

_____

Does the child live with anyone other than the parent/parents? If *yes,* indicate name of person(s) and relationship to child. Include names and ages of brothers and sisters.

_____

_____

Referral/Communication Information

Who referred you to this clinic? _____

Reason for referral: _____

Statement of the child's problem, as you see it: _____

_____

_____

What do you believe caused the child's problem? _____

_____

When was the child's problem first noticed?_____ By whom? _____

(continues)

Figure 8.1. Case History Form for Children.

How has the child's problem changed since it was first noticed? _____

How does this problem affect the child (family/social interactions, school, etc.)?
_____

Have you ever questioned the child's ability to hear normally? If *yes,* explain.
_____

List the dates, locations, and results of previous speech–language and/or hearing evaluations or treatment.
_____

Is the child receiving special services now? If *yes,* where and what type?
_____

Describe any other speech, language, and/or hearing problems in the family:
_____

Birth/Medical History

Were there any problems during pregnancy, labor, or delivery? If *yes,* please explain:
_____

Length of pregnancy: _____ Birth weight: _____

Were there any problems after birth? _____

Did the baby leave the hospital with the mother? If *no,* please explain.
_____

Health History

Has the child had (check appropriate items):

☐ German Measles	☐ Mumps	☐ Bronchitis
☐ High fever	☐ Convulsions	☐ Chicken Pox
☐ Allergies	☐ Ear infections	☐ Myringotomy
☐ Scarlet Fever	☐ Influenza	☐ Tonsillitis
☐ Frequent colds	☐ Tonsillectomy	☐ Adenoidectomy

Describe any other conditions, illnesses, or accidents. Was medical attention necessary?
_____

Is the child taking any medication? If *yes,* please specify:
_____

(continues)

Figure 8.1. Continued.

Developmental History

At what age did the child: babble/coo?_____ say single words?_____ combine words?_____

How does the child communicate most (gesturing, talking, both)?_____

Does the child make sounds correctly? If *no,* which are incorrect?_____

_____

Describe any recent changes in the child's speech:

_____

Have there been any significant events that may have related to the changes in the child's speech? If *yes,* please specify:

_____

How well is your child understood by others? _____

Do you have any concern about the child's speech–language development?

_____

At what age did the child: sit alone?_____ crawl?_____ walk?_____ toilet train?_____

drink from cup?_____ dress him/herself?_____

Does the child tend to favor the right or left hand? _____

Compared to other children of the same age, describe the child's coordination (talking, sitting, standing, running, using hands, etc.): _____

_____

_____

Do you have any concern about the child's motor or physical development?

_____

Educational History

Child's present school: _____ Grade: _____

Preschool/Kindergarten experiences? If *yes,* where?_____

If *no,* who provides/provided care during the day?_____

Describe the child's behavior and performance at school: _____

_____

_____

Does the child receive any special services? If *yes,* please explain:

_____

_____

Do you have any concern about the child's ability to learn? If *yes,* please explain:

_____

_____

(continues)

Figure 8.1. Continued.

Behavioral Information

Do you have any concern about the child's behavior? If *yes,* please explain:

_____

_____

How does the child get along with others (children, adults)?

_____

_____

With whom does the child prefer to play?_____

Additional Questions/Family Observations

What do you hope to accomplish as a result of the communication evaluation?

_____

_____

What questions and concerns would you like to see addressed?

_____

_____

How does the child get along with siblings? _____

Describe the child's areas of strength and special interests or hobbies:

_____

_____

_____

Please provide any other information that you feel might be helpful in evaluating the child's communication skills:

_____

_____

_____

Permissions

In order to help the child, it may be appropriate to send reports to or to contact other agencies or professional practitioners. If we determine this is necessary, we need your permission to do so. Please indicate your permission by signing below.

I authorize and request (clinic name and address) to obtain and/or exchange pertinent medical/educational/communication information. It is understood that all information about the client and the family will be kept strictly confidential.

Name: _____

Signature: _____

Relationship to child: _____

Date: _____

Thank you for taking the time to complete this form. We look forward to working with the child, with you, and with others in the child's family.

Figure 8.1. Continued.

children often fluctuates over time. We will note that clinicians need to determine how representative the child's speech at the time of the evaluation is of his usual speaking behavior. The tape provides a point of comparison with the speech sampled during the evaluation. Finally, the tape provides a sample of the child's speech in a different setting and with different people when compared with that collected at the evaluation.

A Preliminary Phone Call

A phone call to the child's parents (i.e., primary care providers) before the evaluation enables the clinician to prepare the family for the evaluation process. Furthermore, the clinician can address the family's preliminary questions and help them prepare the child for the evaluation itself. This might involve conveying to the child what will transpire (e.g., the clinicians are friendly people who will talk and play with you) and encouraging him to bring several familiar items (such as toys, books, photographs, or other favorite objects) to share with the clinician. Not knowing what to expect and then encountering unfamiliar people in an unfamiliar setting at the evaluation can be potentially frightening for a young child. This fear can be prevented with relatively little effort. In my experience, preparing the family and the child for the evaluation truly has been "an ounce of prevention" resulting in "a pound of cure."

There is yet another benefit of a preliminary phone call to the family that cannot be minimized. Specifically, it is that the clinician conveys to the parents that she cares, is willing and able to help, and that the communicative welfare of the child and the family is important. These benefits are consistent with one of the clinician's major responsibilities as I see it—to help the person who stutters (or is at risk for stuttering) and the family feel realistically better and more optimistic about themselves as communicators and their communication world and future as a result of having interacted with the clinician. This results from serving as a readily available resource of positive support and knowledge, shared planning and helping to achieve fluency success, and conveying and demonstrating a sincere belief in the individual's and the family's potential for communication improvement. In other words, conveying by word and deed that the client and family have a comrade in you, the clinician, is a remarkably empowering experience for our clients. Creating such experiences indeed is our responsibility. The phone call is a relatively small effort that yields potentially large and unfolding benefits. In support of such efforts, Haynes et al. (1992) noted that "the very first contact with a client—the manner in which he/she is treated during a clinical examination—is a crucial determining factor in response to therapy" (p. 26).

ASSESSMENT PROCEDURES

General Considerations

The first face-to-face contact the clinician has with the family of the preschool child often is at the scheduled appointment for the diagnostic evaluation. The parent interview generally precedes a direct observation of parent–child interaction. These two components, however, occasionally are reversed as indicated by the needs of the child. When the child can be separated readily from the parent and when there is a clinician or other responsible adult to interact with the child during the interview, the interview typically is held first. When these two conditions are not present, then the parent–child interaction may be held first to facilitate separation, as will be seen. An important point, however, is that the preschool child should not be present during the initial interview if possible because of two mutually exclusive needs: to talk absolutely candidly with the family members who are present, and to prevent the child from becoming increasingly aware of the observed concern.

To achieve both of these needs, the child must not be present during the interview. Where separation remains impossible, however, I have held parent interviews in the same room with a child who is actively engaged with another child or adult. This scenario is workable but not preferred because both the parents and clinician must attend to the other interaction, thus detracting at least some attention and energy from the interview itself. Peters and Guitar (1991) reminded, however, not to force the child to separate. They advised that it is more important to provide the child a positive association with the treatment experience, even if we are unable to collect all the information we would like. If the child will not separate, they suggested that the clinician talk with the parents about general things in one part of the room while the child plays with toys in another. A short while later, the clinician might suggest moving to an adjacent room with the doors open, leaving the child in view to play with the toys. Sometimes if all must move together, the child will become bored and will gravitate to the toys that are in sight in the original room. Peters and Guitar (1991) noted, and I concur, that children rarely have more than a momentary difficulty separating from the parents.

What follows are general guidelines for conducting a communication evaluation with a preschool child and the family. The proceedings should be tape-recorded for analysis and subsequent retrieval. Videotape recording equipment provides an excellent clinical tool and is increasingly available at reduced cost. I have often said that if I were dropped on an inaccessible island and could bring with me only one diagnostic or clinical tool, I would chose a videotape recording camera, videotape, and monitor. Combined with a clinician's trained eyes and ears and an empathic heart, video equipment proves invaluable. Valuable, but less preferred, is audiotape recording equipment, which cannot capture the visual aspect of communication and its disorders, specifically stuttering. The guidelines that follow should be adjusted as indicated by the child, family, clinician, and setting.

Parent Interview

Preparation

Based on the case history form, initial tape recording, and preliminary phone call, I develop questions that I want to pursue. Typically, I outline for myself in telegraphic form information that I want to receive and provide. In addition, I make a bold reminder to myself to LISTEN. Haynes et al. (1992) provided an excellent chapter on interviewing "do's and don'ts" and methods of improving interviewing skills. I recommend this chapter to all clinicians. In addition to many other valuable suggestions, they warn clinicians to avoid talking too much and providing information too soon. More will be said about this when we address clinician competencies (Chapter 11) and professional preparation and lifelong learning (Chapter 12).

Social Greeting

The initial interview typically is held with the child's parent or parents. Deliberately, I begin with a social comment and positive greeting. Too often, the communication problem becomes the immediate focus rather than the people with whom we are interacting. A social greeting enables clinicians and clients to begin the journey as co-equal participants in a shared process, and helps to establish a social and personal foundation. Before we can respect and respond to each other's role and responsibility as clients or clinicians within the clinical process, we first must value each other as people. The importance of establishing positive rapport cannot be overstated.

Questions and Dialogue

The parent interview consists of many direct and open-ended questions. Their purpose is not to limit the exchange, but rather to provide focus within a flexible, dynamic context. The exchange should be inquiring, supportive, and conversational. After the necessary permission forms are signed and after providing a general orientation as to the assessment process, various areas are probed. These will be addressed now.

Typically, the first questions I ask the parents are why they came to meet with us, and what they hope to accomplish as a result of our meeting. Some parents are taken aback by such questions because they may have become accustomed to professionals' immediate focus on "the problem." The answers to these questions help provide me with an idea of what the parents perceive as their own and the child's needs and objectives, each of which I respond to deliberately before the conclusion of the evaluation. This is essential for at least two reasons. First, by inviting their objectives for the meeting, I am giving the parents an active role in the process from its outset. Furthermore, I do not want to presume that I understand their needs before I inquire about them. Surely, our training and experience help us predict commonalities among families of preschool children who are at risk for stuttering. However, let us not forget that all people and families are different. Asking what their needs are helps also to communicate our interest to understand the child as an individual and the family as a unique communication system. Secondly, we should not assume that the parents are concerned about stuttering. Even if they are, we cannot assume that what the clinician means by "stuttering" is what the parents mean by "stuttering." I have worked with some parents who initially expressed concern over "stuttering," only to discover that their use of the term was a global reference to communication disorders (such as articulation, language, or other area of impairment).

Asking parents the questions noted earlier (why they came and what they hope to accomplish) provides an opportunity for them to begin to explain the nature of their concern. If they haven't already spoken about their concern, I ask for them to discuss the nature of their concern. Whatever word or words they use to describe their concern (e.g., stuttering, stammering, freezing, or other terms), I ask them to elaborate on what they mean when they use that word. Generally I do not use the term stuttering until they do because, as noted earlier, the term is evaluative and is relatively useless without description and qualification. Once they have described their concern, I ask them to discuss, to the best of their memory, the onset and development of the problem they have just characterized. I am interested to know how, when, and by whom the problem was first noticed and how the speech patterns might have changed since the disfluency was first detected (e.g., amount and type of disfluency, remissions, or conditions of predictable fluency or disfluency). Were there any special events in the child's life (e.g., birth of a sibling, death of a relative, language or cognitive leaps, or family tension) that coincided with the beginning of disfluency?

Once the parents have described the communication problem and the surrounding events further, I ask them to describe a typical daily routine. In doing so, I am looking for a description of the family structure and the family's communication interaction. This helps me begin to identify sources of potential communicative pressure at home (e.g., where the child might feel he needs to say things in a hurry so as not to be interrupted, or where the child might be directed not to speak because of seemingly more important events), which will assist me in making specific recommendations later. Williams (1978) noted that it is essential to determine the general atmosphere of pace and tension within a family, which might contribute to the child's development of disfluency. It is equally important, he observed, to determine if the child receives special consideration when he is disfluent that he does not receive when he is fluent. For example, do the parents attend to what he says, limit interruptions, and excuse him for misbehaving only when he is disfluent? In either case (excessive rush and tension contributing to disfluency or overcompensation as a consequence of disfluency), disfluency is being inadvertently precipitated or perpetuated.

Other areas probed include observed patterns (e.g., specific words, situations, people, times of day, or activities) in which the speech fluency is noticeably better or worse. Additionally, how does the child react to the communication context, when fluent and disfluent? How do the other family members react to the child when he is fluent and disfluent? What have the family members done to try to help the child when he is experiencing disfluency and how has the child responded to such efforts? I inquire what the parents believe to be the "cause" of the disfluency. This helps me understand their causal assumptions, which may impact their participation in and confidence regarding the clinical process. Williams (1978) stressed the significance of the language used by the parents to describe why the child is disfluent. Specifically, do they reflect a belief that the disfluency is a symptom of something wrong within the child, or a response by the child to environmental conditions? Furthermore, what is the parents' outlook on the child's communication future? Do they seem more concerned about how the child is functioning and reacting today, or are they more concerned about how the disfluency might impact his life as he gets older? Has the child received any previous communication assessments or intervention?

I ask about whether any other family members have experienced speech–language problems or treatment, all the while exploring feelings and welcoming questions. A significant area to address is any observed awareness or frustration on the part of the child of fluency breakdown. Particularly significant is how the awareness develops and moves from potential neutrality to negativity and frustration. The parent interview itself may take a variety of directions depending on the needs of the parents or child, information presently available, causal assumptions held by and level of participation of the parents, and other factors.

During the parent interview and throughout the assessment process, many other areas are probed. The essential purpose is to gain an understanding of the child's and the family's communication past and present in order to begin to project to the future. Additional areas of inquiry might include birth and developmental history; speech–language, motor, and social development; family history and interactive patterns; social and emotional temperament; and anxiety situational hierarchy (Conture, 1990b; Peters & Guitar, 1991).

Parent–Child Interaction

Valuable information is obtained from observing one or more parents interacting directly with the preschool child. In a university-based speech and hearing center, we observe this directly through a one-way observation window. Where such a facility is not available, the parents and child may interact while the clinician in the same room appears to be busily engaged in some other activity. All the while, however, in fact she is listening intently to the interaction. When limitations preclude such an observation, the clinician may observe the parents and child before the assessment begins, perhaps in the waiting area or in the nearby hallway. In any case, observing the interaction provides a sample of the child's speech behavior with a familiar person (e.g., parents), which then can be compared with that collected with an unfamiliar person (e.g., clinician). Typically, the parents are the persons with whom the child feels most comfortable. Occasionally, however, the relationship between the child and the parents is strained, resulting in increased disfluency being observed in the child's speech.

It is instructive to observe how the child and parents interact with and react to each other. Garrard (1990–1991) presented a useful series of observation worksheets addressing nonvocal and vocal behaviors of the child and parents in addition to the language facilitation strategies provided by the parents. Observed nonvocal child behaviors included attention span, eye contact and joint focus with the conversation partner, receptive language, communication intentions, facial expressions, body movements, cooperative behavior, turn taking, activity initiation, bids for attention, and social play, in addition to vocal behaviors collected during speech–language sampling (e.g., language fluency). Nonvocal parental behaviors included involving the child in play, rapport, warmth and approval, facial expressions, physical proximity, nonvocal responsiveness, pause time, power balance, following child's interests, and nonvocal reinforcement. Vocal parental behaviors included utterance length, appropriateness of prosody, speech clarity, expansions and extensions, topic comments and shifts, repetitions of child's utterance, reference training (e.g., verbalizing child actions and parent actions, labeling objects and events), verbal cues and prompts for child to take a vocal turn, praise, child content, acknowledgment of child interests, confirmation of child comment, chaining to child responses, questions, and types of responses to child's communicative attempts. Parental language facilitation strategies included natural, positive reinforcement to the child's response (verbal—"good," "great," "super;" physical—a smile, pat, hug, clap; or tangible—giving toy, drink, food); physical proximity (parent shares play in close proximity or on general plane with child's); imitations or repetitions of child's words or attempts; expansions and extensions (conversational chaining by adding semantic content to child's utterance); semantic appropriateness (content and vocabulary) for the child; verbal cues or prompts; pausing after conversational turns to encourage turn taking; speech clarity (distinctness, loudness, pronunciation); and warm approval (affection and approval of child through facial or body expressions and confirming verbal responses). Aspects of vocal and nonvocal interaction influence the nature of the exchange between the child and his parents. Observing these and other factors will prove enlightening regarding how language is used and facilitated and how communication including speech fluency is nurtured.

I remember observing a conversational interaction between a father who was a minister and his son who had just turned 3 years old. The father initiated and maintained a number of topics that were all within an abstract, conceptual domain. For example, he spoke of devotion, resurrection, faith, divinity, heaven, and damnation, among others. The boy spoke very little, and responded infrequently to the father's questions of increasing verbal and emotional intensity. When he did speak, the boy's speech was characterized by significantly disfluent speech. Before the end of the assessment, during the period of trial management (a period for using different treatment strategies to determine their relative effectiveness with the child), I explained, demonstrated, and then coached the father in how he might interact with his son about the very same topics while reducing the excessive demand being placed on the boy's developing language, speech fluency, and other aspects of communication. We began with having the boy draw his own picture of the Lord at home, which is called heaven. An artist's representation of Jesus was used to make more concrete the boy's understanding of Jesus as the son of the Lord. Other concepts were discussed with direct connection to concrete objects including birth, death, following rules, and being nice to other people.

Additionally, I illustrated for the father how he can encourage his son to become a more active participant in the conversation. We discussed different types of questions, turn-taking, modeling, and expansion, among other topics. The father indicated that he appreciated my acceptance of the content as important to his family and my willingness to help him convey it more understandably to his son. Over the course of working with the father on three separate occasions focusing on pragmatic language skills with his young son and after subsequent phone contact with the father, the boy's fluency improved significantly, as did the father's interactional skills with his son. The father indicated that what he learned in treatment helped him interact more effectively with other young children in the Sunday School program. The point I want to emphasize is that by directly observing the child interacting with the parent, the clinician gets an idea of the interaction styles, parity of turn taking, and appropriateness of the language model presented to the child. Moreover, the clinician begins to determine how conducive the parent–child interaction is for facilitating the child's speech fluency. Furthermore, the clinician learns about factors that might be addressed with the parents to help them know what they can do to reduce the child's speech disfluency and to facilitate fluency.

Child–Clinician Interaction

Typically, one clinician enters the assessment session and excuses the parents who observe the remaining session if observation facilities are available. If a clinician interacted with the child during the parent interview, it is helpful if that same clinician enters the session now. Familiarity with the clinician from earlier play interaction often facilitates separation. After collecting a speech–language sample between the child and one clinician, it is useful to have a second clinician or other adult enter the assessment session. Doing so enables a comparison of the child's speech across different listener contexts and settings (at home via tape recording, with the parents during the assessment, with one unfamiliar adult, with two or more unfamiliar adults). It is quite possible that limitations unique to the setting might preclude using a second clinician or other adult.

The child–clinician interaction enables the clinician to observe directly the child's fluency and disfluency and the extent to which both are modifiable. Furthermore, the interaction results in a speech–language sample that is as broad based as possible allowing for comparison within and between the various components (e.g., speech sample provided via tape recording, parent–child interaction, and those discussed herein). In other words, I am looking to sample the child's speech fluency control across possible speaking contexts that vary in degree of communicative challenge from least (e.g., uninterrupted conversation) to most (e.g., deliberate interruption and abrupt topic shifts). While the specific speaking tasks and their sequence may vary, typically they include a speech–language sample and structured activities with and without communicative pressure.

Speech–Language Sample Without Communicative Pressure

To gain rapport with the child, I begin with speech–language sampling without communicative pressure. Most clinicians are familiar with procedures for collecting a language sample with a child. In this case, the sample should be of no less than 5-minute duration of the child's talking (approximately 300 words), which might take 10 to 15 minutes of real time. Conture (1990b, 1997) noted that the sample size should be sufficient to permit averaging across several 100-word samples. In most cases, a sample of 300 words or more is adequate and collected with ease. However, for a client who stutters severely, the length of time he would take to produce 300 words may be counterproductive to the goals of the evaluation. In such cases, a sample of between 50 and 100 words may be sufficient, being supplemented at the beginning of scheduled treatment by an additional sample from a larger corpus. The clinician attempts to be minimally directive, both playing and talking with the child whose lead is followed. Objects, toys, and pictures are introduced gradually, but only as needed. Too often, the objects inhibit rather than enhance the conversation between the child and the clinician. The clinician deliberately creates opportunities to converse about events past, present, and future and for the child to demonstrate language (syntactic, semantic, pragmatic, and phonologic) competence. Excellent suggestions are available for facilitating spontaneous talking with young children (Fey, 1986; Garrard, 1990–1991; Haynes et al., 1992). Clinicians need to remember the "child" in childhood language, and that play is a natural context for interacting with children.

Occasionally, however, some children, particularly those who are reluctant to separate from their parents, will not talk with a clinician. Student clinicians have nightmares in anticipation of just such a situation. While a child can learn language with his mouth closed (while refusing to speak) during language intervention, a child's speech fluency cannot be determined under the same circumstances. All is not lost, however. Van Riper (1972) represented the interaction between a clinician and child as an evolving developmental process from solo play, through tangential play and intersecting play, to cooperative play (see Figure 8.2). When a clinician understands the relative stages of play, performance expectations are adjusted accordingly and the child's needs remain the clinician's focus. Van Riper (1972) noted that most adults, including parents, clinicians, and other authority figures, often attempt to get a child to speak by asking questions. Questions are demands, however, subordinating the child to the authority of the questioner who is in control. Similarly, such question-asking techniques in the confines of the treatment room are on the low end of the continuum of communicative naturalness (Fey, 1986), lacking in ecological validity (Muma, 1978), and result in "impoverished samples" (Van Riper, 1972). Furthermore, eliciting speech by questions more likely resembles an interrogation than a meaningful conversation. In contrast, Van Riper (1972) suggested, particularly with reticent children, the following:

> How then should one begin? We suggest that you simply greet the child, then do some simple self-talk, commenting on what you are doing, or perceiving, and with plenty of moments of comfortable silence interspersed, until you have him playing with his box of toys. And then, in the role of adult playmate, you can play with those in your box. Silently at first. No question. No demands. Solo play!
>
> Once the child is comfortable in this activity, you should begin to put some self-talk into your own solo play; first noises (those of trucks, animals, etc.), then single words, then short phrases and simple sentences. All of these refer to what you are experiencing at the moment. Usually the child will begin to follow suit. His noises, his self-talk, begin to flow. Next you should shift to contact play very gradually. Let your toy truck occasionally touch his fire-engine, or help him find a block, or put another one on his toppling pile, or straighten it up a bit so he can make it higher. When you feel the time is ripe in this tangential contact play, begin to accompany it with some noises or commentary, using parallel talking, telling him what he is doing, perceiving, or feeling, again making sure that you have more silence than speech.
>
> From tangential play, you can often proceed rapidly to intersecting play in which your activity becomes a part of his. (Let your truck go over the bridge he has built or feed your doll or toy dog a piece of the play fruit he has put on the playhouse table.) Verbalize what you are doing. Next, seek to achieve cooperative play, assisting him to do the things he is doing. (Have your truck bring to him the blocks he needs to build his tower.) Usually by this time the child is speaking very easily and often copiously, your own verbalizations being primarily confined to reflecting what he has said. From this point onward, the communication can proceed fairly normally and naturally. (pp. 109–110)

Clinicians are encouraged to apply their understanding of the stages of play to procedures that facilitate more spontaneous talking among reticent preschool children. The purpose is to reduce the communicative demand (i.e., pressure) placed upon the child while encouraging verbal exchange in a rela-

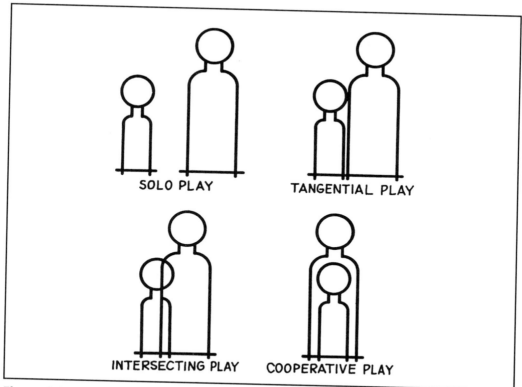

Figure 8.2. Diagram of Interaction Between Clinician and Child. *Note.* From *Speech Correction: Principles and Methods* (5th ed.) (p. 109), by C. Van Riper, 1972, Englewood Cliffs, NJ: Prentice-Hall. Copyright 1972 by Allyn & Bacon. Reprinted with permission.

tively natural context. I remember being invited to do a fluency evaluation of Dawn, a little girl who was 4 years old, at a local health department. I had noticed Dawn's tension as she had been eyeing me, a bearded man wearing a tie. Her parents were not present and the nurse introduced me to her as DOCTOR Shapiro. At this, her tension immediately and visibly turned to panic as, no doubt, she imagined the 6-foot-long syringe or tongue depressor being concealed in my pocket and which she was about to experience. Why else would the nurse have introduced me to her, and then quickly left? Well, the stages of play are useful for a reticent child, but not for one paralyzed in fear. I remember getting Dawn to the soda machine and learning by head nod that she liked orange soda. With permission, I bought the two of us orange sodas and walked out to the parking lot where we sat on the curb and drank soda. I talked, relieving her fear by clarifying that I was not a medical doctor and that my sole purposes were to talk and play with her. While she seemed to believe me (her crying subsided enough to drink soda), she did not want to reenter the building with me where previously she had been treated medically. So we sat on the curb and completed our evaluation as Dawn consumed her orange soda.

In addition to assessing the child's speech behavior, we need to assess the relative valence (positive, neutral, or negative) of his expressions of feelings and attitudes about communication and his communication skills. Most preschool children talk ceaselessly during all waking moments. Of particular concern, however, is when a preschool child develops an overall communication reticence, saying "I don't know," "I can't say that," or just "I can't." I remember another child, Andrew, who was 3 years, 6 months old, who stuttered severely and only spoke when he concealed his face behind his hands, a book, paper, or other object. Assessing the feelings and attitudes of the preschooler without creating awareness on the part of the child regarding concern over speech fluency indeed is a challenge for clinicians. This is done by asking the parents about the child's feelings and attitudes during the parent interview, by observing during the parent–child interaction, and by reviewing the audiotape or videotape recordings made before and during the assessment session. Significant indicators include the child's willingness to talk, amount of eye contact, facial expressions, and nonverbal body language (Guitar & Peters, 1980), all of which might be influenced by multicultural factors. Other indicators include overall degree of tension, speaking volume and rate, spontaneity of response, eye movement, voice quality and pitch, and relative increase or decrease in frequency of total disfluency or of any one disfluency type (Williams, 1978). Another method is probing by the clinician during the child–clinician interaction.

Some of the most useful and sensitive suggestions for talking with children about talking were presented by Williams (1971, 1983). Because these suggestions address more directly school-age children and because school-age children's feelings and attitudes are more frequently affected by the experience of stuttering, my discussion of these suggestions will be reserved for Chapter 9. Peters and Guitar (1991) noted that the feelings and attitudes of the preschool child about speech disfluency range from apparent unawareness of disfluency, to occasional awareness although rarely bothered, to awareness and frustration, to significant awareness combined with frustration and fear. If it is clear that the child is aware of or frustrated about his disfluency, then I will probe the child's feelings further (and my directness will be in direct proportion to the child's observed or expressed awareness).

For example, Tony was a 4-year-old boy who demonstrated noticeable disfluency with concomitant facial, neck, and body tension, yet no reluctance to initiate or respond to a conversational turn. I said to him, "You know, Tony, sometimes when I am tired or get in a hurry, it is a little hard for me to talk." After a brief silence, he offered, "You know, me too! Me too!" I followed up with, "How does that make you feel?" To this, he said, "It makes me feel embarrassed." We talked about his feelings, about how everyone is good at things and has to work at others, and about how people feel when we try our best at things that are difficult to us that seem easy to others. Significantly, Tony related to and extended the probe I offered. He could have not responded during the silence (silence is an essential part of a probe); he could have denied it (offering expressions such as, "Not me. No. That never happens to me."); or he could have been noncommittal ("So?" or "Big deal."). But Tony's response left no doubt regarding his degree of awareness and developing frustration. On the basis of information available from the sources noted earlier and particularly from observing Tony's active participation as a conversational partner, it did not appear that fear or negativity had entered his view of himself as a communicator.

Peters and Guitar (1991) suggested other probes to determine a preschool child's awareness about disfluency. They suggested asking the child if he knows why he has come to see the clinicians, to which some children will be noncommittal, while others might respond forthrightly, "Because I don't talk right." They view this interaction as a possible opportunity to discuss stuttering further and to convey to the child both that he is not alone and that others who also "get stuck on words" have been helped. They also suggested that it might help a child to talk about his stuttering by first telling him about another child who stutters—while using appropriate vocabulary ("getting stuck" or "having trouble on words"). If the child conveys disinterest in talking about stuttering, the clinician might drop the subject initially. Later, the clinician might insert some normal sounding disfluencies in her own speech and first offer a self-comment that sometimes she has trouble getting words out, and later ask the child if he ever has trouble like this. Again, the clinician interprets the child's relative willingness to discuss stuttering and whether or not an opportunity exists to discuss it further. Peters and Guitar (1991) summarized that these and other procedures aimed at assessing and talking with the child about his communication-related feelings and attitudes are intended "(a) to see if the child is accepting of himself and his disfluencies enough to discuss them and (b) to indicate to the child that he is not alone with the problem and, moreover, that we may be able to help him" (p. 165).

Structured Activities Without Communicative Pressure

Once I have a rich conversational speech–language sample, I engage the preschool child in several structured activities that yield elicited verbal responses for analysis. Some clinicians may prefer to begin with structured activities. Generally, I find beginning with conversational interaction to be more successful in building rapport with young children, however. Structured activities may include, but are not limited to, the following:

- Relaying a current event (e.g., birthday, car wreck), holiday (e.g., Thanksgiving, Halloween), or possession (e.g., dog, bicycle). This can be done easily with the carrier phrase, "Tell me about X."

- Explaining a familiar game (e.g., soccer) or activity (e.g., baking a cake, removing a tree with a backhoe, making honey). You might ask, "How do you [*play soccer, make honey,* etc.]?"

- Questions designed to elicit responses on a continuum from shorter (e.g., What is your name? How old are you? What is your favorite TV show?) to longer (e.g., Why do you like that show? What do you do with your brothers? What's your dog like?).

- Repetition of words and sentences of varied length and complexity. While the words and sentences are presented in random order, the clinician is looking to see how increasing linguistic complexity and different phonemic sequences influence the speech fluency. Words range from short and simple (e.g., I, you, got, fish) to longer and more complex (e.g., airplane, cowboy, reported, conversation). Sentences vary likewise from simple (e.g., I like it. That is my dog.) to more complex (e.g., Please sit in your seat. We have two dogs and three cats at home.). As always, these may be adjusted based on the preschool child's age and communication competence.

Williams (1978) suggested other structured activities including naming objects (making one word responses in naming objects on picture cards), making short phrase responses (responding to, "What's going on in the picture?"), and telling a story about a picture (or series of pictures requiring a longer sequential response). As noted in Chapter 7, Ryan (1974) and Ryan and Van Kirk (1971) presented a comprehensive list of structured activities (i.e., Stuttering Interview, Form A) for assessing preschool and young school-age children. These activities included automatic (counting, saying alphabet, singing, reciting poem), echoic (imitating words and sentences), reading (delete for young preschool children), picture naming, speaking alone (clinician leaves room), monologue, speaking with puppet, command speech (client directs clinician), talking with gestures, talking with time pressure (see next section, "Speech–Language Sample and Structured Activities with Communicative Pressure"), talking with drawing, phonemic difficulty (imitating complex words), responding to and asking questions, speaking on telephone, conversational speech, and observation in natural setting. The purpose of all of these activities is to provide the child ample and varied opportunities for structured speech so that the clinician can evaluate what factors tend to relate to fluctuations in speech fluency.

Speech–Language Sample and Structured Activities with Communicative Pressure

Once the speech–language sample and structured activities without communicative pressure are completed, components of both are expanded now with communicative pressure. Communication pressure takes the form of different demands that deliberately challenge the child's ability to remain fluent. The purpose is to determine the relative impact of perceived communicative pressure (including time pressure, linguistic ambiguity, violation of conversational or pragmatic rules) on speech fluency. For example, during conversation with the child, structured activities noted earlier, or other related treatment tasks (games that are appropriate for the child such as drawing, board or card games, and puppet activities), the clinician might begin to rush the activity (by significantly increasing her rate of speech, amount of hand movements and extraneous gestures, or speed of requesting answers), interrupt the child (taking a conversational turn well before the child is about to complete his, or asking a question and then asking a new question before the child finishes answering the first question), demonstrate loss of attention (while the child is relating an event, doing something else that indicates by her action that she is not attending to him), or request that the child say something again (by saying, "I didn't understand that. Would you tell me again?") (Williams, 1978).

The clinician also might make abrupt topic shifts (by introducing a topic prematurely that is unrelated to the child's discussion), overstep the boundaries of the child's linguistic competence (using vocabulary clearly not within the child's semantic repertoire), or introduce deliberate linguistic ambiguity (offering contradictions) or verbal absurdity (such as, "What's this I hear about you sleeping in the garage?" or "How come you make pizza in the bathtub?"). The clinician must remember to share with the parent her clinical rationale for imposing deliberate demands upon the child, particularly when such procedures result in disfluency. Otherwise, the parent might interpret erroneously that the clinician is insensitive or unkind.

Trial Management

The preceding assessment activities enable the clinician to evaluate the child's speech fluency so as to arrive at a diagnosis (see "Diagnosis" section later in this chapter) and to establish a baseline of the child's communication behavior, from which progress in treatment, if necessary, can be monitored (Haynes et al., 1992). As will be seen, the process leading from assessment and evaluation to diagnosis is ongoing and dynamic, not limited to a fixed time frame. Even when treatment has begun, assessment continues and leads to a more precise or refined diagnosis. From the assessment activities, the clinician decides whether or not she feels a more formal evaluation of articulation/phonology and language is necessary. If the child has demonstrated repetition or prolongation of syllables or shows any evidence of awareness of communication concern, frustration, or speech fluency-related communication reticence, the clinician should engage in a brief period of trial management during the assessment session itself. Because the feelings and attitudes related to speech fluency are most frequently in evolution with preschool children, the distinction between fluency shaping and stuttering modification treatment techniques are least clearly defined (compared to that with school-age children and adults). The trial management techniques (different treatment activities to determine relative effectiveness with a particular child) performed during the assessment session and the child's response thereto help the clinician in designing appropriate intervention methods for the preschool child and in offering specific recommendations.

Fluency Shaping

Fluency shaping techniques for trial management include having the child sing a short song and recite a nursery rhyme in chorus with the clinician (both of which are essential for differential diagnosis, as noted in Chapter 4); modeling and impersonating, through puppetry and play, both turtle speech (slow and gentle) and rabbit speech (fast and hard); modeling slow, relaxed, slightly prolonged speech (with slight prolongation on vowels, light articulatory contacts on consonants, while maintaining naturalness in the suprasegmental aspects of speech); and perhaps moving from established fluency in monosyllabic words to polysyllabic words, then to phrases, and finally to sentences.

Stuttering Modification

Stuttering modification techniques include modeling slow, relaxed, prolonged speech; modeling easier versions of the child's stuttering; inserting instances of slight disfluency in the clinician's speech with a self-comment (such as, "Gosh, that was a little hard.") in the context of emotional neutrality, leading to interacting with the child about the clinician's disfluency (such as, "Did you hear the word I just said that was a little hard? What did you think?"); and providing praise to the child for slow and gentle speech (such as, "I love the way you said that. You said wwwell," modeling gentle production of "well.").

POST-ASSESSMENT PROCEDURES

A preliminary analysis of the speech sample is conducted before the post-assessment parent conference in order to present preliminary findings and recommendations. The analyses described later in this section, however, are performed after the assessment session in preparation for the diagnosis that is detailed in the clinical summary report. The purposes of the speech analysis are to quantify (i.e., use numbers, tallies, summary statistics) and qualify (i.e., describe) the speech characteristics along the continuum from speech fluency to disfluency. Common errors are to assess the characteristics of disfluency only (while forgetting that the majority of speech of people who stutter is more fluent than not) and to assume that characteristics of speech disfluency are invariant and static. Rather, we must represent the individual whose communication and speech characteristics are dynamic, highlighting both the fluency and disfluency characteristics in addition to the related feelings, thoughts, and attitudes.

When assessing a preschool child, making a distinction between normal disfluency and incipient stuttering often proves challenging because multiple factors must be considered simultaneously (for example, the frequency, type, and duration of disfluency; Gordon & Luper, 1992a, 1992b), and because once again we are dealing with continuous, multidimensional variables rather than dichotomous, unidimensional ones. Who can distinguish the upper limits of normal disfluency from the lower limits of beginning stuttering? On the basis of behavioral analysis alone, this proves impossible. Our judgment is helped some by assessing the feelings, thoughts, and attitudes as noted, and other factors such as feelings of internal control (Cooper & Cooper, 1995). In the end, there continues to be a critical place for informed and sensitive professional judgment, the value of which cannot be replaced by any isolated assessment technique. Zebrowski (1995) noted that to distinguish stuttering from normal disfluency, clinicians need to be familiar with the behaviors that are salient to making this distinction; be able to observe, quantify, and qualify these behaviors; and integrate this information to judge the likelihood that a child is either stuttering or at risk for stuttering. Therefore, in this section, we will look first at the behaviors that guide our professional judgment in distinguishing between normal disfluency and beginning stuttering. Then we will consider how we quantify and qualify such behaviors. Finally, we will deal with the processes of establishing a diagnosis and conducting the post-assessment parent conference.

Normal Disfluency and Incipient Stuttering

As noted earlier, clinicians often struggle with the distinction between normal disfluency and beginning stuttering. Zebrowski (1994) pointed out that clinicians must determine if the child is stuttering, at risk for stuttering, or normally disfluent. We noted earlier that children who stutter and those who do not demonstrate some similarity in types of speech disfluencies, but exhibit differences in the degree and relative frequency of disfluency (Bloodstein, 1995). All children produce all types of disfluency (including within-word and between-word disfluencies). As a group, however, children who stutter are generally more disfluent overall and tend to demonstrate more within-word disfluencies. In other words, while all children demonstrate whole-word and phrase repetitions, interjections, and revisions (between-word disfluencies), children who stutter tend to demonstrate more part-word (sound or syllable) repetitions and sound prolongations (within-word disfluencies).

Various observational guidelines are useful when distinguishing between normal disfluency and beginning stuttering. One that I have found particularly helpful is the guide presented by Van Riper (1982), which is represented in Table 8.1. He noted that the guidelines are "tentative, incomplete, and unsubstantiated by research" (p. 24) and lacking in item weights. Van Riper's checklist is not directly related to the selection of different treatment strategies and, because of its visual presentation in the form of columns, risks being misinterpreted as discrete rather than continuous variables (for stuttering and normal disfluency). Nevertheless, his guidelines significantly have influenced others that have been developed since (Gordon & Luper, 1992a, 1992b, for a review of six such protocols) and are extremely useful for clinicians and for discussion with parents, teachers, and others.

Van Riper's checklist contains 26 behavioral characteristics that are presented in seven different categories. The categories include: *syllable repetitions* (frequency per word and per 100 words, tempo, regularity, schwa vowel, airflow, vocal tension), *prolongations* (duration, frequency, regularity, tension, voiced, unvoiced, termination), *gaps or silent pauses* (within word boundaries, prior to speech attempt, after disfluency), *phonation* (inflections, phonatory arrests, vocal fry), *articulation postures* (appropriateness), *reaction to stress* (type), and *evidence of awareness* (phonemic consistency, frustration, postponements, eye contact). My own experience has indicated that children with normal disfluency tend to demonstrate relatively effortless, infrequent, and inconsistent syllable (e.g., me–mean) and word (e.g., this this) repetition and occasional prolongation (e.g., sssomething). In addition, increases in both the qualitative (type) and quantitative (amount) characteristics of disfluency, and particularly any evidence of speech-related stress, awareness, or frustration, are indicators of stuttering. More detail will be provided in the next section, "Speech Analysis."

Another set of guidelines was presented by Pindzola (Pindzola & White, 1986) and is represented in Figure 8.3. Like that presented by Van Riper, it is useful for distinguishing between normal disfluency and incipient stuttering, as well as in presenting visual representations to parents, teachers, and other allied educational and health professionals. Pindzola presented 8 categories of auditory behaviors and 3 categories of verbal behaviors, each of which is assessed and marked on the protocol. Auditory behaviors include: *type of disfluency* (interjections; hesitations, gaps, or repetitions; and prolongations or coexisting struggle), *size of the speech unit affected* (sentence or phrase; word; and syllable or sound), *frequency of disfluencies* (repetitions, prolongations, and disfluencies in general), *duration of disfluencies* (typical number of iterations of the repetition, average duration of prolongation), *audible effort* (absence or presence of hard glottal attacks, disrupted airflow, vocal tension, or pitch rise), *rhythm, tempo, and speed of disfluencies* (slow, normal, and evenly paced; or fast and irregular), *intrusion of schwa vowel during repetitions* (schwa not heard or heard), and *audible learned behaviors* (absence or presence of word or phrase substitutions, circumlocutions, or avoidance tactics such as starters or postponers). The auditory behaviors require the clinician or other user of the

TABLE 8.1. Guidelines for Differentiating Normal From Abnormal Disfluency

Behavior	Stuttering	Normal Disfluency
Syllable Repetitions		
a. Frequency per word	More than two	Less than two
b. Frequency per 100 words	More than two	Less than two
c. Tempo	Faster than normal	Normal tempo
d. Regularity	Irregular	Regular
e. Schwa vowel	Often present	Absent or rare
f. Airflow	Often interrupted	Rarely interrupted
g. Vocal tension	Often apparent	Absent
Prolongations		
h. Duration	Longer than 1 second	Less than 1 second
i. Frequency	More than 1 per 100 words	Less than 1 per 100 words
j. Regularity	Uneven or interrupted	Smooth
k. Tension	Important when present	Absent
l. When voiced (sonant)	May show rise in pitch	No pitch rise
m. When unvoiced (surd)	Interrupted airflow	Airflow present
n. Termination	Sudden	Gradual
Gaps (silent pauses)		
o. Within the word boundary	May be present	Absent
p. Prior to speech attempt	Unusually long	Not marked
q. After the disfluency	May be present	Absent
Phonation		
r. Inflections	Restricted; monotone	Normal
s. Phonatory arrest	May be present	Absent
t. Vocal fry	May be present	Usually absent
Articulating Postures		
u. Appropriateness	May be inappropriate	Appropriate
Reaction to Stress		
v. Type	More broken words	Normal disfluencies
Evidence of awareness		
w. Phonemic consistency	May be present	Absent
x. Frustration	May be present	Absent
y. Postponements (stallers)	May be present	Absent
z. Eye contact	May waver	Normal

Note. From *The Nature of Stuttering* (2nd ed.) (p. 25) by C. Van Riper, 1982, Englewood Cliffs, NJ: Prentice-Hall. Copyright 1982 by Allyn & Bacon. Reprinted with permission.

protocol to enter a series of dichotomous or trichotomous judgments of the child's speech behavior (probably normal, questionable, or probably abnormal). Visual behaviors include: *facial grimaces or articulatory posturing, head movements,* and *body involvement.* Visual evidence may be indicative of excessive speaking effort, awareness of a communication problem, adjustment to the disfluency, or relative severity. Finally, 7 historical and psychological indicators (noted following interviews, direct observation, and supplemental tests or questionnaires) include: *awareness and concern* (of child, parents, or significant others), *length of time fluency problem has existed, consistent versus episodic nature of problem, reaction to stress, fears and avoidances* (phonemes, words, or situations), *family history of stuttering,* and *other covert factors.* The auditory and visual behaviors and historical and psychological indicators then are summarized and interpreted in a final section titled "Summary of Clinical Evidence and Impressions."

Another figure that I have found helpful, more for conveying basic information about the development of stuttering than for differential diagnosis, is one that is adapted from a video/film titled *Prevention of Stuttering [Part 1]: Identifying the Danger Signs* (Walle, 1976; see Appendix B). This figure contains less detail than the protocols reviewed earlier, but continues to be effective in helping parents, family members, allied professionals, and significant others visualize fluency and disfluency along a continuum. It is represented in Figure 8.4.

Speech Analysis

Once we are familiar with the characteristics (including behaviors, thoughts, and feelings) that distinguish normal disfluency from beginning stuttering, we can begin to discuss how we analyze what we observe to help us reach a diagnosis and begin to plan treatment if indicated. Parameters of speech fluency that are analyzed include, but are not limited to, the frequency of speech disfluency, type of disfluencies and proportion of each type, duration of instances of stuttering (such as frequency and real time of units that occur in instances of repetition, prolongation, interjection, and other forms of disfluency), rate of speech, and other associated speech and nonspeech behaviors (Conture, 1990a, 1990b, 1997; Peters & Guitar, 1991; Starkweather, 1993; Zebrowski, 1994, 1995). Each will be described briefly now.

Frequency of Speech Disfluency (i.e., Disfluency Frequency Index)

The frequency of speech disfluency refers to the amount of disfluency, regardless of the individual types or relative severity, that is contained within the child's speech. This is a general but important diagnostic measure that indicates the overall extent to which the disfluency disrupts the forward flow of speech. This measure often is used to document the broad effect that treatment has on a person's speech (Zebrowski, 1994). Frequency is reported as a percentage, usually both as an average and a range of disfluency. Using the word as the unit of measure, frequency of disfluency is computed by counting the total number of disfluent words and dividing it by the total number of words spoken (both disfluent and fluent) within the sample collected. Then the resulting decimal is

(text continues on p. 243)

Name _____ Date of Birth _____

Address_____ Age_____ Sex _____

Date of Test _____

Clinician _____

I. Auditory Behaviors

• *Type of Disfluency* (mark the most typical)

Interjections	Hesitations/Gaps or Repetitions	Prolongations or Coexisting Struggle
Probably Normal	Questionable	Probably Abnormal

• *Size of Speech Unit Affected* (mark the typical level at which disfluencies occur)

Sentence/Phrase	Word	Syllable / Sound
Probably Normal	Questionable	Probably Abnormal

• *Frequency of Disfluencies* (compute from speech sample and mark values on continua)

Frequency of repetitions

2%   5%

Probably Normal	Questionable	Probably Abnormal

Frequency of prolongations

1%

Probably Normal	Probably Abnormal

Frequency of disfluencies in general

2%   5%   10%

Normal	Probably Normal	Questionable	Probably Abnormal

(continues)

Figure 8.3. Protocol for Differentiating the Incipient Stutterer. *Note.* From "A Protocol for Differentiating the Incipient Stutterer," by R. H. Pindzola and D. T. White, 1986, *Language, Speech, and Hearing Services in Schools, 17,* pp. 12–15. Copyright 1986 by the American Speech–Language–Hearing Association. Reprinted with permission.

• *Duration of Disfluencies*

Typical number of reiterations of the repetition _____

Less than 2	2 to 5	More than 5
Probably Normal	Questionable	Probably Abnormal

Average duration of prolongations _____

Less than 1 second	1 or more seconds
Probably Normal	Probably Abnormal

• *Audible Effort* (mark those that apply)

Lack of the following items	Presence of the following items
Probably Normal	Probably Abnormal

hard glottal attacks _____   pitch rise _____

disrupted airflow _____   others: _____

vocal tension _____

• *Rhythm/Tempo/Speed of Disfluencies*

Slow/normal; evenly paced	Fast, perhaps irregular
Probably Normal	Probably Abnormal

• *Intrusion of Schwa Vowel During Repetitions*

Schwa not heard	Presence of Schwa
Probably Normal	Probably Abnormal

• *Audible Learned Behaviors* (mark those that apply)

Lack of the following items	Presence of the following items
Probably Normal	Probably Abnormal

word/phrase substitutions _____

circumlocutions _____

avoidance tactics (starters, postponers, and the like) _____

(continues)

Figure 8.3. Continued.

II. Visual Evidence (list behaviors observed)

• Facial Grimaces/Articulatory Posturing: _____

_____

• Head Movements: _____

_____

• Body Involvement: _____

_____

III. Historical/Psychological Indicators (comment on the following based on client and/or parent interviews, observations, and supplemental tests or questionnaires, if any)

• Awareness and Concern (of child; of parents): _____

_____

• Length of Time Fluency Problem Has Existed: _____

_____

• Consistent Versus Episodic Nature of Problem: _____

_____

• Reaction to Stress: _____

_____

• Phoneme/Word/Situation Fears and Avoidances: _____

_____

• Familial History: _____

_____

• Other Covert Factors: _____

_____

IV. Summary of Clinical Evidence and Impressions

_____

_____

_____

_____

_____

Figure 8.3. Continued.

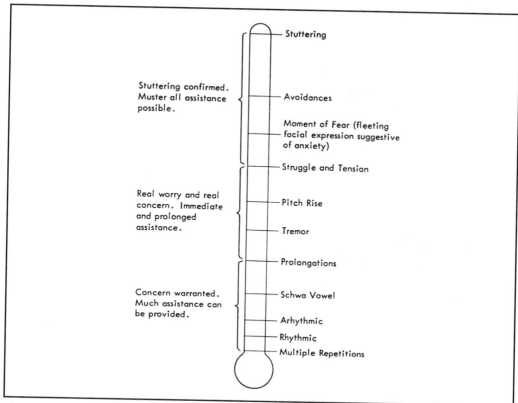

Figure 8.4. The Danger Signs of Developing Stuttering. *Note.* From *Prevention of Stuttering [Part 1]: Identifying the Danger Signs* [Film/Videotape] by E. L. Walle, 1976, Memphis, TN: Stuttering Foundation of America. Copyright 1976 by the Stuttering Foundation of America. Reprinted with permission.

multiplied by 100 in order to convert to a percentage (in order to move the decimal point two places to the right). The syllable can be used as the unit of measure as well. This is done by counting the total number of disfluent syllables, dividing it by the total number of syllables spoken (both disfluent and fluent), and then multiplying by 100. It is critical to use the same unit of measure over time so as to permit comparison for estimation of progress and change. We will assume for most clinical purposes, however, that the word is an adequate unit of measure. In simple form, the frequency of speech disfluency (Disfluency Frequency Index, DFI) is computed as follows:

$$DFI = \frac{\text{Total number of disfluent words}}{\text{Total number of words (disfluent + fluent) spoken}} \times 100$$

To determine the Disfluency Frequency Index (DFI), usually the speech sample being analyzed is of predetermined size or duration. For example, one may figure the number (percentage) of disfluent words in 100 words spoken, in the total number of words produced, or in 1 minute of conversational speech

(Zebrowski, 1995). When reporting the frequency of disfluency as a percentage over 100 words spoken, it is helpful to collect at least one 300-word sample and compute the average and range of disfluency produced (Conture, 1990b, 1997; Zebrowski, 1994). For example, over a 300-word sample, a child may have had 10 disfluent words in the first 100 words spoken, 18 in the next 100, and 8 in the third 100, as follows:

$$\frac{10+18+8}{300} = \frac{36}{300} = .12 \times 100 = \frac{12 \text{ stuttered words per 100 words}}{\text{spoken}}$$

This means that this child demonstrated an average of 12 stuttered words per 100 words spoken (12%), averaged over a 300-word sample. Furthermore, he ranged from 8 to 18 disfluent words per 100 words spoken.

Note that you can easily verify your mathematical accuracy. Figure the Fluency Frequency Index (FFI) by dividing the total number of fluent words by the total number of words (both fluent and disfluent) spoken, as follows:

$$\text{FFI} = \frac{\text{Total number of fluent words}}{\text{Total number of words (fluent + disfluent) spoken}} \times 100$$

Adding the DFI and the FFI together should equal 100%. Using the illustration above, we can figure the Fluency Frequency Index (FFI) by dividing the number of fluent words (264) by the total number of words spoken (fluent, 264; disfluent, 36; total 300), as follows:

$$\frac{264}{300} = .88 \times 100 = 88 \text{ fluent words per 100 words spoken}$$

In this case, 12 (12%) disfluent words per 100 words spoken, plus 88 (88%) fluent words per 100 words spoken, equals 100 (100%) of the words (disfluent + fluent) spoken.

Another way to figure the frequency of disfluency (i.e., Disfluency Frequency Index, DFI) is to analyze a videotape recorded random sample or samples from the child's conversation or other context. This is done in similar fashion. However, one major difference is that the total number of words is not predetermined and therefore must be calculated from transcription (Rustin, Botterill, & Kelman, 1996). The additional procedures involved tend to reduce the interrater reliability of this method of assessing the frequency of disfluency. While transcription is a time intensive process, particularly for novice clinicians, it proves invaluable for understanding the nature of a client's fluency and disfluency. Again, a substantial segment (such as 300 words or 5 minutes) may be analyzed, or separate segments may be pooled into an analysis from which average and range frequency (in numbers or percentages) of disfluency are reported. For example, suppose we have a child who spoke 274 words within the sample, of which 24 words were disfluent. Here is how it looks:

$$DFI = \frac{24 \text{ disfluent words}}{274 \text{ words}} = .0876 = .09 \text{ (rounded)} \times 100 = 9\%$$
$$\text{(disfluent + fluent) spoken}$$

This means that in this sample, the child demonstrated an overall disfluency of 9%. This DFI can be compared to others of similar length (in terms of number of words or duration of talk time). From the comparison, average and ranges can be computed. There is greater variation in this measure as indicated, however, compared to one of predetermined length (such as 100 words, 300 words, and so on).

Zebrowski (1995) summarized that studies comparing children who stutter with those who do not indicate the former to be at least twice as disfluent, with average frequencies of disfluency consistently above 10% of the total number of words or syllables spoken. Similarly, Peters and Guitar (1991) estimated that preschool children who are normally disfluent demonstrate about 10 disfluencies (of all types) in every 100 words spoken. Conture (1990b, 1997) advocated the use of 3 within-word disfluencies per 100 words as a criterion for distinguishing normal disfluency from stuttering. Conture (1990b) justified this criterion by stating that individuals who produce 10 disfluencies of all types per 100 words are likely producing 3 or more within-word disfluencies among these 10. Furthermore, he noted that within-word disfluencies are the type that listeners are most likely to consider as stuttering and are the type of disfluencies that people who stutter produce more often than people who do not.

Zebrowski (1995) indicated that early stuttering often is associated with very high frequencies of speech disfluency (greater than 10% of all syllables or words spoken), followed by a sharp reduction in the frequency over the next 3 to 6 months, continuing to 12 or 14 months from the time the problem was first noticed (Finn et al., 1994; Yairi, 1997; Yairi & Ambrose, 1992a; Yairi, Ambrose, & Niermann, 1993). These same longitudinal studies reported that between 65% and 85% of the children in the studies who stutter recovered without treatment 2 years post-onset. The only distinguishing characteristic of children who did not recover without treatment was a greater amount of disfluency at the beginning and throughout the study (Yairi & Ambrose, 1992a, 1992b). These observations emphasize the importance of early detection of disfluency, promptly conducting the evaluation thereafter, and analyzing speech samples collected at 3- to 6-month intervals after initial contact, all aimed at monitoring the speech fluency of children close to the onset of stuttering or of those suspected to be at risk. Zebrowski (1995) noted other implications of such findings:

> Further, the observation that early improvement and recovery may be the most pervasive developmental pattern calls into question the need for immediate and direct stuttering therapy. Instead, a general strategy of early detection, followed by a six-month period of parent counseling and monthly observation and monitoring of the child's speech may be the most effective and efficient plan. Subsequent decisions to either recycle the child and his family through another period of observation and counseling, or initiate more direct therapy, should naturally be based on the outcome of this initial contact. (pp. 81–82)

Recall the discussion from Chapter 2 in which Yairi (1997) described as a "double-edged ethical dilemma" (p. 73) clinicians' decisions to initiate or delay treatment. He recommended that all young children who are beginning to stutter receive a thorough communication evaluation and subsequent reevaluations combined with parent education about childhood stuttering. He also recommended that those children who have stuttered for more than 14 to 18 months without exhibiting substantial improvement receive a priority for direct fluency intervention.

Type of Speech Disfluency (i.e., Disfluency Type Index)

Another important characteristic to assess is the type of disfluency produced in addition to the proportion of each type. This type of analysis, also referred to as the Disfluency Type Index, indicates what the child is doing that interferes with the forward flow of speech and how what the child is doing changes over time. The Disfluency Type Index (DTI) is computed by using the same sample or samples analyzed earlier for frequency of disfluency. To analyze the individual types of speech disfluency, we divide the number of disfluencies of each individual type (such as part-word repetitions, whole-word repetitions, and prolongations, among others) by the total number of stuttered words. Again, I am electing to use the word as the unit of measure, which I find adequate for most applied clinical purposes. However, clinicians need to be aware that the syllable can be and is used as the unit of measure if an individual clinician so desires. Using the word as the unit of measure, the type of disfluency, or Disfluency Type Index (i.e., DTI), is computed as follows:

$$DTI = \frac{\text{Number of disfluencies of each individual type}}{\text{Total number of disfluent words}} \times 100$$

From the example discussed earlier, let's say that of the 36 disfluent words, 18 contained part-word (i.e., sound or syllable) repetitions, 9 contained sound prolongations, and the remaining 9 contained whole-word repetitions. The number of each individual type (18 part-word repetitions, 9 sound prolongations, 9 whole-word repetitions) is divided by the total number of disfluent words, as follows:

$$\% \text{ Part-Word Repetitions} = \frac{18 \text{ part-word repetitions}}{36 \text{ total disfluent words}} = .5 \times 100 = 50\%$$

$$\% \text{ Sound Prolongations} = \frac{9 \text{ sound prolongations}}{36 \text{ total disfluent words}} = .25 \times 100 = 25\%$$

$$\% \text{ Whole-Word Repetitions} = \frac{9 \text{ whole-word repetitions}}{36 \text{ total disfluent words}} = .25 \times 100 = 25\%$$

This means that the sample of 36 disfluent words contains 50% part-word (i.e., sound/syllable) repetitions, 25% sound prolongations, and 25% whole-word repetitions. Again, to check your mathematical accuracy, you can do two things. Add up the frequencies for each individual type (in this case, 18 + 9 + 9) and it should equal the total number of disfluent words (36). Also, add up the computed percentages for each type of disfluency (50% + 25% + 25%), and that sum should be 100%.

This more narrow form of analysis is particularly important because the frequency of speech disfluency often is so variable both within and between children (Johnson and Associates, 1959, and Yairi, 1981, found that at least one child in their respective studies who did not stutter had at least 25 disfluencies per 100 words). Furthermore, an analysis of the types of disfluency and fluency is an important diagnostic characteristic distinguishing between normal disfluency and beginning stuttering. As noted earlier, while there is a great deal of overlap between children who stutter and those who do not in the types of disfluencies they produce, one significant difference is that those who stutter produce more within-word speech disfluencies (sound or syllable or part-word repetitions, sound prolongations, and those that disrupt the transition between sounds within a word) (Conture, 1990b, 1997; Zebrowski, 1994, 1995). Peters and Guitar (1991) noted the following about normal disfluency:

> Revisions are a common disfluency type in normal children and may continue to account for a major portion of disfluency as the child grows. Interjections are also common, but decline after age three. Repetitions may also be a frequent type of disfluency, especially single-syllable word repetitions of less than two extra units around age 2–3. Repetitions are more likely to involve longer segments (e.g., phrases) as the child grows. (p. 75)

Schwartz and Conture (1988) introduced the Sound Prolongation Index (SPI), which is a measure of one type of disfluency (audible or silent prolongation). Zebrowski (1994) summarized the clinical literature indicating that children with Sound Prolongation Indices (SPIs), or a Disfluency Type Index (DTI) for prolongations, of 25% or more (i.e., 25% of the child's total disfluencies are sound prolongations) are likely to require direct treatment for their stuttering.

Molecular Description of Disfluency

Another important measure of disfluency, in addition to the frequency and type, is a more molecular characterization for individual instances of stuttering. This includes, but is not limited to, duration (real time) and frequency (total number, mean, and range) among others. This is particularly important for measurement of an individual's variation of speech fluency before, during, and after treatment. For example, it was useful for me to be able to document that over a period of 6 months before treatment, Robert, a 4-year-old child, had part-word (sound or syllable) repetitions consisting of between 1 and 9 units of repetition lasting 1 to 19 seconds in duration. Within 4 months of an indirect form of treatment consisting of play intervention and parent counseling, his part-word repetitions reduced to between 1 and 3 units of repetition lasting no longer than 3 seconds. This brief description does not explicitly account for the significant decrease in overall severity measured in elimination of facial and body tension. Reporting the number and duration of repeated and prolonged units provides valuable clinical information for an individual child. A reminder here for clinicians is to account, in the most molecular form possible, for the type and degree of fluency and disfluency. The computations provided earlier for frequency and type only get the processes of analysis and description started. To reflect the nature of the speech itself, we need to document other factors that can be used to describe a child's speech fluency and disfluency over time.

More specifically, tracking changes in a young child's speech fluency can be used to document progression or regression of the disorder. Zebrowski (1995) noted that "increased duration of sound/syllable repetitions (i.e., either overall or with respect to individual repeated units), a slowed rate of repetition, or both, may serve as a valid indication of the progression of stuttering in children" (p. 85). Narrowly describing a child's disfluency is invaluable for monitoring changes in an individual's speech fluency and for contributing to the pool of observations (in addition to those discussed earlier and later) that are considered when making statements of diagnosis. Starkweather (1993) developed this concept and recommended that clinicians measure the duration of all disfluent speech behavior and the total speech time, and calculate the percentage of disfluency speech time. He argued that so much information is added when the duration of stuttering behaviors is measured and compared to the total speech time, which can be used to reliably measure an individual's level of fluency and effectiveness of treatment.

The duration of disfluencies can be used to monitor changes in a child's speech fluency and to measure progression of the disorder of stuttering. It would seem likely, therefore, that differences in the duration of disfluencies (particularly within-word disfluencies) can be used to distinguish children who stutter from those who do not. Zebrowski (1995) cautioned, however, that, "Unfortunately, empirical support for this notion has been inconsistent" (p. 83). In fact, recent studies contraindicate the predictive validity of using duration of within-word disfluencies to compare and distinguish across children. Zebrowski (1994) summarized that little difference was found in the duration of part-word repetitions or prolongations between young children who stutter and those who do not. She summarized, furthermore, that little relationship exists between stuttering duration and a child's age, length of time the child has stuttered, or overall frequency of speech disfluency. These findings, however, do not minimize the significant value of figuring the duration, frequency, and other more molecular measures of individual disfluency for monitoring changes in an individual child's speech fluency over time.

Rate of Speech

Another measure that I have found useful in monitoring an individual's speech fluency and related progress is rate of speech. As the child becomes more fluent or demonstrates fewer disfluencies, rate of speech tends to increase. One may figure the rate of overall speech (both fluent and disfluent words), fluent speech only, or disfluent speech only. The differences found can be attributed to the impact of the disfluency, which should lessen throughout treatment. Rate of speech is calculated by dividing the number of words or syllables spoken (total, fluent, or disfluent) by the talk time in minutes. Again, I am assuming that the word is an adequate unit of measure for most clinical applications.

$$\text{Rate of Speech} = \frac{\text{Number of words spoken}}{\text{Talk time (in minutes)}}$$

When dividing, clinicians need to remember that the talk time (child's talk time only) must be in minutes in order for the result to be an average number of words spoken per minute. For example, if a child spoke the 300 words sampled earlier in 2 minutes and 15 seconds, the clinician must divide as follows:

$$\frac{300 \text{ words spoken}}{2.25 \text{ minutes}} = 133 \text{ words per minute}$$

Remember that 15 seconds is one quarter minute (.25 minutes); 30 seconds is one half minute (.5 minutes). If the clinician has trouble converting the talk time into minutes, she can divide by the total number of seconds and then multiply by 60 in order to convert seconds to minutes, as follows:

$$\frac{300 \text{ words spoken}}{135 \text{ seconds}} = 2.22 \times 60 = 133 \text{ words per minute}$$

Indeed it was instructive for me to be able to report Robert's overall rate of speech increasing from 42 to 129 fluent and disfluent words per minute. Combined with the descriptions reviewed to this point, his increasing rate of speech supported the interpretation that his fluency had significantly improved. Individual methods for figuring rate of speech are in occasional disagreement across the published literature. Note that Williams et al. (1978) recommended the following for figuring rate of fluent speech:

> In counting words in speech samples, count only those words that would have been spoken had the speaker performed no disfluencies. That is, for example, "Uh, when I wuh–wuh–wuh–was 10 years old, I went–I went–I went to New York" is regarded for word-counting purposes as consisting of "When I was 10 years old, I went to New York," a total of 11 words. Count only once each word repeated singly or in a phrase. For example, count "We–we–we went home" as three words rather than five. Do not count sounds or words such as "well," "uh–uh–uh," and the like, which are not integral parts of the meaningful context. In any instance of revision, count only the words in the final form. For example, count "I started to–I went to town and bought some bread" as 8 rather than 11 words, disregarding the false start "I started to." (pp. 260–261)

Clinicians will find that even after reading a variety of standard procedures and selecting one to follow, the process is puzzling at times and individual interpretations and decisions will need to be made. It would be nice if disfluencies were discrete entities. In other words, it would be easier if a word contained only a single instance of disfluency and if the boundaries of words always were clearly marked. In reality, of course, this generally does not happen. The message, therefore, is to be internally consistent (follow the same procedures each time) and account for what you have done and how you have done it. Then your clinical procedures will be both accountable and repeatable.

For purposes of comparison, it is helpful to know what rate of speech is considered to be average or "normal" for children who do not stutter. I have found three studies to be particularly useful for this purpose. Kelly and Conture (1992) found that for boys, age 3 years, 2 months to 4 years, 10 months (mean, or average, age was 4 years, 0 months), the average rate of speech was 153.6 words per minute (standard deviation, 18.3 words per minute), also computed as 177.6 syllables per minute (standard deviation, 18.4 syllables per minute). Kelly and Conture did not report data for girls. Ryan (1992) found that for children of ages 2 years, 10 months to 5 years, 9 months (mean age was 4 years, 5 months), boys' average rate of speech was 128.9 words per minute (standard deviation, 15.6 words per minute), or 164.1 syllables per minute (standard deviation, 20.5 syllables per minute). Girls' average rate of speech was 140.2 words per minute (standard deviation, 10.4 words per minute), or 176.3 syllables per minute (standard deviation, 20.6 syllables per minute).

Pindzola, Jenkins, and Lokken (1989) found that for children (boys and girls combined) who were 3 years old (3 years, 0 months to 3 years, 9 months), the average rate of speech was 140.3 syllables per minute (standard deviation, 14.2 syllables per minute; range, 116–163); for those 4 years old (4 years, 0 months to 4 years, 9 months), the average rate of speech was 152.7 syllables per minute (standard deviation, 17.9 syllables per minute; range, 117–183); and for those 5 years old (5 years, 0 months to 5 years, 9 months), the average rate of speech was 152.2 syllables per minute (standard deviation, 21.8 syllables per minute; range 109–183). Across 3-, 4-, and 5-year-old children, Pindzola et al. (1989) found that the average rate of speech was 148.4 syllables per minute (standard deviation, 18.0 syllables per minute; range 109–183). Their study did not report data for words per minute.

Secondary Characteristics

We also must quantify and qualify other speech and nonspeech factors (associated or secondary characteristics) that both impact and reflect speech fluency. These have been discussed in earlier chapters and in the present chapter under "Normal Disfluency and Incipient Stuttering" (see Table 8.1 and Figures 8.3 and 8.4). The potential list of secondary characteristics is endless. They may include such nonspeech factors as facial tension, head turning, eye movement, grimacing, or body movement. Speech-related associated factors include audible inhalations or exhalations immediately before or after stuttering, pitch rises indicating laryngeal tension, visible oral and neck tension, among others. Preschool children who do not stutter do not show such symptoms. However, such behaviors frequently develop early within weeks or months of stuttering onset. Secondary behaviors may reflect the child's deepening awareness of stuttering, coping mechanisms during stuttering, or attempts to prevent stuttering. Nevertheless, associated speech and nonspeech behaviors are diagnostically significant for distinguishing between stuttering and nonstuttered behavior. Peters and Guitar (1991) noted that while children normally display "tense pauses," such behavior does not appear to be a reaction to the experience of disfluency. They advised, however, that if a child does show what appears to be normal disfluencies (such as single word repetitions) yet consistently displays reactions such as pauses or interjections of "uh" immediately before or during the disfluencies, he should be evaluated carefully.

Severity Rating

Many school systems, clinics, and other facilities require an estimation of relative severity of stuttering. This can be interpreted by the clinician from the assessment components discussed earlier. However, the clinician must remember to keep in mind not only speech behaviors, but related attitudes, thoughts, and feelings. Recall the discussion in Chapter 5 about the woman who presented no perceptible disfluency but continued to interiorize negativity about herself as a disfluent and ineffective communicator. Many useful instruments and protocols are available as well. Haynes et al. (1992) highlighted 22 instruments including diagnostic, severity, and predictive scales for assessing overt features of stuttering (p. 210); 13 instruments including perception/attitude scales and situation/avoidance checklists for assessing covert features of stuttering (p. 213); and three assessment instruments for use with parents of young children who stutter (p. 207).

One instrument commonly used for measuring severity of stuttering is the *Stuttering Severity Instrument for Children and Adults–Third Edition* (SSI–3; Riley, 1994), represented in Figure 8.5. It can be used both with children and adults, has provisions for those who can and cannot read, and measures frequency, duration, and physical concomitants of stuttering. The number of words stuttered and total words spoken are computed during reading and/or conversation. Frequency (percentage) of stuttering is computed by dividing the number of words stuttered by the total number of words spoken and then multiplying by 100 to yield the percentage, which is converted into a task score. The amount of time the client blocks during the three longest disfluencies is averaged and converted into a second task score. Finally, physical behaviors concomitant to speech are rated from *0* to *5* for each of three anatomical areas (*face, head,* and *extremity*). These scores are added to a score (*0* to *5*) for distracting sounds to yield a third task score. The task scores for frequency, duration, and physical concomitants are combined for a total score, which is compared to normative data to yield a measure of stuttering severity (*very mild, mild, moderate, severe,* or *very severe*).

Another instrument for measuring stuttering severity is the "Scale for Rating Severity of Stuttering" (Williams, 1978), represented in Figure 8.6. The scale is a semantic differential containing descriptive statements for *0* (i.e., no stuttering), *1* (very mild), *2* (mild), *3* (mild to moderate), *4* (moderate), *5* (moderate to severe), *6* (severe), and *7* (very severe). The scale is conceptualized as a continuum with equally spaced increments. Van Riper (1982) noted, however, that the different behavioral variables (including stuttering frequency and duration, muscle tensing, and extraneous body movements) do not increase or decrease proportionally for most people who stutter for each scale value. This shortcoming significantly limits the use of the scale to estimate improvement in treatment. To correct for this limitation, Van Riper (1982) revised the severity scale so it can be used as a profile. The revision, the "Profile of Stuttering Severity," is represented in Figure 8.7. Using the profile, the clinician charts separately each of the variables of frequency, tension, duration, and postponement/avoidance. Regular charting enables the clinician to monitor the speech fluency and effect of treatment, thus facilitating planning.

Adaptation and Consistency

We discussed in Chapter 2 the adaptation and consistency effects. Adaptation is the tendency for overall stuttering to decrease with repeated reading or speaking of the same material. Consistency is the tendency for stuttering to occur on the same sounds or words during repeated reading or speaking of the

(*text continues on p. 256*)

SSI-3

Stuttering Severity Instrument–3

TEST RECORD AND FREQUENCY COMPUTATION FORM

Identifying Information

Name _____

Sex M F   Grade _____ Age _____

Date _____ Date of Birth _____

School _____

Examiner _____

Preschool ___ School Age ___ Adult ___ Reader ___ Nonreader ___

FREQUENCY Use Readers Table or Nonreaders Table, not both.

READERS TABLE				NONREADERS TABLE	
1. Speaking Task		**2. Reading Task**		**3. Speaking Task**	
Percentage	Task Score	Percentage	Task Score	Percentage	Task Score
1	2	1	2	1	4
2	3			2	6
3	4	2	4	3	8
4–5	5	3–4	5	4–5	10
6–7	6	5–7	6	6–7	12
8–11	7	8–12	7	8–11	14
12–21	8	13–20	8	12–21	16
22 & up	9	21 & up	9	22 & up	18

Frequency Score (use 1 + 2 or 3) [ ]

DURATION

Average length of three longest stuttering events timed to the nearest 1/10th second

		Scale Score
Fleeting	(.5 sec or less)	2
Half-second	(.5– .9 sec)	4
1 full second	(1.0– 1.9 secs)	6
2 seconds	(2.0– 2.9 secs)	8
3 seconds	(3.0– 4.9 secs)	10
5 seconds	(5.0– 9.9 secs)	12
10 seconds	(10.0–29.9 secs)	14
30 seconds	(30.0–59.9 secs)	16
1 minute	(60 secs or more)	18

Duration Score (2 – 18) [ ]

PHYSICAL CONCOMITANTS

Evaluating Scale

0 = none
1 = not noticeable unless looking for it
2 = barely noticeable to casual observer
3 = distracting
4 = very distracting
5 = severe and painful-looking

DISTRACTING SOUNDS	Noisy breathing, whistling, sniffing, blowing, clicking sounds	0 1 2 3 4 5
FACIAL GRIMACES	Jaw jerking, tongue protruding, lip pressing, jaw muscles tense	0 1 2 3 4 5
HEAD MOVEMENTS	Back, forward, turning away, poor eye contact, constant looking around	0 1 2 3 4 5
MOVEMENTS OF THE EXTREMITIES	Arm and hand movement, hands about face, torso movement, leg movements, foot-tapping or swinging	0 1 2 3 4 5

Physical Concomitants Score [ ]

TOTAL OVERALL SCORE

Frequency _____ + Duration _____ + Physical Concomitants _____ = [ ]

Percentile _____

Severity _____

(continues)

Figure 8.5. SSI–3 Test Record and Frequency Computation Form. *Note.* From *Stuttering Severity Instrument for Children and Adults–Third Edition* (Test Record and Frequency Computation Form, pp. 1–2) by G. D. Riley, 1994, Austin, TX: PRO-ED. Copyright 1994 by PRO-ED. Reprinted with permission.

TABLE 2
Percentile and Severity Equivalents of
SSI-3 Total Overall Scores for Preschool Children (N = 72)

Total Overall Score	Percentile	Severity
0– 8	1– 4	Very Mild
9–10	5–11	
11–12	12–23	Mild
13–16	24–40	
17–23	41–60	Moderate
24–26	61–77	
27–28	78–88	Severe
29–31	89–95	
32 and up	96–99	Very Severe

TABLE 3
Percentile and Severity Equivalents of SSI-3
Total Overall Scores for School-Age Children (N = 139)

Total Overall Score	Percentile	Severity
6– 8	1– 4	Very Mild
9–10	5–11	
11–15	12–23	Mild
16–20	24–40	
21–23	41–60	Moderate
24–27	61–77	
28–31	78–88	Severe
32–35	89–95	
36 and up	96–99	Very Severe

TABLE 4
Percentile and Severity Equivalents of
SSI-3 Total Overall Scores for Adults (N = 60)

Total Overall Score	Percentile	Severity
10–12	1– 4	Very Mild
13–17	5–11	
18–20	12–23	Mild
21-24	24–40	
25–27	41–60	Moderate
28–31	61–77	
32–34	78–88	Severe
35–36	89–95	
37–46	96–99	Very Severe

Figure 8.5. Continued.

FORM 10
Scale for Rating Severity of Stuttering

Speaker _____ Age ____ Sex ____ Date _____

Rater _____ Identification _____

Instructions:

Indicate your identification by some such term as "speaker's clinician," "clinical observer," "clinical student," or "friend," "mother," "classmate," et cetera. Rate the severity of the speaker's stuttering on a scale from 0 to 7, as follows:

0   No stuttering

1   Very mild—stuttering on less than 1 percent of words; very little relevant tension; disfluencies generally less than 1 second in duration; patterns of disfluency simple; no apparent associated movements of body, arms, legs, or head.

2   Mild—stuttering on 1 to 2 percent of words; tension scarcely perceptible; very few, if any, disfluencies last as long as a full second; patterns of disfluency simple; no conspicuous associated movements of body, arms, legs, or head.

3   Mild to moderate—stuttering on about 2 to 5 percent of words; tension noticeable but not very distracting; most disfluencies do not last longer than a full second; patterns of disfluency mostly simple; no distracting associated movements.

4   Moderate—stuttering on about 5 to 8 percent of words; tension occasionally distracting; disfluencies average about 1 second in duration; disfluency patterns characterized by an occasional complicating sound or facial grimace; an occasional distracting associated movement.

5   Moderate to severe—stuttering on about 8 to 12 percent of words; consistently noticeable tension; disfluencies average about 2 seconds in duration; a few distracting sounds and facial grimaces; a few distracting associated movements.

6   Severe—stuttering on about 12 to 25 percent of words; conspicuous tension; disfluencies average 3 to 4 seconds in duration; conspicuous distracting sounds and facial grimaces; conspicuous distracting associated movements.

7   Very severe—stuttering on more than 25 percent of words; very conspicuous tension; disfluencies average more than 4 seconds in duration; very conspicuous distracting sounds and facial grimaces; very conspicuous distracting associated movements.

Figure 8.6. Scale for Rating Severity of Stuttering. *Note.* From "Differential Diagnosis of Disorders of Fluency," by D. E. Williams. In *Diagnostic Methods in Speech Pathology* (2nd ed.) (p. 313), by F. L. Darley and D. C. Spriestersbach (Eds.), 1978, New York: Harper & Row. Copyright 1978 by F. L. Darley. Reprinted with permission.

Scale	Frequency	Tension–Struggle	Duration	Postponement–Avoidance
1	Under 1%	None	Under ½ sec.	None
2	1–2%	Rare but present	Average ½ sec.	Less than 5%
3	3–5%	Usual but mild	Average 1 sec.	5–10%
4	6–8%	Severe	Average 2 sec.	11–20%
5	9–12%	Very severe	Average 3 sec.	21–31%
6	13–25%	Overflow to eyes and limbs	Average 4 sec.	31–70%
7	More than 25%	Overflow to trunk	Longer than 5 sec.	More than 70%

Name: _____ *Joe P.* _____ Date: _____ Speaking Situation: _____ *TAT Pictures*

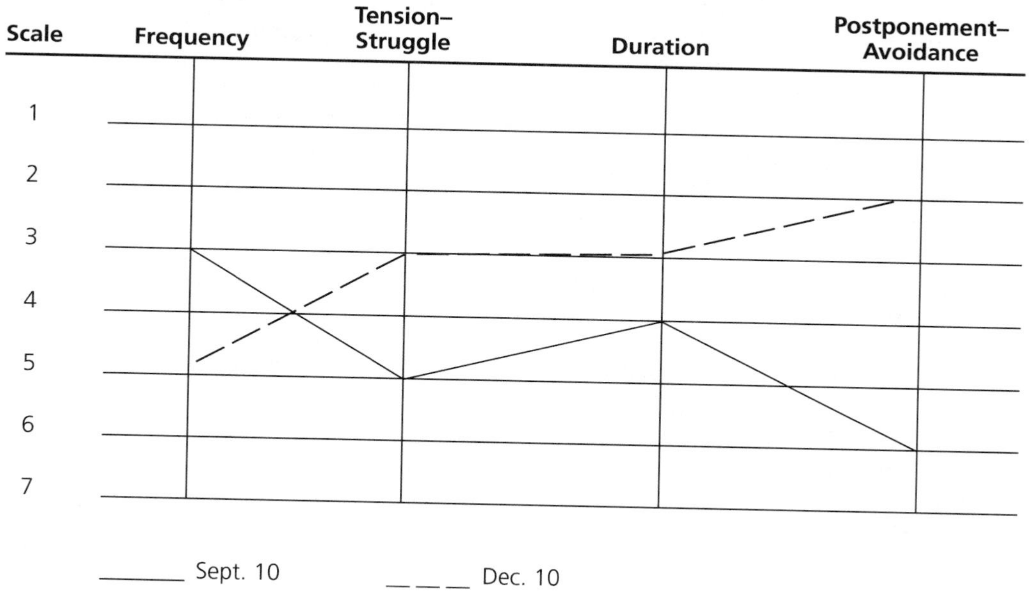

Scale	Frequency	Tension–Struggle	Duration	Postponement–Avoidance
1				
2				
3				
4				
5				
6				
7				

_____ Sept. 10   _ _ _ Dec. 10

Figure 8.7. Profile of Stuttering Severity Showing Changes as a Result of Therapy. *Note*. From *The Nature of Stuttering* (2nd ed.) (p. 201) by C. Van Riper, 1982, Englewood Cliffs, NJ: Prentice-Hall. Copyright 1982 by Allyn & Bacon. Reprinted with permission.

same material (Nicolosi et al., 1996). Both effects, as will be recalled, are demonstrated by people who stutter (as a group). This means that while many show both effects, some individuals who stutter show neither. Zebrowski (1994) noted that children who demonstrate either or both effects may be performing similarly to other children whose behavior has been diagnosed as stuttering. Those who demonstrate neither effect may be unlike others who stutter (as a group), be at risk for stuttering, or be normally disfluent. Because of this within-group variation and because both people who do stutter and those who do not (when considered as 2 different groups) both show adaptation and consistency effects, Williams (1978) advised against routinely collecting adaptation and consistency scores in speech fluency assessments. Williams also cautioned against drawing causal assumptions between adaptation and consistency effects and fear of or anxiety about stuttering. Because of its possible usefulness for differential diagnosis of fluency disorders reviewed in Chapter 4, however, I will highlight the procedures briefly.

Adaptation and consistency can be measured by having the child repeat a short passage or series of sentences five times (readers can read the material orally). Adaptation is calculated by subtracting the number of disfluencies in the fifth recitation from the number of disfluencies in the first, and then dividing this difference by the number of disfluencies in the first. Multiplying this quotient (i.e., the result of division) by 100 creates a percentage. Adaptation measurements of 50% or higher indicate the adaptation effect to be present. Scores greater than 50% indicate greater adaptation; scores lower than 50% indicate that the individual has not significantly reduced the frequency of disfluencies over five recitations (Williams et al., 1978; Zebrowski, 1994).

Consistency is measured by comparing the disfluencies produced in the first three recitations only. Three indices are computed: comparison of Recitations 1 and 2, 1 and 3, and 2 and 3. The indices for each comparison are computed by dividing the proportion of disfluent words in one recitation that also are produced in the second recitation by the number of disfluent words in the second reading. For example, computing the consistency index that compares Recitation 1 and 2, we would determine the percentage of disfluent words in Recitation 1 that also occurred in Recitation 2, then divide that percentage by the number of disfluent words in Recitation 2. The consistency effect is present if the individual exhibits an index of *1.0* or higher. Indices higher than *1.0* reflect greater consistency. Indices less than *1.0* reflect that the individual did not reveal consistency in the location of disfluencies within the recitation (Williams et al., 1978; Zebrowski, 1994).

Other

Finally, when analyzing the speech of preschool children (and that of people of all ages), there are other factors to consider. This is the category of *Other*. We noted when reviewing protocols that we must consider other variables such as the tempo, regularity, rate, relative tension, smoothness of transitions, and physical concomitants, in addition to feelings, thoughts, and attitudes (including avoidances, fears, and feelings of loss of control, among others). There is just so much that can be predicted or described in a chapter such as this. Occasionally I find student clinicians who become flustered when they observe a characteristic that does not fit neatly into any of the categories noted to this point or when the complexity of an individual's speech seems to defy the methods of assessment discussed. I remember a time when one of my student clinicians and I observed a youngster who demonstrated a pattern of final sound or syllable repetition (Like–ike this. This–is is what I mean–ean). The student clinician looked at me absolutely dumbfounded and sternly concluded, "This can't happen!" However, as she learned that day, anything can happen. In time and with the lessons learned from ample experience, the clinical situations that "can't happen" (those that cannot be predicted and those that we never have encountered previously) become the most challenging and instructive, and ultimately the most inviting and rewarding.

Diagnosis

A necessary distinction needs to be made between assessment/evaluation and diagnosis (Haynes et al., 1992). The term "diagnosis" comes from the Greek word "diagignoskein," meaning *to discern* or *to distinguish*. "Dia–" means *to split apart,* and "gignoskein" means *to perceive* or *to know*. Therefore, diagnosis means to identify and distinguish by examination the nature of a problem from among its many possibilities. If a disorder of speech fluency is present, the clinician must determine what type of disorder is operating from among the many possibilities. With respect to stuttering, the possibilities might include that the child is stuttering, is at risk for stuttering, or demonstrating normal speech fluency. If the child is stuttering or at risk for stuttering, then the clinician also must determine if treatment is warranted and recommended and if so, what should be the nature and focus of treatment.

Distinguishing between various possibilities requires absolute familiarity with the person, including how he responds, what he thinks, what he knows. The process of arriving at a diagnosis such as stuttering takes thorough assessment and evaluation, including all of the procedures discussed to this point. Furthermore, the diagnosis is not time bound. This means that the results of formal and informal assessment that contribute to a statement of diagnosis are, of necessity, somewhat tentative. In other words, while we use the best of our professional abilities to make necessary observations and interpretations, we must remain open to the lessons of those things that "can't happen," those aspects of human behavior that only reveal themselves later. Therefore, diagnoses must be robust, yet resilient and thereby responsive to new information.

By implication, diagnoses and the foundation of information on which they stand must be both reliable and valid. Validity reflects the truth, or how closely an assessment actually measures what it is intended to measure. Reliability means that an event is reproducible. Assessment procedures and the diagnoses they yield that are valid will prove to be reliable. The reverse is not necessarily the case, however. Procedures that are reliable are not necessarily valid. For example, at one time it was believed by many that the Earth was the center of the universe. This was a reliable belief. However, Copernicus later proved that such a view did not reflect the truth (was not valid). In fact, he showed that the Earth rotates on its axis and with the other planets in the solar system revolves around the sun (the principle of heliocentric planetary motion). Just because people agree does not mean that they are right (Shapiro, 1987).

Clinicians must follow their clinical wisdom based upon professional training and experience. Too often, when results of standardized instruments challenge the informed professional judgment of knowledgeable clinicians, I see the clinician defer to external forces. Clinicians sometimes assume that external sources of information, by virtue of having been published, profess greater insight than that gleaned from their professional preparation and the most valid diagnostic instruments available, their trained eyes and ears. There always will be a place for professional judgment that occasionally defies training and logic. This part of a professional is what is uniquely human and may be where the head and the heart meet. What I am referring to is respectful of professional knowledge and experience and that which is sensitive, good, empathic, and holds a positive belief in the human potential for learning and change. More will be said about this in Chapters 11 and 12, which address clinician competencies, professional preparation, and lifelong learning. Suffice it now to say that very little "can't happen." Remain open and positive and let's have confidence in our clients, their families, and in ourselves.

Prognosis and Recommendations

In addition to determining a diagnosis, clinicians are responsible for making a statement of prognosis. A prognosis is a prediction of the outcome of a proposed course of treatment for a given client, including how effective treatment will be, how far he can be expected to progress, and how long it will take. Haynes et al. (1992) noted that such predictions have immediate and long-range facets, the purposes of which are to economize therapeutic efforts (focusing on those clients who hold greatest promise for improvement) and to provide families with needed direction. A more positive prognosis with preschool children requires that the intervention take place before the child develops fear and avoidance reactions (before the child internalizes that something is going wrong or that he is losing control over his speech mechanism) and that the parents and others within the child's communication system actively support and participate in the treatment. Haynes et al. (1992) noted several other factors and related questions that must be considered when estimating the child's prognosis for improvement:

- *How long has the child been stuttering?* Children who are younger, specifically whose stuttering is younger, and have relatively little exposure to adverse environmental reactions typically have a more favorable treatment prognosis.

- *What is the nature of environmental reactions to which the child has been exposed?* Children who experience a more positive environmental reaction tend to have a better prognosis. Those who experience penalty imposed from the environment and internalize the negative reaction (such as being slapped, insulted, or humiliated) have a less favorable prognosis.

- *Is the child aware of speaking difficulty?* Reduced awareness and a positive outlook toward communication are associated with a more favorable prognosis. Increased frustration leading to internalization of concern results in a less favorable prognosis.

- *What type of disfluency is the child demonstrating?* Fewer and less involved overt and covert symptoms are associated with a more positive prognosis. When danger signs are frequent and complex (such as exhibiting cessation of phonation, stoppage of airflow, dysrhythmia, tension, fear, or frustration—see Table 8.1 and Figures 8.3 and 8.4), the prognosis tends to be less favorable.

- *How willing and able are the parents to become actively involved?* Effective intervention requires active participation of all members within the family system, leading to a more favorable prognosis.

- *What is the child's overall level of cognitive or intellectual potential?* Those with reduced cognitive or intellectual potential tend to have a less favorable prognosis.

- *Are there any neurogenic or psychogenic factors relating to the onset of stuttering?* Presence of either factor tends to relate to a less favorable prognosis.

All of the information leading to the diagnosis and prognosis is integrated to form the recommendations, which are discussed with the family in the post-assessment parent interview (in the next section). These recommendations will be presented in detail shortly in a later section titled "Treatment."

Post-Assessment Parent Interview

Both the initial and final parent interviews are intended to be conversational and "give and take" in nature. Nevertheless, I have found that the initial conference typically is more heavily one of collecting information from the parents, while the latter is directed toward providing information to the parents. First, we remind the parents of the purposes for the post-assessment meeting: to summarize the results of the assessment, provide recommendations, and discuss any questions that remain. In doing so, I am certain to restate and address the objectives and purposes expressed by the parents in response to my earliest questions (specifically, Why did you meet with us today? What do you hope to achieve as a result of our meeting?). Parents frequently show both surprise and pleasure that I remembered what they had said and that their objectives and purposes were and are sincerely important to me. I invite the parents to interrupt me at any time with questions for clarification or expansion.

In presenting the assessment results, I deliberately begin by providing a summary of the positive aspects of communication that were demonstrated by the child and between the child and the parents. Doing so serves at least two distinct functions. First, being sincerely positive up front establishes, if not reinforces, a positive context within which to approach the communication problem being experienced by the child and the family. Too often, professionals get right to business and describe the characteristics of the child's observed stuttering. I am not suggesting that I hold the parents in suspense, but I do feel it is critical to create by example a positive context within which to proceed with the family. The effect of our model is strong. Families tend to adopt the attitude they perceive from us. Families who seek our help often are vulnerable, if not desperate, and thereby are impressionable. I have observed that when clinicians present "gloom and doom," the family becomes negative and pessimistic. Likewise, by presenting an accurate and realistic picture using positive terminology, particularly for serious conditions, the family tends to be more positive, optimistic, and motivated to accept and participate actively within the recommendations.

There is a second function to providing a summary of the positive aspects of communication that were demonstrated by the child and between the child and parents. After observing the parent–child interaction, often there are characteristics we wish to target for change. To prevent being misinterpreted as criticizing the parents or preaching to them about how to parent, I present a summary of what I have observed that they are doing in conversation that, in my impression, is conducive to supportive language-based interaction and fluency facilitation. Within this positive context, parents are far more receptive to my constructive suggestions for change (incidentally, I am more comfortable in providing them as well). Some may say that I am consuming valuable clinical time, or worse, "beating around the bush." I disagree. I believe that all of us are inclined to do more of what we feel we are doing right, are more receptive to recommendations for constructive change within this positive context, and are more motivated to participate actively within a shared support system. This conveys to the family that the clinician shares their concern and is willing to participate in achieving a solution. This conveys that the burden is shared and that the family is not alone. This message enables the family to feel empowered to approach, negotiate, and participate within the intervention planning and treatment processes. The same will be said later about using a positive approach with older children and adults who stutter and their families.

Then, we summarize in understandable terms the characteristics of the child's fluency and disfluency (i.e., stuttering, if evident) and estimate the relative severity of the latter. In doing so, I have found it helpful for parents if we first review briefly the characteristics of normal disfluency and provide them adequate examples to hear. Peters and Guitar (1991) nicely summarized these characteristics:

> All of the characteristics for this level must be met for the child to be considered normally disfluent. This child will have fewer than 10 disfluencies per 100 words, and they will consist of more multisyllable and phrase repetitions, revisions, and interjections. When the disfluencies are repetitions, they will have two or fewer repeated items per instance of disfluency. The repetitions will be slow and regular. All disfluencies will be relatively relaxed, and the child will seem hardly aware of them and will certainly not be upset when he is. (p. 171)

Even with guidelines as clearly stated as these, clinicians often find it difficult to distinguish between normal disfluency and borderline stuttering. On the surface, any deviation from the description above may be considered evidence of borderline stuttering. Nevertheless, it is challenging indeed to distinguish between a deviation that is attributable to borderline stuttering and that related to variation within each child. It is essential, therefore, for parents to understand the nature of normal disfluency, stuttering and its most common development, and suggestions for environmental intervention aimed at facilitating the development of the child's speech fluency. Furthermore, based on what is known about the symptom intermittency in the earliest stages of the development of stuttering reviewed earlier (Yairi, 1997; Yairi & Ambrose,

1992a, 1992b; Van Riper, 1982), the present meeting with the parents will be the first of no less than several contacts to monitor the child's speech development. I explain to the parents that it is not uncommon for them to experience emotional swings with their child's speech fluency. Just as they might feel, "My gosh, this really is a problem" (when their child's disfluency becomes noticeable and of concern), it might disappear. Likewise, just as they might feel, "Thank goodness, this terrible problem is gone (when the noticeable disfluency has vanished), it might reappear. I encourage parents to listen to other young children engaged in talking to help them hear the range of variation in normal disfluency. The same advice is useful for clinicians.

Once we discuss with parents the nature of normal disfluency, we discuss the nature and development of the child's disfluency using visual representations (Table 8.1, Figures 8.3 and 8.4) and ample examples for them to hear. We invite and address their questions. One of the most common questions is, "What causes stuttering?" I find more often implicitly than explicitly, parents are asking, "Did I cause it?" or a silently pleading, "Tell me I didn't do it. Tell me that even though my child is having trouble talking that still I am a good parent." I take (or create) an opportunity to address, and absolve if possible, the parents' feelings of guilt for real and imagined past sins. I explain that stuttering often is a consequence of an unspecified chain of events, some of which were out of anyone's control. So it is unlikely that the parents or anyone else specifically caused the stuttering to occur. I explain in brief the nature of child development, communication development, and specifically speech fluency development. In simple terms, we discuss the notion of predisposing factors that are not within anyone's control, precipitating factors that may be within our control, and perpetuating factors that indeed are within our control. I discuss the concept of environmental demands that may exceed some children's capacity to remain fluent under certain circumstances. I try to emphasize that we have no control over events that are past, but that there is much we can do together to facilitate the ongoing development of the child's speech fluency and other aspects of communication. We must provide suggestions in such a way that parents feel that the future is within their grasp. Presenting a picture of a child's problem can be disabling unless strategies for improvement in which the parents and families can participate are presented and demonstrated. A discussion of these follows.

A critical part of this meeting with the parents is to present concrete suggestions for parent and family involvement to facilitate the development of the child's speech fluency. I believe these suggestions are critical, not only for parents whose children appear to be demonstrating borderline or more noticeable stuttering, but for those demonstrating normal disfluency as well. Some may ask why I offer concrete suggestions for parents whose children are demonstrating normal disfluency. My response is built on the premise that such knowledge in the hands of parents can only heighten their child's communication development. While specifically aimed at facilitation of speech fluency, the suggestions are conducive to appropriate models of interpersonal communication. Furthermore, we cannot be absolutely sure that the child's speech fluency in the assessment session was representative of that outside (notwithstanding our attempts to sample the child's fluency over time from the preassessment tape recording and parent interview, which are compared to results collected in the assessment session). In other words, realizing that speech fluency fluctuates, providing the parents with information about environments that facilitate fluency contributes to communication development (i.e., "An ounce of prevention is worth a pound of cure.").

In a sense, as speech–language pathologists, we are the parents' teacher. In presenting suggestions, remember that good teachers do at least three things. They tell (i.e., discuss), they show (i.e., demonstrate), and then they coach, critique, and supervise (i.e., direct). Too often we tell the parents what we expect of them, without showing them what we mean or observing them do what we intend to ensure that they understand. Therefore, I always recommend the three Ds (*d*iscuss, *d*emonstrate, and *d*irect). Following presentation and discussion of the suggestions, I model as many as possible with the child (who is not otherwise present during this conference), and then coach the parents as they apply the suggestions they just heard and observed. These suggestions are reviewed in the next section titled "Treatment." After discussion, demonstration, and direction, I recommend several alternative readings. These help the parents better understand communication development and its disorders, including stuttering, and what they can do to help their child. The readings review and expand the suggestions already presented to them. Often the parents' concerns interfere somewhat with how much they can process and remember. The readings reinforce what they learned, saw, and applied during the assessment session. The following readings are among those I recommend: *If Your Child Stutters: A Guide for Parents* (Ainsworth & Fraser, 1989), *Stuttering and Your Child: Questions and Answers* (Conture & Fraser, 1989); *Understanding Stuttering: Information for Parents* (Cooper, 1990b). Furthermore, several videotapes available from the Stuttering Foundation of America are excellent resources for parents (*Prevention of Stuttering [Part 1]: Identifying the Danger Signs; Childhood Stuttering: A Videotape for Parents*). These and other related resources are described in Appendix B.

At the conclusion of the meeting with the parents, we talk about the treatment process as appropriate to the individual child and schedule a follow-up meeting. I tell them to expect a summary report within 1 week. About 2 weeks after our meeting, I make a point of phoning the parents to determine if they have any questions about the evaluation experience, the summary report, or the readings. Furthermore, I discuss with them how well the suggestions are being applied and any observable changes in the child's communication behavior. Beyond the proceedings of this phone call as indicated, I am conveying by my actions that I care about them as individuals and about the family as a communication system. Furthermore, the family sees that they are not alone and that help and understanding are readily available. The door is always open and we wish to model by our behavior open, supportive, and positive dialogue directed to facilitating the fluency of the individual child and the interpersonal interaction among the family members.

TREATMENT

In this chapter, we have discussed general precepts of preschool children and procedures and issues related to assessment (preassessment, assessment, and post-assessment). Now, we turn our attention to considerations of treatment. As noted earlier, it is useful for all parents to understand the nature of communication and its development. Furthermore, it is important for them to understand the factors that facilitate and those that inhibit a child's communication, specifically speech fluency. Therefore, during the assessment session, we discuss, demonstrate, and then direct the parents in how to reduce the counterproductive communicative demands placed on the child while enhancing the facilitators of fluency, and address the feelings and attitudes of all people involved. These suggestions will be addressed first in the present section. Furthermore, we have several contacts with the parents subsequent to the assessment. With the parents of children who demonstrate normal disfluency, we maintain phone contact approximately once per month until the scheduled reevaluation, which is done between 3 and 6 months later. Subsequent to the reevaluation, we have phone contact about every 2 or 3 months for the next year unless the parents wish to contact us in the interim. With parents whose children demonstrate symptoms of borderline or more obvious stuttering, we engage in a period of play intervention with a degree of directness appropriate to the level of awareness being evidenced by that child. While most clinicians prefer treatment sessions of 30 to 45 minutes usually twice or three times per week, I tend to prefer weekly meetings of 1 hour in duration, with particular emphasis on the treatment that is conducted between scheduled sessions (the extraclinical activities focused on transfer). Because of the importance of transfer activities from the very outset of treatment and because of the importance of the parents' role in the treatment process, the parents are engaged with me in the direct treatment experience during a portion of every scheduled meeting. Methods for both parent intervention and direct treatment will be presented now.

Parent Intervention

The parent intervention process addresses three major foci. The first two are the parents' thoughts (i.e., knowledge) and feelings (i.e., emotionally based reactions) about stuttering, their child who stutters, and themselves as parents. The third focus is the parents' behaviors while interacting with their child when he is stuttering and when he is not. The overall objective is to engage the parents in an educational experience so they understand what they already are doing that contributes to the development of their child's speech fluency and other aspects of communication and what needs to be changed. We noted earlier that parents need to be informed and to feel and experience some sense of control. There are few things more worrisome to parents than when their child has a problem that they do not understand and about which they feel helpless. The clinician must respond both to the child's and the family's communication and emotional needs. It has been my experience that the parents' behaviors are more readily changed than either their thoughts or feelings. However, the behaviors they demonstrate often reflect their thoughts and feelings. Furthermore, heightening their awareness of their own behaviors and providing opportunities for behavior change often impact their current thoughts and feelings about stuttering, their child who stutters, and themselves as parents. For these reasons and for instructional purposes in this chapter, the parents' behaviors, thoughts, and feelings will be addressed separately. In reality, however, these three foci often are addressed simultaneously.

Behaviors

A number of behavioral recommendations that deliberately overlap with one another and with the domains of thoughts and feelings will be highlighted and discussed first.

The parents' aim should be to react to and interact with the child without drawing attention to the disfluency. By not drawing attention to the disfluency and by preventing the child from reacting with frustration to the speaking experience, the disfluency will be indirectly controlled, will lessen, and optimally will disappear. Parents know that often children mirror their emotions and facial expressions. As hard as it may seem for the concerned parent, the message here is to respond positively to the content of the child's speech (i.e., what he says) without evidencing any concern or negative reaction to his relative fluency (i.e., how he conveys his message). In no way should this be interpreted that parents need to withdraw emotionally from their child. To the contrary, parents should continue to offer their love and affection to their child in the ways that have become natural for them. Concern over the child's fluency, however, should remain the parents' concern (i.e., which will lessen with the support of the clinician) and should not become the child's concern.

Encourage the parents to be good listeners. I noted earlier that first I highlight the parents' positive behaviors that are supportive of the child's developing communication skills, and thereby those that I wish to target for continuation. For example, we may highlight verbal and nonverbal ways that the parents have offered their support to the child, their appropriately slow rate of speech, or their turn-taking skills with the child, among others. If the parents are reacting inappropriately to the child and his stuttering (such as interrupting the child, filling in the word before the child fully utters it, or telling the child, "Don't stutter. Think about what you say first." I discuss the counterproductive influence that such behaviors can have on the child's speech fluency. However, by identifying their behaviors that are facilitative as well as inhibiting to speech fluency, I suggest with specific examples that they replace the latter with more of the former. Clinicians need to be aware that parents need our support to confront their feelings of guilt for having made, albeit unintentionally, a parental error. We make the point that children are not fragile. In fact, in most cases children are more resilient than parents. Nevertheless, it is never too late to correct mistakes and to do even more of the things they naturally are doing right. Helping the parents know the difference indeed is within the clinicians domain.

Simplify, soften, and slow the daily speech model to which the child is exposed. Reduce other forms of stimulus bombardment (visual, auditory, emotional) to the extent possible within the communicative environment. Often this is a difficult concept for parents to grasp. First, slowing one's own speech model while still sounding natural is difficult. This is an example of where the three Ds (*d*iscuss, *d*emonstrate, *d*irect) are critical. Parents need to know how to provide the child a slow, gentle speech model, just as clinicians need to know how to provide this model for parents. It takes not only slightly prolonging vowels, but softening articulatory contacts on consonants in addition to maintaining normal inflection, juncture, and prosody. Remember, the point is not to draw attention to the speech. Only prolonging vowels often results in a drone that more resembles robotic speech than human speech. To say the least, an inappropriate model such as this calls attention to itself.

Secondly, parents feel frustrated when they believe they are expected to slow their speech all of the time, lest they are hurting their child's speech fluency. They need to realize your understanding that there are times when speech cannot be slowed (such as when the school bus has arrived and will leave if the child doesn't move in a hurry, when the child will be harmed if he doesn't stop his behavior *now,* when Mom or Dad must leave for work *now* in order not to be late, and other instances). Because there are times when speech cannot be slowed, it is helpful for the parents to set aside on a daily basis a special, uninterrupted time for talking with the child. This means that phones will not be answered and faxes will not be sent; just quality, uninterrupted time. When certain events cannot be slowed or prohibit slower, gentler talking, both the parent and the child deal better with the momentary urgency by looking forward to talking together later without interruption. Often I am asked, "How long should this time be?" I respond that both the quantity and the quality of time should be considered, and that the time should be as long as possible. I recommend no less than 30 to 60 minutes. It becomes instructive to see how much or little of parents' time is available to their children. Another frequent question is, "If we set time aside for one child, do we need to do it for all the others?" I believe it doesn't hurt. The point is that the parent should be available without distraction whenever and for as long as possible. "Should we read to the child?" That is a fine activity, as long as the model of speech is appropriately slow and gentle. At least as important is the dialogue about the book that should follow the reading itself, during which each takes turns speaking and the child feels he has the parents' full attention. What is important is for the parent to dialogue with and listen to the child about whatever is currently on the child's mind. I have found that once there is a mechanism in place for focused, slow, and gentle dialogue, most parents find ways to continue this style of interaction throughout many other daily activities in which the two may participate (such as cooking, cleaning up the dishes, making household repairs, or working on the car).

Another aspect that is difficult to grasp is the type and amount of multisensory information that has become so enmeshed into the child's communication environment. In many homes, modern technology has provided us with portable and car phones, beepers, e-mail, fax machines, and so forth, which have only magnified the potential for distraction. Multisensory bombardment continues to be provided by more traditional forms of entertainment (television, radio, and home video players) and time savers (dish and clothes washers, dryers, and microwave ovens). Some may think that I am bashing technology. I am not. I am saying that we as parents (i.e., and clinicians) need to be aware of what consumes our time and energy and what place our children have within these demands. I might add that as a clinician, a user of modern technology, and a parent of preschool and school-age children, I am raising these issues as much for myself as I am for others.

I am reminded of two recent and relevant events. I saw a Bart Simpson cartoon with a family sitting around the television with a caption stating "Family Bonding." The irony is humorous but also of concern, particularly for children who are developing speech fluency and other aspects of communication.

This cartoon became true to life when, during a recent camping trip, I noticed a number of other tent campers sitting under the canopy of stars, yet watching television with their children. I hadn't even realized that there were electrical outlets. What's the point? All people have real demands on their time and energy. At least some resources must be reserved for children who are developing communication skills, particularly those for whom models of slow, gentle, uninterrupted speech are so important.

Give the child as much fluent talking experience as possible. Try to minimize the amount of experience the child has of talking disfluently. We want to prevent the disfluent speech from gaining a foothold within the child's experience. Therefore, we try to manipulate the child's communicative opportunities to increase both the absolute and relative frequency of fluency when compared to that of disfluency. This can be done in a number of ways. First, when the child is fluent, let him speak. As a speech–language pathologist, I know that children learn language and establish patterns of fluent speech both by using and hearing language. Nevertheless, as a parent of a 4-year-old child, I know what it is like when a child seems to speak during every waking moment apparently without taking a breath. Truly appreciating how silence can be golden, I remind myself how important this experience is for my child, both to hear and to use meaningful and fluent speech and language within a supportive, inviting, and reflective environment. This advice rarely presents a problem to parents. When a child is fluent, the parent has no problem knowing what to do—let him speak. When the child is disfluent, however, many parents do not know what to do in order to help their child.

There is much parents can do to help their preschool child when he experiences noticeable disfluency. Again, the purposes are to encourage the experience of speech fluency and to prevent the child from becoming aware of or disturbed over his disfluency. When the child is noticeably disfluent, the parents should try to take their speaking turn a little sooner than they ordinarily do. I am often asked by parents with some alarm, "Do you mean interrupt my child?" This is another concept that is difficult to grasp. I explain that while few people realize it, we all tend to interrupt each other during conversation. I point out to parents, while we are talking, how we tend to take our turns just before our conversational partner is finished with his or her turn. This often comes as a surprise because most people assume that we wait until our partner is finished before we begin to speak. I encourage the parents to become familiar with the conversational patterns between them and their children. Once they realize that they naturally interrupt each other, then they are more receptive to the idea of interrupting a little sooner. Doing so takes the speaking burden off the child momentarily, thus enabling him to hear the slower, gentler speech model from the parents. This relief, combined with an appropriate speech model, often is successful in enabling the child to regain a fluent speech pattern. Sometimes it takes several attempts to achieve the result.

Another common question is, "What do I do if the child continues to be disfluent after I take my turn sooner and model speech fluency?" The next two suggestions are even harder to grasp. We noted earlier that our communicative world is filled with distractions. This is one case for which I recommend a deliberate distraction. For example, the parent may "need" to remove the food from the oven, respond to the microwave beep, or move the clothes from the washer to the dryer. In this case, the distraction is brief, and the conversation continues after having been interrupted briefly. In the interim, the parent models slow, gentle, natural sounding speech. "What if this doesn't work and the child continues to be disfluent?" Then I recommend that the parent move from distraction to a change of topic or activity. The cost for the child (experiencing and becoming aware of noticeable disfluency) outweighs the potential benefit (continuing the conversation). However, I stress the importance of returning to the original topic of conversation after the distraction or the topic or activity shift. In that way, the child is reassured of the parents' interest. The purpose here is to interest the child in something other than talking so that he can regain his fluent speech, after which the parent re-expresses interest and the conversation continues. It should be pointed out that these patterns (i.e., distractions, topic or activity shifts, among others) occur naturally. Therefore, we gain control over a naturally occurring event and use it to the advantage of the child.

Keep the child from becoming aware of his stuttering. Several of the recommendations already mentioned aim to prevent the child from becoming aware of his stuttering. The importance of responding honestly with support and compassion to the child, however, must be emphasized as well. If a child mentions his speech or disfluency, the parents (and clinicians) should not hesitate to verbalize their understanding that we all get stuck at times and to explain briefly and show (by modeling) that speaking slowly helps. Parents and preschool teachers should reflect on the child's feelings while relating to the content of what the child is saying. For example, if the child runs in from the playground and is out of breath and disfluent, the listener may model slower speech saying, "Boy, I can see how excited you are. I want to hear all that you have to tell me."

Reduce the pace of activities and overall tension as much as possible. Slow, relaxed activities are important. A slow, gentle, and natural sounding speech model should be the rule. Again, this is a difficult concept to grasp. Many of us do not realize how tied we are to our racing internal clocks until we attempt to reduce the pace of our speech and overall level of activity. I noted earlier that role-playing helps. Through puppetry within play, the adult and the child may impersonate a turtle who moves and talks slowly and gently, compared to a rabbit who moves and talks fast and hard. I emphasize the importance of directing praise toward the child for what he is doing correctly (while demonstrating slow and gentle speech). When the child's speech behavior is in need of correction, I prefer to create an opportunity within play for the adult to take on the child's disfluent pattern so that she (the adult) might deliberately correct herself or provide an opportunity for the child to correct the adult's speech. The child then receives praise for correcting the adult's speech, initially by evaluating the error (such as, "Too fast. You did that wrong."), then by directing the correction (such as, "Slow down."), and eventually by demonstrating or modeling the correct form (such as, "You have to say it lllike thhhis"). In this way, the child continually receives support for what he does right (slow, gentle speech; correcting the adult, and so forth) while the adult bears the weight of having been corrected, thus conveying to the child indirectly the error behavior, which is corrected into the target form. I believe this is an important message for working with children, particularly preschool children. We need to create opportunities for children to receive praise for and thereby to become aware of all that they are doing right. Children (and the rest of us) naturally become motivated to do more of what they believe they do well. Within play, we create such opportunities for children to succeed and for them to differentiate between the target behavior (slow and gentle speech for which they receive praise) and the error (fast and hard speech for which the parent or clinician receives correction).

Other activities that emphasize slow and gentle speech include "Simon Says." The parent and child can alternate between the leader (Simon) and the follower, giving and receiving orders for various activities including speaking slowly and gently or fast and hard. To help parents establish slow, gentle, and natural sounding speech, it may be helpful to watch and discuss the speech model presented on *Mister Rogers' Neighborhood,* a morning program on many public television stations. Also, it is helpful for parents (i.e., and clinicians) to study their own speech patterns and those of people around them. Parents gain an appreciation for the variety in speaking styles, some of which encourage, while others discourage, speech fluency. Frequently I have observed in developmental daycare and other preschool settings the teacher heightening the children's body awareness through group singing of "Head, Shoulders, Knees and Toes." The pace of this familiar song increases until the children are neurophysiologically unable to coordinate the fine speech–motor movements required of the song and the gross motor movements of touching corresponding body parts. At this point, some children fall to the ground sharing laughter with the teacher. I remember being concerned about a 3-year-old child who was beginning to stutter and who was participating in such activities. The activity was beyond the limits of this child's coordination and, I found, was exacerbating the child's disfluency. After talking with Caroline, the daycare teacher, the activity was replaced with one that was more facilitative to children's motor and speech coordination. Furthermore, on subsequent visits with the child, Caroline's speech became a contraexample (for example, when the clinician deliberately spoke too fast, the child corrected with, "You're talking like Caroline now. Slow down!").

Identify and reduce or eliminate all fluency disrupters. During the assessment, the parents were asked to describe a typical day in the life of their family. As noted earlier, this was intended to identify potential fluency disrupters. An extension of this activity is to talk with the parents about where their child feels comfortable to speak and free of interruption, compared to where he perceives pressure to talk because of impending interruption. This might be an activity that could begin with the clinician, be completed by the parent at home, and then be discussed with the clinician. In many families, mealtime presents potential fluency disruption for children. In these settings, individual family members gather and enthusiastically share what is on their mind (i.e., what they anticipate for the day, or what has happened during the day). Typically, different people talk at once and interrupt one another. This is particularly challenging for a child who is at risk or is beginning to stutter because of the impact that time pressure and perceived impending interruption have on speech fluency. This fluency disrupter can be prevented by establishing a pattern of turn-taking whereby each person waits for the one who is speaking to finish and then takes a speaking turn without interruption. Without drawing attention to the concern of fluency disruption, turn-taking (with no interruptions) can be addressed as a politeness rule (such as, "It is not polite to interrupt. Taking turns is more polite and shows better manners.").

Another common fluency disrupter is demand speech (in which the child must respond to direct questions) or display speech (in which the child is directed to talk for an audience). For example, well-meaning parents might direct the child in front of relatives to tell about his new bicycle, what he wants for Christmas, or a recent joke or riddle. This puts a tremendous and unnecessary burden upon the child whose coordination for speech fluency is evolving. An alternative would be for the parent to relate part of the event, to which the child might independently volunteer more information. Furthermore, if the parents find the child in a situation calling for demand speech, they might help the child by modeling slow, gentle speech and by expanding what the child has already said, again enabling him to participate voluntarily rather than on demand. Another potential fluency disrupter occurs when young children naturally become interested to talk on the phone. The excitement of talking to Grandma and the ambiguity of how she so neatly fits into the phone receiver combines into a frequently unmanageable fluency challenge for the child. Alternative strategies might include sitting with the child who is talking on the phone and coaching him (while modeling slow, gentle speech) about what he might tell his grandmother, thus providing alternative topics for sharing. This tends to reduce the demand placed on the child, enabling him to use more resources for coordination of speech and language fluency. I know in some households with multiple siblings, a ringing phone sets off a mad dash by the children. All rush to be the first to answer the phone. If the child who is beginning to stutter proves victorious, speech fluency potentially is challenged by racing to the phone and competing for and maintaining hold of the phone. Again, turn-taking helps. In such situations, children may answer the phone in a predetermined sequence. Furthermore, the parent may model the phone greeting for the child using slow, gentle speech ("Hello. Who is this please?") before picking up the phone and handing it to him. These simple politeness procedures significantly reduce the demand placed upon the child's capacities to remain fluent.

Another common fluency disrupter is filling young children's schedules too full. Many youngsters are rushed from swimming class, to soccer, to dance, to Leonard's birthday party at McDonald's. Indeed, many children become "chips off the old block." Parents are responsible for filling or overfilling their own schedules. Children, on the other hand, must be guided in making responsible choices. When all of their time is consumed in demanding, albeit creative, activities, little energy remains to meet the demand of speech fluency and other aspects of communication development. A preschool child with whom I worked in play interaction to facilitate speech fluency comes to mind. One day I observed her literally airborne, holding the hand of a baby-sitter who was pulling her out of the preschool setting to rush to her ballet class on the other side of town. Working with the well-intentioned parents, I explained the importance of maintaining a moderate and manageable demand on the child's time, energy, and resources, particularly when a child demonstrates being at-risk for fluency failure. This led into an interesting and candid disclosure from the parents about how complex and overly scheduled they were, and how these factors are causing marital discord. Their intention was to provide for the child, not burden her. Working with the family while focusing on the child's communication development and the family's system of communication resulted in significant insights by and about the parents. Independently, they sought family counseling to study, understand, and alter their lifestyle and communication between themselves as spouses. The parents reported the counseling to be productive. The play intervention with the child, which involved her parents, led to a reduction of disfluency, subsequent monitoring, and eventual dismissal.

There are many potential fluency disrupters. The parents and clinician working together identify them and subsequently reduce, and eventually eliminate, their influence. In addition to the factors already discussed, others include, but are not limited to, the following: inappropriate speech and language models or expectations, rapid speech rates, calling attention to stuttering, punishment for stuttering, time pressure, demand or display speech, interruption, competition, guessing what the child is about to say, speaking immediately after the child stops talking, listener loss, excitement, conflict about discipline, emotional upset, and hectic or unpredictable schedules (Gregory, 1989; Peters & Guitar, 1991; Van Riper, 1973). The list of potential interferences to the child's fluency is endless. Because every family is different, the clinician must help the parents identify both the facilitators and the inhibitors of speech fluency. Doing so is a sensitive task because of the parents' thoughts and feelings, which will be addressed now.

Thoughts and Feelings

If ever a clinician experiences the essence of a therapeutic relationship, it is when she addresses with parents their thoughts and feelings about a child who is beginning to stutter. Discussing this special relationship, Webster (1977) noted that "counseling is not something one does to another person; it is an activity one does with another. Counseling is an endeavor that people engage in together . . . (and) refers to a number of situations in which people communicate" (p. 1). Discussing the unique nature of each person's world and the challenge facing the clinician, Webster (1977) stated:

> Each person exists in a unique and very private world made up of forces that constantly impinge from both inside and outside. The outer forces help to create and shape one's inner world, while internal forces help to create and shape one's perception of the outer world. (p. 3)

A significant challenge facing clinicians when addressing the feelings and attitudes of parents is to understand their inner and outer world. It may appear that one's outer world is more readily understandable because it appears to be more directly observable. However, one's world only can be understood from an appreciation of the inner world and the dynamic interaction between real and perceived internal and external forces. This concept is not unlike those presented in Chapter 5 when discussing personal constructs and family systems. The clinician must work with the parents and other family members to understand their unique interpretation of their world (and specifically the experience of the child's disfluency), the inherent assumptions, and the patterns of communication among the family members. Only when the parents and the clinician become aware of these factors can any belief or behavior be targeted for change.

We discussed earlier how behaviors and thoughts are related. In other words, what one does often reflects what one thinks or assumes, and one's thoughts are confirmed (or challenged, thus requiring revision) by observed behaviors. By discussing with parents their observed behaviors, the clinician has an opportunity to gain insights about the parents' thoughts and their current knowledge base about stuttering. I have come to believe that at worst, most parents are doing their level best. Fortunately, with very few exceptions, parents are trying their best to provide for their children while accommodating life's demands. Most parents who innocently advised their child, "Don't stutter" or "Slow down. Think about what you're saying," did not realize why this is counterproductive. Usually when we talk with parents about the nature and etiology of stuttering, they are eager to adjust their current behavior to help their child. In other words, most of the parents' inappropriate behaviors were based on inaccurate or incomplete information. One of our missions, therefore, is to be a source of information and support for parents.

Sometimes, however, when parents reflect on their well-intentioned errors toward their child and begin to adjust their behavior in order to facilitate the child's speech fluency, feelings of guilt (i.e., emotional regret for having done something wrong) and anxiety (i.e., nervousness and tension) surface. These feelings typically make it difficult for parents to confront their child's stuttering. I discussed earlier the importance of first identifying all of the parents' behaviors that are supportive of and conducive to the child's communication development. Only then, within this positive context, do we discuss possible revisions. Starkweather et al. (1990) noted that they use a similar procedure:

> We begin to alleviate guilt by showing the parents all the correct things they have done to cope with the disorder. All parents have some reactions that are less negative. If they show concern in any positive way or just provide a loving atmosphere, we compliment them on it in order to let them know that their instincts are accurate and have already led them to help the child learn to speak more fluently. If parents are speaking in a reasonably slow rate or taking turns well, we let them know that these things have been helpful. We then go on to suggest other things they might do, some of which they have probably already thought of. This kind of approach is likely to elicit a strong sense of cooperation from the parents in addition to reducing guilt. (pp. 69–70)

Parents' willingness and ability (i.e., readiness) to confront stuttering in their child varies. Some are more accepting and are ready to study and understand the situation and adjust necessary behaviors. Others are loath to confront stuttering, perhaps seeing it as their own failure, thus avoiding or denying it. Among many other things, the rate of recovery without intervention ranges from 50% to 80%, and these figures improve with treatment (Peters & Guitar, 1991). Furthermore, we emphasize that early intervention achieves much success in preventing stuttering. In fact, one of the best prognostic indicators is the amount of time that has elapsed between the onset of the disfluent behaviors and the beginning of intervention. The longer the duration between the identification of disfluency and the beginning of intervention, often the longer it takes to remediate the stuttering. Other prognostic indicators related to a longer duration of treatment for the child who is beginning to stutter are negative reactions of the parent toward the parent's own or the child's stuttering and anything that might make it difficult for the parents to carry out the suggestions provided in treatment (including environmental stress, financial hardship, social problems, an uninvolved parent, and marital discord) (Peters & Guitar, 1991; Starkweather et al., 1990). These and other special considerations were addressed in Chapter 5. Starkweather et al. (1990) added that the consequences of not doing anything are potentially serious enough to warrant a program of management, even if it is one of monitoring (Yairi, 1997; Yairi & Ambrose, 1992a, 1992b; Zebrowski, 1995), being undertaken as soon as possible.

During this period, we invite and address the parents' questions and involve them actively in implementing the recommendations after discussing, demonstrating, and directing them first. These procedures tend to reduce feelings of guilt and anxiety by showing the parents that they have a partner, a comrade, who will work with them to help their child. We identify, explore, and confront as necessary thoughts, feelings and behaviors that might have a negative impact on the child's speech fluency. We remain positive, emphasizing all of the parents' behaviors that are appropriate and monitoring and praising successes. We confront and challenge in a supportive environment. Starkweather et al. (1990) advised as follows:

> When parents have been reacting badly to stuttering, we do not try to underestimate the negative impact those reactions have on the child, but if the parents see these reactions as behaviors they were unaware of, reactions motivated by their love for the child, and accompanied by other helpful behaviors, it is unlikely that they will feel guilty about them. (p. 70)

Identifying and understanding the parents' feelings of guilt and anxiety are essential, as is modification of such feelings. The parents' guilt and anxiety potentially can consume their energy that might otherwise be directed toward implementing suggestions for fluency modification. Furthermore, the child's attitudes toward communication and beginning stuttering are influenced by that of the parent. As the child perceives the parents' verbal and nonverbal tension when the child is disfluent, the child will be inclined to try harder not to be disfluent, thus struggling and forcing as he tries harder, all the while internalizing feelings of guilt for having created unpleasantness for the parents. Cast more positively, and fortunately more frequently, the parents can be helped to understand better their feelings and thoughts about stuttering and their child who is beginning to stutter. With the care of a knowledgeable clinician, both the parents' concerns and the child's symptoms can normalize as all work toward the child's fluent future. The methods for adjusting the behaviors, thoughts, and feelings will be discussed further in the Clinical Portrait at the end of this chapter.

Direct Intervention

The intervention methods discussed so far for a preschool child who is beginning to stutter have been relatively indirect. That is, the clinician works with the parents to manage the communication environment at home and elsewhere in order to achieve a reduction in the child's disfluency and a return to normal fluency. I find it helpful to conceptualize intervention for preschool children as falling along a continuum from *indirect* to *direct*. Indirect approaches do not explicitly or overtly attempt to modify the child's speech fluency. Rather, they focus on the child and the child's communication environment. Such approaches often involve information sharing and counseling with the parents, interacting with the child in a variety of play-oriented activities in which speech is not the obvious focus, and modeling by the clinician and parents of fluent or more "easy" speech for the child. Direct intervention approaches, on the other hand, are characterized by explicit or overt attempts to teach the child how to change his speech or related behaviors, and may or may not be conducted within play (Conture, 1990b; Van Riper, 1973; Zebrowski, 1997).

The methods discussed in this section are of increasing relative directness with respect to the child. They are intended for a child who is beginning to stutter (that is, a child whose amount of disfluency is increasing in frequency, forms are becoming more complex, and behaviors are reflecting increased awareness or establishment of frustration). Peters and Guitar (1991) described the "beginning stutterer" as follows:

> This child is usually between 2 and 8 years of age. In terms of core behaviors, he may exhibit part-word repetitions produced rapidly and with irregular rhythm. He may have vowel prolongations. Some of these core behaviors may contain excessive tension. He may also exhibit blocks. In terms of secondary behaviors, he may have some escape and starting behaviors. This child may be experiencing some frustration because of his stuttering. Finally, he may have a self-concept of himself as someone who has trouble talking, but he usually is not concerned about this. (pp. 273–274)

Within the context of play intervention, the clinician interacts with the child directly with and without the parents present (who participate actively when present). The suggestions reviewed earlier for parent intervention are continued. The direct treatment through play is an addition to parent intervention, not a replacement. The treatment process is becoming more aggressive, yet still relatively indirect as will be seen when compared to that for the school-age child.

Goals

The treatment goals for the preschool child in direct treatment is spontaneous (i.e., normal sounding) fluency and maintenance of a positive attitude toward communication and oneself as a communicator.

Objectives

The objectives for the child in directed play intervention are to establish and transfer fluent speech, to develop resistance to the potential effects of fluency disrupters, to express feelings about communication and oneself as a communicator as appropriate, and to maintain the fluency-inducing effects of treatment.

Rationale

Play and fun create the language of childhood. Intervention with preschool children who are beginning to stutter must be done with laughter. Children want to do more of what they perceive to be successful and fun. It is necessary—but not sufficient—for the clinician sincerely to enjoy working with the preschool child. When the clinician knows and understands what she is doing, feels positive about the child's and the family's potential, and is and has fun, children like the clinician and will work through play with her. Children must like and trust you. Play and fun create trust. Children are mirrors of the clinician's trust, confidence, friendship, and love. All the clinical materials in the world cannot replace a clinician's enjoyment of children and a natural ability to talk with them. I particularly enjoy working with children about whom I am warned to expect behavior problems. These children challenge our professional (i.e., clinical and particularly interpersonal) skills. Although I have had my fair share of healthy challenges, I am yet to find a child who is not manageable. I remain convinced that the behavior of a disruptive child reflects as much the behavior of the responsible adult as it does that of the child. I often remind myself that when we point a finger at a child or anyone else, we have three pointing at ourselves. The procedures that follow are based on the four objectives listed above. Furthermore, the procedures are more direct than those presented for parent counseling, yet less direct than those presented for intervention with school-age children. While a composite is painted here of the preschool child, it is possible that the child's developing symptoms and awareness defy his age. In such a case where the symptoms (behaviors, thoughts, and feelings) are more advanced, the procedures outlined in Chapter 9 for even more direct intervention with the school-age child would be more appropriate, independent of the child's age.

Procedures

Treatment procedures with a brief discussion for each are presented here.

Establish and transfer fluent speech. A first step in establishing fluent speech through play is modeling within a fun context what the child should sound like. How do I do it? We talk. That's all. We talk and I listen to and learn about the child's world. Remember, everybody, even young children, has a story to tell (Shapiro, in press). Let them tell it. Too often clinicians' use of clinical materials hinders rather than helps a child's willingness to talk. Clinicians feel they must be in control, so we talk and we question. It is hard to have a real conversation when we interrogate the child, or when we repeat everything the child said into the tape recorder, or when we write everything down the child said on our legal tablet and clipboard. Just talk, listen, and have fun. In fact, the more listening we do, the more we can take the child's lead. Children see that here they have a big person who does not need to control. In their eyes I can see them thinking, "This is mighty different." Children love to talk. Clinicians may want to review the stages of play discussed earlier in this chapter (see Figure 8.2). Somehow, most adults know how to talk with children when they meet within a social context. They say, "Hey big guy! Those are mighty nifty boots you have on. Mind if I slip them on my feet?" Or they say, "By jingo, you've got the coolest red hair I've ever seen. Do you think I could get mine that red if I used a big red crayon?" But because talking within a professional context is distinguished as "treatment," naturalness and fun, which epitomize the privilege of talking with children, go to the wind. We say things like, "I am Mrs. Smith. I am a speech–language pathologist. Do you know what that is? What is your name?" Or we say, "I am your new speech teacher. Do you know why you are here?" Let's role reverse. If we clinicians were the children listening to the latter, rather stilted, lifeless questions, would we be motivated to talk? If truth be told, I think we'd try to catch some sleep. I think I would hide under the table or throw spit balls because that seems like more fun. What about you?

So what do I do? I play and I have fun. I like puppets a lot. They tend to take the pressure off the child, even though the child is talking for the puppet. We sing songs. If the child is particularly disfluent, we may sing or speak (e.g., nursery rhymes and jingles, among others) in chorus. Throughout the activities, I model slow, gentle, natural sounding speech. Starkweather et al. (1990) described this modeled speech as "naturally cadenced slow-normal speech rate with appropriate melodic contour" (p. 71). We draw and we paint. We play "Simon Says" and we "hide and seek" right in the treatment room. If the child is disfluent, I insert both similar and more gentle disfluencies of the child's form into my speech, sometimes offering a neutral comment about my speech as I go about my play (e.g., "Oops. That was a tough one."). With children, the effect of our model is potent. They see that we and our fun are unaffected with or without disfluency and they follow suit. I remember a 6-year-old girl who put a large ring (from a ring toss game) on my head and said, "You're the King of Laughter." No award or accolade could mean as much to me as what she said. I believe she saw me as fun, able to communicate with her, and inviting of her story. And incidentally, her fluency returned to normal in the process.

An interesting ethical dilemma has arisen on several occasions. Typically, in each scheduled meeting, I work with the preschool child first without his parents, and then I bring them into the session. When the parents are not with me, I encourage them to observe what we are doing from the observation room. (Recall our earlier discussion of observations without observation rooms.) I believe that the child's advantage is served when parents are kept maximally involved and informed. Literally and figuratively, I want to open the door to the parent and family. On several occasions during play interaction, however, a child shared a feeling or an event with me that would not have been shared if the observers had been present. For example, about a father who was clinically depressed and under medical and psychiatric care, the 4-year-old child said, "I don't like my daddy. He scares me. He's mean to me." Another reported, "My mommy is bad. She went to jail." In both of these cases, the parents were observing and expressed alarm at what the children had said. The children's disclosures had a positive outcome, however, resulting in additional productive dialogue between the clinician and the parents and families.

I realize the parents in these cases are the legal guardians and that they, their children, and their family are protected by confidentiality. But what about confidentiality within a family, or a child's right to express a feeling without disclosure to the parent? In some cases where the feelings or events being expressed impact beyond the child's communication or the family as a communication unit, I have made referrals to family counselors, social workers, and social service agencies. But when what is said impacts within our professional domain, communication and its disorders, we neither can prevent nor predict what the child will say or when he will say it. So until children have their own right to confidentiality, discretion and compassion must direct our standing commitment to understanding and helping communicators within families.

For the purpose of transferring fluency to the home and other outside settings, the suggestions provided in parent intervention are continued throughout treatment. Other transfer suggestions are derived from the directed play treatment experience as appropriate for each child. For example, a clinician who is providing specific feedback (such as praise) for the child's fluent speech ("I like that you just used slow, gentle speech"), might have the parent continue this at home (using the three *D*s—discussion, demonstration, and direction). The child's observed disfluency might serve to remind the clinician and parent to continue to praise the fluent speech when observed and to offer correction only indirectly in the form of modeling and expansion. The transfer activities should be emphasized from the very beginning of treatment; hence, the importance of involving the parents and family in all aspects of the treatment experience. The individual transfer activities are limited only by one's imagination and creativity, as long as the recommendations presented for parent intervention are followed.

Indeed it is critical not to single out a child from among other people to slow down. Nevertheless, providing models of slow speech is essential, as are occasional supportive explanations. Consider the following example. A father on a picnic outing by a creek with his 3-year-old son continuously modeled slow, gentle speech, particularly when his son demonstrated noticeable disfluency. Other suggestions implemented by the father, including taking his turn sooner and engaging in gentle distractions, did not prove successful in relieving the child's disfluency. At one point, the father said to the child, "See that yellow leaf on the creek. See how it moves like this (demonstrating a slow, gentle, flowing hand movement from left to right). Let's see if we can talk like the leaf, like this (repeating the hand movement, continuing to model a fluent speech pattern)." The boy said, "Lllike thhhis (gently prolonging initial consonants)?" The father reinforced with, "That's right, just like this." This explanation represents an increase in the father's level of directness in dealing with the child's disfluency symptoms, yet still within an atmosphere of unconditional acceptance and support without any overt or negative judgment. The picnic continued, now in fluent dialogue. About 1 year later, when driving in the car, the father realized that both his rate of speech and that of his son were too fast. As the son's speech was becoming increasingly disfluent, the father commented, "Hold on. We both need to slow down a little" (i.e., as the father modeled slower, natural sounding speech). The son commented, "You mean like the creek?" Having long forgotten the experience from a year ago, the father asked, "What do you mean?" The boy responded with, "You know, daddy, like this" (i.e., moving his hand in the slow, gently flowing, wave-like pattern from left to right, while speaking in a more fluent and gentle, easily flowing speech). "That's right," the dad acknowledged with a laugh. "I had forgotten about that. That's a good thing to remember. Thanks for reminding me," the dad continued while following the child's example for slow, gentle, fluent speech. Children learn and teach by our own example.

Another experience comes to mind. In directed play treatment, a 3-year-old child was provided feedback for using appropriate speech fluency ("I like the way you said that. You used slow, gentle speech"), as discussed earlier. The clinician directed the child to listen to her (i.e., the clinician's) speech and help her slow down when it got too fast. "Sometimes I forget," said the clinician, "and I need a little help from my friends." When the child's speech increased in rate or demonstrated patterns of noticeable disfluency, the clinician assumed a rapid rate with some noticeable disfluencies, thus inviting the child's correction. As discussed earlier, the purpose here was to provide the child ongoing support for what he (the child) was doing right, and for the clinician to wear the weight of correction when necessary (i.e., when the child's speech rate or disfluency increased), thus conveying the correction to the child indirectly. Again, the rationale is for speaking to continue to be a fun, positive experience. The parents were included in this experience during directed play and carried it over to the home setting. They reported that on several instances when they (i.e., the parents) forgot to focus on fluency, failing to provide models of slow, gentle speech, and the child reminded them, "You're talking too fast," or "Slow down!" Note that the child had never been directed to "slow down," but internalized the correction and generalized it to the speech behavior of others. Again, children learn and teach by our example.

Here's another example. We have emphasized the importance of slow, relaxed activities to regulate speech fluency. What happens when the activities run out and when bedlam strikes? This happened to one family recently while they were taking a road trip of 10 hours. There were two children in the family, one of whom was a 4-year-old boy who demonstrated beginning stuttering. His speech fluency remained under control within slow, relaxed activities. When the activities ran out, as did fluency control, the mother suggested, "Let's sing songs. How about 'Itsy Bitsy Spider?'" At that she began to sing, thus regulating a slower, gentle pace. The children joined in chorus, followed by their own selections. Slowing down the overall pace through song reestablished a comfortable speech model for all. This activity led to others (such as "I Spy" and guessing games) within which slow, gentle speech was used. Remember that suggestions for transfer such as these are in addition to the recommendations given earlier for parent intervention. In essence, every waking moment holds the potential for speech fluency facilitation and transfer.

Develop resistance to the potential effects of fluency disrupters. Once fluent speech is established and is being transferred to the home and other outside settings, we increasingly work to develop resistance to fluency disrupters, or buffering mechanisms (Van Riper, 1973). In other words, the test of any treatment is how well its effects are maintained when the conditions that formerly resulted in stuttering are systematically reintroduced. Other tests include transfer (already discussed) and maintenance of fluency, in addition to the feeling of fluency control. I find it best to conceptualize fluency challenge as falling along a number of continua. Fluency challenge is least present when the recommendations given for parent intervention are followed continuously and greatest when they are not followed at all. We might consider the recommendations separately and reintroduce fluency challenge for each.

One example already mentioned involved rate of speech. To establish fluency, we seek to model slow, gentle, natural sounding speech as much as is reasonably possible, in addition to that within special uninterrupted family time already discussed. We noted that along the way, when the child's rate or disfluency increases, we model the contraexample (fast, hard speech), inviting the child's correction in order for him to reestablish more appropriate speech patterns. Once speech fluency is established, and is being transferred and maintained, we may deliberately demonstrate contraexamples, or barbs (Conture, 1990b), more frequently. These barbs enable the child to gain experience withstanding potential fluency interrupters, thus minimizing their impact. Similarly, we may reintroduce interruptions and deliberately violate other conversational turn-taking conventions (by abruptly shifting topics or appearing distracted when the child is talking).

A major goal here and throughout, however, is to ensure the child's success. No positive aim is served by the child's failure. The clinician's responsibility is to ensure that the child is and remains successful. We already reviewed the motivating impact of success. If the child fails to succeed, then the learning step taken with the child between where you are (e.g., modeling slow, gentle speech always) and where you want to go (e.g., deleting the clinician's model of slow, gentle speech) is too great. You may delete your model for 1 minute during every 5- or 10-minute interval, systematically increasing both the frequency and duration of the periods with no deliberate model. Eventually, the child will maintain slow, gentle, natural sounding speech in the context of no deliberate model, interruption, listener loss, increasing audience size, demand and display speech, and other challenging contexts. Sometimes it is helpful to remind the child in advance to remember to use slow, easy speech even when the clinician "forgets." That way, the child will not be confused about why the clinician's manner of speaking has changed, and he will expect increasing and deliberate challenge. The challenge of remembering to use slow, easy speech can and should become another fun game between the child and clinician and parents.

Encourage expressions of feeling about communication and oneself as a communicator, as appropriate. One of the hallmarks of the preschool child who stutters or those who are demonstrating beginning stuttering is the absence of deep emotional involvement. Part of his emotional neutrality reflects the absence of a long and potentially painful history of fluency failure. Another part reflects the positive, accepting, nurturing response the child receives—when he is fluent as well as when he is disfluent—from his parents and all others who function within the child's communication system. Whether the child is emotionally neutral toward his speech, or better yet, overtly positive about the communication experience, is critical and a significant distinguishing characteristic of the preschool child. Our job as clinicians, and that of other communicators within the child's environment, is to make sure that the child's attitude toward communication and himself as a communicator remain positive. We do this by being open, accepting, and nurturing toward the child about his speech and all other areas of potential; by being receptive and responsive to the child's affective expressions; and by creating opportunities for the child to express feelings and to be supported for having done so.

To understand the significance of such a positive, nurturing communication context, I recommend to clinicians and parents that they record a video sample of their interactions with the child. Reviewing the videotape for both verbal and nonverbal factors invariably proves enlightening. We might take particular notice of the comments directed to the child. Are the comments emphasizing what the child is doing correctly and what you sincerely believe he can do ("You can do it. I know you can. Fantastic! What you just said was great slow, easy speech. You are always such a good artist. You know so much about dinosaurs.")? Or are they focusing on what the child is doing wrong, is not doing, should or should not be doing, and can't do ("Stop that now. If you do that one more time . . . Sit in your chair. Put that down. No, that's not right. I already told you how to do that.")? One of the few things that makes my uvula steam (and I don't get upset often) is when I observe clinicians verbally reward children with, "Good boy!" or "Good girl!" when a child has done something correctly, but then fail to offer a verbal reward when the child has shown his best effort but did not succeed. This concerns me for several reasons. First, this communicates to the child that he is a good person when he succeeds and implies that he is bad when he does not. What ever happened to receiving honest recognition for doing your best, whether you win or lose? Furthermore, I recommend showing unconditional positive regard for the person ("That a boy! Way to go."), consistent recognition for the sincere effort ("That was a dynamite try. Hang in there. I'm so glad you are doing your best work."), and more discriminating feedback for the relative accuracy of the response ("Oops. That was a tough one. Why don't we try it with our slow, easy speech, like this," offering explanation, demonstration, and then supportive coaching). A scenario that invites constant correction and behavioral management might present a level of difficulty that is too challenging and might not be appropriately structured for the strengths, needs, and interests of the individual child. If this occurs, consider a lower level on the hierarchy or continuum of difficulty.

How inviting are we to the child's expressions of affect? Do we create opportunities for the child to offer expressions of feeling or preferences and then support him for having done so? When we give the child a choice, do we honor his selection? As noted earlier, asking a child, "Do you want to come with me?" or "Do you want to look at these pictures with me?" invites a choice of two implied alternatives, *yes* and *no*. When the child says, "No!" and we coerce the child into coming or looking, we have not honored the child's selection. Furthermore, we convey to the child that his expression of preferences will not be taken seriously anyway. Recall discussion earlier about how to phrase questions differently so that the child's alternatives are supportive of the treatment objectives. When a child sincerely confesses, "I don't want to do that," do we listen and respond having considered the child's perspective, or are we locked into our own perspective (Moses & Shapiro, 1996; Shapiro & Moses, 1989)? Preschool children generally are not intricately aware of how or what they feel. When they offer behavioral outbursts or emotional tantrums, do we assume that they are intentionally disruptive or that they have received poor parenting? One little disfluent boy told me from my knee, "Everybody is always mad at me. Everybody blames me." Indeed these were significant expressions, as the parents were inadvertently triangulating the boy into an unstable marital relationship, vacillating between obsessive concern over his fluency and excessive criticism of most other behaviors. The concept of triangulation was reviewed in Chapter 5. Yes, it is true that not all disruptive or emotional expressions are symbolic and that some behaviors are downright and brilliantly manipulative. But what I am saying is that we have to listen and be able to hear the child's message which often is overlaid and rather indistinct from his feelings. To do so, clinicians must understand their own feelings, strengths, and needs, both personally and professionally, so as to shift perspective and to assume the internal world of the child. These and other clinician competencies will be discussed in Chapter 11.

Maintain the fluency-inducing effects of treatment. Once the child is speaking fluently both inside and outside the clinical setting with a variety of speakers, with and without potential fluency disrupters—all the while accepting of himself as a communicator—we begin to reduce the time spent in directed play treatment. If sessions are weekly, they may move to every 2 weeks, then once per month. Assuming that the achievements are maintained, we schedule abbreviated reevaluations every 2 or 3 months for the first year in addition to maintaining phone contact and receiving audiotapes monthly during the interim. During the reevaluations, we sample and analyze the child's speech and interview the parents. Reevaluations decrease in frequency over the following year. Should the child regress or should the parents wish to discuss the child's or the family's communication needs, they are welcomed back at any time.

 ## Clinical Portrait: Amy Stiles

Selected Background Information

Amy* was 3 years, 10 months old when she was referred by her parents for a speech–language evaluation because of her "stuttering." Both Mr. and Mrs. Stiles attended the scheduled evaluation, reporting that "sometimes when Amy speaks she will stutter. She gets real upset." Amy's disfluencies first were noticed by the parents about 1 year prior to the evaluation when she told a little boy, "I–I–I am Amy," reportedly resulting in laughter from the boy. Regarding Amy's speech fluency, the parents reported fluctuation with long periods of remission and apparent awareness leading to frustration by the child, evidenced by her stopping midsentence and stamping her feet. Amy had no previous speech–language intervention. Amy's birth, developmental, and medical history was without complication. She had no siblings and her family history for communication problems was negative. Because of financial hardship, Amy's family lived with her maternal grandmother. Mr. Stiles was employed as a manual laborer in a factory. Mrs. Stiles was not employed outside of the home.

Abbreviated Speech–Language Analysis

An analysis of Amy's conversational speech revealed an average rate of 140 fluent words per minute, or 152 words per minute when figuring fluent and disfluent words. These rates represent a low average rate of speech. Most of Amy's speech was characterized by relatively effortless, gentle articulatory transitions of even rate with normal sounding suprasegmental features (such as pitch, juncture, and loudness). Disfluencies across the conversations were characterized by whole-word (what–what) and part-word (the–they) repetitions and occasional sound prolongations (lllot), which did not interrupt the motor sequence, intended message, or communication effort. Based on samples of 100 words in length, Amy's overall disfluency averaged 9%. Part-word repetitions accounted for 54% of the total disfluencies and were characterized by no more than 3 units of repetition per instance. Whole-word repetitions comprised 36% of the disfluencies and again revealed no more than 3 units of repetition per instance. Prolongations, 10%, were gentle and fleeting, not exceeding 1.5 seconds in duration. The only secondary characteristic observed was occasional, inconsistent tense eye blinking during the prolongations. No disfluencies were observed during song or choral recitation of nursery rhymes. More frequent disfluencies were noted on repetition of longer, more complex words (such as *celebrate* and *incubator*). Before attempting to repeat *incubator*, Amy expressed, "My mouth is getting tired." Symptoms suggesting the beginning of communication interference included the high proportion of within-word disfluencies, slight increase in disfluency in conversations with unfamiliar people and with increased linguistic demand, infrequent eye tension, and her

---

*All clinical portrait names have been changed to protect confidentiality.

comment about "getting tired." All other aspects of assessment (both informal and standard-ized) revealed age-appropriate speech (that is, articulation and phonology) and language (semantics, syntax and morphology, and pragmatics) development. All parameters of voice and hearing were within normal limits.

Recommendations

Because all other aspects of Amy's speech, language, motor, cognitive, and social development were within normal limits, Amy's disfluency was considered to be of "borderline" concern. I elected parent intervention as a form of prevention with ongoing monitoring to ensure stabil-ity in the development of Amy's speech fluency. Suggestions for parent intervention were reviewed with the parents at the time of the evaluation, followed by the clinician's demonstra-tion of the techniques and then coaching the parents in using the techniques with Amy. The parents were given supportive reading material, told that the summary report would follow within 7 to 10 days—at which time they should call me—and scheduled for reevaluation in 6 weeks. In addition, a supportive letter (represented in Figure 8.8) was sent immediately fol-lowing the evaluation.

Follow-Up

Subsequent analyses of Amy's speech and parental reports for 6 months indicated that parent intervention was effective in stabilizing and reducing Amy's speech disfluency. However, the parents elected to have Amy participate in children's presentation at their Kingdom Hall, the house of worship of the Jehovah's Witness faith, which proved to have a significant and dele-terious effect on Amy's speech. This experience was discussed in advance, described as demand and display speech, and therefore discouraged. The presentation involved a number of pre-school children individually going to a microphone and telling about a poster depicting a religious theme. Fortunately, the parents audiotape recorded the program, from which Amy's presentation was analyzed, as summarized in the following paragraph.

Amy spoke 62 words, of which 36 contained one or more types of disfluency, over a 90-second duration. Her overall rate of speech in this context was 41 words per minute (compared to 152 words per minute in the assessment setting), revealing an overall disfluency of 58% (fig-ured by dividing the total words spoken by the number of stuttered words); compared to 9% in the assessment setting. Rate of speech was irregular, revealing both instances of even tran-sitions and silent and audibly tense pauses of up to 6 seconds in duration.

Forms of disfluency included part-word repetition (e.g., A–A–Adam; 66%), which con-tained up to three instances of uneven and audibly forced repetition; whole-word repetition (snake–snake–snake; 20%) of up to 3 units of repetition; and sound prolongations (EEEEEve; 6%) that contained audible voiced and unvoiced struggle and vocal fry without pitch rise. Addi-tionally, unlike that demonstrated in the assessment context, Amy's speech contained broken words (Ca–*silent pause*–in, A–*silent pause*–bel), combined repetition with tense prolongations (f . . . f . . . for), interjection of prolonged syllables (uuum) and phrases (yyyou know) unevenly spaced of up to 3 units of repeated interjection, and word (picture, um, poster) and phrase (that's it, that's what it is about) revision.

These selected data in this context indicate a significant decrease in Amy's fluency; increase in the observed types, complexity, and frequency of disfluency; and serious interfer-ence in her effectiveness as a communicator. In response only to her presentation, the audience applauded in empathic relief.

Treatment Snapshot

Because of the significant reduction in Amy's speech fluency subsequent to the presentation, she was enrolled in direct fluency treatment for the ensuing year, which utilized play both as a context and a medium for exchange. Following the suggestions described earlier in this

May 30, 1997

James and Susan Stiles
21 East Main Street
Sylva, NC 28779

Dear Mr. and Mrs. Stiles:

It was my pleasure to meet with you and your daughter, Amy, on Tuesday, May 27. Indeed, you are a beautiful and supportive family.

My assessment of Amy's speech is that she is in an early stage of the development of stuttering. Having seen evidence of her frequent repetitions during the evaluation, I feel that it is a critical period in that so much can be done now in order to prevent the disfluencies from becoming chronic.

This type of disfluency generally is most effectively treated by the parent, with advice from a speech–language pathologist. For this reason, I do not recommend scheduled direct treatment at this time. As we discussed at our meeting, I feel that the following suggestions will assist you to increase the likelihood that Amy's speech continues to develop without serious increase in the amount or type of her disfluency.

I feel that you are doing an excellent job in managing the disfluency which is observed and in being "good listeners." I recommend that you continue the same approach with the following additions. First, try to provide Amy with models of slow, simple speech. Gradual slowing probably will be less obvious and more natural for you. Second, whenever possible, reduce any pressures on her to speak quickly or fight against interruption. If members of your family and friends can refrain from interrupting her, that should be helpful. Third, if Amy has a sudden occurrence of disfluency either when excited or in a hurry, try to get her interested in something else besides talking, so that she does not have much experience with serious disfluency. Then later, when she is less excited, you might ask her about what she was telling you. Fourth, try to keep her from being aware of the disfluency. If she mentions it to you, however, don't hesitate to tell her that you know that we all get stuck on words at times. Suggest by showing her that trying to say them slowly or easily may help.

I hope that these suggestions prove helpful and that you have had an opportunity to begin reading *If Your Child Stutters: A Guide for Parents* and *Stuttering and Your Child: Questions and Answers*. Both of these books I loaned you from the Stuttering Foundation of America, in addition to their videotape (*Childhood Stuttering: A Videotape for Parents*), should reinforce and expand upon our conversation and recommendations. I look forward to speaking with you soon regarding these suggestions and future considerations.

If you have any questions, do not hesitate to give me a call at the Western Carolina University Speech and Hearing Center. You will find the phone number at the top of this letter. Again, thank you for meeting with us and for sharing your commitment to Amy's communication development.

Sincerely,

David A. Shapiro, Ph.D., CCC–SLP
Speech–Language Pathologist
Faculty Supervisor

Figure 8.8. Follow-Up Letter.

chapter, the parents both (that is, the mother consistently, the father inconsistently because of schedule conflicts with work) observed the first half of each session and participated directly in the latter half. Puppetry was used as one of many different materials to differentiate between "slow, easy" and "fast, hard" speech. Amy was provided frequent verbal rewards for remembering her slow, easy speech. Correction of the clinician's puppet was used initially to remind Amy indirectly to use a more fluent pattern, and eventually to challenge Amy's fluency control. She was told by the clinician's puppet, for example, "Sometimes when I get excited to talk with my friends, I forget to use slow, easy speech. Will you help me remember?" Then, the clinician deliberately inserted noticeable disfluencies ("What is going to ha–ha–ha–happen?"), to which Amy's response systematically increased over time in steps or levels of challenge. The same error will be used for illustration here, but in reality, both the errors presented by the clinician and the response expectation of the child vary, as follows:

- Initially Amy offered, "Slow down!"

- Then, she was asked, "What do you mean?" To this Amy explained, "Bird, you have to put a little stretch in that."

- Still later, Amy was asked, "Would you show me how to do it?" Hearing the clinician's error, Amy was observed at one point to subvocalize the correct form of the clinician's error (clinician said "ha–ha–ha–happen," to which Amy subvocalized, or mouthed without sound, hhhappen). She then offered in slow, gentle speech, "Hhhappen."

- The clinician challenged, "Do you mean 'ha–ha–ha–happen?' " To this, Amy both critiqued the clinician's error ("No, that's not right.") and offered the corrected form ("What is going to hhhappen?").

- Then the clinician offered, "Do you mean, 'What is going to hhhappen?' " To this, Amy offered, "Yes, that's it." Then the clinician rewarded and reauditorized the correct form, "Oh, thank you. What is going to hhhappen. So, what is going to hhhappen?"

These few steps indicate how within the context of play intervention using puppetry, the response expectation for the child moved from identification of the error, to analysis of the error (what aspect was wrong), explanation of how to correct the error, internalization of the corrected form, demonstration of the correct form, correction (response analysis) of the contraexample, reinforcement (response analysis) for the corrected form, and coaching the clinician for the correct form. Just as I have discussed the importance of telling (discussing), demonstrating, and then directing (coaching and critiquing) when teaching a child or parent a new behavior, here the child is "teaching" the clinician within an opportunity created by the clinician. After completion of this sequence, the clinician created opportunities to model and expand the topic of discussion while using the correct form of the word that the child "taught" the clinician how to say correctly. A sequence such as this shows how the response expectation of the child can be increased systematically within the context of play.

Follow-Up and Epilogue

Directed play intervention worked effectively in helping Amy both regain control of her speech fluency and remain positive about communication and herself as a communicator. Furthermore, regular conferences with the parents combined with their active participation in all aspects of the treatment process enabled them to understand and contribute meaningfully to the treatment process. After having worked with the family for 1½ years (6 months in parent intervention only; then 1 year in direct treatment), Mr. Stiles received a transfer to Atlanta, GA, a distance of 150 miles. For a short time, the family commuted from Atlanta in a most unreliable vehicle. Then, Mrs. Stiles, Amy, and her newborn sister came to live with Amy's maternal grandmother just so the family could receive fluency treatment. I remained concerned about the family being apart (between Cullowhee, NC, and Atlanta, GA). When they moved to

Atlanta, I investigated treatment options there, although none were possible for the family because of the financial expense involved. We maintained phone contact nearly monthly for the next year, during which time the family continued to send audiotapes of Amy's speech. Having followed the family for 2½ years, we lost contact for about 18 months. One day, a tall girl whom I barely recognized knocked on my door. Amy had grown so in stature and maturity that, for the moment, it was hard to remember the kid I had worked with a year and a half ago. I was thrilled to hear her speech fluency. We promised to exchange letters by audiotape, which we did for several months following. She told me about Chinese cooking, Girl Scout cookie sales, and her little sister whom she described as "a pain." Happily, Amy's rate of speech stabilized between 170 and 180 words per minute without a trace of noticeable disfluency. The only concern was a defective /r/ production, which was receiving attention at school. Here's to good stories, happy endings, and committed families.

Central and Guiding Intervention Assumptions

Before ending this chapter, I want to return briefly to the principles that have guided our discussion to this point and that continue to serve as a basis for constructing and critiquing treatment. These are the intrafamily (personal constructs, family systems), extrafamily (interdisciplinary teaming and multicultural awareness), and psychotherapeutic (fluency shaping and stuttering modification) considerations.

Intrafamily Considerations

Fortunately, all members of the Stiles family maintained, in their thoughts, feelings, and behaviors toward and about Amy, the assumption that she is communicatively able and will communicate more fluently. This personal construct shaped the way the parents approached and participated in the treatment experience and the way Amy continued to view herself as a communicator. Fortunately, throughout her experiences, which potentially contributed to increased demands placed upon her (such as presenting at Kingdom Hall; moving to, from, and back to Atlanta; the birth of her sister; financial hardship; and going to school, among others) and with the ongoing and positive support of her parents, Amy did not need to reconsider or revise the way she thought about herself. Although occasionally challenged, Amy continued to predict her future as she had always known her past, one of love, nurturing, and encouragement. Similarly, the Stileses continued to function as a family unit. Every event that affected one of its members affected, in some way, each other member. This was seen not only in Amy's fluency, but in all other family matters. When times seemed at their darkest (e.g., during miscarriages, loss of employment, and the seemingly ongoing repair of the family truck), the family pulled together the most and pooled resources. Both the family's view of Amy as a communicator and the networking of communication within the family were considered always in the planning and evaluation of treatment.

Extrafamily Considerations

For different reasons (distance traveled, family preference), there was relatively little involvement of an interdisciplinary team. Only when treatment was considered in the Atlanta region, did I contact other professionals. However, the records provided by the family were complete, ensuring my understanding of Amy's and the family's history. The family's involvement in the Kingdom Hall and other activities of the Jehovah's Witness faith provided a significant focus in their life and a source of emotional, social, and spiritual support, particularly during challenging times. I respected their faith and learned by their example. Furthermore, as the clinician, I needed to be sensitive to and understand their faith in the design of treatment (not recognizing common holidays, birthdays). And while the importance of not engaging Amy in demand or display speech in the Kingdom Hall seemed so obvious to me, the parents' view toward their faith and their connection to others within the congregation needed to temper my concern over the parents' not following the advice that was provided.

Psychotherapeutic Considerations

Finally, as reviewed previously, fluency shaping and stuttering modification treatments are least distinct for preschool children who are beginning to stutter. Parent counseling and direct treatment reflected an appreciation of both sets of assumptions. For example, providing more opportunity to talk when fluent and less when disfluent, structuring communication environments, establishing fluency and increasing challenge in small steps, and building resistance to potential fluency disruption all have roots in fluency shaping considerations. Remaining positive about and toward the child as a communicator, not showing parental upset or frustration when disfluency occurs, creating opportunities for expression of feelings and support for having done so, engaging the child in making choices about the treatment experience, and constructing treatment within a play context originate from stuttering modification considerations. However, these distinctions overlap. They become clearer as the stuttering enters the child's view of himself as a person and as a communicator within a social context. Such clarity will be discussed when we address school-age children who stutter, in the next chapter.

CHAPTER SUMMARY

This chapter reviewed a variety of strategies for assessing and treating preschool children. In doing so, two major points were emphasized. First, distinguishing between normal disfluency and incipient stuttering requires analysis of the child's behaviors, thoughts, and feelings, and ultimately a professional judgment on the part of the clinician. Second, intervention with preschool children and their families requires an understanding of the communication environment, full support and involvement of all members with the communication system, and identification and elimination of potential precipitating and perpetuating factors.

We noted that preschool children are in a period of intense development, are insightful, vary in their apprehension of the clinical setting, engage in play and fun which represent the language of childhood, and have a story to tell. Pre-assessment procedures for preschool children include completing a case history form, obtaining and reviewing an audio- or videotape recording of the child interacting with his family or other members of the household, and making a preliminary phone call to address the family's initial questions and to help prepare the child for the evaluation. Assessment procedures include a parent interview, a parent–child interaction, a client–clinician interaction, and trial management. The parent interview is a conversational sharing of information between the clinician and parents. The parent–child interaction is observed by the clinician who gains a better understanding of how the child and parents interact with and react to each other. The client–clinician interactions are designed to enable the clinician to observe directly the child's fluency and disfluency and the extent to which both are modifiable. These include speech–language sampling and structured activities with and without communication pressure. Trial management provides the clinician an opportunity to use different treatment activities to determine their relative effectiveness with a particular child.

Post-assessment procedures for preschool children include a thorough analysis of speech and language skills, leading to statements of diagnosis, prognosis, and recommendation, all of which are summarized in a post-assessment parent conference. Speech analysis addresses the frequency, types, molecular description, rate, secondary characteristics, severity, and adaptation and consistency of the child's disfluency. A diagnosis is an integration of all information available to determine if the child is stuttering, at risk for stuttering, or demonstrating normal speech fluency. If the child is stuttering or at risk for stuttering, then the clinician must determine if treatment is warranted and recommended, and if so, what should be the nature and focus of treatment. Before making treatment recommendations, the clinician makes a statement of prognosis, which is a prediction of the outcome of a proposed course of treatment. Treatment recommendations may take a variety of forms and are discussed with the parents and other family members.

Treatment for preschool children always includes family intervention and may include direct intervention. The goal of parent intervention is the prevention of stuttering by engaging the parents in an educational experience that allows them to understand what they already are doing that contributes to the development of their child's speech fluency, as well as what needs to be changed. Behavioral recommendations include: (a) reacting to and interacting with the child without drawing attention to the disfluency, (b) being good listeners, (c) adjusting (by simplifying, softening, and slowing) the daily speech model to which the child is exposed, (d) maximizing the child's experience with fluency and minimizing that with disfluency, (e) preventing the child from becoming aware of his stuttering, (f) reducing the pace of activities and overall tension, and (g) identifying and reducing or eliminating fluency disrupters. Other suggestions were discussed for helping parents understand and adjust, if necessary, their thoughts and feelings about their child and his stuttering. For cases in which stuttering more clearly is indicated and direct intervention is warranted, the treatment goal for preschool children is achievement of spontaneous fluency and maintenance of a positive attitude toward communication and oneself as a communicator. Four objectives were addressed, including establishing and transferring fluent speech, developing resistance to the potential effects of fluency disrupters, encouraging expressions of feeling as appropriate about communication and oneself as a communicator, and maintaining the fluency-inducing effects of treatment. Specific suggestions were presented for achieving each objective. The chapter ended with a clinical portrait of Amy Stiles, a girl who was 3 years, 10 months old, with whom the assessment and treatment considerations were applied and discussed.

Chapter 8 Study Questions

1. Normally developing children create opportunities for themselves to use and develop language by interacting verbally with adults. How might stuttering in young children affect their development in speech and language and other areas?

2. We noted that there is a fine and invisible line between normal disfluency and incipient stuttering. How would you as a clinician make that distinction and what factors must be considered? What aspects of making this distinction are concrete, and what is the role of professional judgment?

3. We reviewed several precepts of preschool children. How does an awareness of the nature of preschool children impact the assessment and treatment processes?

4. Preassessment, assessment, and post-assessment procedures provide much valuable information that is analyzed by the clinician. What components of this information do you feel are most important? How do you feel each element contributes to the important decisions being made by the clinician?

5. What recommendations do you have for preschool children who are stuttering, at risk for stuttering, or demonstrating normal speech fluency?

6. Results of recent longitudinal investigations of untreated stuttering patterns in preschool children (Finn et al., 1994; Yairi, 1997; Yairi & Ambrose, 1992a, 1992b; Yairi et al., 1993) indicated that severe disfluency tends to lessen after 2 or 3 months of onset (boys' stuttering tended to persist longer than that of girls), followed by an increase in chronicity from 14 to 18 months after onset. Between 65% and 85% of the children recovered without treatment within 2 years of onset. What impact do these findings have on the assessment and treatment processes?

7. Chapters 5, 6, and 7 reviewed intrafamily, extrafamily, and psychotherapeutic intervention considerations, respectively. What impact do these factors have on the assessment and treatment of preschool children and on interactions with members of the family system?

Unit III

◆ ◆ ◆ ◆ ◆ ◆ ◆ ◆ ◆ ◆ ◆ ◆ ◆ ◆ ◆ ◆ ◆

Assessment and Treatment Strategies with People Who Stutter: A Life Span Perspective

Chapter 8
Preschool Children: Assessment and Treatment

Chapter 9
School-Age Children Who Stutter: Assessment and Treatment

Chapter 10
Adolescents, Adults, and Senior Adults Who Stutter: Assessment and Treatment

Chapter 9

School-Age Children Who Stutter: Assessment and Treatment

♦ ♦ ♦ ♦ ♦ ♦ ♦ ♦ ♦ ♦ ♦ ♦ ♦ ♦ ♦ ♦

General Precepts About School-Age Children Who Stutter   294

Preassessment Procedures   295

Assessment Procedures   296

General Considerations   296

Parent Interview   296

Teacher Interview   297

Child Interview   298

Speech–Language Sample Without Communicative Pressure   301
Structured Activities Without Communicative Pressure   304
Speech–Language Sample and Structured Activities with Communicative Pressure   304

Trial Management   305

Fluency Shaping   306
Stuttering Modification   306

Post-Assessment Procedures   307

Speech Analysis   308

Frequency of Speech Disfluency (i.e., Disfluency Frequency Index, DFI)   308
Type of Speech Disfluency (i.e., Disfluency Type Index, DTI)   308
Molecular Description of Disfluency   308
Rate of Speech   308
Secondary Characteristics   309
Severity Rating   309
Adaptation and Consistency   309
Feelings and Attitudes   309
Other   309

Diagnosis   309

Prognosis and Recommendations   310

Post-Assessment Interview with the Parent, Teacher, and Other Participants   311

Treatment   312

Goals   312

Objectives   312

Rationale   312

The Changing Needs of the Child   312

Intrafamily Considerations   313

Extrafamily Considerations   314

Psychotherapeutic Considerations   314

Procedures   315

Increase and Transfer Fluent Speech   315

Construct a "safe house" within which fluency blossoms, children (and clinicians) grow, and magic happens   315

Invite treatment objectives from the child   316

Create opportunities for the child to experience fluency success   317

Heighten the child's awareness of his speech fluency; Make the child's speech fluency (and only then, disfluency) the object of study   318

Develop or improve use of fluency facilitating techniques during instances of stuttering   321

Transfer fluency facilitating techniques to extraclinical settings   326

Develop Resistance to Potential Fluency Disrupters   327

Engage the child in activities with gradually increasing degrees of competition   327

Reintroduce direct fluency challenge   327

Address the situations on the top rung of the child's communication hierarchies   328

Prepare for relapse: Relapse happens!   328

Establish or Maintain Positive Feelings About Communication and Oneself as a Communicator   329

Prepare the child for the likelihood of being teased; Empower him with constructive strategies to withstand the potential ill effects of teasing   329

Help the child maintain positive thinking about communication and himself as a communicator   330

Talk with the child in positive ways; How we talk with children powerfully influences what they think about themselves   331

Maintain the Fluency-Inducing Effects of Treatment   333

Help the child become his own clinician   334

Decrease the frequency of scheduled treatment   335

Maintain regular maintenance checks of decreasing frequency for at least 2 years post-treatment   335

Build in regular, child-initiated benchmarking   336

Deliberately revisit the past   336

Reexamine the child's personal construct   337

Integrate treatment changes within the communication system   339

Working with School-Age Children Who Stutter and Have Concomitant Language or Phonological Impairment   340

Concomitant Disorders   340

Effects of Concomitant Disorders   340

To Treat or Not To Treat?   341

If *Yes,* Where Do I Begin?   341

Sequential Vs. Concurrent Intervention   342

Blended Intervention Approaches   343

General Principles   343

Working with Parents   344

Access to Parents   344

Respecting the Primary Role of Parents   345

Meeting Parents' Needs   346

Working with Teachers and Other School Personnel   348

Build Rapport and Establish Colleagueship with Teachers   348

Banish Elitism—All Colleagues in Education Are Equal   349

Provide Teachers with Strategies To Facilitate Fluency in the Classroom   351

Advocate for all children, particularly a child who stutters   351

Provide the child with more opportunity to speak on days when he is fluent,
less when he is more disfluent   351

Expect the child to participate in regular assignments, but provide flexibility
and support when adjustments need to be made   352

Shift perspective to see through the eyes of the child who stutters   353

Provide all children, particularly those who stutter, regular support for their daily victories   354

Prevent singling out a child who stutters   354

Clinical Portrait: Thomas Wells   355

Selected Background Information   355

Abbreviated Speech–Language Analysis   355

Recommendations and Objectives   356

Treatment Snapshot   356

Follow-Up and Epilogue   358

Central and Guiding Intervention Assumptions   358

Intrafamily Considerations   358

Extrafamily Considerations   358

Psychotherapeutic Considerations   359

Chapter Summary   359

Chapter 9 Study Questions   362

I watch as my child struggles with his words so much like I have done time and time again. He doesn't have a clue what to do. But he gets through it. Listeners are compassionate. He is very young. He has not missed anything for lack of speech. His awareness is growing. So I wonder how long will it be till others are not compassionate, till they move on to the next person cause they didn't know he was trying to talk, till they figure he just doesn't know what to say, till he's not cute enough for folks to go out of their way to meet him half way.

He needs to learn now what to do. He needs to learn to bring his techniques, however simple, into all of his speech, not just to impress his speech therapist. He needs one or two ways that work, to empower him to face his world with confidence.

I want it now for him. Not after embarrassment rips his confidence away. Not after he throws his dreams away. Not after he gives up dreaming. Not after he thinks he can't talk. Not after his hopes and dreams quit sprouting. Cause that might turn his words inside, words which can't come out. Not after he gives up.

I want it now. While he believes he can talk. While he believes others will listen. While he knows good things can happen. While he's still the master of his world.

I want someone to help him, someone who knows what to do.

(FROM THE MOTHER OF A 7-YEAR-OLD BOY WHO STUTTERS.
Subsequent to this letter, both the boy and his mother enrolled in fluency intervention.)

In the previous chapter, we addressed preschool children and their families. Specifically, we looked at general precepts about preschool children, assessment procedures (i.e., preassessment, assessment, and post-assessment), treatment procedures (i.e., parent intervention and direct intervention), and a clinical portrait of a preschool child and her family. In the present chapter, we will consider school-age children who stutter. Following a structure similar to that used in the last chapter, we will look first at general precepts, then assessment and treatment procedures and related considerations (working with children who stutter and have concomitant language or phonological impairment, and working with parents and teachers), and conclude with a descriptive clinical portrait of a school-age child who stutters. In doing so, we will emphasize the following points:

- School-age children who stutter must understand the nature of their own speech fluency and be in control of it before effecting reduction in disfluency.

- Clinicians must manage not only the behavioral characteristics of speech fluency, but what each child thinks and feels about communication and himself as a communicator as well.

- Effective intervention requires an understanding of the child's communication environment and active participation of the child, his family, and others in all aspects of treatment planning, implementation, evaluation, and follow-up.

GENERAL PRECEPTS ABOUT SCHOOL-AGE CHILDREN WHO STUTTER

The following observations can be made about school-age children who stutter. Again, such observations tend to be from a bird's eye perspective, one that emphasizes group trends. Conture (1990b) aptly noted, "Stutterers don't enter your clinical doors in a group; they walk in as individuals" (p. 61). In other words, an individual school-age child or other person who stutters may or may not show similarities to group trends. We noted in Chapter 8 that similarities between an individual and group trends (such as demonstrating adaptation and consistency effects) may indicate just that, similarity, or predictability of behaviors. When one's behavior is not similar to group trends, that might imply that one is unlike others who stutter as a group, is at-risk for stuttering, or is demonstrating normal disfluency. Distinguishing among these alternative diagnoses is the clinician's responsibility. Conture (1990b) noted, "Individual behavior varies around the group's central tendency (for example, mean), and it is not at all unlikely that one particular stutterer may show very little consistency (or minimal adaptation) but still be a stutterer and need your services" (p. 61). The same could be said about any other individual characteristic when considered in isolation and compared to that of a group composite. With this caution in mind, we look now at general patterns of school-age children and of those who stutter (Conture & Guitar, 1993; Haynes et al., 1992).

- School-age children who stutter no longer are beginning to stutter. Typically, their gentle repetitions and prolongation have progressed into struggling with, avoiding, and disguising disfluency and combating frustration and fear (Haynes et al., 1992). Peters and Guitar (1991) characterized the "intermediate stutterer" as follows:

  > The intermediate stutterer is usually between 6 and 13 years of age. Thus, he is typically in elementary or junior high school. He is exhibiting part-word and monosyllabic repetitions and vowel prolongations that contain excessive tension. He is also exhibiting blocks. In terms of secondary behaviors, he is exhibiting escape, starting, and avoidance behaviors. The avoidance behaviors may include word substitutions, circumlocutions, and avoidance of certain speaking situations. This child is also experiencing frustration, embarrassment, and the beginning of fear related to his stuttering. Finally, he has a definite concept of himself as a stutterer. (pp. 331–332)

- Similarly, a longer time since onset of stuttering has elapsed for school-age children than for preschool children. While some children begin to stutter in school, most who enter the first grade have stuttered 1 or more years. The additional habit strength of the stuttering acquired from cumulative experience of increasing duration presents a less favorable prognosis and, therefore, unique treatment concerns (Conture & Guitar, 1993).

- School-age children are developing increasing independence from their parents, and are spending more time with children and adults other than their primary care providers, siblings, or relatives. However, they continue to be dependent upon parents for guidance, physical care, transportation, and primary needs (Conture & Guitar, 1993).

- School-age children, while becoming increasingly independent from parents, are becoming increasingly dependent on their peers for their social, emotional, and academic development. The child is introduced to and begins to participate in peer pressure, criticism, and social conformity (Conture & Guitar, 1993).

- While becoming less willing to accept advice, direction, and guidance from adults, particularly their parents, school-age children are increasingly influenced by school personnel, one of whom is the speech–language pathologist. Whereas many preschool children are referred for communication assessment and/or treatment by their parents, school-age children most often are referred by school personnel (Conture & Guitar, 1993). Many children tend to associate the speech–language pathologist with other school personnel who, in some cases, may be penalizing or disturbing listeners. Furthermore, children may associate speech–language pathologists with authority figures (because often the child has no choice about entering treatment), thereby potentially undermining a trusting relationship (Haynes et al., 1992).

- Generally, school-age children are reluctant or unable to verbalize internal feelings and lack the insight to analyze a problem objectively in order to establish alternative solutions (Haynes et al., 1992).

PREASSESSMENT PROCEDURES

The assessment procedures for the school-age child are similar to those for the preschool child. The reader is encouraged to refer back to those in Chapter 8 now. Before the assessment procedures begin, the parent (i.e., primary care provider) completes the case history form represented in Figure 8.1 in order to provide the clinician an understanding of the child's developmental and medical history; family structure; communication strengths and limitations; and onset, development, and current perspectives regarding the communication problem. The parent is asked to make an audio- or videotape recording of the child engaged in family interaction so that the clinician can sample the child's speech in that setting and begin to understand the communication dynamics within the family. Again, the clinician makes a preliminary phone call to help prepare the child for the evaluation, to address the parents' questions, and to convey the clinician's support and commitment.

The other people with whom the child spends much of his day need to be involved in preassessment as well. Children who stutter often are identified from communication screening in the schools or are referred by the classroom teacher. If the teacher has not already conveyed preliminary observations, he or she should be invited to do so and to provide a tape recording of the child talking in the classroom setting. Again, this gives the clinician another opportunity to see how the child's speech fluency varies by setting and other communicative demands. Typically the clinician to whom the child is referred is employed by the school system, thus giving her an ideal opportunity to observe the child within the classroom before the assessment procedures commence. This provides the clinician with a preliminary impression of the child's communication and social skills.

ASSESSMENT PROCEDURES

General Considerations

Most assessments of school-age children who stutter are conducted by the clinician employed in the schools. The assessment procedures as discussed here reflect that assumption. Unlike other clinical settings where different interviews and observations are conducted at the same scheduled appointment, assessments conducted in the schools often require several different appointments. The appointments scheduled generally include a parent interview, teacher interview, and child interview, in addition to observing the child interacting in as many different settings as possible (the tape recordings provided by the parent and teacher prove invaluable here). The proceedings should be tape-recorded for review and analysis. As noted in Chapter 8, videotape is preferred but audiotape still provides valuable information.

Parent Interview

Based on information received from the case history form, initial tape recordings, the preliminary phone call, and other interactions, the clinician outlines in advance for herself questions and other topics to pursue for clarification or expansion. Because interviews typically are scheduled when school is open, thus conflicting with work and other parent responsibilities, it is common for only one parent to attend the conference. In some cases, clinicians will schedule appointments after school hours to accommodate the parents. After a social greeting, the clinician invites the parents to share what they hope to achieve from this meeting. Although school personnel most frequently initiate the referral, parents often respond with an expression of concern (for example, "I want to know what we can do to help Billy when he stutters. I want to make sure we are doing the right thing."). The parents' response to my initial question conveys the parents' view regarding their child's and their own needs and objectives. The clinician then shares her overall purpose for such a meeting in order to orient the parents, being sure to relate directly to the parents' statement of objective. The clinician explains that she is interested to learn more about the child's communication past and present and how the family members communicate with one another to help the child and understand his communication environment outside of school.

Once the parents elaborate the nature of their concern, I ask them to discuss to the best of their memory the onset and development of the problem that they just described. Many of the questions asked of parents of school-age children are the same as those of preschool children, discussed in Chapter 8. Additional questions address how the child's communication skills affect his school experience including friendships, academic performance, and other factors. As noted when discussing the preschool child, the parents' description of a typical day in their household helps the clinician understand the family structure and communication dynamics and identify sources of possible communication pressure and inadvertent penalty. Williams (1978) addressed developing a profile from the parents of school-age children who stutter, as follows:

> Generally you will want to obtain the parents' views and attitudes about the stuttering problem now and the effect that they perceive it has had on their child. Reflected in their attitudes will be hints about the way the child has been treated in the family. Examples of questions that may be asked include: Why do you believe that he continues to stutter? How serious a problem is it to you or to him? How do you handle it and how do you think it should be handled by other people? In what ways do you feel it has affected your child? What kind of child is he now? In what ways do you think he would be different if he had not stuttered? How does he get along with boys and girls his own age while in school or playing? To what degree has his stuttering influenced his relationship with children or with adults (teacher, grandmother, others)? How has it limited what he has achieved socially or educationally? How much help does he need in meeting new situations or new problems? What special allowances do you think he should receive because of his stuttering? How independent is he in comparison with other children? How has he reacted to his stuttering? How has he reacted to your help and concern about it? Questions such as these provide a picture, albeit somewhat cloudy, of the ways in which the parents have reacted to their child as a "stutterer"; and it often provides an overview of the way in which he may be reacting to himself. (pp. 68–69)

Teacher Interview

The child spends a substantial portion of each day with his teachers who observe and interact with him regularly. Teachers know their children—all of them. In our excitement to help a child who stutters, we clinicians must be sensitive to the demands placed upon teachers to meet all of the regular and special needs of all of their children. Teachers provide a valuable and ready source of information as long as we remain interested in and supportive of helping teachers achieve their instructional mission as well. More will be said later in this chapter about how to work with teachers as partners in the intervention process.

Just as we want to learn how the child is functioning in the classroom setting, the teacher wants to understand stuttering and what can be done about it. Again, I recommend inviting the teacher to express what she would like to achieve from the meeting so that her needs are heard, met, and thereby treated as important. Just as we build relationships with children who stutter and their families, we need to nurture relationships with our professional colleagues including teachers. Many of the same questions presented to parents also could be presented to teachers, thereby guiding the discussion with them as well. Other questions might address the child as a communicator in class and the teacher's feelings about and reactions to the child (such as, What is the child's communication like in class? How does he seem to feel about his stuttering and himself as a communicator? How does his stuttering impact his classroom participation, academic performance, and overall progress? How does the child interact with other children? Is the child experiencing any teasing? If so, to what extent and how does he handle it? How does the teacher feel about the child's stuttering and how does it affect the classroom? Does the teacher feel comfortable meeting the instructional mission while accommodating the child's individual communication needs?) (Peters & Guitar, 1991).

Child Interview

After the necessary permission forms are signed, the clinician schedules through the teacher a relatively convenient time to meet with the child. When possible, I recommend that the child be given at least two alternative times from which to select his preference. We need to show by word and deed that he is important to us. Just as we appreciate being given alternatives from which we might accommodate our busy schedules, so does the child (as well as parent and teacher). The child is busy and has preferences too. Too often, children are pulled without consideration from their favorite activities (e.g., playground, art, gym, music), those that contribute significantly to building the child's positive self-concept and feeling of accomplishment (see Figure 9.1). Sometimes schedule conflicts are unavoidable. However, the child's schedule, needs, and preferences should be considered.

When meeting with the child, the clinician must convey her sincere interest in the child as a multifaceted person, not just as one who stutters (Guitar, 1997). How can we learn about the child as a person without first addressing his interests, talents, hobbies, family relationships, and friendships? Likewise, the clinician must present herself as an interesting person too, one who is inviting yet reflective, and positive and nurturing by nature. Intervention with people who stutter is about building relationships. How can we hope to convey our sincere interest in the child as a person, when seemingly within the same breath as having just introduced ourselves, we are asking the child to describe his problem? It does not take long to establish a foundation, but the time spent is irreplaceable. No dwelling will stand for long without a foundation. Building a foundation and working with a child who stutters is a form of counseling. "Simply stated, counseling involves talking *with* another person" (Williams, 1983, p. 35). Talking *with* does not mean talking at, below, around, or above. It means helping a child to see more clearly what he is good at and the nature of all of his fluency. From this positive and informed framework, the child can explore what he is doing that results in speech fluency and what he is doing differently that results in speech disfluency. We help the child make this distinction and guide the child in how to do more of what he is already doing that results in speech fluency. Focusing first on the speech fluency defuses the child's defenses, which more often than not have risen to the surface and are consuming the child's energies to control or deny their existence. The child comes to feel in control and successful in being able to do more of what seemed so elusive.

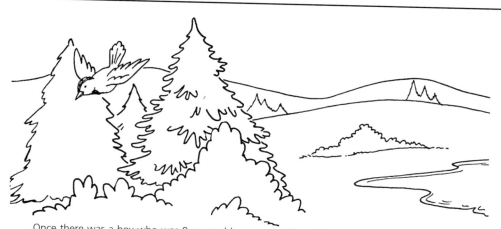

Once there was a boy who was 9 years old. He was not unlike many other children. He usually was happy and lived with his parents, sister, and brother in a house surrounded by a forest that had lots of streams and even a few lakes.

The boy had many friends to play with. His best friend, though, was Buddy, a funny looking dog that had long black, white, and brown hair all over its body and always a wet nose. Buddy and the boy were friends for a long time, in fact, ever since Buddy was a pup and the boy was 3 weeks old. As they grew together, they took many long walks in the woods, and they even fell asleep together in the sun by the stream. Everyone knew when they saw the boy that Buddy was not far away.

One place you would not see Buddy was in school. The boy had many other friends in school, though. He especially enjoyed playing with Billy on the playground and in gym, art, and music. These were the boy's favorite times in school because he felt that he was good at what he did. He could kick the ball higher and farther than most other children; he could run very fast; and he could climb the ropes almost without using his feet. Music was fun too because the boy liked to sing.

But the boy often did not like going to school because it was hard for him to talk in class. The boy stuttered, and he knew it. Even when he knew the answer to a question, he would not talk because he was sure the children would laugh when he tried to speak.

One time, even the teacher laughed. When the boy tried to take his turn reading out loud, he simply could not say the words. He knew the words, but the sounds just wouldn't come out. Sometimes, trying so hard, the boy sounded like a little grizzly bear.

When the teacher said, "You do know how to read, don't you?" or "You do have a name, don't you?" (when the boy could not say his name), the children laughed. Only Billy never laughed. Billy was the boy's friend.

The boy acted like a good sport, but inside he cried. It hurt to be teased so much. He was a smart boy too. He always got good grades—usually 90 to 95 in all of the subjects, but a 65 in oral reading. That hurt too.

One thing the boy especially did not like was being pulled from the playground, gym, art or music to go to speech class. These were activities in which the boy felt normal—almost like the other children.

Over the years, the boy worked with many different speech therapists. They usually were nice. There was one that the boy did not like because she always told the boy to read. The boy knew he couldn't read out loud. Why didn't the speech therapist know that? He surely wished he could be playing with Billy or with Buddy. One time, it was so hard for the boy to keep trying to read to the speech therapist that he started to cry and ran out of the room. That was the last time he went to that speech therapist.

One day when the teacher talked to the boy's parents about how hard it was for the boy to talk in class and how unhappy it made the boy feel, the boy's parents decided to take him to a different speech therapist after school. The boy thought that might be a good idea—he didn't like to stutter one bit. "Wouldn't it be wonderful," he thought, "to be able to talk to anybody, just like talking to Buddy?" He never stuttered when he talked to Buddy.

(continues)

Figure 9.1. A Way Through the Forest: One Boy's Story With a Happy Ending. *Note.* From "A Way Through the Forest: One Boy's Story With a Happy Ending," by D. A. Shapiro, 1995, March, *The Staff,* pp. 2, 7. Reprinted with permission of the publisher (J. B. Westbrook/Aaron's Associates).

Anyway, the new speech therapist was a man. He didn't tell the boy to read. In fact, he didn't tell the boy to do anything. He asked the boy what he wanted to do. "This is surely different," the boy thought. The boy said that he'd like to walk by a stream, just like he does with Buddy. So that is what they did. Sometimes they talked, and sometimes they didn't. The boy felt that he found another friend. In a funny way, it was like being with the boy's grandpa. The boy and his grandpa often took long walks. That made the boy feel special. Sometimes they talked, and a lot of times they just listened to the stream and walked. That was what the boy was doing with his new speech therapist.

Time passed, as did Buddy, Billy, the boy's grandpa, and the new speech therapist. Although it has been over a quarter of a century since the boy's last walk with the speech therapist, this boy remembers it well. If they could walk together again and "if words could make wishes come true," these would be the boy's words of thanks, and among the thoughts he would dream possible for other children who stutter.

Thank you for listening rather than talking.

Thank you for asking me to share my thoughts and desires, rather than demanding that I read out loud, or fit into a program that didn't fit me.

Thank you for being so interested in my feelings and for reminding me of all the things that you thought I could do so well, rather than reminding me of what I already knew I could not do.

Thank you for helping me to speak more gently by guiding me in what to do, rather than by directing me in what not to do.

Thank you for talking to me in words that I understood, rather than sounding professional.

Thank you for your patience, understanding, and support, rather than showing me frustration when I did my best, but couldn't succeed.

Thank you for being so enthusiastic and for knowing that at worst, I always did my best.

Thank you for helping my teachers understand stuttering and know how best to deal with it in class.

Thank you for reminding my parents of all of the many things that they did right.

Thank you for caring. With your help, they were all positive that the boy could find his way through the forest. They were right.

The boy reminds other children, parents, and speech–language pathologists that things that are most meaningful and difficult to achieve often take a long time to accomplish, and those that are seemingly impossible might take a bit longer.

Remain positive. Admit honestly to when and what you don't know. Know when to seek help. Recognize feelings for what they are and are not. Continue to believe in yourselves and the healthy process of constructive change. You're in good company. Good luck.

Figure 9.1. Continued.

This experience is a gateway to the child's emotions, which often are expressed in laughter or, less frequently, tears.

This section addresses how to provide school-age children such an experience by providing them guidance in what to do, rather than in what not to do. Providing guidance in what to do (what I am recommending) helps the child become focused on fluency, or disFLUENCY. Directing the child more in what not to do focuses on disfluency, or DISfluency. The child comes to see that his talking, like other behavior, is controllable. My experience has been that by providing the child guidance in how to do more of what he already is doing that facilitates fluency heightens his awareness of what he is doing right, helps him feel in control of his fluency, and brings a positive outlook and peak motivation to the experience. Within this framework, much of the disfluent speech literally drops away. The residual disfluency is addressed directly, however, within the positive framework already established.

The reader may sense my concern that much of the intervention for people who stutter (children and adults) focuses on eliminating the disfluency (directing a person in what not to do), rather than in facilitating the fluency (discussing, demonstrating, and directing/coaching in what to do). This may seem to some as just a semantic quibble. It is not. To me, this distinction is at the very heart of successful intervention and working with people who stutter. It seems that many clinicians, albeit sincere and well meaning, tend to focus on what the client should not do because that (i.e., what the client is doing wrong, or what is not facilitative to fluency) is so readily apparent. What seems puzzling to clinicians is knowing what the client is doing right (i.e., facilitative of fluency) and therefore what the client needs to do more often to increase the fluency, thereby effectively eliminating the disfluency. In other words, what the client should not do is clearer than what the client should do. This discussion neither ignores that fluency and disfluency are multidimensional, complex variables, nor is intended to criticize clinicians. Significantly, however, the majority of clinicians holding master's degrees have expressed a lack of confidence in treating people who stutter and a need for direction in planning and implementing such treatment (Mallard, Gardner, & Downey, 1988; Healey & Scott, 1995; Manning, 1996; Williams, 1971). This general attitude is not surprising given changes in certification requirements by the American Speech–Language–Hearing Association no longer requiring academic and clinical experience specifically in the area of stuttering (this area of training is being de-emphasized or eliminated; Manning, 1996; Starkweather & Givens-Ackerman, 1997) combined with a discouraging and unfortunate influence of instructors expressing "that treatment for fluency disorders was rarely successful and that the student would be well advised to concentrate on those clients who were more likely to make progress" (Manning, 1996, p. 142). As a result, "many clinicians actively avoid, or at the very least, are anxious about, the possibility of working with children and adults with fluency disorders" (Manning, 1996, p. 142; see also Conture, 1990b; Silverman, 1996). The implications of the changes in ASHA's certification requirements and training standards will be discussed in Chapter 12.

Meeting with the child serves several functions. We already discussed the importance of establishing a foundation as mutually interested and interesting people. The clinician conveys her understanding and acceptance of the child independent of the child's speech fluency. The clinician is interested in observing the child's speech directly to determine: the degree to which it is affected by structure, linguistic complexity, and communicative pressure; the degree to which it is modifiable; and the relative developmental level of the child's behaviors, feelings, and attitudes. This speech sample collected will be used for analysis and comparison to others collected from different speaking contexts. For the sake of organization, the initial interaction between the child and the clinician will be discussed in terms of speech–language sampling and structured activities with and without communication pressure.

Speech–Language Sample Without Communicative Pressure

While inquiring about the child as a person and relating to his experiences, the clinician collects a speech–language sample of no less than 300 words (Conture,

1990b, 1997), or approximately 5 minutes of the child's talking (approximately 10–15 minutes of real time). As noted in the last chapter, the purpose is to develop a corpus from which to assess the child's communication skills, including speech fluency. Once the clinician and the child have established a foundation as people with lives and interests, they may talk about their respective roles within the school. The clinician might ask the child about his friends, favorite subjects, and classroom activities. Deliberately steering the conversation toward the communication experience, the clinician asks the child how he feels about his communication skills. If an anchor is needed, the clinician may ask the child to evaluate himself on a scale from 1 to 10 for different interests and talents already discussed (such as basketball, spelling, art, and others) and then for talking skills. This invites a frank, open, accepting conversation about the child's beliefs regarding what he feels he does relatively well versus poorly; his assessment of himself as a communicator; what he feels helps him to talk better; and related thoughts and feelings.

Williams (1971) indicated that school-age children vary widely in the consistency of their stuttering and the degree to which their feelings and attitudes have been affected by the stuttering experience. Furthermore, while adults often talk with children who stutter about stuttering or not stuttering, they rarely talk about talking, how we talk, and different ways of talking. The child will come to see that both fluency and disfluency represent different ways of talking and the consequence doing things differently. Such a realization invites the child to make choices and helps him to realize that ways of talking potentially are controllable. Among the purposes of the initial meeting are to collect the child's current ideas and assessments and to begin to present the child with alternatives to consider. The child begins to talk about talking and to think about his own thoughts about his speech and himself as a communicator. The clinician guides the discussion while assessing the child's behaviors, feelings, and attitudes.

Within the process as described, many different topics are addressed. The child's level of awareness guides the directness and the content of my questions. The child may be asked why he feels he is meeting with the clinician and what he hopes to get out of the meeting. The child's response will begin to indicate his level of awareness or concern. If the child responds with, "I don't know," the clinician may do some gentle probing ("What do you think? What did your teacher or parents tell you about why we were meeting?"). If the child responds with, "I don't talk well," or " 'Cause I stutter," these responses need to be probed further ("What do you mean?"). In any case, the clinician should be careful not to manipulate what the child says (i.e., not to put words into the child's mouth), all the while encouraging free expression without penalty or judgment. Peters and Guitar (1991) noted that children may respond reluctantly to invitations to express feelings because adults have inadvertently rejected or negated their feelings by such comments as, "You don't need to feel that way" or "Why do you let it bother you?" Expression of feeling requires a trusting relationship that may take several meetings to establish. Indeed, the clinician should not confront the child immediately with alternative interpretations; rather, she should nurture the child's expression while actively listening and clarifying as appropriate to help both better understand the child's thoughts. Depending on the child's level of awareness, he may be asked when his stuttering was first noticed, how it has developed and changed over time, why he believes he talks this way, what he does to make talking easier, how others (such as family, teachers, friends, and others) react to his stuttering, where and with whom talking is relatively harder and easier, and how he feels about the way he talks and about himself when he talks that way.

Others recommend different strategies to gain similar knowledge about and from children within the context of conversational exchange. Williams (1978) suggested that the clinician needs to understand the child's view of the talking world and his place in it. She needs to learn the child's views regarding his verbal interactions at home and at school, specifically his perception of the different people's reactions and how he feels about the experience of stuttering. To do so, Williams (1978, pp. 69–70) recommended a series of questions, summarized here as follows:

- *"Whom do you like to talk to?"* The clinician might ask, "Whom do (and don't) you like to talk to at (home, school, and other settings)? Who likes (doesn't like) to talk to you at (home, school, and other settings)?" Each reply might be expanded by asking, "Why do you think this is so?"

- *"Who talks the most?"* These questions include, "Who talks the most (the least) at (home, school)? Whom do you talk to the most (the least) at (home, school)? Whom does your (father, mother, brother, teacher) talk to the most (the least)? Why?"

- *"Who interrupts?"* "Who interrupts the most (the least) at (home, school)? Who interrupts (father, mother, brother) the most (the least)? Whom do you interrupt the most (the least) at (home, school)? Why?"

- *"Who are good talkers?"* "Who is the best (poorest) talker at (home, school)? Why?" If the child has mentioned himself directly, the clinician might follow-up with where the child puts himself on the scale from best to poorest talker at (home, school).

- *"When do you want to talk well?"* "Are there times when you want to talk extra well? Where? Why? Are there times when you don't care particularly how you talk? Where? Why?"

- *"When do you want to talk more than you do?"* These questions include, "When would you like to talk more than you do at (home, school)? When do you want to talk less than you do? Why? Do you think other children feel this way too?"

- *"Who listens?"* The clinician might ask, "Who pays the most (least) attention to you when you talk at (home, school)? What do you like listeners to do when you talk to them (for example, look down, look at you, smile, interrupt, talk for you)? Who does what you like (don't like) at (home, school)? Why do you think they do it?"

Questions such as these are intended to facilitate the conversational exchange, not to inhibit or overly structure it. Depending on the child's unique experience (stuttering behaviors, feelings, attitudes, willingness to share, and other factors), the conversation may go in a number of different directions. As already noted, the sample is intended to foster a supportive, trusting relationship and will be used for subsequent communication analysis.

Structured Activities Without Communicative Pressure

After collecting a rich conversational sample, I engage the school-age child in a number of more structured activities that yield elicited responses for subsequent analysis. Again, we are comparing the child's communication skills, including speech fluency across speaking contexts, for assessment and differential diagnosis (i.e., to determine if a disorder of fluency is present, and if so, what type). Unlike the procedures for the preschool child reviewed in Chapter 8, those for the school-age child will include a sample of reading if the child is a reader. In kindergarten or first grade, as children are first learning to read, observed disfluency may represent more language disfluency than speech disfluency. In other words, the assessment of speech fluency within reading may be confounded by the reading difficulty as well as the demand placed upon the child to remain fluent.

Ferreting out the speech disfluency that is independent of the influence of reading presents a challenge for clinicians. The same challenge is encountered when assessing older school-age children (or adults) who have a reading disability. In such cases, the clinician compares the speech fluency within and between reading samples, as well as between reading and conversational and other more structured tasks. With these cautions, I have found it useful with older school-age children to sample their speech during reading as many as three different passages. One should be easy, or below the child's reading ability; one at his reading level; and one deliberately above his level. When selecting a fairly challenging passage, I use one of the phonetically balanced passages (e.g., *Arthur, the Young Rat,* which contains 180 words; found in Williams et al., 1978, p. 276) not only to sample speech fluency but also to screen for articulation errors or phonological processes.

Other structured activities are similar to those reviewed in the last chapter, as follows:

- Telling about a current event, holiday, or possession

- Explaining a process or procedure, such as a familiar game or activity

- Responding to questions requiring answers of differing length and complexity

- Repeating words and sentences of varied length and complexity

- Commenting on pictures (by naming objects, making short phrases in response to "What's going on in the picture?" and telling stories)

- Others reviewed previously (such as automatic speech, echoic speech, speaking alone, monologue, talking with puppet, command speech, talking with gestures, talking with phonemic difficulty, and talking on telephone, among others)

Speech–Language Sample and Structured Activities with Communicative Pressure

Once the speech–language sample and structured activities without communicative pressure are completed, different talking activities are entertained with communicative pressure. The purpose is to assess the relative impact of perceived communicative pressure (of time pressure, linguistic ambiguity, and violation of conversational rules, among others) on the child's speech fluency. Some activities already completed that may have involved some communicative pressure are reading a difficult passage, repeating long and complex words, and responding to questions about speaking experiences at home or at school that might be emotionally loaded for a particular child. Other activities with more distinct and deliberate communicative pressure might include playing games in which time pressure is a part of the competition (for example, games in which each player must be the first to verbally identify something, or in which a finite time, of say 30 seconds, is allowed to complete a verbal description). Other pressured activities might involve: rushed behavior (in which the clinician increases her own rate of speech, hand and overall body movements and extraneous gestures, and speed of requesting answers; or directs the child to "hurry up"), interruptions (which involve taking a conversational turn before the child has completed his, or asking a question and then asking another before the child finishes the answer to the first), loss of attention (which involves doing something else when the child is relating an event), or requesting the child to say something else (such as, "I didn't get that. What did you say?").

Other challenges are offered by abruptly shifting topics (such as, introducing a topic prematurely that is unrelated to the one being discussed by the child), overstepping boundaries of the child's linguistic competence (using vocabulary that is too complex or addressing topics that are conceptual and out of the child's experiential domain), introducing linguistic ambiguity (contradicting things said by the child or clinician), or introducing verbal absurdity (saying things that border on foolishness, such as addressing the child by the wrong name, talking about a pictured girl as "he," or telling the child a joke where the punchline makes no sense). Similarly, the child may be asked to tell a joke, an experience during which linguistic demand is high. All the while, the clinician must be sensitive to the child's feelings and inform him, when and how appropriate, as to why she is engaging in speaking activity with deliberate communicative pressure. Incidentally, engaging in such pressure is particularly important when the child presents no observable sign of speech disfluency. Such pressure increases the demand placed upon the child's ability to remain fluent, thus eliciting disfluency when it is not otherwise observed.

Trial Management

The assessment activities discussed to this point enable the clinician to evaluate the school-age child's speech fluency, related attitudes and feelings, and other aspects of communication, in order to arrive at a diagnosis. Furthermore, the data collected provide a baseline of the child's communication behavior from which progress in treatment can be monitored. From the information collected, the clinician decides whether more formal evaluation of articulation or phonology and language is necessary. If the child demonstrates symptoms of disfluency (during the speaking activities or during elicitation) or behaviors suggestive of negative attitudes, thoughts, or feelings associated with communication, then the clinician engages the child in a variety of trial management techniques based on principles of fluency shaping and stuttering modification. The management techniques become increasingly differentiated for school-age children (compared to those for preschool children) because the stuttering behaviors and related feelings and attitudes are likely to be more developed. These techniques that are used during the assessment session (or phase, if over more than one session) help the clinician determine the child's responsiveness to different treatment strategies, thus contributing to the design of specific recommendations.

Fluency Shaping

Fluency shaping techniques include engaging the child in singing a short song and reciting a riddle or poem in chorus with the clinician. As noted earlier, these activities are essential for differential diagnosis. One would expect a child who stutters to demonstrate consistent fluency during singing (except perhaps when initiating a new passage or bar following a pause) and choral speaking or choral reading. If the child does not, the clinician must entertain the possibility that another fluency disorder is operating. Other fluency shaping techniques include establishing fluency (using slightly prolonged vowels, soft articulatory contacts on consonants, and natural suprasegmental features) through modeling, choral speaking, using mechanical devices (such as delayed auditory feedback machine, or metronome) or other externally driven methods. For children demonstrating more involved symptoms of disfluency, the clinician may first establish a fluent syllable and systematically shape it into increasingly longer and more complex units such as monosyllabic words, polysyllabic words, phrases, and, eventually, sentences. This can be done first by imitation, then moving to delayed imitation, and elicitation through picture cards, and ultimately moving to more spontaneous forms. The clinician provides verbal praise and other forms of positive reinforcement as a consequence to and contingent on a fluent utterance.

Stuttering Modification

One of the major objectives of stuttering modification is to learn that there are different ways to stutter. One can stutter hard or soft, long or short, loud or quiet, tense or relaxed, or frustrated or calm, among others. We want the child to experiment with us and thereby to realize that *talking is something that we do; it doesn't just happen.* Both fluency and disfluency are the consequence of something that we do differently with our speech apparatus. There are many ways to help the child achieve this discovery. In trial management, we use several different procedures and gain an impression of the child's relative responsiveness to the methodology. These and other methods will be used at a later time in scheduled treatment, should it be recommended. For example, we may use any of the following methods, among others:

• *Model slow, relaxed, prolonged speech with soft articulatory contacts* ("Wwhy donn't wwe llook at thhat picture nnext?").

• *Model easier versions of the child's stuttering in a modeling and expansion format* (*Child:* "That that that i–i–i–i–s muh–muh–muh–muh–my buh–buh–buh–boo–k." *Clinician:* "I ssee thhat bbook iis yyours. Hhow about iif wwe take a llook aat iit?").

• *Demonstrate easy and eventually hard disfluencies in the clinician's speech.* First offer descriptive, emotionally neutral self-comments (*Child:* "Gosh, that was a little hard.") and later invite the child's comments and assessment (*Clinician:* "What did you think about that one?" *Child:* "That was wild. Was that a real one?").

- *Identify instances when the child uses gentle speech onset with light articulatory contact, then describe what he did* ("You really used slow, gentle speech when you said the *b* in bboy. You barely touched your lips together and that was great"), and offer positive visual and verbal feedback for successful or otherwise sincere efforts (the clinician will have a positive facial expression and say something like "Yes!" in a bold voice). This procedure is intended to do two things: to heighten the child's awareness of the fluent speech that he already possesses (both how much and what types); and to model for the child how to identify his fluency, describe what he did, and offer positive feedback (three steps that at first the clinician does for the child, and eventually the child will do for himself).

- *Provide the child with one or two behaviors on which to focus, providing activities that he can do.* For example, the clinician may model slow and gentle speech, pointing out that the two behavioral foci are *slow* and *gentle*. These two will enable the child to focus his energies, thus maximizing positive change in his speech. More will be said about this in the section on treatment.

- *Explore and support the child for expressions of feeling related to stuttering or himself as a communicator.* Given the school-age child's experience with disfluency and degree of emotional involvement, the discussion about feelings and attitudes tends to be more direct than that with the preschool child, but less direct than that with the adult.

- *Engage the child in a discussion of where and with whom he would expect his speech to be more fluent and less fluent and related feelings.* This type of hierarchy can be started in the assessment session, continued in the interim before treatment, and discussed and completed in the initial treatment sessions. This activity can be conducted with significant others as well, including teachers and parents, among others. Essentially, this activity is one of several that facilitates transfer from the beginning and helps individualize treatment.

POST-ASSESSMENT PROCEDURES

Once the clinician has collected a speech–language sample, engaged the child in more structured activities—first without and then with communication pressure—and collected her preliminary impressions, it is time to analyze the results more thoroughly. She needs to do the following:

- *Represent both quantitatively (using frequency counts, means, ranges, or other summary statistics) and qualitatively (narrowly describing) the nature of the speech fluency and disfluency across speaking contexts and time.* This includes behaviors, feelings, thoughts, and attitudes. The reader may want to review the descriptive protocols discussed in Chapter 8.

- *Represent the other characteristics of communication* (language fluency in terms of syntactic and morphologic, semantic, pragmatic, and phonologic and articulation competence).

From the information collected so far, the clinician conducts an analysis from which she makes statements of diagnosis, prognosis, and specific intervention recommendations, in addition to referral to other professionals as appropriate. These results are conveyed to the significant parties during individual or group meetings (involving parents, teachers, or other professionals on the Pupil Planning Teams) and summarized within a report.

Speech Analysis

Analyses on the speech samples collected from preschool children, discussed earlier, are conducted on the conversational and structured speech from school-age children. These will be reviewed briefly here. The reader is referred back to the section on "Speech Analysis" in Chapter 8 for a detailed discussion of analysis procedures and examples. The analyses, assuming the word to be the unit of measure, include the following:

Frequency of Speech Disfluency (i.e., Disfluency Frequency Index, DFI)

This is a general measure of the amount of disfluency, without consideration to the individual types or relative severity, that is contained within the child's speech. Reported as a percentage, the DFI is computed by dividing the total number of disfluent words by the total number of words spoken (both disfluent and fluent), and then multiplying the resulting decimal by 100 to achieve the percentage. The frequency of speech disfluency typically is reported as a percentage of 100 words spoken, averaged over samples of 300 or 400 words.

Type of Speech Disfluency (i.e., Disfluency Type Index, DTI)

This measure identifies the individual proportions for each type of disfluency. It is computed by dividing the number of disfluencies of each individual type by the total number of disfluent words, and then multiplying by 100.

Molecular Description of Disfluency

This includes the duration and frequency (reported in terms of total, mean, and range) of the most prominent or otherwise significant forms (particularly within-word disfluencies).

Rate of Speech

This is a measure of the number of words spoken per minute. The more a person stutters, the more his rate of speech is reduced. As treatment decreases the degree and amount of disfluency, rate should steadily increase and approximate normal standards. Rate is computed by dividing the number of words the child has spoken by the child's talk time in minutes. We noted in Chapter 8 that it is helpful for purposes of comparison to know what rate of speech is considered average or "normal" for children who do not stutter. Peters and Guitar (1991) reported that in Vermont, school-age children who were 6, 8, 10, and 12 years old demonstrated the following ranges in syllables spoken per minute: age 6 years, 140–175; age 8 years, 150–180; age 10 years, 165–215; and age 12 years, 165–220. Data for rate of speech in words per minute were not available.

Secondary Characteristics

The secondary or associated characteristics, both speech-related (such as audible inhalations or exhalations, pitch rises, oral and neck tension) and non-speech-related (such as facial, head, eye movement or tension), are quantified and qualified. These may reflect the child's developing awareness of stuttering, coping mechanisms during stuttering, or attempts to prevent stuttering.

Severity Rating

This is an assessment of the child's relative degree of stuttering involvement considering a variety of speech and nonspeech factors. Use of the *Stuttering Severity Instrument–Third Edition* (SSI–3, see Figure 8.5), *Scale for Rating Severity of Stuttering* (see Figure 8.6), the *Profile of Stuttering Severity* (see Figure 8.7), or other severity instruments helps standardize assessment of relative severity of a speaker's stuttering over time and across speakers. However, the information provided by such instruments proves to be confirmatory, if not redundant, with the other quantitative and qualitative information collected.

Adaptation and Consistency

This measures the degree to which an individual's disfluency resembles that of people who stutter (as a group). Specifically, with repeated recitation of the same material, adaptation is the tendency for overall stuttering to decrease; consistency is the tendency for stuttering to occur on the same sounds or words.

Feelings and Attitudes

This assessment is pivotal to a clinician's understanding of a client's stuttering experience. It is an assessment of the degree to which a speaker is experiencing covert involvement related to the experience of stuttering. Haynes et al. (1992) reviewed 13 available protocols. Peters and Guitar (1991) noted, and I concur, that "the most reliable measure of the child's feelings and attitudes is your [the clinician's] judgment" (p. 178).

Other

This is an open category that invites assessment of tempo, regularity, relative tension, smoothness of transitions, physical concomitants, in addition to any other overt or covert features not yet reported.

Diagnosis

From the assessment and evaluation of all information available, the clinician makes a statement of diagnosis regarding the child's communication skills. This is where she determines the nature of the child's speech fluency and disfluency, stating whether he is demonstrating stuttering, is at-risk for stuttering, or is demonstrating normal disfluency (in addition to interpreting the child's competence in language, articulation and phonology, and voice). If the child's disfluency is observed and of concern, the clinician distinguishes between stuttering and other disorders of fluency. In any case, the clinician must establish if treatment is warranted and recommended, and if so, what should be the nature and focus of the intervention. As already noted, the experience of arriving at a diagnosis is dynamic, and continues to respond to new information as it becomes available.

Prognosis and Recommendations

The child's prognosis for improvement in the area of speech fluency is derived from a variety of sources. These include the assessment and evaluation results, child's response to trial management, a clinician's professional experience with other school-age children who stutter, and the relevant clinical literature. On these bases, the following factors suggest a more positive prognosis (Haynes et al., 1992):

- *No previous unsuccessful treatment.* An absence of treatment seems more conducive to success than a history of treatment failure.

- *A cooperative family system.* In effective systems, family members, particularly parents, are willing to participate in a program of family counseling and to assume an active role in the treatment process.

- *Cooperative interdisciplinary team members, including teachers and allied professionals.* The more the team members work together and communicate, the more potent the treatment effect.

- *More severe stuttering pattern.* Although it may appear counterintuitive, school-age children with more severe stuttering tend to have a better prognosis; those with milder stuttering tend to show little improvement.

- *More positive self-concept of the child.* The more the child views himself as an effective, or potentially effective, communicator and the more actively engaged he is in all aspects of the treatment process, the more positive the treatment outcome.

- *No other significant problems.* Other problems that may hinder progress include reading difficulty, learning disability, and academic difficulty independent of stuttering.

- *Other available resources.* Other resources include skill in athletics, music, scouting, biking, and so forth.

- *Regular and relatively intensive treatment.* Some clinical literature (Andrews et al., 1983; Haynes et al., 1992) indicates a greater amount of treatment (three or four contacts per week) to be predictive of a more positive treatment outcome. As I will discuss in the treatment section, I have found that so many contacts with a clinician tend to build communication dependence rather than independence. I have found that the more regular the treatment (i.e., weekly) and the more emphasis there is on transfer activities from the very beginning of treatment (such as engagement of the child and others in treatment that occur between scheduled sessions), the more positive the treatment outcome and more the child develops communication independence.

The information leading to the diagnosis is combined with prognostic indicators as indicated. These factors are integrated with intrafamily, extrafamily, and psychotherapeutic intervention considerations, all of which play a major role in designing treatment recommendations. Intrafamily considerations focus on the way the child views himself as a communicator who is successful or potentially successful (personal construct) and the extent to which members of the family system communicate openly, support each other, and sincerely participate within the clinical process (family systems). Extrafamily considerations address how the members of the interdisciplinary team communicate openly and contribute to the integrated fluency intervention program (interdisciplinary teaming), and multicultural factors that might impact planning for, conducting, and interpreting the treatment experience (multicultural awareness). Psychotherapeutic considerations are those that tend to individualize the treatment plan based on the relative degree of involvement of both overt and covert factors and seek to establish objectives that are appropriate to each individual (fluency shaping, stuttering modification). Together, this pool of information yields informed treatment recommendations.

Post-Assessment Interview with the Parent, Teacher, and Other Participants

In clinical settings, post-assessment conferences are held immediately after the evaluation. In school settings, however, these conferences generally are scheduled by subsequent individual appointments and group meetings of the Pupil Personnel Teams. In any case, the purposes are the same: to summarize the results of assessment, provide recommendations, and discuss any questions that remain. It always is helpful to address the needs and concerns raised by the parents and teachers, and to begin by expressing positive observations about the child's communication skills and about the adults' interactions with the child. This positive tone in which results are summarized and discussed, even for serious concerns, sets the style of interaction among all involved. Be negative and the intervention experience will be problem focused and one of repairing the child's and the family's communication deficits. Be positive, realistic, and optimistic about designing strategies, achieving communication improvement, and working toward realizing fluency potential and the intervention process will become solution and strategy focused where all work together and support one another.

In the post-assessment conferences, I summarize in understandable terms the characteristics of the child's fluency and disfluency. Some of the information that is reviewed for the parents of preschool children regarding the development of speech fluency and the nature of developmental stuttering is reviewed for parents and teachers. Again, protocols that help visualize the development of disfluency (see Figures 8.3 and 8.4, Table 8.1, Appendix B) prove helpful during our conversations. I try to address their questions about causality by summarizing what we know about predisposing factors and the importance of identifying and controlling for precipitating and perpetuating factors. I offer recommendations, remembering the importance of not just telling, but discussing, demonstrating, and directing/coaching. Various resources that review and expand on the points made within the conferences are recommended to the parents and teachers. These resources include the booklets mentioned in Chapter 8, in addition to "A Way Through the Forest: One Boy's Story

With a Happy Ending" (Shapiro, 1995; Figure 9.1); "A Guide for Parents of Children Who Stutter" (from the National Stuttering Project); and pamphlets and videotapes from the Stuttering Foundation of America (*Pamphlets:* "If You Think Your Child is Stuttering," "Turning On to Therapy," "The Child Who Stutters at School: Notes to the Teacher," "How to React When Speaking with Someone who Stutters;" *Videotapes: Childhood Stuttering: A Videotape for Parents, Therapy in Action: The School-Age Child Who Stutters*). Additional information about these and other resources and the sponsoring organizations will be found in Appendix B.

TREATMENT

Thus far in the present chapter, we have characterized school-age children and reviewed a variety of assessment procedures. Now we take a look at an integration of treatment procedures addressing the behaviors, thoughts, and feelings of school-age children who stutter.

Goals

The treatment goals for the school-age child who stutters are spontaneous or controlled fluency and establishment or maintenance of a positive attitude toward communication and oneself as a communicator.

Objectives

The objectives for a school-age child who stutters are to establish or increase and transfer fluent speech, to develop resistance to potential fluency disrupters, to establish or maintain positive feelings about communication and oneself as a communicator, and to maintain the fluency-inducing effects of treatment on communication-related behaviors, thoughts, and feelings.

Rationale

On the surface, the goals and objectives for the school-age child who stutters sound similar to those for preschool children. While spontaneous fluency and a positive attitude about the communication experience and oneself as a communicator are common goals to both groups, the treatment procedures differ based upon the changing needs of the child and the intrafamily, extrafamily, and psychotherapeutic considerations.

The Changing Needs of the Child

Typically, school-age children who stutter no longer are beginning to stutter. A longer time has elapsed since the onset of stuttering for school-age children than for preschool children. Increased personal independence is paired with greater dependence on peers and others within the social and educational context. School-age children become aware of and attend to how they are perceived by others. This social consciousness takes the form of peer pressure, criticism, and social conformity. School-age children who stutter have an additional factor that operates in how others perceive them and how they perceive themselves. Their developing independence and concomitant need for control over their lives is met with an increasing challenge. Stuttering, by nature, is experienced as a loss of control, the antithesis of the social perception children who stutter are attempting to manage. This internal conflict experienced by the school-age child who stutters forces an adjustment to how he perceives himself and what he predicts about himself. This conflict often is experienced as disequilibrium, frustration, feelings of helplessness, and despair. For these reasons, the clinician's skill in talking with children about talking and related feelings is of utmost importance. The clinician is uniquely suited to help reduce the child's burden through understanding and sharing, and to help him find a way through the forest.

Intrafamily Considerations

The school years are critical in the development of a child's personal construct, or what he thinks and expects about himself as a person and a communicator within a social context. Not surprisingly, the school years also are critical in the development of the child's stuttering. It is unusual for a school-age child to be unaware that he stutters. During these years, the overt speech behaviors often are seen to increase in complexity and consistency. The component feelings and attitudes are in transition as well. The clinician must come to understand both the overt (directly observable aspects of the child's speech fluency and disfluency) and the covert (internalized feelings and attitudes about communication and oneself as a communicator) features of communication. The clinician's challenge is heightened if not masked by the child's reluctance or inability to verbalize internal feelings, particularly to an adult in authority. In other words, the clinician must determine the child's unique personal construct, which is evolving, thus appearing imprecise and often ephemeral. My own observations and experiences have indicated that a major distinction between providers of effective and ineffective treatment is the extent to which a clinician shifts to and works from within the child's framework and personal perspective (i.e., the child's personal construct) (Moses & Shapiro, 1996; Shapiro & Moses, 1989). This means that the clinician must internalize the child's reality, yielding shared understanding, insight, and acceptance.

The school-age child's family is critically important to the success of treatment. The more the family members are aware of, participate in, and provide support for the treatment experience, the more the child internalizes and habituates the fluency facilitating controls and maintains a positive attitude about himself as a communicator. In a clinical or university-based speech and hearing center, direct meetings with one or more parents tend to be more frequent. Within such an arrangement, I structure each treatment session in order to work individually with the child and then with the family members present. In the school setting, however, such regular and direct involvement of the parents proves more difficult. For this reason, the clinician must find ways to keep the family aware of, involved in, and communicating about the treatment experience. This means scheduling meetings with parents as frequently as possible, adjusting the time of treatment to accommodate the parents, phone calling, exchanging letters and tape recordings, and so on. The point is that family members continue to be essential to successful treatment, although access to them may prove more difficult in school settings. While designing methods to include them in the treatment process, the clinician must remain sensitive to the child's need for increasing independence. Thus, the child must understand why their involvement is so important and the parties must negotiate methods about which all are comfortable.

Extrafamily Considerations

The interdisciplinary team is available to the clinician of school-age children who stutter. In addition to working with the parents, the clinician works regularly with the teachers who are critical members of an interdisciplinary team. Together, they see that the communication needs of the child are met and the objectives of treatment are carried out in the classroom setting. More will be said later about working with classroom teachers. School-based clinicians have the luxury of easy access to other allied educational (learning disability and other special education specialists, psychometrists, psychologists, principals, counselors, psychotherapists, and others) or medical (physicians, nurses, physical and occupational therapists, and others) professionals as needed. The child's educational and multicultural experiences influence the content of the treatment experience and become part of the work addressed in the clinical and classroom settings.

Psychotherapeutic Considerations

We already noted that with preschool children, there is relatively little distinction between stuttering modification and fluency shaping procedures. With the school-age child whose stuttering and associated thoughts and feelings are evolving, this distinction becomes increasingly apparent. Many clinicians, however, feel uneasy about how to design a program, and how to know whether it should be slanted more toward fluency shaping or toward stuttering modification. As noted in Chapter 7, the decision to design treatment more in one direction than the other has relatively little directly to do with the severity of the child's stuttering behavior. Rather, a program oriented more toward stuttering modification is indicated when the child avoids or otherwise attempts to conceal his stuttering, demonstrates upset or embarrassment because of the stuttering, feels negative about communicating or himself as a communicator, experiences intentional or inadvertent punishment in any settings because he stutters, and demonstrates a positive response to stuttering modification techniques during trial management. A program oriented more toward fluency shaping is indicated when the child stutters openly without trying to hide or conceal it, does not avoid speaking, exhibits a neutral or mildly negative attitude about communicating and himself as a communicator, and demonstrates a positive response to fluency shaping techniques for trial management. As can be seen, behaviors often coexist with feelings, attitudes, and thoughts. Children who demonstrate more severe stuttering behaviors often show avoidances and negativity as well. This is not always the case, however. Therefore, it is the openness with which the child stutters and the involvement of his feelings and attitudes that help guide the design and relative structure of treatment. In fact, because many of the child's attitudes are evolving, neither course is clear cut, arguing for an approach for combining fluency shaping and stuttering modification. We also noted earlier that when fluency shaping and stuttering modification are compared, fluency shaping tends to be more efficient in changing speech behaviors, while stuttering modification is more effective in reducing fears and changing attitudes as well as strengthening generalization.

Because school-age children vary remarkably, intervention planning must be individualized. Guitar and Peters (1980) noted that the child of 6 or 7 years old, for treatment purposes, often is more like the preschool child in terms of borderline or incipient stuttering. On the other hand, the child of 12 or 13 years may be more like the adolescent or adult who stutters. As I noted in the last chapter, I have worked with children as young as 3 years old whose stuttering behaviors, thoughts, and feelings were severely involved, and adults whose stuttering behaviors, thoughts, and feelings represented only a minor nuisance, if that. While children who stutter may have some experiences in common, their differences remind us that each must be considered individually in all aspects of intervention.

Procedures

An integration of procedures for school-age children will be discussed with respect to each objective. Although the objectives are presented in a logical order for instructional purposes, in reality they are multidimensional and overlapping.

Increase and Transfer Fluent Speech

The first major objective with school-age children who stutter is to help them increase the amount of fluent speech and to transfer the fluency facilitating techniques learned to extraclinical settings. To do so, different but related procedures addressing the child's thoughts, feelings, and behaviors are utilized, as follows:

Construct a "safe house" within which fluency blossoms, children (and clinicians) grow, and magic happens. A clinician's treatment room must be a safe house, a retreat, a place where "a kid can be a kid" and where communication and communicators feel nurtured and secure. The clinician's role in facilitating and maintaining the child's speech fluency and positive perception of himself is absolutely critical. In an environment where the child feels unconditional positive regard and understanding, he will express himself freely, fluently or disfluently, and should not feel even a hint of penalty. Thankfully, in most cases the clinician establishes an environment to which the child relates as being similar to that at home. Unfortunately, however, there are cases where the clinician is the only person the child encounters who presents a nurturing experience in which the child believes that somebody believes in him. We reviewed in Chapter 5 that some families have circumstances that overshadow the child's need for support and tangible expressions of encouragement and love. The potential influence of school personnel, particularly the speech–language pathologist whose interactions with children are within individual or small group meetings, is profound.

How is a safe house established? I believe the strategy varies with each clinician and with each child. Through our actions and by what we say, we express and demonstrate that the child is important to us as a person. We focus on all of his abilities first, and only within that positive context do we provide him with proactive strategies with which to increase his capacity to remain fluent. The child is shown that he is fluent most of the time and that he possesses the ability to be fluent even more often. We create opportunities for the child to succeed; we design treatment so as to prevent failure; and we guide the child to fluency accomplishments that he could not even imagine possible. We believe in the child and we help him grow. Recall how important our sincere belief in the child is as a predictor of his fluency success (Daly, 1988). This belief and this sincerity must come from within the clinician. We encourage the child's success, and we help the child see beyond predictable setbacks to future success. Increasing fluency does not occur in a straight line; it is more of a jagged profile. The child advances and then plateaus, if not regresses, until subsequent advances. We help the child understand the treatment process and his role and progress within it. We believe in the child. We accept his questions. We understand his self-doubts. We are there as an advocate, a coach, a cheerleader, a score keeper—a friend.

Reflecting on the importance of feeling "safe" with a clinician, Dell (1979), a speech–language pathologist, recalled his experiences as a school-age child who stuttered:

> The school clinicians did accomplish several very important things. They provided a place where I could come and talk, where no one would laugh at me or scorn me, where I felt free to communicate even if I did stutter. What a great feeling that was! My dog was the only other living creature with whom I felt that way. Here was a place where I could learn something about my stuttering, that mysterious thing that no one else ever mentioned. I needed a safe place where I could touch it and confront it. All of these benefited me a great deal as a young boy. . . . But most valuable of all was the gift of caring. They cared! I was made to feel some worth as a human being despite my stuttering. Because of this experience, stuttering did not destroy my self-concept the way it does in many young stutterers. The caring and warmth I received from my school clinicians helped me stay together as a person. (p. 9)

Invite treatment objectives from the child. Within the safe, supportive environment, invite the child to talk about and share his objectives, what he wants and hopes to achieve as a result of treatment. There are several valuable purposes in doing this. First, we want to learn the child's perspective and, in so doing, learn about his level of awareness with respect to his stuttering. Children's responses to what they hope to achieve range from general ("To talk better.") to specific ("To be able to say my *B*s and *G*s without getting tight in my mouth"). In either case, appropriate follow-up inquiries may ask the child to elaborate what he said and why he does what he just described. This helps the clinician understand the information with which the child is operating. Another reason for asking the child for his objectives is to convey that the child's input is important to the clinical process. From the beginning, the child needs to see that his participation will be taken seriously and will be encouraged. I remember a 10-year-old boy who stuttered. When asked what he hoped to achieve or what he wanted to improve, he responded with, "You're supposed to tell me. I'm just a kid." When I explained that inviting him to share his wants and needs is a first step in helping him understand the treatment process that combines our ideas and skills, he responded with a smile, "Cool. Nobody ever asked me that." Recall from Figure 9.1 the boy's reaction of surprise when asked by the clinician what he (i.e., the boy) wanted to do in treatment. Another boy recalled how much he appreciated his fourth grade teacher asking him privately how he (i.e., the boy) felt he would like to have his stuttering handled in class. The message to the child is that his active participation and input are essential, without which the process cannot succeed.

One early activity serves multiple purposes. Specifically, designing hierarchies that contain speaking situations listed in increasing order of perceived or anticipated difficulty helps individualize the treatment experience, facilitates transfer of fluency to outside settings, and helps the child discuss objectives and related feelings and attitudes. The child is asked to think about those situations in which he would expect his speech to be fluent. Common situations include speaking alone, to a pet, with family, or with close friends. Then he is asked to consider those in which he would predict his speech to be disfluent, those that he anticipates with a measure of dread. These often include speaking to groups of increasing audience size, unfamiliar people, persons of the opposite sex, and so on. Such hierarchies may be detailed further to include lists of speaking situations or contexts (home, classroom, stores), conversation partners (mother, father, siblings, friends, teachers, or principal), content of the conversation (conversing with parents about the family pet may be easier than explaining why the child broke the garage window after having been told four times not to play near the garage door). Generally, these assignments are begun with the clinician and expanded by the child and family outside of the treatment session. The expansion then is discussed between the clinician and child. The hierarchies represent a working plan, a best guess of anticipated difficulty, and as such guide the order with which extraclinical situations are targeted for fluency facilitating control. However, the hierarchies are neither static nor permanent. They need to be discussed regularly for possible revision. It is quite possible that tasks that the child anticipated would be easy were in fact harder than expected; those anticipated with dread might have been accomplished with relative ease. The purpose of establishing hierarchies is to increase the level of speaking challenge in minimal steps to ensure the child's successful use of fluency facilitating controls in extraclinical settings. Furthermore, the hierarchies individualize the treatment experience and emphasize the importance of the child's active participation from the outset of treatment.

Create opportunities for the child to experience fluency success. The beginning of treatment builds upon what was established during the assessment and evaluation and trial management. Typically I begin treatment with a short fluency shaping exercise such as choral speaking or choral reading. Once the child is comfortable following my speech model during choral speech, I vary the volume of my speech. By reducing my volume, I allow the child to attend more to his speech and feel in control. Eventually, I reduce my volume further to approximate lipped speech and ultimately cease modeling, but then return to modeling before the child experiences disfluency. This takes practice for the clinician. When done correctly, the clinician's and child's speech is synchronized and balanced, thus preventing the child's disfluency. I do this to establish a foundation whereby the child can feel, without reservation, "you know what, I CAN be fluent." This is the first of an endless number of attempts to create opportunities for the child to amass a foundation of successful speaking experiences. I want to begin to immerse the child in successful speaking. We mentioned that a child's personal construct is a prediction of his future based on his past. If he experiences regular fluency failure, then he will predict or anticipate that he will stutter. Likewise, by beginning to create a foundation of fluency success, the child will begin to anticipate the same in his future ("I can do it. I know I can. I was fluent yesterday and this morning. Maybe I can be fluent again this afternoon in reading class."). You may call this *I Can* Therapy. Treatment brings children from feeling unable ("I can't") and helpless and powerless ("Why is this happening *to* me?") to feeling able ("I think I can. I can. I know I can.") and powerful and in control ("When I stutter, I am doing something other than what I should be doing. When I use my controls, I know I can blast those stutters. I am in control."). What this means is that by creating opportunities for the child to experience fluency success, we help him replace the self-doubts and negativity he has acquired from fluency failure with confidence derived from a realistically positive attitude toward himself as a potentially more fluent and independent communicator. Throughout the treatment experience, we increase the fluency challenge in minimal steps to ensure success. If the child does not succeed, then the actual challenge between where we are and the intended next step is greater than we realized.

In addition to collecting data regularly on relative fluency (specific data related to the objectives, such as self-corrections, gentle onsets, soft contacts, and slow rate), I collect data on the verbal comments the child makes about himself as noted above. It is interesting to note how feelings are reflected in what children say about themselves and how what they say changes over the course of successful treatment. Such changes are seen in tandem with improvements in speech fluency. Changes in speech behaviors and comments reflecting feelings and attitudes all are observable and reportable. When the frequency (or percentage) of positive and negative self-comments are plotted over time, increases in speech fluency often coincide with significant increases in the positive statements about one's ability and control over fluency; decreases in speech disfluency often coincide with decreases in negative statements about one's ability and control over fluency. I record these data among others over time as a valuable measure of treatment efficacy and as a visual representation with which to discuss the child's progress and by which to help maintain his motivation.

Heighten the child's awareness of his speech fluency. Make the child's speech fluency (and only then, disfluency) the object of study. After creating opportunities for the child to experience fluency success, the clinician and child focus on and analyze together the behaviors, feelings, and thoughts that characterize what both described as "speech fluency." Initially, the clinician excitedly identifies when the child demonstrated fluent speech ("That's it! You just used your slow, easy speech!"), models what he did ("You said, 'Wwhere ddid yyou ggo?'"), and describes (using appropriately slow, gentle speech model) what was done and encourages continuation ("Tthat wwas grreat. You were really gentle on 'Wwhere.' Llet's see if yyou ccan kkeep thhat up. I knnow you can."). The clinician and child discuss the placement of the articulators and proprioceptive feedback (literally how they felt; e.g., "The lips were nicely rounded on the *w* without any pushing."). Affective feelings are discussed as well ("It felt easy and gentle. It wasn't hard to say because I remembered to be slow and gentle.").

Once the clinician and child are comfortable with this arrangement in which the clinician identifies, models, describes, and elicits from the child subsequent feedback and feelings, the clinician gradually shifts responsibility the child. To do this, the clinician might identify when the child used particularly slow, gentle speech by saying, "That's it! You just did it again!" followed by a leading question, "What did you do?" The child describes what he did ("I remembered to use slow, easy speech."), after which the dialogue further describes (a) which sounds in which words were affected, (b) proprioceptive feedback, and (c) affective reactions. Ultimately, the child becomes increasingly responsible by identifying instances of speech fluency, describing what he did while continuing to use an appropriate speech model, and offering a description of proprioceptive feedback and affective reactions, to all of which the clinician offers praise, appropriate speech models, and support ("You're really becoming aware of your slow, gentle speech. That's great. It surely sounded slow and gentle to me when you said the *g* in girl. Keep it up!").

Such activities heighten the child's awareness of his more fluent speech and convey that he already possesses within his speech much of what he needs to do even more often. The child gains a feeling of control within this type of positive approach. This approach helps the child become increasingly aware of all that he is doing right, necessary proprioceptive feedback, and affective reactions. This approach is naturally reinforcing, in that children (and adults) gravitate to wanting to do more of what we feel we can do well. This is not a minor point. I have observed many treatment sessions in which the clinician focuses on the child's disfluency, directing him not to tense, not to look away, or not to talk so fast. In the next section, I will propose how to establish fluency facilitating control. Suffice it here to say that heightening the child's awareness of when and where he is fluent, what he does to be fluent, proprioceptive feedback, and affective reactions goes a long way toward paving a more fluent future. Surely, as will be seen, I deal directly with the residual disfluency; however, a positive approach such as this is more motivating and generates internalized feelings of success and control, especially when compared to a traditional treatment, which initially focuses on disfluency, what one is doing wrong, and relearning how to talk.

We have stressed the importance of treatment that occurs between the scheduled meetings of the clinician and client. One of the predictors of treatment outcome is time in treatment (Andrews et al., 1983). One critical dimension of treatment that facilitates speech fluency and builds communication independence is designing outside assignments with the child that will be done regularly between treatment sessions. At first the clinician offers more initiative in designing assignments for the child. Eventually, the child participates increasingly in designing the specific activities. As always, the assignments must be presented in such a way that the child is clear about what is to be done and why. The task must be specific (including what will be done, when, how often or how many times, how will it be documented, and other details) and must be one that will ensure success for the child. As stated earlier, no constructive purpose is served by the child failing to succeed.

To ensure success, we use the three *D*s (*d*iscuss, *d*emonstrate, *d*irect/ coach). I might add here that generally I do not ask the child to do a task outside of the treatment room unless he has already mastered it with me within the treatment setting. An ideal early assignment, which actually might be initiated in the assessment or evaluation meeting, is to identify one word that was spoken fluently and to describe telegraphically characteristics of the experience including the setting, listener, and feelings. At first, the child might make note of one word per day. This means that at each weekly treatment session, after a brief social update, the child will review his progress between sessions and thereby will review no less than seven fluent words that were spoken fluently. While the child is focusing on what was said and how it was said, he describes and thereby internalizes the nature and process of fluent speech production, the very purpose of this stage in treatment and the follow-through assignment.

After some experience with an assignment such as this, the child increases the performance expectation to once in the morning, once in the afternoon; then to morning, afternoon, and evening. Some may increase the frequency or duration of the intervals during which the child focuses on fluency. In order to increase the frequency with which school-age children and adults focus on fluency, I work toward having them associate their fluent speech (or other related treatment assignment) with a frequently occurring activity. For some people, eating or snacking occurs frequently, often around other people; therefore, fluency becomes associated with anything edible. The association is unique to each person who stutters. However, the purpose is to internalize and habituate the process of speech fluency and to heighten the child's awareness of his fluent speech and related thoughts and feelings. The importance of this expanding and positive experience in building a fluent future and adjustment of one's self-concept cannot be overstated.

Forty years ago, Williams (1957) expressed similar concern regarding the negative or problem focus of traditional treatment on stuttering and trying not to stutter, as follows:

> The therapy procedures which appear to be most widely employed use the 'stuttering' as the point of reference. The subject is asked to study his stuttering, to change his stuttering, and to control his stuttering. . . . The speaker is trained, in a sense, to keep his eyes on the stuttering and to work to reduce and minimize it. (pp. 394–395)

Furthermore, Williams (1957) recommended that people who stutter be directed to focus on the nature of speech fluency and how to do more of it, as follows:

> From the point of view of the present discussion, it is suggested that the speaker be asked to take his eyes off the stuttering and to look instead toward the total process of talking. There are obvious advantages in looking in the direction in which one is attempting to go instead of continually glancing backward in an effort to work away from something one calls his 'stuttering.' The degree to which one does more things that most speakers do will be the degree that he does more things that most speakers do! This, it seems, can be considered a more meaningful use of the term 'improvement.' Certainly it is more meaningful than striving for 'improvement in stuttering.' The goal, then, is not to reduce or to stop something called 'stuttering.' It is to change the way the speaker talks, so that he does more and more things that most people do when they talk. (p. 395)

Williams (1957) argued that one who stutters develops a "point of view" about stuttering that affects and permeates his behavior as a communicator. A person who stutters tends to believe that stuttering is an independent entity, whether residing inside or outside of the speaker, that must be controlled, lest it will control the speaker. In other words, a person who stutters comes to be fearful that stuttering will happen "to him," failing to see that stuttering, in part, is a behavioral process created by the speaker. Behaviors are purposeful actions that are observable and modifiable. Williams advised that people who stutter become more observant of "normal" speakers and more aware of normal speech production, including the fluency and disfluency. This same advice might as well be offered to clinicians and others. From this heightened awareness, the person becomes more aware of what he is doing as he talks that most speakers do and do not do. Treatment procedures, therefore, should not focus on stopping or controlling an entity called stuttering; rather, "the changes should be in the positive direction of doing more things that normal speakers do" (p. 397).

Develop or improve use of fluency facilitating techniques during instances of stuttering. Fluency facilitating control is proactively built upon a foundation as described to this point. Such a foundation is characterized by a safe, supportive environment in which the child and clinician actively work and interact together; where objectives are designed and planned with the child; where the child is immersed in speaking experiences that highlight fluency success; and where the child has become aware of the nature of his speech fluency and that of other speakers. By this time, the child understands that both fluent speech and disfluent speech are consequences of what he is doing, albeit differently. From a clear understanding of the behaviors that result in fluent speech, the child is guided in how to do these behaviors more frequently and consistently. Concrete examples and analogies are provided to help the child internalize the motor sequence and proprioceptive feedback that facilitate speech fluency. For example, the clinician and child vary the form of disfluency, as discussed in Chapter 7 and earlier in the present chapter. The child again sees the connection between his behaviors (i.e., what he does) and the characteristics of his speech. This helps the child feel control by breaking old stereotyped habits. The child can stutter more fluently, with less abnormality. By heightening the child's awareness of what he does when he speaks, he can elect to change what he does.

Once stuttering is significantly and voluntarily varied (in degree of tension, loudness, frequency, speech rate, and types), then we discuss that there are two ingredients that are necessary and sufficient to eliminate the behaviors of stuttering. Granted, stuttering is more than a behavior (with respect to feelings, attitudes, and thoughts). If one speaks sufficiently slowly (i.e., reduced or minus rate; − rate) and gently (i.e., reduced or minus tension; − tension), one cannot stutter. In other words, Slow + Gentle = No Stuttering. If one stutters, either one is attempting to speak too fast (i.e., + rate) for the requirements of the motor coordination or there is tension (i.e., + tension) somewhere within the speech apparatus. An increase in rate often triggers a compensatory reaction of increased tension. Likewise, an increase in tension often triggers a compensatory reaction of increased speaking rate.

While I do not make this observation the cornerstone of treatment as do a number of behavioral programs, I do believe that this observation provides two appropriate foci for the school-age child who stutters. That is, we look to identify a few targets for the child, behaviors that he can do, that will have a pervasive and positive effect on his speech fluency. With appropriate models as described, working to speak sufficiently slowly and gently (with the suprasegmental features of speech naturalness) often gives the child such constructive targets. Focusing on what the child can and will *do* is in contrast to targeting behaviors that the child will *not do* (for example, do not look down, do not interject, do not repeat, do not break words, do not tense the lips). We discuss, demonstrate, and direct/coach the characteristics of slow and gentle speech. The child puts these characteristics into his own words and we design a system to evaluate such features on a regular basis.

Another illustration, represented in Figure 9.2, often helps the child visualize and internalize the component concepts. I used to ask the child to visualize a milk bottle (the type with the foil seal, the first original "pog"). However, since milk delivery to most homes is bygone, I ask children to visualize a full 1-gallon cider jug fresh off the shelf, or an old water cooler bottle. What happens when we attempt to flip it over, upside down, and pour into a glass too quickly? The child explains that the liquid doesn't come out too well. It comes out in blurps and blobs, a whole bunch at one time, nothing at another, with lots of air getting stuck inside. We compare that visual image to taking the bottle and slowly and confidently tipping it over, ever so gently. What happens then? The child explains that it all comes out slowly, steadily, consistently, and evenly. The comparison to the speech process becomes obvious. Excessive rate and ten-

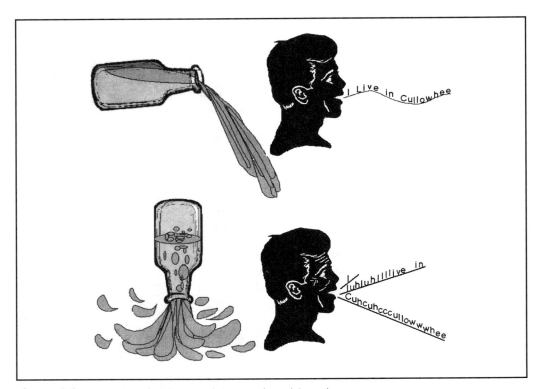

Figure 9.2. A Simple Befuddling Truth in Vessels and Speech.

sion interfere with the forward flow of speech. In contrast, slow, gentle, evenly and regularly produced movement facilitates natural sounding, continuous, and forward moving speech. The visual analogy described here to represent the process of speech fluency, to my surprise, was articulated by William Shakespeare:

> I wouldst thou couldst stammer, that thou mightst pour this concealed man out of thy mouth, as wine comes out of a narrow-mouthed bottle; either too much at once, or none at all. (cited in Carlisle, 1985, Post-Preface)

The procedures and activities described to this point help the child become more aware of what he does when he speaks fluently. I believe this awareness is essential in order to heighten the frequency of speech fluency, thus decreasing the frequency of disfluency. Increasing the frequency first paves the way for addressing directly the residual disfluency within a much more successful and overall positive context. Furthermore, I find this approach to be far more efficient than targeting elimination of each disfluency, only to need subsequently to instate parameters of speech fluency and naturalness.

We noted earlier the importance of increasing the child's awareness in order to facilitate change. It is interesting to discover how many people who stutter are not aware of what they do when they stutter. They know when a stutter has occurred, but describe the experience only in the most global terms. As the child's awareness increases, it is not uncommon to see dramatic, albeit temporary, increases or decreases in fluency. These anticipated changes must be discussed with the child (and adult, as will be seen) in order to prepare him for their occurrence. Otherwise, left unprepared, the child will view an immediate increase in fluency as a "cure," leading to unrealistic expectations regarding his fluency and the process of intervention. Similarly, immediate decreases lead the child to believe that his speech was damaged, that he was better off without treatment. Both interpretations are equally unfortunate. The fact is that the dramatic change reflects the child's heightened awareness; no more, no less. The child needs to realize that quick fixes are misleading; meaningful change usually takes hard work.

Why do dramatic changes occur at this point? I explain to the child that it is kind of like being told about a big, blue elephant standing on all fours with his ears flopping and his big, blue trunk curled in front of himself, and being told *not* to think about or visualize it. When we become aware of and visualize our speech patterns, it is hard *not* to think about it. Thinking about speech affects how we speak. When I talk with student clinicians in class about interjections as a type of speech disfluency and they ask questions and interact in class, they become aware of how many interjections naturally occur in their speech. Typically, when they try to suppress the occurrence of interjections, the opposite effect occurs, and interjections vastly increase in frequency. So, the child needs to anticipate that an increased awareness of speech patterns, fluency, and disfluency is a necessary first step in effecting change. However, immediate but temporary changes often are observed and must be understood.

There is another outcome of heightening the child's awareness of his speaking behavior. While initially aware only globally of his disfluency, the child may come to see that many of his blocks (i.e., fixed or oscillatory postures) are inappropriate articulatory postures with respect to the intended targets.

For example, if one were to block on the initial sound in the word *boy*, you would expect a bilabial posture. However, if the child were to lock into an open mouth posture, this is inappropriate for the intended bilabial target. Similarly, if a child blocks on the initial sounds in words beginning with certain vowels (*eye*, *elephant*, *apple*, and so forth), you would expect an open mouth posture. However, if the child were to demonstrate a locked bilabial posture (with lips tense and together), this posture is inappropriate for the intended target. Occasionally, I have developed rules with children who demonstrate such patterns of inappropriate targets. When children's disfluency takes the form of a fixed posture, they are to do the following. First, they are to ask themselves, "Am I in the right posture? Are my articulators where they should be?" If the answer is "yes," then they are to soften the contacts of the articulators. If "no," then they are to release the posture, move to the appropriate posture, and gently initiate the first sound in the series with soft contacts. This may sound simple on the surface, but it is challenging for the child and profound in its impact. So often, children exert tremendous effort to get through an inappropriate posture before they can focus on softening the appropriate contacts in the target sounds. I say to the children, "If you're going to get stuck, get stuck in the right position!" I would prefer that the child use his resources to establish soft contacts on appropriate targets rather than potentially exhaust such resources on an inappropriate target.

Typically in conversation, we work to establish more fluent speech with slightly reduced and more regular rate, softened articulatory contacts, gentle onsets, and continual, gentle airflow. This process adds slight prolongation to potentially difficult sounds. As noted before, establishing slow, gentle, normal-sounding speech takes practice for both the clinician and client. Each vowel and consonant will be stretched and softened. Common errors include stretching only vowels (it is harder to stretch and soften consonants) and pausing between words. Some worry about the increase in the number of prolongations, or the slight distortion that occurs on stops and affricates as a result of slowing and softening. I am not concerned about this. I find that establishing such a pattern of speaking in conversation greatly eliminates much of the existing disfluency. What remains of the disfluency (i.e., prolongations, stop and affricate distortion) gladly will be addressed directly.

Another common outcome of slow, gentle speech is an overall increase in rate of conversational speech. This may seem counterintuitive to some. In other words, how can slower, more gentle rate result in a faster rate overall? Typically, disfluent speech is irregular in rate and rhythm. While our ear may perceive the speech of a person who stutters to be too fast, computing rate of speech often reveals that one's speaking rate is below average (defined loosely as 150–180 words per minute). Slowing the speech transitions, softening articulatory contacts, and using natural-sounding suprasegmental features results in speech that is more evenly and regularly produced, thus resulting in greater overall speech output per unit of time (that is, rate of speech). I remind children of the popular fable about the tortoise and the hare. In it, the slow, careful tortoise overcomes great odds and the fast, sly, and cunning hare to achieve unprecedented victory. The moral, therefore, is that slow and gentle wins the race.

As noted, most of the intervention is done within a conversational context. When we establish slow, gentle speech patterns, Van Riper's techniques (1973) prove useful, as follows:

- *Cancellation:* completing the word in which a block has occurred, and then saying the word again, this time with a slower and more gentle production in place of the block; thus, modifying the form of a block *after* it has occurred.

- *Pull-out:* changing or modifying the form of the disfluency *while* the disfluency is ongoing.

- *Preparatory set:* changing the form of the disfluency *before* the word in which it would be contained is spoken; thus, in the anticipatory stage.

These forms of modification were discussed in detail in Chapter 7 (see Figure 7.1). Guitar and Peters (1980) indicated that the pull-outs and preparatory sets are preferred over cancellations because children tend to find it easier to replace a new form of stuttering for an old form by following the clinician's model. I agree that the clinician's models are essential. We noted that the clinician regularly inserts disfluency into her own speech and models different ways of varying the disfluency. Also, the clinician models ways to vary the child's disfluency by internalizing his forms and demonstrating alterations, followed by discussion that includes the child's assessment. Nevertheless, I have found that cancellations provide the child with a simpler, more concrete task ensuring success, particularly when the disfluency is more involved or advanced. When cancellations are used, I find that children are relatively rapid (when compared to adolescents and adults) in their transition to using pull-outs and then to preparatory sets. Every step of treatment is supported by regular activities between the scheduled meetings.

In establishing fluency facilitating techniques, treatment often is a combination of different therapy forms. Treatment often combines modified forms of airflow therapy (maintaining a continuous, gentle, and natural-sounding airflow), relaxation (systematic reduction in specific and general sites of tension), and cognitive restructuring and visualization (developing visual imagery to facilitate cognitive imaging of slow, gentle speech patterns), among others. For example, you will recall from Chapter 8 the description with appropriate hand movements of a slow moving creek given to a preschool child. This child altered his speech pattern to approximate the gentle flow of the creek, and subsequently recalled the analogy to alter the speech pattern of his conversational partner. With the school-age child, I combine such cognitive imaging with a modified relaxation technique. For example, I might direct the child to close his eyes with me, and visualize a calm, relaxing image of the child's choosing. We discuss the image, clarifying the similarities and differences within our minds' eye, all the while using slow, gentle, natural-sounding speech. To use the creek example for illustration, we describe the leaf that is floating down the stream in our imagination. We discuss the slow and gentle movement of the leaf and the support given to it by the water. Initially, the clinician initiates discussion and clarification. To a lesser degree than with the adult, the child comes to initiate occasional turns discussing the leaf and the movement of the water, while using appropriately slow and gentle speech. Ultimately, the child will internalize such cognitive imaging and modified relaxation techniques and use them as needed to reestablish his fluency control. As always, the child is supported and receives praise for his active participation in the treatment process (specifically to this relaxation and cognitive visualization exercise).

Transfer fluency facilitating techniques to extraclinical settings. All of the procedures that have been discussed to this point for increasing the child's frequency of fluent speech also emphasize transferring fluency facilitating skills to outside settings. These purposes are accomplished by emphasizing the child's active role in all aspects of treatment, tailoring activities to the individual child, focusing on the child's successes, and incorporating activities and experiences that the child can internalize and thereby carry with him wherever he goes (defined here as the essence of transfer). For example, establishing a safe house deliberately nurtures and helps a child feel secure. The success of this objective may be measured, not only by how the child feels when he is with the clinician, but how the child internalizes such feelings when he anticipates being with the clinician. Inviting objectives from the child emphasizes the importance of the child's participation in treatment and helps tailor the process to the individual. Similarly, creating opportunities for fluency success and heightening the child's awareness of his speech fluency enable the child to be proactive and successful, ingredients that foster heightened motivation and create natural transfer. The fluency facilitating techniques are derived logically from an understanding of the process of communication and one's role as a communicator; help the child internalize the motor sequence and proprioceptive feedback; and address the child's related feelings, thoughts, and attitudes. Particularly important are the activities designed with the child that are completed regularly outside of the treatment setting and emphasize fluency success. We discussed treatment activities that become extraclinical assignments, including designing communication hierarchies and describing with increasing frequency the characteristics of fluent words spoken. Similarly, following discussion, demonstration, and directing/coaching, other aspects of treatment are continued outside including use of fluency facilitating controls. All the assignments to be completed outside are specific in terms of where, when, how often, and how they will be documented (typically in a small clinical notebook), criteria for success, and so on.

Another significant aspect of treatment that emphasizes transfer of fluency facilitating control is the conversational context within which most of the treatment is conducted. With few exceptions, the fluency facilitating techniques are addressed within the context of conversation, rather than beginning at the sound level, moving to monosyllabic words, polysyllabic words, phrases, and sentences. There are times when individual words are analyzed for relative fluency and disfluency components. However, most of the clinical exchange is conducted within conversation, a medium that is both portable and transferable to any extraclinical setting. Using slow speech transitions with gentle onset and natural-sounding suprasegmental features within conversation, combined with the regular assignments for extraclinical practice (home, school, other conversational contexts and speaking partners), facilitates the child's reliable fluency facilitating control. No less important, transfer is strengthened by (a) pointing out what the client already is doing that facilitates speech fluency, (b) encouraging an increase of the speech fluency already demonstrated, (c) providing strategies for the client to do rather than focusing on what not to do, (d) building social and situational hierarchies, (e) monitoring regularly by the clinician and client, (f) engaging in regular assignments and monitoring by the child outside of the treatment setting, (g) designing specific objectives and assignments to ensure success, and (h) modeling consistently to encourage self-monitoring.

Other activities that encourage transfer include bringing friends into treatment, discussing speech with friends in treatment and in the classroom, implementing specific assignments in class, and self-monitoring in class and at home. One major factor emphasizing transfer is the child's active involvement in and ownership of the treatment process from the very beginning.

Develop Resistance to Potential Fluency Disrupters

While strengthening fluency facilitating controls, the child also needs to develop resistance to old fluency disrupters. Several of the procedures already discussed, particularly those under transferring fluency facilitating techniques to extraclinical settings, promote the child's resistance to fluency disruption. Others of a behavioral nature will be discussed here; those with a primary affective focus will be discussed in the next section. Dell (1979) emphasized the importance of heightening the child's awareness of his speech fluency and developing resistance to fluency disrupters:

> We need to find ways for showing the child how fluent he is most of the time. Too many of these children think only about their stuttering. The only words they remember are those they stutter upon. We want them to shift their attention to their abundant fluency. We need to increase the amount of the child's fluency while at the same time helping him build a tolerance for and a defense against those fluency disruptors that face him everyday. If we can design our therapy to accomplish these goals we will not need to worry much about the child's occasional mild disfluencies. (p. 39)

Engage the child in activities with gradually increasing degrees of competition. We have emphasized the importance of conducting treatment within a conversational context. The earliest activities have little, if any, perceptible degree of competition. They are simply discussions about various topics of interest to the child. Eventually, activities with increasing degrees of competition are used. These might include games in which participants are playing against each other (such as board or card games), those in which each participant needs to be the first to respond in order to advance, or those in which deliberate time pressure increases the demand on the child's capacity to remain fluent while increasing rate of speech (e.g., increasing the number of fluent sentences spoken during a 1-minute interval timed with a sand filled egg timer). Individual clinicians and children will determine the activities based upon their preferences.

Reintroduce direct fluency challenge. Much of the treatment experience to this point has focused on eliminating environmental stimuli that created excessive demand upon the child's capacity to remain fluent. To develop the child's resistance to fluency disruption and to increase the strength of their fluency facilitating controls, these stimuli need to be reintroduced gradually, ensuring that the child's fluency does not break down. In other words, we deliberately challenge the child's fluency control by deliberately talking too fast, interrupting him, asking a question and then asking another before the child has finished responding, making abrupt topic shifts, among other disruptions. However, we only provide fluency challenge to the point at which the child remains successful. If the child's fluency begins to fail, then we back off, discuss the experience with the child, and try to design with the child smaller steps that will ensure fluency success. Dell (1979) stated the importance of reintroducing direct fluency challenge this way:

> You can also begin to put the child under more stress now that he is talking easier but we never put more stress on him than he can handle successfully. If we start increasing the communicative stress and he begins to have some bad stuttering, then we stop and talk about it and see if we can't solve some of his difficulty. If after returning to the stressful communication he is still not able to handle it, we drop the task for the moment and return to this activity at a later date. This rarely happens in our experience. After a number of these retrials he should be desensitized enough to handle the stressful situation. (p. 82)

Address the situations on the top rung of the child's communication hierarchies. The communication hierarchies were designed with the child to help individualize the treatment process, to engage the child actively in that process, and to organize the extraclinical speaking activities and assignments. The clinician and child regularly reassessed the hierarchies and adjusted them as appropriate. At this point, the child should be conversing in situations and contexts, with partners, about topics, and under the circumstances described in the hierarchies that represent the most difficult level of challenge for the child. This might involve calling a girl on the phone, talking to a sizable group of children with the teacher and principal present, or talking with one's parents about misdeeds that were forewarned. Whatever the experiences are, the child should feel good about his accomplishments and about his increasing ability to resist fluency disruption.

Prepare for relapse: Relapse happens! One way to prepare for relapse, the partial or total regression to pretreatment speech patterns, is to talk with the child about the likelihood of its occurrence. The worst thing for a child to experience is the surprise yielding defenselessness and helplessness that come when one is not prepared for relapse. While the likelihood of relapse with children who successfully complete formal treatment is far less than that for adults (Manning, 1996; Peters & Guitar, 1991; Starkweather et al., 1990), children need to be prepared nevertheless. Discussing this possibility with children, the clinician reminds the child of his progress in treatment and uses appropriate visual analogies to help the child understand. For example, when talking with the child about relapse, I refer to the tool box that we might keep in our car. We don't expect to use these tools often. In fact, we may never need them. Nevertheless, it gives us confidence to know where they are and how to use them should the need ever arise. Similarly, the child may never relapse. Yet he needs to feel confident and be reminded that he has the necessary tools, the fluency facilitating techniques, if he needs them. The clinician and child may role-play a scenario of relapse to help the child prepare for its occurrence. Similarly, the parents, teachers, and others also should be informed of its likelihood so no one is surprised. Treating relapse as a probability, rather than a remote possibility, will enable the child to respond constructively with minimal interference. Manning (1996) recommended a "buddy system" to help prevent relapse and otherwise support the child from the potential ill effects of such an experience. He suggested that when entering a new and challenging speaking situation outside of the treatment setting, "the presence of someone who understands the dynamics of the situation can have a powerful supporting effect. If the clinician or parent is not there, the presence of a speech buddy may be extremely beneficial" (p. 133).

Establish or Maintain Positive Feelings About Communication and Oneself as a Communicator

The child's positive attitude about communication and himself as a communicator is critical for increasing and maintaining speech fluency. In a reciprocal arrangement, one's attitude affects one's speech fluency; one's speech fluency affects one's attitude.

Prepare the child for the likelihood of being teased. Empower him with constructive strategies to withstand the potential ill effects of teasing. It is not uncommon for children with exceptionalities, particularly stuttering, to encounter teasing or ridicule. Without being prepared with behavioral and cognitive coping devices, children may experience frustration and humiliation, which over time may negatively impact their self-concept (i.e., personal construct) and their motivation to continue to monitor their speech fluency. Ramig and Bennett (1995) recommended a number of strategies for clinicians to help prevent such negativity. These included the following: (a) empowering children to alter their reactions to teasing. This is done by helping children understand why others tease, why children react, and how to stop reacting; (b) brainstorming ways children can react to teasing (e.g., ignoring the teaser or saying such things as, "Yes, I stutter" or "Would you like to know more about stuttering?"); (c) talking about possible consequences of each response to teasing; (d) role-playing teasing and selected responses. This helps children understand and communicate their feelings and alter their response pattern. Ramig and Bennett recommended the following analogy to help children confront teasing:

> Teasing is like playing basketball. The child who teases throws the ball into your court. You have two options: tease back and throw the ball into the teaser's court or respond assertively and keep possession of the ball. When you react with a hurtful comment, you throw the ball back into the "teaser's" court. He or she now has possession of the ball and can continue to tease you. If, however, you stop reacting and keep the ball by responding in ways that take care of yourself, you take control of the situation. If you do this often enough, you take the "thrill of teasing" away from the "teaser" and "steal the ball." (p. 143)

Similarly, Manning (1996) emphasized the importance of role-playing teasing and alternative responses, thus providing the child opportunities for becoming desensitized to expected taunts and insulting comments, expressing anger and frustration, and adopting more comfortable response alternatives. Furthermore, Manning discussed humor as a significant clinical device. With respect to the experience of teasing, Manning indicated that humor may help defuse or redirect the potentially hurtful comments by acknowledging the obvious and directing the comments of others back to them, as follows:

> For example, the child may say: "Yes, as a matter of fact I do stutter. But what you said was stupid and mean." In addition, depending on the circumstances

and possibly the size of the children involved, the child may want to add, "And tomorrow I might no longer stutter but you may still be stupid and mean." Alternatively, in response to other children imitating a child's moment of stuttering, he may say something like: "Look, if you're going to stutter you ought to learn how to do it correctly. Prolong the first sound like this and add a little more tension. If you get really good at it and you're brave enough, try it with me in class tomorrow." (p. 137)

I remember a brilliant technique used by a child some years ago (B. Baxley, personal communication, 1985). He responded to teasing by telling his taunters something of this sort: "You may call me names but, in fact, I'm the lucky one. I get to go to Ms. Baxley's speech room. She's got alligators in there. I bet you didn't know that. She lets us feed them and play with them. Too bad you can't go." When the bullies asked how they could get to see the alligators, the boy responded with, "Only kids who stutter get to play with them. Too bad you can't." For the remainder of the year, the children who had been teasing no longer did, hoping that their good behavior would warrant reconsideration, thus enabling them to see the alligators. The clinician helped the boy turn a situation that was to be avoided (i.e., stuttering, going to the speech room) into an enviable opportunity (i.e., leaving class to play with alligators and other interesting creatures).

Even with the best preparation to withstand the effects of teasing and ridicule, the experience nevertheless often hurts to a certain degree. Clinicians are reminded of the importance of providing unconditional acceptance and support to their clients who stutter, and in maintaining a safe house to which the child can seek refuge at any time. The clinician is uniquely suited to help the child retain a positive self-image and to work within the family system and the interdisciplinary team to provide opportunities for the child to receive support and reminders of all that he does so well.

Help the child maintain positive thinking about communication and himself as a communicator. Another aspect that must be confronted in order to establish or maintain positive feelings about communication or oneself as a communicator is negative thinking. Negative thinking inhibits fluency facilitating control among children who stutter and increases the likelihood of relapse. Manning (1996) noted the following:

> The attitude and cognitive aspects of the problem, often in the form of negative self-talk, are likely to take the lead in the progression of relapse. As elements of avoidance and fear begin to multiply and increasingly influence the speaker's decision making, overt stuttering will not be far behind. (p. 241)

Indeed, treatment as described helps the child maintain positive thinking. By focusing on, understanding, and increasing the child's fluent speech; by creating opportunities for the child to succeed; by involving the child in all aspects of the treatment process; and by attending to and supporting the child's related feelings and attitudes; the child moves from feeling unable ("I can't; I'm never going to be able to talk right.") to able ("I just used a gentle stretch again. I think I can do this. I know I can.") and from feeling out of control ("Why is this happening to me?") to being in control ("I just self-corrected. I know I can catch those blocks before they catch me."). Daly (1988) addressed the importance of positive self-talk in combining negative thinking and learned helplessness and in producing self-assurance and fluency success.

Ramig and Bennett (1995) recommended that clinicians help children recognize their thought patterns and help them assume responsibility for how they react to teasing, thus recognizing that how they think affects what they do. For younger children, Ramig and Bennett recommended that the clinician help the child identify "put downs" (hurts from the outside) and negative thinking (hurts from the inside), and replace "stinkin' thinkin'" (thoughts that hurt) with "friendly thinkin'" (thoughts that help). To establish a change in the thought process with older children, Ramig and Bennett recommended designing three columns—what the child says to himself (I can't talk right.); trigger thoughts (I should be able to talk right.); and the thought without the negative spin (I am doing the best I can today.).

The value of positive thinking and cognitive coaching is indisputable. Nevertheless, as noted, I have found that creating opportunities for children to experience directly fluency success powerfully alters their thought process in a positive direction, cementing their personal construct as effective communicators. In other words, nothing succeeds like success itself. Therefore, my best advice for clinicians working with children who stutter is to design treatment as described, while at the same time helping them cope in constructive ways with teasing, maintain positive thoughts about communication and themselves as communicators, and express their feelings within a supportive and nurturing context.

Talk with the child in positive ways. How we talk with children powerfully influences what they think about themselves. While developing independence from parents, school-age children are becoming increasingly dependent on others outside of the home for social and emotional development. What this means is that children are having experiences with an expanding variety of people, thereby confirming or challenging the impressions children have developed about themselves on the basis of interactions with family. In other words, children are vulnerable. Children's impressions about themselves and their own personal constructs are in evolution. The Golden Rule is taught most powerfully during the school-age years. How we talk with children, particularly children who stutter, is critically important to helping children establish or maintain positive feelings about communication and themselves as communicators.

You might say that children, like the rest of us, are sensitive both to the medium (how we talk with them) and the message (what is conveyed or received). From a communicative standpoint, the medium and the message (Finkelstein, 1968; McLuhan, 1964; McLuhan & Fiore, 1967; Merrill & Lowenstein, 1971) are inseparable yet dynamically interrelated. The best intentioned verbal expression of support (i.e., the message) will only be as effective as the way in which it is expressed (i.e., the medium) and the degree to which the child honestly believes and relates to what is being shared. To heighten the likelihood that the message intended translates into the message received, the clinician can help the child understand directly why he is being given expressions of support. This is done by maintaining the child's active participation within the treatment process, helping the child to be keenly aware of what he is doing well, and ensuring that the message is compatible with the child's personal construct. The child must own his success. This means that he must begin to internalize the positive support received. In other words, if the child has had nurturing experiences and has internalized such a positive impression of himself, expressions of support from the clinician will "fit" or will be compatible with what the child thinks about and thereby expects for himself. Conversely, if the child has developed negative impressions about himself (e.g., I am so bad at this. I always fail. I just know I am going to fail again.), all of the positive expressions of support will fall short, unless the child is given deliberate opportunities to succeed, to be responsible for and keenly aware of his success, and to hear ongoing expressions of sincere and justifiable support from a nurturing clinician.

In other words, the clinician must be aware of, as well as sensitive and responsive to, the child's developing personal construct. A building is only as sturdy as the foundation upon which it stands. We cannot begin the construction process (i.e., building the fluency) without first taking stock of the foundation—the child's beliefs, thoughts, and attitudes about himself within a social context—some of which was built before we arrived. How do we assess and influence the degree to which the child's thoughts about himself are positive, while at the same time work to increase the child's fluency? Specifically, this is influenced by how we talk with children and what we say, and the opportunities we provide for children to experience successful control of their speech and to believe in themselves.

There are many wonderful illustrations of how to talk with children in positive ways (Dell, 1979, 1993; Peters & Guitar, 1991; Van Riper, 1973). In my mind, Dean Williams was the master of how to talk with children about talking. In his many publications and workshops, Williams demonstrated how to discuss *with* (not talk *to* or *at*) children their beliefs about what they believe is wrong, what they believe helps them talk better, and what their feelings are about talking (1983). Once this is determined, children need information about what talking involves and what they can do to talk the way they want to talk. Williams explained, as follows:

> The talking that is done is structured around an active process of directing observations as the children are experiencing the ways they are talking and then of helping the children evaluate and re-evaluate their interpretations of those observations. The goal is to assist the children explore the reality of what they are doing and to introduce and demonstrate the alternatives they have for change. (1983, pp. 35–36)

In other words, the clinician helps the child understand his own thoughts, beliefs, and feelings, and become empowered to effect change. Understanding what the child believes is wrong and what he can do to talk better assists the clinician in knowing what information to provide and how to provide it. Furthermore, whatever explanation the child offers, whether vague ("I don't know.") or specific ("Words get hooked in my throat on little fish hooks."), the child's beliefs deserve consideration because they influence what he is doing to overcome the stuttering as he perceives it. Williams explained as follows:

> Regardless of the reasons given by a child, they deserve and require respectful discussion with the child; not from a perspective of implying that the idea is

silly or that it is wrong or that it is unimportant, but from the standpoint of listening, of questioning, of thinking out loud with the child what it means—of sharing with the child his dilemma. No conclusions need be drawn at the time. If the child seems to be confused or frightened by his uncertainties the clinician can reflect these or similar feelings by stating something like, "It's confusing isn't it?" Or, "It's kind of scary to not have any idea what's wrong isn't it? You're trying to talk and all of a sudden things just go whambo!" (1983, p. 37)

Williams explained that children's beliefs create strong motivation for the way they behave. The child who believes that his words are caught on fish hooks will push harder to release the words from the hooks. Williams warned that changes in the way a child behaves should not be attempted without considering the motivations and beliefs that prompt the behavior. Otherwise, even if changes are accomplished, they are likely to be unstable unless corresponding changes occur in the child's motivation and beliefs. Discussing a similar notion earlier, we stated that the clinician must be aware of the child's developing personal construct in order for the clinician's expressions of positive support to have an ultimate impact.

In much of Williams' work, the clinician is advised to help children understand their beliefs about talking, stuttering, and themselves as communicators, and that what they are doing is plausible based on their beliefs. In other words, the clinician needs to help the child understand that both stuttering and more fluent talking are both the consequence of things that the child is doing differently. Once the child understands this difference, he has a choice, a conscious decision. Williams stated the following:

> This results in his learning that he has a choice. This is the goal of obtaining congruence between what a person intends and the way he behaves. . . . The child should possess the basic orientation that talking smoothly involves an active doing process to be learned—with the acceptance of the mistakes that accompany any learning. (1983, p. 45)

Furthermore, the school-age child who stutters is "a pretty 'normal kid' who may get tangled up at times when he talks—but that if he does, he can change what he is doing and talk the ways he wants to talk" (Williams, 1984, p. 40). Stated differently, by providing the opportunities described (helping the child understand his own thoughts, feelings, and attitudes; talking and providing feedback in candid, supportive, nurturing ways; and enabling the child to experience fluency success and control over his communication), the child discovers that stuttering is, in part, the consequence of a decision he is making. There are alternatives. He has choices. This discovery is a remarkably empowering experience for the child.

Maintain the Fluency-Inducing Effects of Treatment

Of the different aspects of treatment (including the establishment or increase of speech fluency, transference of fluency facilitating controls to extraclinical settings, and maintenance of fluency after the completion of treatment), maintenance has proven to be the most challenging (Manning, 1996; Peters & Guitar, 1991; Van Riper, 1973). Possible explanations are many. I noted earlier that school-age children with a more severe stuttering pattern tend to have a more positive prognosis for treatment outcome. It seems that from a cost and benefit perspective, those who stand to benefit the most are more willing to invest greater energy and other resources into the treatment experience. Similarly, as children develop increasing degrees of fluency control, their stuttering problem becomes less handicapping, thus moving from being a central issue in their life (one of foreground) to a more peripheral issue (one of background). Consequently, the continuing effort and vigilance that are required for long-term maintenance may come to be perceived by the person as less important or less worth the effect (Cooper, 1977; Manning, 1996; Perkins, 1983, 1984). Manning stated that, "The problem will no longer be a major one for the person, and he may decide to devote his finite time and energies to issues in his life that he considers more important" (p. 242). The loss of motivation in the terminal stages of treatment is a reality of consequence. Just as transfer of speech fluency must be addressed from the outset of treatment, safeguards for maintenance of fluency after the completion of treatment must be addressed directly and early. Specific suggestions follow:

Help the child become his own clinician. Maintenance of speech fluency originates at the beginning of formal treatment, not at the end, and continues throughout the treatment process. One way to facilitate both transfer and maintenance of speech fluency is to involve the client in all aspects of decision making in treatment and deliberately to shift responsibility for intervention from the clinician to the client. Initially, the clinician invites the client's ideas but is relatively assertive for establishing objectives, designing procedures and assignments, providing feedback, and monitoring speech production and progress. Over time, the client needs to assume increasing degrees of responsibility for these and other related activities. I discuss with my clients, including school-age children, that our shared objective is to reach the point where we put me (the clinician) out of a job. We want the child to become his own clinician, so that he monitors and regulates his own speech behavior, therefore no longer needing the clinician to serve in this capacity. Left unchecked, it is easy, particularly for novice clinicians, inadvertently to establish a dependence of the client on the clinician. In Chapter 11, we will discuss clinicians' needs and the importance of clinicians being self-aware in order to address the needs of their clients. All clinical activities from the very beginning (including making decisions about treatment times, inviting input for treatment objectives, designing hierarchies, and describing and increasing the nature of existing fluency) are intended to heighten the client's ownership of the treatment process and its outcome. Frequently when I prepare student clinicians for working with people who stutter, these clinicians assume the posture of the "great provider," intending to apply their knowledge by telling clients what they need to achieve, by when, and how it will be done. Rarely do clinicians consider the importance of inviting clients to participate in these critical decisions. Sometimes the best way we can provide to our clients is to invite or elicit from them their own views. That way, the client is a responsible participant from the very beginning and the process is one of shared responsibility.

I use a very similar process when teaching student clinicians in their requisite courses. They, like our clients, unfortunately have become accustomed to a reactive or relatively passive role in the learning process. When I invite students to share what they hope to achieve as a result of taking the course, how they would like to achieve it, and what their related questions might be, I am greeted with dumbfounded expressions and quizzical confessions of the sort, "Nobody ever asked us that before," or "I never thought about that before." Just as we hope to sow the seeds of life-span learning and ongoing professional development (i.e., maintenance of professional skills, which is addressed in Chapter 12) early in one's professional career, similarly we invite and expect our clients to participate actively and with increasing independence in the intervention program to facilitate their ownership of the process and internalization of self-monitoring and self-regulating skills, thus maintaining speech fluency. The more likely these skills are to be internalized and habituated, the more likely they will continue after the completion of formal treatment.

Decrease the frequency of scheduled treatment. Once the affective, behavioral, and cognitive objectives for treatment have been met (and the client is using fluency facilitating skills independently and assuming responsibility for his communication), the frequency of scheduled direct treatment is decreased. The client thereby becomes increasingly responsible for managing his communication, monitoring progress, and maintaining consistent levels of speech fluency. Essentially, this is a weaning process, one in which the client increasingly becomes his own clinician. Meetings with the clinician become maintenance checks, wherein the clinician serves the role of an active listener as the client summarizes, evaluates, and projects. I must underscore the importance of the client internalizing the self-evaluating and self-monitoring skills, while assuming increasing levels of treatment responsibility and communication independence. The young driver of a standard shift vehicle is very conscious at first of which gear he is in and all of the individual elements of a larger motor process. Ultimately, the process becomes internalized, habituated, and thereby synchronized. The driver evaluates, monitors, and adjusts as needed. While the parallel to maintaining speech fluency may be somewhat distant, the ultimate objectives are similar. The person who stutters becomes increasingly responsible for coordinating and adjusting the synchronized process of speech fluency and maintaining these skills for the long haul.

Maintain regular maintenance checks of decreasing frequency for at least 2 years post-treatment. As the frequency of scheduled treatment decreases, the importance of regular maintenance checks increases. As noted, the client becomes responsible for reporting, evaluating, monitoring, and adjusting. Initially, the maintenance may be once monthly, moving to once bimonthly, every 4 months, 6 months, 1 year, then 2 years. I noted earlier that the risk of relapse typically is greater for adults than for children and for those whose pretreatment level of fluency is less severe. Manning (1996) indicated that some type of follow-up is necessary for most clients. He recommended, therefore, that change be viewed as a long-term process, that clients have the option of returning for treatment in some form for as long as they need it, and that follow-up visits not be viewed by clinician or client as an indication of failure. Rather, follow-up should be anticipated as "a natural and acceptable part of the process of change" (p. 240). He indicated, and I concur, that most clients do not require a return to intensive treatment, and that generally individual follow-up, group treatment sessions, or support group meetings enable clients to continue making progress.

Build in regular, child-initiated benchmarking. A related activity that I have found useful with both children and adults for maintaining speech fluency is benchmarking. This means reassessing where one is, where one wants to be, and addressing any discrepancy. A few examples will help illustrate its usefulness.

A child who can do five sit-ups is working toward being able to do 10. He has increased from one by adding one additional sit-up per week to the daily exercise routine. By continuing to add one per week, the child should achieve his goal in 5 weeks. The child benchmarks by reassessing his progress on a weekly basis with respect to a long-term goal, making adjustments as necessary. Many of us know the increasing challenge of keeping off the extra pounds. We step on the scale every day. Seeing that we are 170 pounds and that we wish to be 165, we establish a goal of dropping 1 pound per week for the next 5 weeks. We monitor every day, but we benchmark (by stepping on the scale and reassessing current weight, projected weight, and effectiveness of current strategy) every Saturday morning.

Maintaining speech fluency is not much different. Begun at the early stages of treatment and continued throughout, we have our client benchmark with respect to each individual objective. Once we get to the stage where maintenance of fluency receives primary focus, the client benchmarks the present level of fluency-related behaviors, thoughts, and feelings with respect to pre- and post-treatment levels and previous long-term projections. With decreasing, albeit regular, frequency (weekly, monthly, bimonthly, and so on), the client reassesses his present level of functioning and determines if it is consistent with earlier projections. If so, the client internalizes the reward for maintaining communication progress. If not, the client interprets the discrepancy with respect to relevant circumstances and designs a realistic, specific strategy for change. For example, if the regularity of self-monitoring speech fluency has slipped, the school-age child may commit himself to disciplined, focused self-monitoring during group reading and show-and-tell activities at school. If he comes to experience the thoughts of inability or helplessness, he may revisit the strategies used previously in treatment to document and focus on successes and reestablish ways of positive thinking. As mentioned above, these are the times when follow-up visits with the clinician in a supportive and nurturing environment are useful. Likewise, ongoing support and involvement from parents, teachers, and others within the child's communication system help maintain the long-term benefits of treatment.

Deliberately revisit the past. Sometimes wishing not to relive the past helps motivate one to maintain speech fluency. Those whose stuttering is most severe often are more committed to the change process. As we work toward maintenance of speech fluency, I prepare a client to view a videotape of his pre-treatment communication. I do this with two objectives in mind. First, I want to celebrate with the client his accomplishments, which are so well deserved. Second, I want to increase his motivation to maintain the level of speech fluency that has been achieved. In other words, I want the client to revisit concretely how he spoke previously so that he will reaffirm his commitment to himself to do his utmost to avoid returning to pre-treatment levels. This is a hard thing for a client to do and must be done with sensitivity and support. The focus of discussion before, during, and after returning to times past is, "Look at all of the things (i.e., forms of disfluency) that you have left behind."

While the clinician sincerely intends a positive focus, some clients nevertheless are disturbed when they are faced with the reality of how they spoke previously. There is a delicate balancing act here. We want to help clients remain focused on the positive aspects of change, while at the same time deliberately presenting the sometimes shocking reality of the past. We want to encourage maintenance of fluency change and all of the constant vigilance and work it entails by recognizing and rewarding improvements (using positive reinforcement, which increases the likelihood of fluency by presenting a pleasant or satisfying consequence) and by recreating the reality of pretreatment stuttering (using negative reinforcement, which increases the likelihood of fluency by presenting an unpleasant, unsatisfying, or painful consequence). In other words, we want to reward the client for progress, but we also want him to redouble his commitment never to speak like he used to again. We want him to recall just how painful it was to be out of control and to experience communicative helplessness in order to heighten motivation never to experience that again. Memories of a cold winter without firewood may be poignant enough to prevent ever being without firewood again.

Reexamine the child's personal construct. We have discussed that one's personal construct is a composite of thoughts, feelings, and attitudes about communication and oneself as a communicator. Personal constructs serve as a filter through which one views his world, interprets his role within it, and thereby comes to anticipate events that are compatible with or similar to those past. In order for affective, behavioral, and cognitive changes to be maintained after the conclusion of treatment, these changes must be integrated with one's personal construct. Many clinicians and researchers have asserted that we are far more knowledgeable about how to help people who stutter become fluent than we are about how to help them maintain that fluency (Bloodstein, 1995; Cooper, 1977; Van Riper, 1973). I agree. At the same time, I argue that one explanation for this ongoing state of affairs is that not enough attention is being paid to aspects other than observable behavior (i.e., level of speech fluency); that is, what people who stutter think and how they feel about themselves as communicators. Unless those who stutter feel secure with the changes and feel that the changes "fit" with who they are and are becoming, indeed the changes will not last.

Consider the parallel with overeaters. We have a friend who over the last 2 years dropped and then regained over 100 pounds. While Janet was losing the weight, she received ongoing social support for visible progress. In time, social support lessened as people became accustomed to and therefore anticipated Janet's relatively slim appearance. Behaviors only last as long as they are integrated within one's personal construct, however. Janet continued to "feel" obese. She enjoyed the novelty of reduced weight and the praise she had received. But throughout, she felt overweight, like an impostor who would be found out. Her new behaviors that included altered eating patterns and reduced weight were not integrated with how she felt and what she thought about herself as a person. Consequently, old eating patterns gradually returned as did the extra pounds.

The feelings and attitudes of school-age children, including those who stutter, are in evolution. Clinicians must look within the child to understand how he sees himself. Those who stutter are coming to view themselves as "stutterers." Knowing the experience of fluency failure, many children internalize this experience and come to expect the same. One of the advantages of working with children is that they literally have not lived long enough for the roots of stuttering to have taken hold impenetrably. Even when life events fertilize the growth of stuttering, the roots can grow just so quickly. This is not to minimize the significance of the stuttering experience for the individual child. How do we change the child's expectation? How do we change this course of development? The answer to these questions is this: We flood the child with successful fluency experiences. We show him that he already possesses much fluency and the skills necessary to be fluent even more often. We involve the child actively in the treatment process and the related decisions, as we do the parents, teachers, and others. We create opportunities to provide the child with so much data indicative of his success and inherent potential that he has no choice but to look at those data within the context of how he views himself. Indeed the clinician's role is to help the child interpret these data and to address the discrepancy with how he feels and what he thinks about himself.

Furthermore, the clinician must help the child know how to use the fluency. Just because the child is becoming fluent doesn't mean that he automatically knows how and when to speak in socially appropriate ways. The clinician may need to work with the child to build pragmatic fluency, knowing what to say within situational constraints. Using language follows a variety of social scripts. Taking turns is a social script. Speaking at home requires a different social script, involving a different set of situational constraints, than speaking at school. Similarly, we will see that adults who become fluent may need to learn the social scripts for dating, interviewing, socializing, working, and parenting. The point is that we need to help children feel fluent and internally in control of their communication (by owning their fluency and feeling comfortable with it), and then to help them use their speech in pragmatically appropriate ways that are both internally and externally rewarded (ways that facilitate transfer and maintenance).

Manning (1996) supported the concept that maintenance of speech fluency must be multidimensional and address not only behavioral features, but affective and cognitive ones as well. He stated:

> Relapse may occur, not only in terms of fluency level, but more important, in the direction of the pretreatment attitude and cognitive features of the syndrome. Just as the assessment of this syndrome must be multidimensional, the maintenance of success is multidimensional as well. Concentration on a single feature, such as the level of fluency, excludes the cognitive features of the syndrome that those who are doing the stuttering perceive as critical. (p. 238)

To help clients maintain affective and cognitive changes that are critical to maintenance of speech fluency, clinicians must help the client feel comfortable with and accept his new role and possibilities as a communicator. When adjusting to the new role, Manning (1996, p. 243) noted, the person who stutters must come to view himself "as something beyond an individual who stutters," and must "evolve as a person and form a new paradigm, a new view of himself and his possibilities." Manning also summarized that those who have been most successful in maintaining their fluency have made changes in their lifestyle throughout the treatment process. Through this process of adjustment, some people who stutter report feeling less than fully comfortable with their fluency, feeling that they are deceiving others, waiting for their disfluency to return. In short, "They do not feel like themselves. Their new fluency and all the responsibility for self-management that goes with it have changed the self they had grown used to." Again, treatment must work toward maintaining affective and cognitive changes in addition to the directly observable speech fluency behaviors.

Integrate treatment changes within the communication system. We established previously that clinicians need to help people who stutter adjust to behavioral, affective, and cognitive changes that come with increased fluency and heightened communicative independence. Similarly, clinicians also need to help listeners adjust to the "new" speaker. In other words, conversational partners are adjusting their expectations in response to changes with the person who stutters. We noted earlier, particularly in Chapter 5, that changes affecting one person also affect all others within that person's communication system. As the person who stutters achieves fluency and becomes inclined to speak more assertively and take more communicative risks, conversational partners must adjust to different expectations. These adjustments take time and support.

Clinicians can be particularly helpful to those within the communication system (such as family, teachers, and classmates) by providing support in the form of helping them understand the nature of the changes that are occurring and ways that they can react constructively to those changes. In most cases, the clinician helps the conversational partners continue to feel needed but in different ways. Family members who have become accustomed to speaking for a child who stutters will need direction regarding when and how to allow and encourage him to speak for himself. Teachers who have become used to altering assignments to prevent penalizing a child who stutters will need guidance in learning how to include the child and what to expect of him. Friends who have protected and "looked out" for a child who stutters will need to know how to behave differently. All well-meaning people in the child's environment will need to continue to feel needed within the revised "rules" or expectations. Manning (1996) noted that successful treatment of people who stutter will impact others. "If these other people in the client's life fail to understand and recognize the nature of progress, they will be less likely to provide positive reinforcement for these changes, and to some degree, long-term progress will be less likely to occur" (p. 243). People within the larger communication system of the person who stutters will need to shift their perspective and adjust their roles.

As logical as this sounds, some conversational partners resist this change. Expectations based on precedent are hard to change. Listeners report feeling that the stuttering has become viewed as part of one's personality. Change takes time and focus, both of which might be rare commodities among those adjusting to people who stutter. Other pressures occasionally placed on children who stutter inadvertently impede change. For example, pressure is often placed on the speaker following treatment to demonstrate much improved or even perfect fluency ("How awful, after all of this time and effort and money and he still stutters!"; Manning, 1996, p. 244). Any observable stuttering may be viewed as a sign of failure by the child who stutters or his listeners. Indeed, clinicians help facilitate change by helping the participants know what to expect, how to respond, and otherwise how to contribute actively and meaningfully to the change process. The integrated and overlapping processes of treatment, transfer, and maintenance indeed are multidimensional and dynamic.

WORKING WITH SCHOOL-AGE CHILDREN WHO STUTTER AND HAVE CONCOMITANT LANGUAGE OR PHONOLOGICAL IMPAIRMENT

Concomitant Disorders

Many children who stutter also have concomitant speech or language impairment; many have concomitant speech *and* language impairment. Estimates suggest that of all the children who stutter, about one third can be expected to demonstrate articulation or phonological problems (Bloodstein, 1995; Conture, 1990b; Manning, 1996; Peters & Guitar, 1991). Of the children studied by Louko, Edwards, and Conture (1990), 40% who stuttered also displayed delayed and atypical phonological development, compared to only 7% of the control group (who were normally fluent and demonstrated a similar profile). Others conducting similar investigations have reported that fluency and articulation impairment co-occur among school-age children as much as 58%, compared to 2% to 6.4% of the school-age population who do not stutter yet demonstrate articulation impairment (Conture, 1990b; Manning, 1996). The co-occurrence of stuttering and language impairment is not as well documented, in part because the co-existing impairment may only become apparent after the fluency has improved (Conture, 1990b; Manning, 1996; Ratner, 1995). Furthermore, Conture (1990b) noted that although other problems (such as voice, hearing, psychosocial adjustment, cerebral palsy, and cleft palate) have not been noted to co-occur with school-age children who stutter in greater frequency than with those who do not, all children should be evaluated for such problems before treatment, and treatment should be designed for each child individually. While it is not uncommon for children who stutter to demonstrate concomitant disorders (Nippold, 1990; Wall & Myers, 1995), assessment and treatment techniques that are both sensitive and responsive to potential interference across the disorders only recently have received attention in the literature (Peters & Guitar, 1991; Ratner, 1995).

Effects of Concomitant Disorders

There are at least two significant issues that clinicians must confront when working with children who have or are suspected to have coexisting communication problems (Manning, 1996). First, some children who are being treated for speech—language disorders have become more disfluent or have begun to stutter as a consequence of treatment (Conture, 1990b; Ratner, 1995; Starkweather, 1997). Conture (1990b) suggested that the risk of stuttering onset is increased if a child is being treated for severe articulation impairment or unusual phonological problems. Furthermore, treatment for articulation or language impairment may disrupt speech fluency if the children are placed in treatment too early (i.e., before the child is capable of producing sounds correctly with relative ease), or if the treatment experience places communicative demands upon the child for speech sound or language comprehension or production that exceed the child's finite (i.e., individually defined) capacity to produce fluent speech (Conture, 1990b; Manning, 1996;

Starkweather, 1997; Starkweather et al., 1990). Conture (1990b), noted the following:

> We have noticed this association between positive change in language and increases in speech disfluency to be particularly apparent in children around five to six years of age. We are not sure what this means or its long-term implications for recovery from disfluency. We are inclined to speculate that increases in the length and complexity of verbally expressed languages increase the opportunities for instances of disfluency to emerge and is probably a natural byproduct of improved but still unstable expressive language skills. (p. 105)

Secondly, there is a "trading" relationship among fluency, language, and phonological skill within a child. In other words, demands in a variety of domains can result in fluency breakdown (Starkweather, 1997; Starkweather et al., 1990). Ratner (1995) noted that, "Efforts to remediate areas of deficiency are likely to exacerbate patterns of fluency failure. . . . This situation places the clinician in a planning dilemma—how to improve skills in one domain without further compromising skills in another" (p. 182).

To Treat or Not To Treat?

To treat or not to treat? That is the question often facing informed speech–language pathologists. Manning (1996) noted that the issues that must be addressed are complex; yet the answer often is *yes*. Because articulation and language problems often require long-term treatment, initiation of fluency intervention often cannot wait until the articulation and language problems are resolved because of the significant social, emotional, and educational consequences that would result (Ratner, 1995). Furthermore, waiting to begin fluency intervention is contraindicated by the efficacy data suggesting the importance of early intervention.

If *Yes,* Where Do I Begin?

Once the clinician has decided to begin intervention, then she must decide which disorder (stuttering, articulation, or language) deserves more immediate attention. About children who stutter and demonstrate a delay in language, Conture (1990b) indicated the following:

> Therapy oriented to modification of language seems most appropriate if the child's speech disfluencies are of a physically easy, relatively short duration and consist mainly of part- and whole-word repetitions. . . . Conversely, therapy should probably be more oriented to modification of stuttering if the speech disfluencies are associated with visible and audible signs of physical and psychological tension, and are relatively longer in duration and of a sound prolongation (audible and inaudible) type. (p. 106)

About children who stutter as a consequence of articulation treatment, Conture (1990b) noted that "these children need experience with speaking in a physically relaxed, relatively slow-paced atmosphere where communication is made an enjoyable, interesting, and shared activity" (p. 107). In such cases, phonetic placement or other forms of direct remediation of the child's speech fluency and articulation are secondary. The primary objective is to convey to the child that speech and communication can be fun and can be done in a physically relaxed, unhurried manner. Similarly, Conture (1990b) noted that children who stutter and demonstrate an articulation impairment should be helped to "develop a physically easier, less hurried or rushed means of initiating and maintaining speech rather than very careful, cautious, physically precise, and overarticulated productions of sound" (p. 108). Deciding which impairment is to receive relatively more immediate or substantive focus essentially is a question of which exceptionality is more primary, which is secondary, and so forth. This entails also an appreciation for how intervention in one area of exceptionality may impact other exceptionalities.

Sequential Vs. Concurrent Intervention

Ratner (1995) approached the challenge of establishing therapeutic goals and priorities somewhat differently. She indicated that depending on the associated impairments, the clinician must decide whether to address the problems sequentially or concurrently. Sequential treatment plans have the advantage of being able to achieve a level of success in one area before tackling another. For example, the clinician may decide to heighten a child's expressive language formulation skills before addressing his fluency facilitation skills. However, whether fluency or language/phonology is addressed first, the child's capacity to remain fluent will be challenged by the demands experienced when language/phonology receives primary focus. Ratner (1995) indicated that concurrent intervention for fluency and other communication disorders attempts to address fluency within the lowest level of phonological and linguistic demand. For example, about sequential intervention for children who stutter and demonstrate a language disorder, Ratner (1995) noted the following:

> Particularly given documented trade-offs between expressive syntax and fluency . . . , the premise that all fluency therapy for children should introduce fluency skills at carefully graded levels of linguistic demand is all the more important when both expressive language and fluency are impaired. Fluency-facilitating activities should actively avoid requiring the child to produce utterances beyond those that are comfortably within the child's expressive grammatical repertoire. (p. 182)

In such cases, the areas of the child's relative language competency should be used as initial fluency practice targets. Ratner recommended that such competencies as well as activities and structures that place significant demand on the child be determined on an individual basis. For children who stutter and who present a phonological impairment, Conture, Louko, and Edwards (1993) piloted a concurrent methodology using a fluency shaping protocol with indirect phonological intervention. The clinician is cautioned to avoid any overt correction of the child's speech. This is consistent with fairly wide-spread advice against providing children direct feedback regarding accuracy of their articulation. The reasoning behind this advice is that doing so would place additional demand (communicative or emotional) on the child's capacity to remain fluent.

Nevertheless, Manning (1996) advised that clinicians should feel free to model fluency facilitating techniques in their own speech, and should determine each child's response to linguistic and emotional demands both inside and outside the treatment setting.

Blended Intervention Approaches

Goals for fluency intervention can be incorporated or "blended" into other remediation activities (such as phonology) (Ratner, 1995). For example, while practicing articulation targets, children in Conture et al.'s (1993) pilot program were encouraged to speak slowly, adjust rhythm and rate, decrease interruptions, increase the pause time between conversational turns, and adopt an overall relaxed manner of speaking. However, as Manning (1996), Ratner (1995), and others have pointed out, blended intervention may not be advised when the articulation or language intervention focus stresses, and thereby disrupts, the fluency system. In such a case, a sequential form of treatment would be advised; a stable level of progress in one area should be achieved before the clinician addresses another.

General Principles

General principles that can be used for designing intervention for children who stutter and have concomitant disorders were presented by Ratner (1995) and expanded by Manning (1996). First, phonological and linguistic processing create heightened demands on the child's finite capacity to maintain fluent speech. Second, clinicians should design treatment in such a way as to minimize such demand. This is done by moving from articulation and language activities that the child has mastered to those that involve minimally increasing articulatory and linguistic challenge. Third, specific feedback, particularly negative feedback, about the child's speech efforts or accuracy of articulatory and linguistic targets should be avoided. Withholding such feedback will slow articulatory and linguistic growth, but will reduce the demand placed upon the child's capacity to remain fluent. Fourth, based on an understanding of the child's concomitant disorders and his unique capacities to withstand communicative demand, clinicians will need to design treatment individually.

Manning (1996) noted that such principles are useful not only for children who stutter and have concomitant disorders, but for all clients. All treatment should be designed with an understanding of the child's unique capacities and responses to incoming and increasing demands. Furthermore, clients should be "pushed to the upper ranges of their ability" with full support, acceptance, and nurturing in order to impact significantly their fluency disorder. Manning's (1996) conclusion applies to all children, as follows:

> The clinician working with young fluency-disordered children should be able to help the child to learn to easily produce difficult sounds or new grammatical structures without introducing the idea that they need be concerned or frightened or should struggle with their speech. It is possible to model a smooth and flowing manner of speech production while also giving the child a real sense of command over himself. (p. 131)

WORKING WITH PARENTS

No one more profoundly influences a child than his parents or other primary care providers. Because of this influence and the dynamic interaction between members of a communication system, the importance of actively engaging the parents within the intervention process is indisputable. In Chapters 5 and 8, we discussed these influences and the importance of working with parents. The few additional comments here will focus on the uniqueness of working with parents of school-age children who stutter.

Access to Parents

For a number of years in my work at a university-based speech and hearing center, I have enjoyed the luxury of relatively easy access to the parents of my school-age clients who stutter. With few exceptions, at least one parent actively participates in a part of every scheduled treatment session and in the activities that are conducted regularly between scheduled sessions. I have never forgotten, however, from the years I worked as a school-based speech–language pathologist, that such regular access to parents is rarely possible in school settings. What this means is that direct meetings with parents, albeit less frequent, take on even greater significance for the clinician, who is challenged to develop other mechanisms to inform and engage parents within the intervention process. Others have addressed such mechanisms, including specially scheduled meetings that accommodate the parents' schedules, phone calls, newsletters, memos, and so forth (Dell, 1979; Manning, 1996; Peters & Guitar, 1991; Ratner, 1995). In other words, maintaining active interaction with the parents and involving them in the treatment process are key objectives. To these ends, the quality of such varied forms of interaction with parents takes on additional meaning; indeed such quality cannot be replaced by an increase in quantity.

Families often have special circumstances (see Chapter 5) that reduce their ability to attend scheduled meetings during the hours of school operation. In addition, cultural considerations (see Chapter 6) might influence the parents' willingness to participate in the intervention process or the child's ability to follow through with assignments outside of the clinical setting. It must not be assumed that such lack of attendance, participation, or follow-through necessarily equates with a lack of interest or concern. Manning (1996) and Ramig (1993) pointed out that parents have many priorities (such as work schedules or financial considerations) that understandably may be regarded as more important than their child's speech fluency. Other limitations may exist. In mountainous, rural, or poor urban areas, some families may not be reached by telephone, some may be functionally illiterate, or some may not speak English. Particularly when there is only one parent at home, some families may not be able to afford services and some may not be able to transport the child to treatment (Manning, 1996). These and other circumstances may interfere with the child's or parents' participation in the intervention process.

Respecting the Primary Role of Parents

A brief but significant caution is in order. In our commitment to help children transfer and maintain the effects of treatment on their speech fluency, we solicit the help of others, particularly parents, outside of the clinical setting. I am concerned, however, that at times the degree and type of involvement proposed for the parents may not reflect an awareness of and sensitivity to their unique role. In other words, the parent is not the clinician in absentia. The parent is the child's primary source of guidance, support, and nurturing. This is not to say that the parents cannot or should not be critically involved in all aspects of the treatment process. Indeed, they should. However, in considering and designing methods for the parents to contribute to the intervention process, clinicians must be mindful of the parents' more primary roles.

An example might help illustrate my concern. Most clinicians would agree that parents often are inclined to provide their child with verbal feedback about the relative correctness (i.e., fluency) of the child's speech. It is hard for parents to watch their children make errors. Typically, parents (i.e., and clinicians) remember to provide feedback when disfluency is observed. In such cases, therefore, the feedback frequently provided is one of correction ("No, that's not quite right. Try slowing down a little; Oops! You forgot the gentle stretch; Wait a minute. Let's remember to talk like the turtle."). Without advice from the clinician, well-meaning parents inadvertently create a situation in which the child becomes reluctant to talk, knowing that he is facing certain correction. In other words, while the parents believe they are being helpful, they are inadvertently penalizing the child for talking. The child ceases to participate in family conversations and the parent or child become emotionally upset.

Let's cast this a little differently now. To prevent a setback, we can discuss with the parents the importance of keeping verbal interaction a fun, happy experience and of encouraging the child to develop his own communication independence. One method that encourages both of these objectives is to provide the child with positive feedback. That is, we need continually to point out to the child all that he is doing right. All of us are inclined to do more of what we feel we are doing well. Showing the child that he is succeeding will encourage him to be a more active conversationalist; constantly correcting him will close him down thus becoming less verbally assertive. Some parents will say, "But he is so disfluent. Listen to the way he struggles." Such disclosures remind us that we need to show (discuss, demonstrate, and then direct/coach) parents that even when the child is highly disfluent, much, if not most, of his speech is fluent. The fluency is what we want to highlight. In fact, the child's disfluency should serve as an additional reminder to the parents to compliment the child's fluency ("You said that great! That was really gentle. You remembered to use your slow, easy speech just now when you said 'ttthat.'"). Other parents will say, "Sure, I can give feedback for the fluency, but I'm not doing anything about the disfluency." This is where modeling and expansion comes in.

I explain to the parents that a good way to correct the disfluencies is to show the child by example how to talk more slowly and gently. When the child is disfluent, his parents may use the word that the child spoke disfluently in a different but related sentence while using slow, gentle speech. For example, if the child says, "I cuh–cuh–cuh–can't find the duh–duh–duh–dog," the parent might respond with, "You cccan't ffffind the dddog. I bbbet hhhe'll be bbback sssoon to bbbe fffed." Taken together, the parent is being encouraged to compliment the child on all aspects of his speech that are slow and gentle, and to model and expand the child's sentence during instances of disfluency. Furthermore, it is helpful for the parents to demonstrate ongoing models of slow, relaxed speech for the child. In this way, fluent speech is encouraged and modeled, all within a positive framework, one in which the child develops or maintains his active role and independence as a communicator. Other suggestions discussed in Chapter 8 for parental intervention apply here as well (be good listeners; simplify, soften, and slow daily speech models; reduce the pace of activities and overall tension; identify and eliminate interruptions). The reader may want to refer back to Chapter 8 to review these suggestions, or review other resources discussed in Appendix B.

Meeting Parents' Needs

To this point, we have addressed how parents can help respond to the communication needs of their child. In most cases, the child's welfare is the parents' primary concern. We cannot overlook, however, that parents have needs of their own. Like that of the children, parents' needs are behavioral, affective, and cognitive. We have addressed the parent's behavioral needs (i.e., what the parents can do to help their child establish, transfer, and maintain speech fluency). But meeting the parents' needs does not end there.

Many parents have intense feelings about their child's stuttering. Some feel responsible, some feel helpless, some feel resentment. Many parents are not precisely aware of how they feel. Parents experience multiple demands upon their time and energy; thus, many do not afford themselves the "luxury" of focusing on, understanding, or addressing their own feelings. Dell (1979) recommended that clinicians provide parents "an opportunity to unburden themselves of some of their pent-up feelings of frustration, guilt or anxiety resulting from their child's stuttering. . . . The parents need to talk and talk freely" (p. 88). Parents so often are advised by well-meaning peers and professionals not to worry about their child's stuttering. We noted in the last chapter that "worry" is a factor in most parents' job descriptions. Telling them not to worry is not only useless advice, it reflects neither an understanding of nor a sensitivity for the parent as a person. Dell (1979) suggested asking parents general but leading questions combined with active listening and reflective speech. Such techniques help parents see that we are interested in and relate to their story and encourage them to talk further. For example, the clinician might say, "Tell me about Johnny. What are some of his strengths and weaknesses, his likes and dislikes, and so on." When the parent talks about the development of the child's speech and particularly stuttering, the clinician asks about what they think might have caused it and what they are doing to help the child when he stutters. Dell suggested the following as a lead-in for parents to express their feelings:

> I'll bet you've had lots of advice from relatives and friends? It seems that every-
> one is an expert on the problem of stuttering and they all feel that you are not

using the right methods to cure his stuttering. People love to give advice to us about our children." (1979, p. 89)

Combined with leading expressions and reflective listening, clinicians must be tolerant, if not nurturing, of silence. Without such constructive silence, parents often are unable to unburden themselves and share their feelings and clinicians are unable to gain insights about our clients and their families.

Such interactions with parents often reveal their feelings of guilt. Some parents conceal their feelings of guilt by appearing calm and confident. However, when provided the opportunity, many parents express somewhat emotionally loaded feelings of accusation from society or self-condemnation for their child's stuttering. Dell (1979) emphasized the importance of alleviating the parents' feelings of guilt, even when parents have done things that are harmful to their child's fluency, because such feelings impede the parents' ability to follow the clinician's guidance and facilitate the child's fluency. Also, the parents' feelings of guilt often are communicated to and affect the child. The child may feel that he is at fault for causing the parent distress and may become even more reticent to talk. Clinicians can alleviate such feelings of guilt by accepting and supporting the parents' expressions of feelings and insight, yet providing more accurate information about communication, stuttering, and strategies available for intervention. In other words, we cannot change what has already passed. However, the clinician is a source of support and a resource of information, the combination of which alleviates the parents' fears by knowing that both the burden of stuttering and the commitment to successful intervention are shared.

The clinician also must meet the parents' cognitive need, or need for knowledge. That is, parents' actions, what they typically do or say to help the child while he is stuttering, reflect what they think or know about communication and stuttering. One of the first questions parents ask is, "What causes stuttering?" An implicit request is, "Tell me I am not the cause of it. Tell me that I am O.K. as a parent even though my child stutters." Again, we need to determine the parents' beliefs and assumptions, offering support for all the parent might be doing that facilitates fluency. At the same time, we must provide information that reflects our collective knowledge base in these areas and offer constructive suggestions for intervention and change that will facilitate the child's fluency. These discussions, however, must be responsive not only to the child's needs, but to the parents' ability to understand the information provided and to contribute meaningfully to the intervention process. Most parents are willing and able to contribute to the intervention process and help with follow-through activities at home. We must remain mindful of the multiple and pressing demands experienced by parents.

One parent, however, stands in my memory as a reminder of the importance of understanding and responding to the parents' cognitive needs and abilities. When I was a clinician based in the schools, one of the young boys who was receiving fluency intervention caught a persistent cold. We learned that he had been bathed in a nearly frozen creek during the winter. With ongoing encouragement from the school personnel, the mother took the child to a physician who prescribed medication. Unable to read, albeit well-meaning, the mother fed the entire 10-day dosage to the child at one sitting. When we called to inquire about the boy's extended absence, this story surfaced. Does this mean that a parent such as this cannot or should not be involved in the intervention process? Indeed not. But it does mean that the information provided and expectations for participation in the intervention process must be tailored according to one's relative competence and need for knowledge. It became apparent that this mother was receiving instruction in parenting skills from Social Services. We helped her understand the importance of basic pragmatic language skills, specifically conversational turn-taking. She helped us at home by implementing rules for turn-taking, thus minimizing the demand placed on the child's capacity to remain fluent. Indeed, this experience provided me (and other school personnel) with insight about the boy, his home, and the nature of the communication system within which the boy functioned. This knowledge helped us communicate with and meaningfully involve the boy's mother and tailor methods for transfer and maintenance of fluent speech.

WORKING WITH TEACHERS AND OTHER SCHOOL PERSONNEL

School personnel, particularly teachers, play a key role in the management of school-age children who stutter. Many of the suggestions discussed earlier for parents also apply to classroom teachers. Excellent instructional materials are available with constructive suggestions for teachers and intervention in school-based settings (Cooper, 1979; Cooper & Cooper, 1991; Dell, 1979; Manning, 1996; Ramig & Bennett, 1995).

Build Rapport and Establish Colleagueship with Teachers

Most teachers know their children so well, even before the school year begins, that they proactively seek appropriate information when they anticipate working with a child who stutters. Nevertheless, before we can expect teachers to help contribute to our communication mission with children who stutter, we first must establish rapport with teachers as colleagues in education. One way to do so is by initiating an initial meeting with the teacher. If at all possible, invite from the teacher her preferred times or at least give several options from which the teacher might choose. Again, this shows our respect for the teacher's time-consuming responsibilities. The purpose of the meeting not only is to exchange information so that the teacher can help us achieve the child's communication objectives. We must be mindful of the teacher's instructional mission as well, and determine how we can help her achieve that mission, particularly with our children who stutter. In other words, clinicians inadvertently may communicate that they want to receive instructional support from teachers without regard to providing the same to teachers.

Every professional in the school believes that his or her specialty is critically important. Therefore, mutual respect and support must rule. In the initial meeting, teachers often ask about the nature of stuttering in general, and with more specific regard to the child who now is in her classroom. At the same time, clinicians should inquire about the curriculum and the teacher's objectives and related plans. The classroom (and the curriculum) provides an excellent context to facilitate transfer and maintenance of speech fluency. There is no reason why the clinician cannot apply the fluency facilitating techniques to discussions of the content being addressed in the classroom. Teachers appreciate our interest in their work and individual missions. In fact, the degree of commitment shown by some teachers to support the fluency intervention process is a direct reflection of that shown by clinicians toward the curriculum and classroom activities. Dell (1979) noted the importance of an initial meeting with the teacher. He indicated that there are too many distractions during recess or in the teachers' lounge for good communication. After such a meeting, however, subsequent interactions typically can be less structured and even held in passing.

Manning (1996) noted that the character of the relationship between a clinician and a teacher will depend partly on the model used for service delivery in the schools. In a consultative model, for example, the clinician works through the teacher and parents to help the child. In a collaborative–consultative model, the clinician works with the child on an individual basis and collaborates with the teacher and parents in planning activities for transfer and maintenance of fluency into the child's world and daily activities. In a pullout model, children are taken out of the classroom and are seen individually or in small groups by the clinician. The first two models are more conducive to creating long-term change for the child in addition to professional interaction and a sense of colleagueship between the teacher and clinician (Gregory, 1995; Manning, 1996).

Providing communication workshops is another strategy for building rapport and colleagueship between clinicians and teachers and involving school personnel in the communication intervention experience. This is easy for clinicians to do (after the initial experience) partly because of the instructional brochures and pamphlets in addition to audio- and videotapes that are readily available from the Stuttering Foundation of America and the National Stuttering Project, among other organizations. Teachers typically have a weekly faculty meeting held after school. I always have found teachers and administrators highly receptive to my willingness to present such a workshop. This is an excellent time to build teachers' understanding of the nature and treatment of children who stutter, in addition to those with other communication exceptionalities. I have found that video clips from actual treatment easily hold teachers' attention and generate rich questions and lively discussion. Also significant is the clinician's willingness to share not only what she knows, but a glimpse of what she does. By example, this invites such sharing among all teachers and provides an excellent opportunity for clinicians to express interest in what teachers know, what they do, and how the clinician can learn from and help the teacher.

Banish Elitism—All Colleagues in Education Are Equal

Elitism is thinking that one is part of a superior or privileged group. Clinicians, particularly those who are itinerant, run the risk of inadvertently communicating a sense of elitism. Clinicians are in short supply. Clinicians hold a master's degree (with some exceptions specific to individual state and licensing laws). Clinicians often receive a pay supplement or differential for serving the needs of those with exceptionalities. Clinicians work with fewer children. Itinerant clinicians are in an individual school for less time than classroom teachers, guidance counselors, and other school personnel. Clinicians generally do not do bus duty, hall duty, cafeteria duty, and other such chores. The list of frequent distinctions between clinicians and teachers goes on. However, the beauty of working in the schools is that all educators are colleagues in the same bunker. All within the educational team seek to help children achieve their full potential. That is our mission. Nothing more; nothing less. Nevertheless, some teachers have expressed understandable resentment when itinerant clinicians assume that their time is in shorter supply and communicate that their instructional needs should take priority. How do we prevent acting or being perceived as elitist? We become an indistinguishable part of the educational team. We volunteer to do all the things that teachers do, even those that they get stuck with. I recommend that we volunteer to do bus duty, cafeteria duty, sit through faculty meetings, and chaperon school events, among others. I remember visiting and eating with teachers in the teachers' lounge. It is amazing what you can learn from and about teachers by just listening. I even contributed to the "sunshine fund," the kitty of money that was used to recognize significant events in teachers' lives (birthdays, weddings, anniversaries, births, deaths, and others). Even though I circulated to three schools, I enjoyed birthday cake as much as anyone else. More than that, I enjoyed being associated as a member of the educational team. I still maintain some of the friendships that were forged during my first position in the schools 20 years ago.

Since that time, I have held several positions. The most recent position in the schools was under contract with the university with which I was employed. In other words, while employed by a university, I established a speech–language–hearing program in a local school district, coordinated related services, and supervised the practicum experiences of student clinicians from the university. For these services, the university was reimbursed by the school for my time (two days per week). One day, I was approached by the principal, who invited me to chaperon the annual sixth grade trip to New York City. He explained that I was one of several teachers who were chosen both by students and teachers to go on this 3-day trip. Flattered as I was to be an indistinguishable part of the educational team, I responded, "Sure, I'd love to." It was not long before I remembered that the university was paying me to provide assessment and treatment services to the school, not walk the streets of the Big Apple. Anyway, the principal and superintendent officially made their request of my supervisor at the university. All agreed that if I were willing, the school's request of me would be supported and my time during those days would be spent on the school trip. To say the least, a fun time was had by all. I remember more than a little chagrin expressed by my senior colleagues at the university that I would be willing, no less interested, to engage in such an activity. My purpose in sharing this anecdote is to convey how important it is for clinicians to function as educational colleagues in the schools.

Provide Teachers with Strategies
To Facilitate Fluency in the Classroom

We noted earlier that teachers provide a pivotal role in helping children who stutter transfer and maintain the positive effects of treatment. Within an educational context in which all professional colleagues are equal, learn with and from each other, and strive to hold paramount the needs of all children, teachers and other educational personnel welcome and are receptive to our suggestions for facilitating fluency in the classroom. Teachers frequently ask questions such as, "When and under what conditions should a child who stutters be expected to recite in class?", "Should you talk with him about his speech or ignore it?", "What should you do if the other children laugh at or tease him?" (Williams, 1971, 1979). A few suggestions for teachers follow (Dell, 1979, 1993; Manning, 1996). Readers may wish to review the recommendations for additional reading and other resources found in Appendix B.

Advocate for all children, particularly a child who stutters

Advocating for a child means showing understanding, being available to the child, and rewarding what she or he recognizes as progress in behavioral or affective change (Manning, 1996). This advocacy, like that provided by the clinician, parents, and others, can powerfully reduce the potentially handicapping influence of stuttering. Teachers need to feel sincerely positive about the child who stutters and communicate that feeling to him and others. Negative reactions toward and discomfort about a child who stutters most likely reflects a lack of experience and understanding on the part of the teacher. Clinicians can help provide information and instructional materials to help teachers understand the nature and treatment of stuttering. By understanding and being a part of the intervention process, teachers are in a better position to help the child transfer and maintain the positive effects of treatment. Furthermore, the teacher more likely will have and communicate a positive attitude toward the child as an effective communicator who is working toward self-improvement.

Provide the child with more opportunity to speak on days when he is fluent, less when he is more disfluent

Stuttering, particularly in the early stages of development, tends to be cyclic. In other words, it comes and goes with long periods of remission. In fact, there is some evidence to indicate that early stuttering is situation or context specific. The child may be relatively fluent in most situations, but may be more disfluent on the playground, or in the lunchroom. As stuttering becomes more firmly established, the child demonstrates disfluency in an increasing number and variety of situations with increasing consistency (i.e., reduced intermittency). Therefore, while the intermittency is frustrating both to the child and to teachers, parents, and others around him, it is a positive indication of its incipiency.

By understanding the cyclic nature of stuttering, teachers can encourage the child's participation by calling on him more and providing more opportunities for him to speak on his fluent days. As discussed in the last chapter, providing opportunities for fluent talking experience helps the child remain positive about communication and the prospects for treatment (Dell, 1979). Conversely, the teacher may reduce the frequency of the child's participation by calling on other children first on days in which he is relatively disfluent. Manning (1996) noted that as teachers understand the effect of time pressure and other stimuli on stuttering, they may be inclined occasionally to call on a child unexpectedly or early in the class, when stuttering is less likely to occur. After being called on, the child can relax somewhat and be more attentive to classroom activities. Similarly, teachers may call on a child who stutters when the anticipated response is relatively short, particularly on those days when the child's fluency is more challenged. As always, an open, positive interaction between the child and his teacher is critical for building an understanding of what will or did happen and enabling the child to discuss his stuttering openly, thus receiving an avenue of ongoing encouragement and support.

Expect the child to participate in regular assignments, but provide flexibility and support when adjustments need to be made

Teachers frequently find themselves in a dilemma when considering how much verbal participation to expect from a child who stutters. Should a child who stutters be expected to recite a poem or book report or read aloud in front of the class or should the child be excluded to avoid embarrassment? Dell (1979) reviewed that there is no easy or clear-cut solution. On one hand, forcing a child who stutters to embarrass or humiliate himself seems unnecessary, if not unfair, yet granting special privileges (such as handing in a written report instead of doing an oral report, presenting to the teacher alone, or not doing the assignment) may result in teasing from the other children and a loss of confidence and self-respect. In other words, expecting a child with leg braces to run the 50-yard dash along with the other children and maintaining the same performance expectation and evaluation criteria seems inflexible, insensitive, and unresponsive to a child's unique strengths and limitations. There is no easy solution. One solution would be to talk with the child privately to discuss this dilemma, thereby conveying understanding and support. The teacher might inquire about how this challenging situation has been handled in previous classes and about the child's preferences. Similarly, the child's parents, clinician, and teachers might be involved in a meeting with the child present in order to problem solve together. Importantly, the teacher conveys her concern for the child's feelings and her commitment to understand and support the child. The discussion should be positive in nature, based on all of the child's significant abilities. All children have strengths and limitations. No pity or sympathy should be conveyed or tolerated. Just as some children need extra help in other areas (such as math, reading, eye sight, or physical activity), the teacher and others are interested in and supportive of discovering ways to ensure the child's continued success.

Furthermore, a variety of strategies might be considered. First, oral reading or presenting an oral report or recitation might be addressed directly with the clinician in the treatment setting first, thus enabling the child to use the classroom setting as an ultimate transfer context for fluency facilitating control. This experience might follow similar transfer activities conducted at home or among friends. Second, the clinician and child may design some instructional aids (e.g., an outline of topics distributed or projected to the class, charts, or tangible materials) that might direct the immediate attention away from the child, thus reducing the demand placed upon the child. Third, the child may engage in some audience participation, again to reduce the immediate demand at least momentarily. Fourth, we know that stuttering tends to reduce somewhat as audience size decreases, and to disappear when reading or speaking in chorus (in unison) with someone else. Therefore, teachers may consider having the children participate in group activity whereby each child may present to smaller groups of children. Similarly, teachers may consider having children recite or read orally in unison as appropriate, preparing the child to read in unison with groups of decreasing size and ultimately alone.

Manning (1996) acknowledged the importance of both preventing children who stutter from escaping school assignments and responsibilities and of making adjustments as indicated. Rather than excluding children from class presentations or plays, he suggested helping teachers understand that such children typically do not stutter when they play a role, speak with a dialect, or sing. Therefore, if children who stutter are reluctant to participate in a speaking part in presentations or plays, teachers may consider involving them in nonspeaking or nonverbal parts. Again, there are no simple solutions. Each strategy must reflect an understanding of the child's strengths and needs, expectations with the classroom context, and both sensitivity and creativity of the teacher. Most importantly, the strategy implemented will be jointly decided so that the child realizes the positive support he is being provided and thereby the burden is lessened by virtue of it being shared.

Shift perspective to see through the eyes of the child who stutters

When a teacher indicates not understanding stuttering or not knowing how to respond to a child who stutters, a reminder to shift perspective might help. For example, teachers often ask, "Should I fill in for a child when I know the word he is trying so hard to say?" or "Should I continue to look at the child when he is struggling so miserably? I don't want him to think I am staring." When seeing from the child's perspective, solutions might become more apparent. Generally, I recommend not filling in for the child, yet continuing to look at him as one would any other conversational partner. Filling in the word may seem expedient, helping the child in the short run. However, think about how the child will come to feel in the long run, knowing he failed and that the teacher had to talk for him (e.g., "I couldn't even say my own words. Ms. Brown had to say it for me"). Also, looking away again might seem expedient until one considers the child's perspective (e.g., "Was it that bad? Did I look so grotesque that the teacher couldn't bear to look at me any longer?"). Teachers should be encouraged to treat children who stutter as "normally" as possible. This means continuing to function as an active listener, conveying appropriate eye contact (although not a staring contest), and patiently waiting for the child to finish what he is saying. As with parents, teachers might be reminded by a child's disfluency to reward evidence of speech fluency and any indication of treatment progress, and to model and expand occasional words that the child spoke disfluently in slow, gentle, relaxed speech. It is important for children to feel that they have as much time as they need to express themselves and that their teacher is sincerely interested in what they have to say and confident in their ability to say it.

Provide all children, particularly those who stutter, regular support for their daily victories

Throughout this chapter, I have stressed the importance of serving as a resource for the classroom teacher. This means helping her understand the nature of stuttering and how to manage the child's communication in the classroom, and involving her within the treatment process. The more a teacher understands and contributes to the intervention process, the more a child stands to gain in transfer and maintenance of speech fluency. As discussed earlier, to help "teach" the teacher, the clinician must use the three Ds (discuss, demonstrate, direct/coach). Manning (1996) noted that as the teacher recognizes that a child is electing to participate in class despite his stuttering, the teacher may reward that event while it is occurring or after its completion, verbally or nonverbally. When a teacher is involved in the intervention process, she will know when and how to respond when a child adjusts his tense and fragmented speech into a more gentle, forward-flowing pattern. She also will recognize when he transfers a fluency facilitating technique (such as cancellation or pull-out) from the treatment setting to the classroom. Furthermore, the teacher will be pivotal in rewarding these events when they occur in other school settings such as the playground and lunchroom, among others. Importantly, when the teacher recognizes these seemingly small events as personal victories (Manning, 1996), indeed she will recognize and reward their occurrence, thus facilitating the intervention process and cementing the child's positive self-image.

Prevent singling out a child who stutters

In their attempt to protect a child who stutters, teachers may be inclined to speak to the class to build their understanding and acceptance of stuttering. This is not all bad, but must be handled with care. Consider the following statement of a teacher to her class: "We all know that Johnny tries as hard as the rest of us. We know that he stutters and therefore let's show him our undivided attention and patience." Such expressions may be well meaning, but invite ridicule from other children and embarrass the child who stutters and bring unnecessary attention to him. Cast differently, the teacher may do any of the following: First, establish classroom-wide rules against interruption. All children will have a chance to speak (to initiate or respond) without being rushed, but interruption will not be permitted. Secondly, demonstrate a pattern of active listening in which the teacher paraphrases or verbally confirms what each child has said so as to reward, clarify, and encourage the effort. This way, when such restatement follows the response of the child who stutters, he will not feel singled out. Furthermore, such a response is much more affirming than simply ignoring a stuttered response or reacting with silence, thus communicating that what was said by the child who stutters was unimportant. Paraphrasing and clarifying what children say is a valuable instructional tool for the classroom. Third, accept and positively reward the contributions of all children. The teacher should not look tense, uncomfortable, or alarmed when a child verbally contributes to the classroom activity, including those who stutter. Teachers need to be aware of the forms of feedback they provide, both verbal and nonverbal. Finally, address exceptionality as a topic of instruction.

Stuttering can be discussed as one of many exceptionalities. The children may talk about their interests and strengths and acknowledge the area or areas in which each is working toward self-improvement. Likewise, the child who stutters may talk about his strengths (e.g., he can run the 50-yard dash in 6.9 seconds, a school record) and interests (e.g., sports, photography, nature and wildlife), and indicate that his area of self-improvement is speech fluency. He might choose to share his speech-related objectives and how he is transferring his fluency skills to the classroom. Different school professionals may be invited to talk about exceptionality. For example, the speech–language pathologist may talk about stuttering in addition to other communication disorders; special educators may address learning exceptionalities; the nurse may address diseases, syndromes, and sensory impairments. In this day of heightened appreciation of human diversity, all efforts to build understanding, and thereby acceptance of each other, are consistent with our collective educational mission—to enable each person to become all he or she is capable of and to learn with and from each other in the process.

 ## Clinical Portrait: Thomas Wells

Selected Background Information

Tommy* was 9 years, 1 month old when he was referred by his parents and school-based speech–language pathologist for a communication evaluation because of "severe stuttering." Only Mrs. Wells accompanied Tommy to the evaluation and reported that, "His speech gets better and then worse. Now it is so bad that he gets mad, cries, and says, 'I can't talk. I'm choking.'" Reportedly, Tommy demonstrated average to early developmental milestones and unremarkable birth and medical history. Tommy's disfluency first was noticed when he was 3 years old. Its onset was gradual, without any significant co-occurring events. Having been told to "ignore it" and that "he would outgrow it," Mr. and Mrs. Wells did not seek professional advice until Tommy entered kindergarten. Since that time, he has been enrolled, dismissed, and subsequently re-enrolled in school-based intervention. Treatment had focused on a modified fluency shaping approach in which Tommy received a token for use of slow and gentle speech. The parents reported being informed of his progress but otherwise uninvolved. Tommy was an above-average student in the fourth grade who reportedly felt "singled out" because of having to leave class to go to the school clinician and because of teasing he was receiving. Tommy resided with one older brother and both parents. Family history for communication disorders was negative. Mrs. Wells was a teacher. Mr. Wells was a professor at a community college.

Abbreviated Speech–Language Analysis

Tommy's communication was analyzed from a variety of tasks including conversation, reading, structured and unstructured play activities, imitation of words and sentences, and responses to questions. Tommy's speech rate revealed an average of 98 fluent words per minute in conversation and 79 in reading, both significantly below average. Conversational speech ranged from 6% to 16% disfluency, averaging 14 disfluent words per 100 words spoken. Types of disfluency, based on samples of 100 words spoken, included part-word repetitions (sound or syllable repetitions, 47%), whole-word repetitions (6%), audible sound prolongations (20%),

---

*All clinical portrait names have been changed to protect confidentiality.

inaudible sound prolongations (13%), word and phrase interjections (10%), and word and phrase revisions (4%). Tommy spoke up to 20 fluent words between disfluencies. However, rhythm and phrasing were irregular. Part-word repetitions (e.g., luh–luh–luh–luh–like) contained up to 7 units of repetition per instance; whole-word repetition contained somewhat less (i.e., up to 3 units of repetition per instance). Audible and inaudible sound prolongation ranged from 2 to 17 seconds, the former containing pitch rise indicative of significant laryngeal tension, both containing rapid eye blinking, facial tension, and irregular, horizontal movement of the head. Interjections ranged from 1 to 6 units per instance; revisions were 1 unit per instance. Reading proved more difficult than conversation, as did repetition of longer words and sentences than shorter ones, and responses to questions that were longer and more complex than shorter and simpler ones. The only other secondary characteristic than those already noted was aversion of eye contact during disfluency. No disfluency was observed during song or choral speaking or choral reading. All other aspects of assessment (informal and standardized) revealed age appropriate speech (articulation and phonology) and language (semantics, syntax, pragmatics). All parameters of voice (except the instances of laryngeal tension noted) and hearing were within normal limits. Tommy's response to trial management combining fluency shaping and stuttering modification during the evaluation was favorable, if not dramatic. Tommy candidly discussed his feelings and frustration about stuttering and significantly reduced the relative frequency and severity of his disfluency.

Recommendations and Objectives

Based on the results of the evaluation, the positive influence of trial management, and the ready support of his family, Tommy was recommended to receive direct intervention for 1 hour per week. The objectives were as follows:

- To heighten Tommy's awareness of his fluent speech.

- To increase the frequency of Tommy's fluent speech.

- To establish fluency facilitating control during instances of disfluency.

- To transfer fluency facilitating techniques to extraclinical settings and to maintain the effects of treatment.

- To heighten Tommy's understanding and thereby acceptance of himself as an effective communicator.

- To invite, encourage, and expect Tommy (i.e., and his parents) to participate actively in all aspects of the treatment process (including planning clinical and extraclinical activities, implementing activities, evaluating effectiveness of procedures, and follow-up and revision, as appropriate).

- To provide a forum for candid, supportive dialogue and shared problem solving.

Treatment Snapshot

Treatment began by establishing a social, human connection between Tommy and the clinician. The clinician learned that Tommy was an avid coin collector, photographer, swimmer, and biker. To Tommy's surprise, the clinician then invited Tommy to share what he hoped to accomplish as a result of the intervention process, during which the clinician listened and took notes about Tommy's ideas and verbally rewarded Tommy for his many instances of gentle fluency. At one point, Tommy broke out into an awkward laughter. The clinician inquired, "What's so funny?" noticing that Tommy's eyes were watering with emotion. Tommy explained, "No one ever asked me what I wanted to do. I was always told what I was going to do. They think we're just dumb kids. And I thought you were going to correct my stuttering, not tell me I was doing great." This gave the clinician an opportunity to explain the nature and process of treatment. "In other words," the clinician explained, "you're going to learn first that most of your speech is fluent. And there seems to be no reason why you can't, with my help and a lot of work, learn to do more of what you already are doing when you are fluent. You will see that being fluent and disfluent aren't things that happen TO you, but are results of things you DO differently." "You mean, I CAN be fluent?" Tommy asked. "Why not? While I cannot promise, we learn to do lots of things by setting our mind to it. We learn to ride a bike. We learn to swim. We learn to use a camera. Why can't we learn to speak just as fluently as you do even more often?" the clinician responded. Tommy continued, "You're saying that I have a choice? I can be fluent or disfluent?" "That's a big part of it," the clinician added, "You'll see."

The clinician explained that because most of Tommy's speech was fluent, fluency seemed like a good place to start. Indeed, because Tommy's conversational speech ranged from 84% to 94% fluency, why not first work to increase Tommy's control over his fluent speech, thereby increasing its frequency? Rather than direct him NOT to blink, NOT to repeat, NOT to interject, and so forth, this strategy provided Tommy guidance in what he CAN DO, and what he CAN DO MORE OFTEN. This presented a positive, optimistic, empowering foundation. By doing so, Tommy increasingly took control over his speech by adopting foci (such as slowness and gentleness) that have a pervasive effect on his communication. Within such a positive foundation, remaining disfluencies then were addressed directly (e.g., "Hey, wait a minute! What happened there?"). The focus was on what Tommy CAN DO, rather than on what he CANNOT DO. Using these procedures and others discussed in this chapter, most of the major forms of disfluency virtually disappeared.

To establish a slow, gentle speech model, the clinician engaged Tommy in a choral reading exercise, during which the clinician faded her speech volume, but returned before Tommy became disfluent. Again, Tommy laughed with delight. Initial treatment activities were used to design speaking hierarchies and to describe narrowly the fluent experience. Assignments were designed to be completed at home on a daily basis, following the procedures used in treatment. At first Tommy focused on what it felt like to be fluent when talking to his dog (the lowest or easiest end of one hierarchy), and reported in a little speech notebook one fluent word he spoke in the morning and one in the afternoon (specifically, the word, perceptual and proprioceptive feedback, and the surrounding circumstances). These activities continued up the hierarchy of perceived difficulty and increased in frequency and performance expectation.

One activity that Tommy particularly enjoyed was role-playing an announcer for a swimming competition. A videotape-recorded swim meet was played with the volume turned off. Tommy sportscasted the event, demonstrating his use of fluency facilitating control and his knowledge of swimming. One day, the clinician videotape-recorded Tommy in the role of the sportscaster, so that the two could review and critique it, particularly attending to the speech fluency that was maintained as the rate of speech increased (toward the end of the meet).

Tommy's mother was involved in the last quarter of every 1-hour treatment session. His father attended less regularly, but was involved nevertheless. At each session, Tommy explained to his mother what he had accomplished. The clinician helped Tommy keep the discussion focused on his successes and maintain a positive attitude about successes he was yet to achieve. On infrequent occasions, Tommy's brother, special friends, teacher, and school speech–language pathologist (with whom Tommy continued to receive treatment, with the clinician's support provided) attended the sessions. In general, discussions addressed Tommy's successes and the importance of providing praise for Tommy's fluent speech and ongoing models and expansions using slow, gentle speech. Tommy's behaviors, feelings, and thoughts were addressed directly, as were those of the other participants.

Tommy demonstrated increased fluency and successful use of fluency facilitating controls inside and outside of the clinical room. He reported feeling more in control of his speech as well as experiencing more enjoyment of the communication experience. At the top of his hierarchy, Tommy successfully used his controls when speaking to the class, to the principal, and when on the phone. His teachers reported marked increase in his willingness to participate and the speech fluency with which he did so. His parents reported that the recommendations provided enabled them to feel that they could actually support his communication needs, resulting in his increased fluency at home and away with family and friends. Others reported to the parents and teachers having noticed Tommy's significant improvement.

Follow-Up and Epilogue

Treatment continued for less than 2 years. During the latter stages, frequency of direct treatment was reduced steadily, requiring increased vigilance on Tommy's part to transfer and maintain fluency. Tommy's fluency facilitating techniques were challenged deliberately by the clinician in the treatment setting, and by his parents, teachers, and the clinician in the home and school settings. Eventually, Tommy was dismissed with an explicit welcome to return anytime.

Follow-up continued for 2 years after treatment concluded. Tommy's rate of speech in conversation and reading had stabilized between 150 and 160 fluent words per minute. His frequency of disfluency remained no greater than 1% (one disfluent word per 100 words spoken). Tommy reliably adjusted his oral posture to facilitate fluency before the block occurred (preparatory sets), although occasionally he needed to perform the adjustment while the block was occurring (pull-outs). The only remaining disfluency, therefore, was gentle prolongation of fleeting nature, lasting no greater than 1 second. These behavioral data, combined with self-reports indicating positive feelings and thoughts about himself as a person and as a communicator, and reports from parents, teachers, and friends of maintained fluency success all revealed significant and maintained fluency progress.

Central and Guiding Intervention Assumptions

Again, let's briefly return to the assumptions that are central to designing and critiquing intervention. These are the intrafamily (personal constructs, family systems), extrafamily (interdisciplinary teaming and multicultural awareness), and psychotherapeutic (fluency shaping and stuttering modification) considerations.

Intrafamily Considerations

Feelings of isolation and negativity brought on by his stuttering were beginning to influence Tommy's personal construct of himself (as a person and as a communicator). That Tommy remained conversant about such feelings, however, was a positive prognostic indicator that his feelings still were in evolution. Treatment was designed from a positive perspective, accentuating Tommy's understanding of and control over his fluent speech. This control and internalized experience of success then was applied to his disfluent speech. Tommy learned and insightfully expressed that fluency and disfluency both were consequences of his actions, a realization which provided Tommy a deliberate and responsible choice. Tommy's family was consistently supportive, adjusting aspects of their interaction and discipline to cast Tommy and his older brother in a positive and constructive light. The parents were welcoming of support and constructive suggestions, even when these necessitated behavioral and attitudinal change on their part. They willingly shifted their assumed posture from the clinician in absentia (i.e., correcting and charting Tommy's disfluency, and reminding him to do his speech homework) to Tommy's advocate at home, thereby praising him for his frequent use of gentle speech and self-corrections; providing ongoing models of slow, gentle speech; offering correction only by example (demonstrating models and expansions of words on which Tommy was disfluent, rather than telling him what to do); and identifying and eliminating sources of interruption and time pressure. Most importantly, the family members were supportive of Tommy's strengths and needs and rallied to participate in and support each other through the intervention process. The parents and brother were as candid in expressing feelings of uncertainty as they were in receiving praise and constructive suggestions.

Extrafamily Considerations

The teacher and other school personnel were key figures in helping Tommy transfer and maintain his speech fluency. Specifically, the classroom teacher, specialty teachers (of physical education, art, and music), school-based speech–language pathologist, and principal, among others, understood what Tommy was trying to accomplish and were active on the treatment team, contributing meaningfully to the decisions within the intervention process. These school personnel also felt relatively comfortable in responding to Tommy and adjusting to meet his needs. Significantly, all members communicated regularly among each other, thus feeling involved, informed, and supported in helping meet Tommy's needs, while also feeling valued for possessing unique areas of expertise and for handling multiple, and occasionally conflicting, responsibilities. The most significant multicultural (i.e., diversity) consideration was Tommy's age and stage of development. All participants in the intervention process acknowledged Tommy as a person whose thoughts, feelings, and behaviors as a communicator were evolving. Other factors of diversity addressed or acknowledged during intervention were the professions held by Tommy's parents, and the unique interests of Tommy and his family, which were discussed and valued during the treatment process.

Psychotherapeutic Considerations

Tommy's feelings as a person and as a communicator were becoming negatively influenced by the experience of stuttering. Therefore, in order to help Tommy preserve his personal construct, treatment combined fluency shaping and stuttering modification techniques. Tommy was provided opportunities to gain control over his fluency and thereby generalize these methods to instances of disfluency (fluency shaping), while participating actively in all aspects of the treatment process, discussing his thoughts and feelings about communication and himself as a communicator, and becoming increasingly responsible to function as his own clinician (i.e., stuttering modification). Significantly, the people in Tommy's communication system (including parents, teachers, and friends) all participated in planning, implementing, and evaluating the treatment process, all with Tommy's communication-related behaviors, thoughts, and feelings in mind. Tommy became empowered to realize that fluency and disfluency each represented active and deliberate choices available to him. Perfection was never a goal. Rather, Tommy set out to achieve as much control over his communication skills as he could, treating his errors (disfluency, temporary communication-related setbacks) as constructive stepping stones to learning. Within this positive, constructive, and integrated communication system, Tommy achieved significant gains that have been maintained over the test of time and life experience.

CHAPTER SUMMARY

This chapter presented a variety of strategies for assessing and treating school-age children who stutter. First, each child who stutters must understand the nature of his own speech fluency and be in control of it before effecting reduction in disfluency. Second, clinicians must manage not only characteristics of speech fluency, but also what the child thinks and feels about communication and himself as a communicator. Third, effective assessment and treatment require that the clinician understand the child's communication environment and that the child, his family, and others participate actively in all aspects of treatment planning, implementation, evaluation, and follow-up.

School-age children who stutter typically have been doing so for some time. They are developing independence from their parents, while spending more time with children and adults outside of their family structure. Furthermore, school-age children are becoming increasingly dependent on their peers and influenced by school personnel, yet frequently are reluctant or unable to verbalize internal feelings and lack insight to analyze a problem objectively in order to establish alternative solutions. Based on these observations, the potential influence of a speech–language pathologist on school-age children who stutter is profound.

Preassessment procedures include completing a case history form, obtaining and reviewing an audio- or videotape-recording of the child, and making a preliminary phone call to or contact with the parents, teachers, and others. Assessment procedures include a parent interview, teacher interview, child interview, and trial management. The parent and teacher interviews are conversational exchanges of information in order to understand the child in a variety of communication settings. Because of potential schedule conflicts during the school day, these meetings often are held before or after regular working hours. The child interview is an opportunity for the clinician to convey her sincere interest in the child as a multifaceted person, not just as one who stutters. The interactions with the child enable the clinician to observe directly the child's speech fluency and disfluency and the extent to which his speech is modifiable, and to gain a better understanding of the child's thoughts, feelings, and attitudes that may relate to his stuttering. The child interview contains speech–language sampling and a variety of structured activities with and without communicative pressure. The clinician uses different forms of fluency shaping and stuttering modification treatment during trial management in order to determine their relative effectiveness with the particular child. Post-assessment procedures for school-age children include a thorough analysis of speech and language skills. This analysis leads to determination of diagnosis, prognosis, and recommendations, all of which are summarized in subsequent meetings with the child, parents, and teachers. Speech analyses for school-age children are similar to those reviewed in the last chapter, including the frequency, types, molecular description, rate, secondary characteristics, severity, and adaptation and consistency of the child's speech disfluency. The diagnosis integrates all of the information available to determine the nature of the child's speech fluency and disfluency and whether or not treatment is warranted and recommended. If intervention is indicated, the clinician estimates the child's prognosis for improvement within a proposed course of treatment. Treatment recommendations vary with each child, particularly with respect to intrafamily, extrafamily, and psychotherapeutic considerations, and are discussed with all parties involved.

Treatment goals for school-age children who stutter are spontaneous or controlled fluency, as well as establishment or maintenance of a positive attitude toward communication and oneself as communicator. Specific and comprehensive treatment strategies were presented, discussed, and applied for the purpose of achieving four objectives: (a) establishing or increasing and transferring fluent speech, (b) developing resistance to potential fluency disrupters, (c) establishing or maintaining positive feelings about communication and oneself as a communicator, and (d) maintaining the fluency-inducing effects of treatment on communication-related behaviors, thoughts, feelings, and attitudes. Increasing and transferring fluent speech involves constructing a "safe house," inviting treatment objectives from the child, creating opportunities for the child to experience fluency success, heightening the child's awareness of his speech fluency, developing or improving use of fluency facilitating controls during instances of stuttering, and transferring fluency facilitating controls to extraclinical settings. Developing resistance to potential fluency disrupters involves engaging the child in activities with gradually increasing degrees of competition, reintroducing direct fluency challenge, addressing the situations on the top rung of the child's communication hierarchy, and preparing for relapse (Relapse happens!). Establishing or maintaining positive feelings about communication and oneself as a communicator involves preparing the child for the likelihood of being teased and empowering him with constructive strategies to use during such times, helping the child maintain positive thinking about communication and himself as a communicator, and talking with the child in positive ways. Finally, maintaining the fluency-inducing effects of treatment requires helping the child become his own clinician, decreasing the frequency of scheduled treatment, implementing regular maintenance checks of decreasing frequency for at least 2 years post-treatment, building in regular child-initiated benchmarking, deliberately revisiting the past, reexamining the child's personal constructs, and integrating treatment changes within the communication system.

Other suggestions were provided for working with children who stutter and have concomitant language or phonological impairment, and for working with parents and teachers. Working with children who stutter and have other concomitant communication impairments requires that clinicians understand the effects of concomitant disorders; address the questions of, "To treat or not to treat?" and "If yes, then where do I begin?"; and decide between sequential, concurrent, and blended approaches. Working effectively with parents involves access to parents, respecting the primary role of parents, and meeting parents' needs. Working effectively with teachers and other school personnel requires building rapport and establishing colleagueship, banishing elitism, and providing teachers with strategies to facilitate fluency in the classroom. Such strategies include: (a) advocating for all children, (b) providing the child who stutters with more opportunity to speak on days when he is fluent and less when he is disfluent, (c) expecting the child to participate in regular assignments but providing flexibility and support when adjustments need to be made, (d) shifting perspective to see through the eyes of the child who stutters, (e) providing all children regular support for their daily victories, and (f) preventing a child who stutters from being singled out.

The chapter ended with a clinical portrait of Tommy Wells, a 9-year-old boy, in order to apply and discuss the assessment and treatment suggestions in addition to intrafamily, extrafamily, and psychotherapeutic intervention considerations. In doing so, we discussed selected background information, an abbreviated speech–language analysis, recommendations and objectives, a snapshot of treatment, and a follow-up and epilogue.

Chapter 9 Study Questions

1. This chapter began with a review of general precepts about school-age children who stutter. How might the factors reviewed impact the clinical process involving the child, parents, teachers, and others?

2. We discussed preassessment, assessment, and post-assessment procedures primarily as conversational exchanges of information for a variety of purposes. What is the significance of using the medium of conversation, and how does that medium impact the process and products of assessment?

3. Assessment and treatment of school-age children who stutter are multidimensional and dynamic processes. How do the processes relate to and impact each other? In working with school-age children who stutter, what are the demarcations of assessment and treatment? In what ways might assessment continue into treatment? How is treatment begun during the period of initial assessment? What do you feel are the necessary tasks and competencies for effective assessment and treatment?

4. We have addressed the significant impact of intrafamily, extrafamily, and psychotherapeutic considerations on the intervention process. How do these factors affect assessment and treatment with school-age children who stutter? What similarities and differences are there in the influence of these factors on intervention with school-age children compared to preschool children?

5. Clinicians must be aware of a number of considerations when working with school-age children who stutter and have concomitant language or phonological impairment. What do you believe are the critical issues to be addressed in assessing and treating such children? How can what we know about the trading relationship between components of communication be used to the child's advantage in designing intervention?

6. Many strategies were reviewed for working effectively with parents and teachers. What do you feel are the most critical ingredients for effective clinical interaction with these people? What might parents and teachers hold to be the most important elements of effective interaction with speech–language pathologists? How will the knowledge you gained from this and previous chapters impact your interactions with parents and teachers? How will this knowledge influence the design and implementation of workshops you will present for these audiences?

Unit III

◆ ◆ ◆ ◆ ◆ ◆ ◆ ◆ ◆ ◆ ◆ ◆ ◆ ◆ ◆ ◆ ◆ ◆ ◆

Assessment and Treatment Strategies with People Who Stutter: A Life Span Perspective

Chapter 8

Preschool Children: Assessment and Treatment

Chapter 9

School-Age Children Who Stutter: Assessment and Treatment

Chapter 10

Adolescents, Adults, and Senior Adults Who Stutter: Assessment and Treatment

Chapter 10

Adolescents, Adults, and Senior Adults Who Stutter: Assessment and Treatment

◆ ◆ ◆ ◆ ◆ ◆ ◆ ◆ ◆ ◆ ◆ ◆ ◆ ◆ ◆ ◆ ◆ ◆ ◆

General Precepts About Adolescents, Adults, and Senior Adults Who Stutter   367

Precepts Common Across These Three Groups   368

Precepts About Adolescents   368

Precepts About Adults   370

Precepts About Senior Adults   371

Preassessment Procedures   375

Case History Form, Audio- or Videotape Recording, Preliminary Phone Call   375

Preassessment Conference   376

Assessment Procedures   382

General Considerations   382

Client and Family Interview   383

Preparation   383

Social Greeting   383

Questions and Dialogue   384

Speech–Language Sample Without Communicative Pressure   387

Structured Activities Without Communicative Pressure   389

Speech–Language Sample and Structured Activities with Communicative Pressure   391

Trial Management   392

Fluency Shaping   392

Stuttering Modification   393

Post-Assessment Procedures   394

Speech Analysis   395

Frequency of Speech Disfluency (i.e., Disfluency Frequency Index, DFI)   395

Type of Speech Disfluency (i.e., Disfluency Type Index, DTI)   395

Molecular Description of Disfluency   395

Rate of Speech   395

Secondary Characteristics   396

Severity Rating   396

Adaptation and Consistency   396

Feelings and Attitudes   396

Other   396

Diagnosis   397

Prognosis and Recommendations   397
  Prognostic Musings   397
  Prognostic Indicators with Adolescents, Adults, and Senior Adults   399
  A Prognostic Caveat—Chronic Perseverative Stuttering Syndrome   402
  Recommendations   405
Post-Assessment Interview   405

Treatment   407
  Goals   407
  Objectives   407
  Rationale   408
    Intrafamily Considerations   408
    Extrafamily Considerations   409
    Psychotherapeutic Considerations   410
  Procedures   410
    Increase and Transfer Fluent Speech   411
      Establish the treatment setting as a "safe house" where clients and clinicians
        learn with and from each other and, as a consequence, grow together   411
      Invite treatment objectives from the client   412
      Create opportunities for the client to experience fluency success   412
      Heighten the client's awareness of his speech fluency; Make the client's
        speech fluency (i.e., and only then, disfluency) the object of study   414
      Develop or improve use of fluency facilitating techniques during instances of stuttering   415
      Address thoughts, feelings, and attitudes directly   416
      Transfer fluency facilitating techniques to extraclinical settings   417
    Develop Resistance to Potential Fluency Disrupters   417
      Introduce direct fluency challenge   418
      Revisit and advance toward the top rung of communication hierarchies   418
      Prepare for relapse: Relapse happens!   418
    Establish or Maintain Positive Thoughts and Feelings About Communication
      and Oneself as a Communicator   420
      Treat teasing and relapse as probabilities rather than possibilities; Empower clients
        with constructive strategies to withstand the potential ill effects of teasing and relapse   421
      Help clients maintain positive thinking about communication and
        themselves as communicators   422
      Talk with clients in positive ways; Help clients understand
        how they speak, think, and feel about themselves   424
    Maintain the Fluency-Inducing Effects of Treatment   424
      Help the client become his own clinician   424
      Decrease the frequency of scheduled treatment   425
      Maintain regular maintenance checks of decreasing frequency
        for at least 2 years post-treatment   425
      Institute regular, client-initiated benchmarking   426
      Deliberately revisit the past   426
      Reexamine the client's personal construct; Be sure the changes
        are integrated into the client's personal construct   427
      Integrate treatment changes within the communication system   431
      Respect the primary role of the conversational partners and help support their needs   432

Clinical Portrait: Bill Rice   434

>   Selected Background Information   434

>   Abbreviated Speech–Language Analysis   434

>>   Conversation   434

>>   Reading   435

>>   Word/Sentence Repetition   435

>>   Other   435

>   Trial Management   435

>   Recommendations, Goals, and Objectives   436

>>   Recommendations   436

>>   Goals   436

>>   Rationale and Procedural Approach to Goals   437

>>   Objectives   437

>>   Rationale and Procedural Approach to Objectives   438

>   Treatment Snapshot   438

>   Follow-Up and Epilogue   440

>   Central and Guiding Intervention Assumptions   441

>>   Intrafamily Considerations   441

>>   Extrafamily Considerations   441

>>   Psychotherapeutic Considerations   442

Chapter Summary   442

Chapter 10 Study Questions   445

I have been a stutterer since I was five years old. I am now 61 years of age. Although I have learned to live with it, I would like very much to be cured. I have retired from the city of Asheville after 36 years of service. My children are all grown and on their own. So I feel that now I could give this problem my full time. It would the greatest thing in the world to be able to talk fluently. Do you think it would be possible to talk with you about this problem?

(FROM A CLIENT'S LETTER OF INITIAL CONTACT.
This man achieved controlled fluency after 2 years of treatment. Presently, he orders for his
wife in restaurants, introduces himself on the golf course, and lay reads in church,
the three most challenging yet appealing objectives he set for himself.)

The previous two chapters addressed preschool children and school-age children who stutter. Specifically, we looked at general precepts of these children, assessment and treatment strategies and related considerations, and descriptive clinical portraits. The present chapter, which concludes Unit III, uses a similar format to study adults who stutter. Specifically, we will consider what it means to be an adolescent, adult, or senior adult; how to assess the communication of an adult who stutters; and how to design and implement treatment with such individuals. We will consider how stuttering impacts the behaviors, thoughts, and feelings of adults who stutter, and will conclude with a clinical portrait of one man's intervention experience. In doing so, we will make the following points, among others:

- Adults who stutter must understand, be in control of, and thereby increase their speech fluency before they can effectively reduce their disfluency.

- Clinicians must help adults who stutter manage not only the behavioral aspects of stuttering, but the more central thoughts and feelings about communication and themselves as communicators as well.

- Effective intervention must consider and be responsive to intrafamily (personal constructs and family systems), extrafamily (interdisciplinary teaming and multicultural awareness), and psychotherapeutic (fluency shaping and stuttering modification) factors.

- Change is realistic, desirable, and possible at any age across the life span.

- Intervention with senior adults who stutter is a positive, inviting, and enlightening opportunity.

GENERAL PRECEPTS ABOUT ADOLESCENTS, ADULTS, AND SENIOR ADULTS WHO STUTTER

This section addresses what it means to be an adolescent, an adult, or a senior adult. We will entertain commonalities first before addressing each group separately. As always, such patterns represent group trends and may or may not relate to a particular individual who stutters.

Precepts Common Across These Three Groups

• *Typically, adolescents, adults, and senior adults who stutter have been doing so for a number of years.* This is a logical conclusion based on observations such as those of Andrews (1984) who indicated, "Most children begin to stutter before they are of school age and virtually none, unless they become brain damaged, begin after puberty" (p. 11).

• *The stuttering behaviors, thoughts, and feelings tend to increase in complexity the longer one stutters.* However, there are many adults whose stuttering symptoms are described by both the speaker and listeners as "mild." Nevertheless, Peters and Guitar (1991) described the "advanced stutterer" as follows:

> The advanced stutterer . . . will be either an adult or high school student. In terms of core behaviors, he will exhibit any of the following: part-word repetitions that contain excessive tension, vowel prolongations that have excessive tension, and blocks. In terms of secondary behaviors, he may exhibit escape behaviors, starting behaviors, postponements, word avoidances, and situation avoidances. The advanced stutterer will evidence frustration, embarrassment, and fear relative to his stuttering. Finally, he will have a definite self-concept of himself as a stutterer. (pp. 215–216)

• *Age of the stuttering is thought to be more significant prognostically than age of the person who stutters* (Conture, 1990b; Daly, Simon, & Burnett-Stolnack, 1995). This means that the older the stuttering (the longer one's history of stuttering), the less favorable the treatment prognosis. However, I will argue later that this often is not the case. We will discuss significant communication improvements experienced by adults and senior adults who, for the first time in many years, are able to focus on themselves, their communication, and self-improvement. As a consequence, there apparently is no externally imposed limit to their potential progress including establishment, transfer, and maintenance. The extent to which they wish to progress (and implicitly, the extent to which they are willing to invest in the process of self-improvement) is individually defined and, indeed, an active and constructive choice.

• *People who stutter, particularly those who have lived the longest, have stories to tell.* Stories and dialogue provide a real (i.e., not artificial) and meaningful (i.e., ecologically valid) context for human interaction that promotes through modeling the very communication skills we are trying to establish with adults who stutter (Shapiro, in press). Conversation, therefore, provides an ideal context for clinical interaction and for all participants to learn with and from each other.

Precepts About Adolescents

• *Adolescence is the period of transition between childhood and adulthood.* This transition and others that characterize the life cycle were discussed in

Chapter 5. Adolescence theoretically begins with the physical and emotional changes accompanying puberty, and ends when the adolescent becomes more independent and self-sufficient, typically leaving home or starting a career. Adolescents no longer consider themselves to be children, yet may recognize that they are not quite adults (Schwartz, 1993). Conture (1990b) noted that adolescents' mood swings and struggle with independence are similar to an approach–avoidance conflict (Sheehan, 1958, 1970, 1975). One minute adolescents want freedom and disassociation from parents, while seemingly in the next minute they are asking for their parents' advice and support. Similarly, they seem to want the freedoms and privileges of adulthood while occasionally refusing the responsibilities that come with them. Just as adolescents are challenged to group themselves as children or adults, so are speech–language pathologists who have grouped adolescents who stutter with older children (Conture, 1990b) and with adults (Peters and Guitar, 1991) when considering intervention.

• *Adolescents have been classified on the bases of both the age of one's stuttering (the amount of time an individual has experienced stuttering) and one's chronological age* (Schwartz, 1993). For example, by referring to "advanced stutterers" and grouping adolescents with adults who stutter, Peters & Guitar (1991) used the amount of time individuals have stuttered as a basis of classification. In grouping adolescents with older children, Conture (1990b) distinguished between children and adults, thus suggesting adolescence as a transition between childhood and early adulthood. Discussing these observations, Schwartz (1993) suggested that we view adolescence as representing characteristics of both younger children and adults, and as a series of transitions from "early adolescence" to "later adolescence." Others have classified adolescents who stutter on the basis of chronological age. Bloodstein (1995) classified younger adolescents (late elementary school and junior high school) in Phase 3 in the progression of stuttering development, and older adolescents (high school and beyond) and adults in Phase 4.

• *Adolescence, with or without stuttering, is a confusing period for an individual and his family* (Andrews & Andrews, 1990; Schwartz, 1993). I remember vividly the moment when I realized just how difficult it was going to be to raise a set of parents—my own. The changes experienced and pressures perceived by adolescents are significant and real. These include rapid physical growth, sexual maturity, conflicts between dependence and independence, development of self-confidence and interpersonal skills, search for personal identity and ultimate meaning, group loyalty, and career choices (Haynes et al., 1992). For these and other reasons, adolescents often are overloaded with personal concerns and therefore do not always welcome clinical intervention. Daly et al. (1995) discussed the difficulties in getting adolescents to commit to the intervention process, and recalled Manning's (1991) recommendation that a clinician who successfully convinces a teenager who stutters to enroll in fluency intervention should receive a large bonus.

• *Adolescents often demonstrate a strong desire to be like and liked by others, and not to appear in any way to be frail or insecure.* Revealing that one stutters, even if help is needed and desired, may be perceived by the adolescent as such an indication of frailty. Indeed, Conture (1990b) cautioned that the last thing teenagers may want is to touch, see, feel, and discuss their speech, the very thing that is bothering them most and the expressed objective of the speech–language pathologist. Some adolescents have been sent for intervention without their consent; others may be growing weary of continued treatment. Some will mask their true feelings with a "No big deal" appearance or message, concealing their feelings, thoughts, and attitudes. Discussing these observations, Haynes et al. (1992) recommended a straightforward approach whereby the clinician acknowledges the pressures on the individual, discusses the successes experienced by others, and addresses the academic, social, and economic penalties that result from communication impairments such as stuttering.

• *While occasionally appearing stalwart and confident to a fault, adolescents are remarkably vulnerable.* We will discuss again the importance of building meaningful rapport where the clinician and client are sincerely interested in each other as people; where the treatment room is a safe house; where the client feels free and without penalty to express himself; and where the clinician is herself, offering sincerity, confidentiality, personal commitment, ongoing positive regard, and deliberate opportunities for systematic fluency success. Haynes et al. (1992) advised clinicians to explain the assessment and treatment processes thoroughly, to encourage questions, to listen without judgment to criticisms of parents or school officials, and to discuss the results of intervention with the adolescent who stutters before talking with the parents or school personnel.

Precepts About Adults

• *Distinguishing between the end of adolescence and the beginning of adulthood is an inexact science at best.* Adulthood begins when the individual becomes relatively independent and self-sufficient, typically coinciding in mainstream United States with leaving home or starting a career. We discussed in Chapter 5, however, how other cultures often do not separate emotionally or geographically. For our discussion, adulthood will be assumed to represent the working and/or parenting years, the end of which signifies the beginning of senior adulthood. In other words, adulthood is assumed to begin approximately between 18 and 21 years of age and end between 55 and 65 years of age.

• *Stuttering is thought to be fully developed in adulthood* (Haynes et al., 1992; Manning, 1996; Peters & Guitar, 1991). Cooper and Cooper (1995), however, reported that for many people who stutter, adolescence and adulthood represent "the beginning of a decline in the severity and significance of the disorder" (p. 125). Others have indicated that it is not known for certain whether people who stutter become more or less disfluent as they age (Bloodstein, 1995; Manning & Shirkey, 1981; Rosenfield & Nudelman, 1991). Nevertheless, Haynes et al. (1992) represented stuttering in adulthood as follows:

> Speech interruptions are more complex and characteristically compulsive; fears and apprehensions become chronic; avoidance, disguise, and negative attitudes hamper and distort the individual's relationships with others. At this stage, a speech breakdown is not simply a response, it is also a stimulus—the problem has become cyclic and self-reinforcing. Clinicians agree that the treatment of stuttering at this advanced stage is complicated—but far from impossible. (p. 222)

Precepts About Senior Adults

• *General Definition:* For this discussion, senior adulthood will refer to those years after one has completed his or her career, when the adult children are grown and on their own. We think of this period as beginning roughly between 55 and 65 years of age. In Chapter 5, we referred to this period as one of review and integration in which we see shifting generational roles, maintaining one's own and the couple's functioning and interests during physiological decline, exploring new family and social role options, supporting the more central role for the middle generation, making room in the system for the needs and wisdom of the older generation, preparing for and dealing with the loss of a spouse, siblings, and peers, and preparing for one's own death.

• *Age:* Senior adulthood is a time of aging and later development. The "graying of America" refers to the increase in the elderly population, particularly those 85 and older. In the United States, people 65 years and older constitute the fastest growing segment of the population. Representing only 4% of the population in 1900, people 65 years and older today represent over 12% and are projected to represent 22% of the population by the year 2030. In other words, between 1990 and 2030, the population of people aged 65 and over will double, from 32.2 million to 64.4 million (MacNeil & Teague, 1987; Myers & Schwiebert, 1996; Rakowski & Pearlman, 1995). This population has been characterized as representing three different stages, namely the young-old (age 65–74), middle-old (75–84), and old-old (85 and over) (Hartke, 1991; MacNeil & Teague, 1987; Rakowski & Pearlman, 1995; Scheuerle, 1992). The "oldest old," those 85 years and over, represent the fastest growing segment of all. In 1990, people 85 years and older represented 1% of the total population and 12.6% of the over-65 population; by 2030 they will represent 5% of the total population and 22% of the over-65 population (Rakowski & Pearlman, 1995).

• *Race and Ethnicity:* People 65 years and older represent a particularly diverse and heterogeneous group. While nationally about 86% of people over 65 years are White, the minority population of elderly is growing faster than Whites. This more rapid growth of the Nonwhite elderly population is projected to continue from a present percentage of 14% to 20% by 2010, and is partially attributable to higher fertility rates among African American and Hispanic populations relative to Caucasians. In other words, between 1990 and 2030, the population of Caucasians over 65 years old will grow 92%, compared with 247% for older African Americans and 395% for older Hispanics. Nevertheless, the proportion of Caucasians over 65 years old compared to those of other races will continue to be higher because African Americans and other minorities continue to die more frequently than Caucasians from illness and disability. Such higher morbidity and mortality among African Americans reflect longitudinal disparity in education, employment, and income, all of which limits access to and use of health care (Rakowski & Pearlman, 1995). Rakowski and Pearlman (1995) added that by age 75 years, mortality rates are lower for African Americans than for Caucasians. They explained as follows:

> Black Americans who survive middle age may have better coping resources or even a hardier and more resilient biology in later life than whites. Blacks who survive to old age appear to have informal sources of support within their

families and communities that help them cope better than whites with stressful health situations. (p. 489)

• *Sex:* Chances of surviving to senior adulthood are related to a person's sex. In 1995, life expectancy at birth was 72 years for men and 79 years for women. By 2030, life expectancy should increase 3.4 years for men and 3.3 years for women. The gender gap in life expectancy shrinks somewhat once people reach the age of 65 years. Men who turn 65 can expect to live another 15 years; women can expect an additional 19.4 years. Because of longer survival rates among women, the population of the "oldest old" primarily is female. For example, in 1989, the ratio of people between 65 and 69 years was 84 men to 100 women; those over 85 years old were 39 men to 100 women (Rakowski & Pearlman, 1995). Similarly, most older men (75%) remain married until they die, while nearly half (49%) of women over 65 years are widowed (MacNeil & Teague, 1987; Myers & Schwiebert, 1996; Rakowski & Pearlman, 1995).

• *Geographic Distribution:* People over 65 years old are not evenly distributed across the United States. The greatest proportion of senior adults in this country (more than 17%) live in Florida. In 1989, 52% of the total population of people over 65 years lived in nine states: California, New York, Florida, Pennsylvania, Texas, Illinois, Ohio, Michigan, and New Jersey (Rakowski & Pearlman, 1995). This is significant because speech–language pathologists in these states will be expected to respond to a greater than average demand for intervention services for this population. Similarly, several smaller states have relatively high proportions of people over 65 years (e.g., Rhode Island, 14.8%; Arkansas 14.8%; West Virginia, 14.6%; Connecticut, 13.6%; Maine, 13.4%) (Rakowski & Pearlman, 1995). Clinicians in these states will face greater than average demand for intervention from senior adults as well.

• *Communication Problems:* Demographics including number and proportion of people over 65 years and geographic patterns become particularly significant when prevalence of communication disorders among the elderly is considered. Shadden (1988) reviewed estimations that 8 million older Americans have a speech, language, or hearing disorder. While 20% of the total population of individuals with speech–language impairments is 65 years or older, this proportion will climb to 39% by the year 2050. Similar proportional increases are being seen in the hearing impaired population. While those 65 years or older represent 43% of the hearing impaired population, this proportion will climb to 59% by 2050. Shadden (1988) noted that senior adults with communication impairments represent an underserved population. Furthermore, the implications for demands and necessary competencies for service delivery to persons over 65 years who have a communication disorder are profound (Beasley & Davis, 1981; Myers & Schwiebert, 1996; Shadden, 1988).

• *Fluency, Stuttering, and Aging:* There continues to be a relative paucity of clinical literature on older adults and senior adults who stutter. Manning and Shirkey (1981) indicated that while stuttering most often first appears in childhood and continues to develop with the individual through adolescence and adulthood, "Stutterers in their middle- and late-adult years, however, have received very little attention" (p. 175). In fact, Manning and Shirkey noted that Van Riper and Freund, both familiar with American and foreign literature, reported being unaware of a single article concerning the nature of stuttering in older individuals. While there has been some interest expressed over the last two decades on older individuals who stutter (MacFarlane, Hanson, Walton, & Mellon, 1991; Manning, Dailey, & Wallace, 1984; Peters & Starkweather, 1989), studies continue to address primarily younger people who stutter. The literature that does exist tends to indicate that the older the stuttering, the less favorable the prognosis for intervention (Conture, 1990b; Daly et al., 1995). In fact, there is general agreement that prognosis for a successful outcome for older people who stutter is relatively poor when compared to that of younger people who stutter (Bloodstein, 1995; Manning & Shirkey, 1981; Peters & Guitar, 1991; Van Riper, 1982). The literature on older speakers, both those who do and those who do not stutter, also indicates an interesting paradox. Manning and Shirkey (1981) noted:

> The available information indicates that older nonstutterers have more fluency breaks during the decades of their sixties and seventies. In addition, much of what we have discussed suggests that older stutterers are likely to experience a decrease in stuttering behavior during these same years. (p. 183)

Specifically, people who do not stutter increase in disfluency as they reach senior adulthood, particularly in the forms of interjections, whole word and phrase repetition, and revisions or incomplete phrases in the absence of any obvious tension (i.e., referred to as between-word, formulative, supramorphemic, or "normal" disfluency). During the same years, people who stutter tend to demonstrate a decrease in stuttering behavior, particularly in breaks between sounds or syllables, visible tension during the breaks, and pauses with cessation of air flow or voicing between small linguistic units (i.e., within-word, motoric, coordinative, or "stuttered" disfluency) (Benjamin, 1988; Manning & Monte, 1981; Manning & Shirkey, 1981; Rosenfield & Nudelman, 1991; Yairi & Clifton, 1972; Van Riper, 1982). Explanations for these apparently paradoxical trends abound. Nevertheless, the following summary remains current and deserves attention:

> What little we know about the nature of stuttering in older persons suggests that there may be a decrease in the number of people who stutter. There may also be a decrease in the severity of stuttering for those who continue to stutter. (Manning & Shirkey, 1981, p. 185)

These findings demand that we take a closer look at several critical aspects of stuttering and people who stutter. As indicated, clinical wisdom holds that treatment prognosis is directly and positively related to age of stuttering (i.e., the younger the stuttering, the more favorable the prognosis; the older the stuttering, the less favorable the prognosis). If research addressing older people who stutter continues to substantiate reductions in stuttering and the number of people who stutter, then we must reconsider these prognostic assumptions. Perhaps, as Manning and Shirkey (1981) indicated, "It may be that stutterers are at least as likely to recover from stuttering during the last few decades of life as they were during the teenage years" (p. 185). My work with senior adults who stutter indicates that factors other than age of stuttering are at least as relevant when estimating prognosis for improvement in fluency as a consequence of treatment. For these reasons, the nature and efficacy of treatment for older people who stutter must receive a more careful and optimistic review.

• *Multiple Perspectives and Intervention:* Ripich (1991) emphasized the importance of considering multiple perspectives when engaging in research or intervention with the "elderly." In fact, the heterogeneity of this vast population commands us to reconsider our assumptions. Bengtson and Schaie (1989) noted the following:

> To think of the later years of life as having a "course"—a set of complex developmental movements, not just a downward trajectory in function or competence—is a relatively new idea in human experience. . . . Prior to the mid-twentieth century, most characterizations of aging in Western thought reflected the theme of inevitable and irreversible loss. (p. vii)

Bengtson and Schaie (1989) indicated that two major events force us to shift our perspective on aging from a time of loss and decline to one of inviting and enlightening opportunities. The first event is the change in human demographics related to age and social activity. During the last century in the United States, life expectancy for females has increased from 41 years for those born in 1900, to nearly 80 for those born in 1980. Retirement for males has become a much more common period of life. In 1900, only 22% of those still living after 65 years were out of the work force. By 1980, 89% of those 65 and older were no longer working, and life expectancy for men aged 60 rose to 75 years. Furthermore, age composition has changed dramatically in the United States. In 1900, those over 65 years numbered 1 in 22, compared to 1 in 9 in 1980. The second event was the significant increase since 1940 in research and public awareness regarding both normal and pathological changes with age, revealing heterogeneity in social functioning and responses to biopsychological processes of aging. Moreover, "multidisciplinary research has contributed to the notion of a complex trajectory of human development past the middle years, seen in both decrements and adjustments to biological, psychological, and social competencies after young adulthood" (Bengtson & Schaie, 1989, p. viii).

Indeed, working with senior adults who stutter has provided me with at least several insights. Senior adults are not necessarily any more like each other than are children and adolescents. As noted earlier, notwithstanding the value of understanding group trends, senior adults enter the treatment experience one at a time, not as a group. Furthermore, senior adults who stutter have proven to me that change is realistic, desirable, and possible at any age across the life span, and intervention with such persons is a most positive, inviting, and enlightening opportunity.

• *Adjustments and Intervention:* Highlighting the diversity among the population of senior adults, Haynes et al. (1992) noted that some older clients may present some special problems requiring clinicians to make behavioral adjustments in treatment while others may need no special handling. They advised clinicians to be alert to fatigue, disorientation, failing eyesight, and hearing loss, and to structure, organize, and pace clinical procedures to ensure understanding. They indicated that, "Following standard procedures may not be as important as providing an environment in which the person is able to perform at optimal level" (p. 21). Furthermore, clinicians should expect and invite the clients to share their own story. Haynes et al. (1992) noted that because of feelings of uselessness or disintegrating health, older clients may need to talk to a clinician as a listening audience about past accomplishments or medical concerns.

Indeed, Hooper (1996) suggested that clinicians not only should expect clients and family members to tell "what grandma was like before," they (i.e., clinicians) should facilitate such a process by encouraging use of photographs, pictures, stories, videos, and other memorabilia from a past work or home life. Furthermore, she advocated for clinicians and other service providers to identify and understand the client's belief systems as they relate to the condition being treated; views of power and control specifically with respect to service delivery; and differences in professional, family, and client point of view, communication style, and abilities. Doing so helps "to enhance a positive therapeutic alliance" (Hooper, 1996, p. 45). Similarly, Shapiro (in press) expressed the importance of encouraging people who stutter, particularly adults, to share their own story and for clinicians to learn about their clients from these stories, as follows:

> People who stutter have stories to tell. Some of their stories are sweet, some of them are not sweet. The stories shared between people who stutter and their clinicians provide a web, a network, a system of communication that connects the participants in the clinical process to each other in a shared focus that transcends time and place. The stories, some of which are yearning to be told, also provide a basis of commonality and dialogue between clients and clinicians. Stories convey a message or a lesson. Stories told within the clinical context are no exception. However, no less significant within the clinical context is the actual telling of the story. Telling, sharing, and exchanging stories express hope, trust, courage, and faith. These entities are not given. They are earned and nurtured by the clinician. They express the client's developing belief that the world of communication can improve, that good things can happen to good people, and that good things can become even better.

PREASSESSMENT PROCEDURES

The assessment procedures for adolescents, adults, and senior adults are similar. Where significant differences exist, they will be highlighted.

Case History Form, Audio- or Videotape Recording, Preliminary Phone Call

Several weeks before the assessment appointment, the client completes the case history form represented in Figure 10.1. This form provides the clinician information about the client's developmental, medical, and educational history; family structure; communication strengths and limitations; and onset, development, and current perspectives about the communication problem. Because this form is somewhat generic (i.e., it requests information that would be appropriate for other speech and language disorders), the clinician may get an idea if the presenting fluency disorder is stuttering and if other communication disorders co-occur. The client is asked to make an audio- or videotape recording of himself while engaged in family interaction to help the clinician assess his relative speech fluency in that speaking context and begin to understand the communication dynamics within the family or partnership. As noted before, the clinician makes a preliminary phone call to help prepare the client and his family for the evaluation, to address preliminary questions, and to convey from the outset the clinician's support and commitment. When possible, the clinician is encouraged to provide the client at least two alternative times for the assessment appointment. These procedures establish mutual respect, joint decision making, and shared ownership from the beginning of the clinical process.

Significant others with whom the client communicates should be involved in assessment-related experiences to the extent possible and appropriate. Indeed, the longer we live, the more our lives affect and become affected by those family and friends with whom we interact closely. Many adolescents are referred by their classroom teachers or parents. If these individuals (i.e., teachers and parents) have not already provided preliminary observations and impressions, they should be invited to do so and to provide a tape recording of an interaction with the client from their respective settings. Adolescents are encouraged to complete the forms and preassessment procedures themselves but parental help is welcomed. Adults and senior adults often discuss, if not decide, with their spouses or families the prospect of pursuing fluency assessment. Helping to prepare all members of this significant therapeutic alliance and addressing their questions, therefore, is critical. Hooper (1996) reported one client as advising, "If you want to help me, help my family" (p. 43). Indeed, Hooper recommended intervention from a family, rather than individual, perspective and distinguished between "primary kin" (i.e., spouse, children, and siblings) and "secondary kin" (i.e., others who may function as family, such as friends and neighbors). Hooper noted that secondary kin "may provide as much, or more, quality of life and happiness for the older adult as the primary kin. They often provide support in tandem with other family members" (p. 44).

Preassessment Conference

Another procedure that I have found useful with prospective clients and their families, particularly with adolescents, adults, and senior adults, is a pre-assessment conference. Sometimes, inquiries from these individuals or their families or friends about assessment or treatment seem somewhat tentative, if not reluctant. Such reluctance results from a variety of reasons (e.g., discouragement with previous treatment, anticipated pressure from professionals to enroll in treatment, pressure or ambivalence from family or friends, misinformation, embarrassment, or fear). In such cases, I invite a preliminary conference in which the clinician interacts informally with prospective clients and their families. This is not a time for structured assessment. Rather, it is a meeting of people, as people, to discuss in a positive, inviting context the questions of our prospective clients and their families and the preliminary aspects of the presenting concern.

Furthermore, the clinician observes the communication dynamics among the family members; the family has an opportunity to learn about communication, its disorders, and the nature of intervention. I believe firmly that clients

(text continues on p. 380)

Please complete this form as completely as possible. Feel free to add information on the back or on additional sheets.

Person completing this form: _____ Date: _____

Identifying Information

Name:_____ Date of birth: _____

Social Security #: _____ Medicaid/Medicare #: _____

Gender: _____ Race: _____

Home address: _____

Home telephone #: _____ Work telephone #:_____

Occupation/Employer: _____ Education: _____

Physician: _____

Address/Phone: _____

In case of emergency, contact:_____

Address/Phone: _____

Family Information

Marital status (e.g., unmarried, married, separated, divorced): _____

Name of spouse: _____ Date of birth: _____

Occupation/Employer: _____ Education: _____

Name, age, and relationship to client of all people living in client's home: _____
_____

Do you have children not living with you? If *yes,* indicate name, age, and address:
_____
_____

Referral/Communication Information

Who referred you to this clinic? _____

Reason for referral: _____

Describe the problem you are having with speech, language, and/or hearing: _____
_____
_____

What do you think caused this problem? _____

How does this problem make you feel about yourself? _____

How has this problem changed since it was first noticed? _____
_____
_____

(continues)

Figure 10.1. Case History Form for Adults.

How has this problem affected you (e.g., family/social interactions, occupation, education)?

_____

_____

_____

What specific communication situations present difficulty for you?

_____

_____

Have you ever sought professional advice about your communication problem? If *yes,* list dates, locations, and results of previous evaluations and/or treatment:

_____

_____

_____

_____

_____

Have any relatives had a communication problem? If *yes,* explain:

_____

_____

_____

Medical and Health History

Describe any illnesses, injuries, operations, or other health problems you have or have had:

_____

_____

In what way might these experiences contribute to your communication problem?

_____

_____

Have you been hospitalized in the last year? If *yes,* explain:

_____

List all prescription and nonprescription medication used over the past year:

_____

_____

_____

(continues)

Figure 10.1. Continued.

Have you ever had a neurological examination? If *yes,* indicate date, location, and result:

_____

_____

Vocational History

In order of earliest to most recent, list the dates and locations of your past employment:

_____

_____

Additional Questions and Family Observations

What do you hope to accomplish as a result of the communication evaluation?

_____

_____

What questions and concerns would you like to see addressed?

_____

_____

What factors (such as family, home, or work) do you feel are influencing your speech?

_____

_____

Describe your areas of strength and special interests or hobbies:

_____

_____

Please provide any other information that you feel might be helpful in the evaluation:

_____

_____

_____

Permissions

In order to help you, it may be appropriate to send reports to or to contact other agencies or professional practitioners. If we determine this is necessary, we need your permission to do so. Please indicate your permission by signing below.

I authorize and request (clinic name and address) to obtain and/or exchange pertinent medical/educational/communication information. It is understood that all information about the client and the family will be kept strictly confidential.

Name: _____

Relationship to client (if not client him/herself): _____

Signature: _____ Date: _____

Thank you in advance for taking the time to complete this form. We look forward to working with you and others in your family.

Figure 10.1. Continued.

and their families make the best decisions when they are fully informed and involved. That is central to the purpose of the preliminary conference—to help the client and the family decide whether they wish to pursue a diagnostic assessment. Other avenues of intervention are available and indeed more appropriate for some (such as fact finding, reviewing literature or instructional videotapes for the public about stuttering, or reading personal accounts of successful adults who stutter and have had positive treatment experiences). It is very important to me that the client experience no pressure. Too many clients report having previously experienced pressure by prospective clinicians in addition to receiving unrealistic promises, only to have their hopes dashed. As a consequence, precious years pass until the client even envisions pursuing treatment again.

Starkweather (1993) discussed the importance of preventing clients from experiencing the placebo effect. Starkweather explained that the stuttering severity of some people is strongly attributable to the desperation they feel to find relief, as follows:

> When the stutterer believes that he has finally found, perhaps after years of unsuccessful treatment, something that is really going to help him, the desperation gives way to relief, and, since the desperation was causing all or some part of the behavior, the behavior diminishes or disappears. The emotional high that some stutterers feel as they begin a program that they believe in advance will finally resolve their problem may itself have a direct effect on muscle activity levels. (p. 163).

I support the importance of understanding and preventing a placebo effect in fluency assessment and intervention. Furthermore, I agree that our discussion of treatment options and their potential for success needs to be "realistic" and that we ought "not sell [y]our therapy too much." However, I do not agree that we should present a "pessimistic perception of how successful therapy is going to be" (Starkweather, 1993, p. 163). Clients deserve an opportunity to learn from a clinician who is positive yet realistic within an inviting, supportive, interactive context where they feel understood and secure. Within such a conference, clients directly experience the clinician's competence and interpersonal skills. I find that after a conference of this sort, the client and family are more fully prepared and, with few exceptions, elect to pursue the assessment appointment, now with confidence and heightened understanding.

I remember conducting a preliminary conference with a young man of 16 years and his parents. Having been through a variety of fluency shaping programs without elimination of noticeable stuttering, the family conveyed feelings of shared failure and related frustrations. Essentially, they were "shopping" for other approaches. They expressed frustration that previous treatment seemed to work as long as the young man was "plugged in," but once he left the treatment setting he was no more fluent than before. I took this to mean that they were displeased with the relative lack of transfer of fluency shaping techniques (i.e., delayed auditory feedback, or DAF) and his lack of relative communicative independence. They were intrigued to learn that some therapies address the cognitive and affective aspects of stuttering in addition to the observable behaviors, individualize the design of treatment, involve all members of the family system as active participants in the treatment process, require active participation between all treatment sessions, and emphasize the importance of increasing fluency as a vehicle toward decreasing disfluency. Also, they were intrigued when encouraged not to make a treatment decision, but rather to leave and discuss their options as a family and to feel welcomed to call if I might be of help. Indeed they called, and achieved their shared objectives over the next 18 months of scheduled treatment.

I remember another preliminary conference, this time with a man in his 60s who stuttered and his wife. He recalled a history of intermittent treatment spanning more than 50 years. Treatments included immobilizing one side of his body and crawling to stimulate compensation in the contralateral cerebral hemisphere, engaging in elocution exercises, receiving psychotherapy and medication, and undergoing hypnosis. They too were intrigued with another approach that maximized their participation in all aspects of the treatment process in order to facilitate communication independence. Abbreviated differential diagnostic procedures indicated that the man indeed stuttered, and that he possessed the ability to speak more fluently. He discussed being denied promotions because of his stuttering, which had a negative impact on his retirement. The man's wife discussed all of the compensations she and their sons made to minimize the impact that his stuttering had on the family (e.g., she always ordered in restaurants for the family, she or the sons answered the phone, and so on). At this, I asked them to consider if they wanted to "open a can of worms." This was not to discourage them, but to invite them to think seriously about the positive effects that his increased fluency would bring and the impact such changes would have on each other and on their lifetime of adjustments. Some of the effects of stuttering would be irreversible. Specifically, the man had retired; his working years were over. I knew that once he experienced speech fluency and communication independence, he would think about how different his retirement would have been had he been more able to receive his promotions.

This family, like so many others, pursued the assessment appointment and subsequent treatment. During the first day of treatment, as the man was participating in modified fluency shaping techniques (i.e., choral reading with the clinician who reduced and systematically eliminated her speech model), the man exclaimed, "Tell me why! Why couldn't I do this 40 years ago? Why couldn't I do this while I was still working?" We recalled together the "can of worms" and how some tender issues surface and need to be addressed as a part of the change process. Talking candidly with the couple and their adult sons in advance helped them make a joint and informed decision about pursuing treatment, and helped prepare the family for the shared problem solving and adjustments that would be necessary at tender moments of discovery such as these. This man's treatment lasted 2 years, during which time he established communication independence (exhibiting controlled fluency with minimal noticeable stuttering) and mastered the speaking challenges he established for himself that were at the top of his individualized hierarchy—ordering for himself in a restaurant, introducing himself on the golf course, and lay reading in church.

ASSESSMENT PROCEDURES

General Considerations

Interacting with adolescents, adults, and senior adults within a supportive, nurturing, conversational context provides an ideal opportunity to invite and dialogue about the client's story. Indeed, it often seems that those who have lived the longest have the richest tales to tell. For years, student clinicians and practicing speech–language pathologists have told me that when I am engaged in assessment or treatment with people who stutter, it looks like we are just talking. Indeed we are, with a shared focus, mission, and bond. I noted earlier that the conversation creates a context for the clinician to model appropriate speech and communication skills and for the client to practice these skills within a medium of conversational dialogue that is relatively natural and therefore generalizable to the client's extraclinical communication settings. The importance of involving the client's family and significant others in the decisions and procedures related to the clinical process cannot be overstated. Doing so facilitates changes experienced by both the client and significant others, all of which are brought about by improvements in the client's fluency. Working with and within families ensures that the change process will be productive and constructive.

Assessments of many adolescents who stutter are conducted by the clinician employed in the schools. In these cases, the sequence of procedures is similar to those outlined in Chapter 9 (i.e., interviews with parents, teachers, adolescent; observations of adolescent interacting in as many different settings as possible; and critique of audio- or videotape interactions in extraclinical settings). Readers may wish to review these procedures in Chapter 9. Haynes et al. (1992) noted that assessment of older students who stutter is even more challenging than that of younger students because of denial of the problem, lack of cooperation, and lack of motivation. Indeed, adolescents present unique and often predictable challenges. Nevertheless, the passages being experienced by many adolescents are real, confusing, and somewhat frightening for them. Recognizing and understanding such passages from the individual adolescent's perspective is a critical skill for clinicians, one which transforms the treatment setting into a safe house and enables the adolescent to feel understood and secure. This does not mean "swinging" with the adolescent, attempting to be "cool," or otherwise relinquishing one's professional role. It does mean, however, that clinicians must avoid preconceptions of or stereotyping adolescents and interact with each from the perspective of an open mind. Clinicians must realize that stereotypes of adolescents are no more just than adolescents' preconceptions or stereotypes about speech–language pathologists. Many adolescents are remarkably supportive, cooperative, and motivated. Adolescents, like clients of all other ages, present opportunities to rally, use, and improve our own clinical skills.

The remainder of this discussion on assessment procedures will assume that adolescents (i.e., young adults), adults, and senior adults are being seen at a clinical facility other than that provided in schools. Adolescents are grouped with other adults for discussion purposes because the main emphasis at these ages is on the effect that stuttering has had on their lives and the ways they have learned to react to it. Also, with few exceptions, people of this age who stutter serve as the primary informant for assessment purposes (Williams, 1978).

Client and Family Interview

Preparation

Before the interview and based on preliminary information (including case history form, tape recordings, phone calls, allied medical or educational records, etc.), I prepare myself a telegraphic outline of information that I want to receive and that which I want to provide. As always, I remind myself in writing to listen and to facilitate an opportunity for the client's story to unfold. This outline helps me to organize my thoughts and procedures, thus enabling me to focus more attention on the client and to the dialogue between us. The outline, however, must never be used inflexibly. We must adapt and adjust continuously to the needs, questions, and concerns of those with whom we are interacting. The proceedings should be tape-recorded (i.e., videotape is preferred) for later review and analysis. The clinician is interested to observe the adult's speech directly and determine how it is influenced by structure, linguistic complexity, and communicative pressure; how it is modifiable; and the relative developmental level of the client's behavior, feelings, and attitudes. The speech sample collected will be used for analysis and comparison to others collected from other speaking contexts.

Social Greeting

The interview should begin with a social greeting. I feel strongly that before we can interact effectively within a professional domain, we must recognize and respect each other as people. In the last two chapters, we discussed the importance of establishing a foundation as mutually interested and interesting people. The clinician seeks to understand and conveys her acceptance of the adult and his family, independent of the stuttering. In the old days, establishing a personal foundation was referred to as "establishing rapport," a critical first step in the clinical process. It seems that today, with our fast pace, modern pressure, and unavoidable accounting of "patient contact hours," something risks being lost. We might be inclined to get right to business, to use clinical time "efficiently." We might ask questions immediately about the problem (e.g., "So, tell me about your stuttering"), rather than to connect as people (e.g., "Did you find the clinic O.K.?" or "What do you think about this crazy weather?"). We discussed the importance of intra- and extrafamily considerations in designing assessment and treatment. Occasionally, such "small talk" leads to discussion that helps us understand one's assumptions about oneself and communication (personal construct), one's family structure (family system), previous treatment or professional contact (interdisciplinary teaming), or unique cultural or personal views (multicultural awareness). While the clinician structures the assessment context, there is no replacement for talking and communicating with the people and families we are trying to know, understand, and serve. At this point, permission forms and releases are signed, and the client is provided a general orientation of the assessment process. The clinician explains that she is interested to learn more about the client as a person and as a communicator and about the network within which the client interacts. To do so, she explains, she will be asking a number of questions about the client's communication experiences and related feelings and engaging the client in a variety of speaking tasks. Each of the procedures, which will be audio- and videotape recorded, will result in speech samples that will be analyzed for speech fluency and communication competence. The results of this analysis, including a diagnosis and related intervention recommendations, will be discussed in a closing interview at the end of this meeting, and will be followed by a written report detailing the items discussed.

Questions and Dialogue

The assessment of adults who stutter primarily is an interview consisting of many direct and open-ended questions. Readers will recognize parallels in the interview presented here with those presented in earlier chapters. After social "ice breakers" in which we have established a conversational context, a series of questions is begun that address the client's and family's general orientation to the assessment experience, followed by those that address the past (onset and early development, causal assumptions, family history, previous treatment), present (experience with the problem educationally, socially, vocationally; variability, learned responses; feelings and attitudes of self and others), and future (outlook toward change, inherent motivation and priority) with respect to communication and the communication impairment (Peters & Guitar, 1991; Williams, 1978). It is important to remember that the questions that are asked and discussed should reflect a dialogue (an exchange of information, thoughts, and feelings), not an interrogation. The extent to which such an interaction is conversational reflects one of the distinctions of a seasoned clinician. The clinician learns about the client's background by asking, responding, commenting, probing; all the while exercising an invisible but effective balance between conversational structure and clinical flexibility. The first general orientation questions are as follows:

• *Why have you come to meet with us today?* A related question is, What do you hope to achieve as a result of our meeting? Responses to these initial questions provide me with an idea of what the client perceives as his own needs and objectives, to each of which I respond directly before the conclusion of the evaluation. Furthermore, these initial questions invite the client's participation in the clinical process from the very beginning and communicate the clinician's interest in understanding and serving the client as a member of a communication system. We must remember also that clients are referred for many reasons. We cannot presume that we know our clients' needs before we ask about them. Even if they are referred for "stuttering," we cannot assume that they and we mean the same thing by the word "stuttering." The clinician then shares her overall purpose and a general orientation to the assessment process, being sure to relate directly to the client's or family's statement of objective.

• *When you use the word X* [stuttering, stammering, hesitating], *what do you mean?* The questions noted earlier (regarding why he came and what he and his family hope to accomplish) provide an opportunity for the client to begin to explain the nature of his concern. If he has not already done so, I ask the client to discuss the nature of his concern and to elaborate on whatever words he used to describe his concern. As noted before, generally I do not use the word stuttering until the client does because the term is evaluative and is relatively useless without description and quantification.

From these questions of general orientation, we move to those that help us learn about the client's communication past, as follows:

• *Describe the best you can when and how your stuttering began.* How did it develop or change over time? Once the client has described his concern, I ask him to describe the onset and development of the problem he has just characterized, highlighting any patterns or changes that have been noticed. The clinician should try to determine the source of the client's information. Specifically, does he recall its onset, or is he relying on reports of parents or other family members? We noted that family reports, while well meaning, often contain errors of memory and association. Patterns of late or abrupt onset may need to be investigated for the possibility of neurogenic or psychogenic disfluency or other disorders of fluency (discussed in Chapter 4). Peters and Guitar (1991) noted that events associated with changes in the stuttering (such as job changes, or family or personal events) might be precipitating or perpetuating factors and therefore might require more focused attention.

• *What do you think caused your stuttering?* What did your parents or other family members believe caused your stuttering? The discussion of causal assumptions often is easily tied to previous questions about onset and development. These causal assumptions can reveal the attitudes and beliefs that the client has held about his stuttering and about himself as a person and as a communicator. The clinician will better understand the client's personal construct once she appreciates his assumptions about his stuttering and the general orientation with which he operated in growing up and from which he has attempted to cope with the problem (Williams, 1978). Responses to these questions also have implications for the client's motivation. For example, if stuttering is viewed as a divine punishment, efforts to change may be viewed as conflicting with one's religious beliefs (see Chapter 6). Similarly, clients who assume that stuttering is inherited or caused by a psychological disorder will be relieved and thereby motivated to learn other causal interpretations and to gain the clinician's assessment that he possesses the ability to speak more fluently (Peters & Guitar, 1991). Clinicians need to understand the client's causal assumptions and relative accuracy of information, thereby determining what can and should be changed.

• *Have you ever had previous treatment for stuttering?* If so, for how long and what did it involve? What did you feel were most and least helpful aspects? Williams (1978) underscored that the client's attitudes and beliefs about previous treatment experiences will affect directly the way he responds in future treatment. Therefore, Williams advised that the clinician determine the degree to which it left him with discouragement and negative ideas about himself and his stuttering that must be addressed directly for present treatment to be successful. Furthermore, the clinician needs to determine what the client expects from treatment and from the respective roles of the clinician and client within the process. From an understanding of the client's past treatment experiences and related attitudes and beliefs, the clinician will be in a better position to facilitate the design and implementation of effective intervention.

• *Does anyone else in your family have a communication impairment?* Does anyone else in your family stutter? Peters and Guitar (1991) indicated that determining if other family members stutter may help the clinician understand the factors that influence the client's attitudes toward himself and his communication skills.

From questions such as these that inquire about the client's past experiences, we move to those that investigate the client's perceptions of how his stuttering has impacted his experience educationally, socially, and vocationally.

• *How would you describe yourself as a communicator?* How do you think others would describe you as a communicator? It is important to determine whether the client acknowledges his communication strengths and the extent to which he perceives stuttering as a central part of himself. Similarly, it is important to see how he views himself as being perceived by others. Lasting change in fluency intervention must be based on a foundation of communication strengths. Therefore, one of the first steps of treatment must help the client recognize and identify with his strengths as a communicator. Such questions also help assess the degree to which stuttering might be interiorized. There are times when the client perceives his stuttering as far more intrusive than do his listeners. In such cases, clients need to appreciate his listeners' perspective in order to realize and build on their communication strengths.

• *How is your stuttering affecting you at the present time?* Responses to this question often provide insight into the factors that motivated the client to initiate or return for treatment. For example, one woman indicated that her stuttering is worst at her work where she felt she had been passed over for promotions because of her stuttering. By pursuing intervention, she wished to eliminate any question over her competence to ensure professional advancement. Another client, a physician in his 40s, indicated that his stuttering rendered him unable to give oral depositions in court. This man wished to pursue his fluency; otherwise he would relinquish his position as chief psychiatrist.

• *Where and with whom would you expect your speech to be best (where do you experience no disfluency)?* Where and with whom would you expect your speech to be worst (where do you to experience significant disfluency)? What strategies do you use in each of these situations to help keep your speech as fluent as possible? Responses to these questions have direct implications for treatment. They provide the clinician a picture of the client's perceptions and attitudes about his speaking experience outside of the treatment setting and his current use of fluency facilitating controls versus tricks (postponements, avoidances, and word substitutions, among others). Designing communication hierarchies such as these helps tailor treatment to the needs of each individual, facilitates the process of transfer from the very beginning, and engages the client actively within the clinical process.

• *How have your educational, social, or vocational activities been affected by your stuttering?* How would your participation in these activities have been different had you not stuttered? As to the questions indicated above, responses to these questions reflect the client's beliefs and attitudes about ways that his stuttering has interfered or facilitated his progress in life experiences. This information can be used in treatment planning, particularly with respect to establishing hierarchies for transfer of fluency facilitating controls, and can indicate the need for appropriate referrals (interpersonal counseling, psychotherapy, and vocational counseling).

Finally, the clinician needs to assess the client's outlook on the future and the extent to which he sincerely believes that he possesses the ability to change his communication behavior.

• *How do you see your communication skills as affecting your future (including school, career, retirement activities)?* A related question might be, How would improvement in your communication skills change your life? By discussing topics such as these, the client offers a glimpse of his feelings, thoughts, and attitudes toward stuttering in addition to his personal degree of motivation to change this condition. The clinician might ask, "On a scale of *1* to *10*, where would improving your fluency fall as one of your life's priorities?" In order for an adult to improve his speech fluency permanently, the change must be among one of his top priorities in life and he must have the support of those within his family system. However, for an adult to be unable to project how reducing his stuttering would change his life is not necessarily an indication of lack of motivation or a negative prognostic indicator. Some people have stuttered for so long that they cannot even imagine how their communication might be improved. Many of my adult clients have confessed that they even stutter in their dreams. One aptly said, "Stuttering is all I have ever known." For some, it is as though their motivation has enabled them to approach and knock on the door of fluency, yet they have no idea what is on the other side of the door. For these adults, their dreams begin to take form as they experience fluency success and communication independence within individualized treatment.

• *What are your feelings about enrolling in fluency intervention?* What would you expect from such a prospect? What are your family's feelings about your interest in pursuing fluency intervention? These questions likely overlap with some addressed earlier. They seek to determine how the client's motivation might be affected by others around him, and the extent to which the family members might be actively involved in the treatment process. As noted earlier, the client's inability to articulate his idea of treatment structure and outcome is not necessarily a negative indicator.

• *Thinking about yourself as a communicator, are there any other questions you have or topics you think we should address?* As discussed earlier, the interaction should reflect a dialogue whereby the client has asked questions that he feels are pertinent. A follow-up question such as this again invites the client to participate actively and to share any additional thoughts that might have surfaced during the process of interaction.

Speech–Language Sample Without Communicative Pressure

When meeting with an adult, the clinician must demonstrate sincere interest in the adult as a multifaceted person who also is a member of a communication system. The client not only is someone who stutters; he is someone with interests, talents, hobbies, family relationships, and friendships. In short, he is someone with a life story. Before addressing aspects of the person's communication skill and experiences, the clinician has an opportunity to convey a powerful message regarding her interest in knowing, understanding, and relating to the person who has come for help. Meeting as people first creates a foundation upon which a solid clinical relationship can be built. It does not take long to establish this foundation, but the time spent building this foundation with the client is invaluable and irreplaceable. Relationships are built on shared interests and sincere feelings of mutual respect. Clinical relationships are no exception.

I am working with a man in his 50s who, in addition to working in a precision tool and die plant, is an expert carpenter and wood worker, maintains a farm, likes to travel, and particularly enjoys fine food—and, he stutters. We have a lot in common. We always seem to have a home repair project ongoing at any given time; we always seem to be returning from or planning a trip; and we always have a recent tale of the best or worst meal we just experienced. I have sought his advice on numerous occasions regarding the fixes I find myself in when tackling home repairs I know I should not have attemped. We respect each other; we like each other. Why do I mention the farm? Because he enjoys a frequent laugh on my account given my lack of experience in this area. Just as Eskimos know snow, he knows cows. I feel accomplished that I can distinguish a cow from a pig. I enjoy learning from his experience, particularly in those areas about which I am unfamiliar. We talk and we laugh. We laugh at ourselves and, occasionally, at each other. His wife is a dignified and delightful woman who is involved in every treatment session. She recently commented how much she appreciates that we have interests in common other than our communication focus, and indicated that this, in part, is one causal explanation for his significant communication success when compared to previous treatments. Are our commonalities so deep, so significant, that we become kindred spirits or bonded to one another? Hardly; but meaningful relationships often are based on sharing life's simple things, the simple joys and occasionally life's disappointments. Does this mean that clinicians and clients must be friends in order to work effectively with one another? No again; but relationships are built on those commonalities from which people often come to care for and about each other as people. Does this mean the fluency and stuttering take a back seat? Absolutely not. Our commitment to understanding and improving communication is the primary focus and that bonds our relationship. All of the commonalities we share only contribute to our foundation as caring, interested, and committed people, a foundation on which a meaningful and constructive clinical relationship is based.

The interview questions discussed in the previous section, in addition to the clinician's sincere interest to become familiar with the client as a person, create an ideal opportunity to collect a speech–language sample (i.e., without communication pressure) from the client. As noted in the last chapter, the sample should be no less than 300 words (Conture, 1990b, 1997), or 5 minutes of the client's talking (approximately 10–15 minutes of real time). This sample provides one of the bases to assess the client's communication skills including speech fluency. Such conversational interactions invite candid, open, accepting exchanges about the adult's beliefs regarding what he does relatively well versus poorly, what he does to speak as fluently as he can, his self-assessment as a communicator, and his thoughts and feelings that have resulted from or been affected by the experience of stuttering. While often thinking about stuttering or not stuttering, adults rarely think or talk about talking, how we talk, and different ways of talking.

The client will come to see that fluency and disfluency both represent different ways of talking and the direct consequence of doing things differently. Coming to realize that stuttering is not something that happens to you, but something you do, implies that speech is potentially controllable; thus the adult has choices to make. When sharing his ideas and assessments and receiving alternative ideas to consider, the adult begins to think and talk about talking in different and positive ways. He begins to consider his own thoughts about his speech and himself as a communicator. Invariably, the adult begins to question ways he has viewed himself as a person including social, educational, and vocational choices he has made. In some ways, conducting assessment and treatment with adults who stutter and their family is like opening Pandora's Box. Neither the clinician nor the client knows exactly what lies inside. However, a relationship has begun in which each is committed to the other to pursue the journey together, discovering communication-related behaviors, thoughts, feelings, and attitudes, all the while working, learning, and growing together. More specifically, the conversational sample is intended to foster a supportive, trusting, engaging relationship and will be used later for subsequent analysis.

Structured Activities Without Communicative Pressure

After collecting a rich conversational sample as described, the clinician now engages the adult in a variety of relatively structured activities to yield elicited responses. These are used for subsequent analysis and comparison across speaking contexts in order to assess and differentially diagnose the individual's communication skills including speech fluency. In other words, in addition to assessing the individual's competence in parameters of speech sound production, language, and voice, we are determining if a fluency disorder is present, and if so, what type. The following activities are among those used:

• *Reading.* For readers, typically three different passages are used (i.e., below, at, and above one's reading level). Easy passages might include the morning newspaper; moderate passages include one or two different phonetically balanced passages, such as *My Grandfather,* reproduced by Duffy (1995, p. 95) and Shipley and McAfee (1992, p. 121), among others, and *The Rainbow Passage* (Fairbanks, 1960, p. 127); difficult passages include a page from a difficult statistics textbook or *The New England Journal of Medicine.* The phonetically balanced passages contain all of the sounds in the English language and thereby provide an opportunity for screening articulation and phonology as well as speech fluency. People who stutter typically become more disfluent as the level of reading difficulty increases. However, the clinician must be mindful that assessment of speech fluency may be confounded by one's reading competence. This means that while the clinician interprets the influence of increasing linguistic demand on speech fluency (i.e., imposed by more difficult reading passages), she must also ferret out the linguistic disfluency that reflects inadequate reading skills (e.g., those with a reading disability or bilingualism).

• *Recalling and describing events, holidays, possessions.* The client is asked to describe both simple/concrete and complex/abstract events and things. Theoretically, the former imposes less demand on the individual's ability to remain fluent than the latter. For example, to elicit simple or concrete recall, the clinician might ask the client, "If I were to visit your home or work, what would I see?" In comparison, to elicit complex recall, the clinician might ask about a technical aspect of the client's work (e.g., "I understand that the plant where you work makes tool and dye equipment for the production of zippers. What is the process that results in a finished zipper?").

• *Word and sentence repetition.* The clinician prepares on her outline words and sentences of increasing length and complexity. When asking the client to repeat them, however, the clinician presents them in random order, thus not conveying the pattern inherent to the task (i.e., increasing length and complexity). The clinician then looks for a relationship between length/complexity and fluency. Typically, the simpler or shorter words and sentences impose less demand and therefore result in less disfluency than longer or more complex items.

• *Questions and answers.* The client is directed to respond to questions requiring answers of differing length and complexity. Again, for people who stutter, shorter/simpler questions and answers frequently are associated with greater fluency than those that are longer/more complex. One explanation is that the former imposes less linguistic demand than the latter. For example, answers to, "What is your favorite X [*television show, food, sport*]?" often are less disfluent than those to, "Which presidential candidate do you feel had a more convincing economic policy and why?" There are predictable exceptions, however. Most people who stutter report that responding to, "What is your name?" is one of the most difficult fluency challenges. This question, while both simple and concrete, provides no alternatives (i.e., if your name is David, you cannot respond with Susan), thus superimposing a type of demand speech over a relatively simple linguistic demand. I believe that is why answering the phone is so difficult for so many people who stutter (i.e., there are few alternatives to "Hello," combined with internalized time pressure). Similarly, other questions whose surface structure reflects less demand (i.e., shorter/simpler) often result in more disfluent responses when other factors produce greater demand at an underlying or deep structure level. For example, questions that elicit emotional, affectively awkward, politically polarized, or otherwise "off limit" responses tend to impose more demand than that predicted from the surface structure of the question alone (e.g., "What's going on in this picture?" when presented a picture of sexually suggestive or explicit content; "How much money do you make?," "Are you voting as a Democrat or Republican?," "What do you think of the gender gap today?"). These and other factors must be considered when identifying patterns and variability of stuttering.

• *Other.* There are a number of other relatively structured activities that clinicians might use. These include commenting on pictures, naming objects, telling stories, automatic speech, echoic speech, speaking alone, monologue, command speech, talking with gestures, talking with phonemic difficulty, and talking on the telephone.

Speech–Language Sample and Structured Activities with Communicative Pressure

After the clinician completes the speech–language sample and structured activities without communicative pressure, she then engages the client in different activities with deliberate communicative pressure. By doing so, the clinician is looking to determine the effect of communicative pressure (e.g., time pressure, linguistic ambiguity, and violation of conversational rules) on the adult's speech fluency. Some of the activities already completed deliberately contained differing degrees of communication pressure. Also, some of the questions and discussion might have addressed aspects of the adult's communication past, which evoked sensitive issues and tender memories.

For example, I remember clearly a man who was 63 years old at the time of the diagnostic assessment. Addressing questions about how his parents and family responded to him when he stuttered, the man recalled the physical abuse he incurred as a child. Describing vividly and emotionally what his father's hands looked like as they reached for him when he stuttered, the man articulated how his father either beat the boy's (i.e., the adult client's) head on the barn door or submerged his head into a barrel of water until he promised he would not stutter again. The man showed us the remaining scars on his forehead. I remember while listening to this human tragedy, the two student clinicians each had a tear running down their cheek. Interestingly, as I write these words years later, my own eyes still water as I share this man's experience. Indeed, his treatment was interdisciplinary, and it included his wife, friends, a psychiatrist, and psychiatric social worker, among others. The point is that the nature of the conversation itself during the assessment imposed an emotional demand on the man's ability to remain fluent.

Other activities involving deliberate, albeit less emotional, communicative pressure include rushed verbal and physical behavior (the clinician increases her rate of speech, hand and overall body movements and extraneous gestures, speed of requesting answers and responding; and directs the client to "hurry up"), interruptions (the clinician takes a conversational turn before the client has completed his, asking a question and then asking another before the client finishes answering the first), loss of attention (the clinician does something else when the client is relating an event), or requesting the client to say something else (the clinician says, "I didn't understand that. What are you trying to say?"). Other deliberate verbal challenges include abruptly shifting topics (introducing a topic prematurely that is unrelated to the one being discussed), overstepping boundaries of intellect or experience (using words about topics that are unfamiliar to the adult), introducing linguistic ambiguity (contradicting things said by the client or clinician), or verbal absurdity (treating foolish statements as if they are legitimate; e.g., addressing the client by the wrong name, making deliberate errors in topics discussed or pictures described, or telling a joke with a punch line that makes no sense and asking the client if he understood it). The clinician also may direct the client to tell a joke, deliberately creating a high linguistic demand on the client. The clinician must remain sensitive to the client's feelings and inform the client as to why she is engaging in activities that might seem odd or rude. These activities are important even when the adult client is not showing observable signs of disfluency. By increasing the demand on the adult's ability to remain fluent, the activities may elicit disfluency when otherwise it is not apparent. As stated earlier, such pressure may affect the fluency of different clients in unique ways.

Trial Management

The activities described so far enable the clinician to evaluate the adult client's speech-related fluency, feelings, thoughts, and attitudes, in addition to other aspects of communication, and to arrive at a diagnosis. The data also provide a baseline of the client's communication behavior from which the effects of treatment can be measured. Furthermore, the data help the clinician determine if more formal evaluation of articulation or phonology and language is necessary. If the adult demonstrates observable disfluency or negative communication-related attitudes, thoughts, or feelings, the clinician engages in trial management techniques based on fluency shaping and stuttering modification. Trial management, a necessary part of the evaluation process, enables the clinician to help the client directly by exploring and adjusting his behaviors, thoughts, and feelings (i.e., heretofore, the clinician has been assessing and evaluating, deliberately without providing speech-fluency related assistance), to determine the client's responsiveness to different and specific treatment strategies, and thereby to design specific treatment recommendations.

Fluency Shaping

The clinician should engage the client in a variety of fluency shaping techniques for the purposes of differential diagnosis and determining the client's relative responsiveness to such techniques. For example, I often engage the client in singing, choral speaking (such as reciting the Pledge of Allegiance, a poem, or some other familiar verbal passage) and choral reading. People who stutter should demonstrate consistent fluency during such experiences, except when initiating a new passage or bar of music following a pause. If the client does not demonstrate remarkably improved fluency, the clinician should consider the possibility that some other disorder of fluency is operating. Manning (1996) noted, "These fluency-enhancing activities can provide highly dramatic results, and such instantaneous improvements tend to have the effect of making anyone who uses them an 'expert' on how to help people who stutter" (p. 146). The clinician must communicate why she is using such techniques and the fact that their effect is temporary at best, to prevent the client from gaining inappropriate expectations.

The activities are extremely useful, however, to enable the client to "feel" fluent speech directly, sometimes for the first time. Doing so often has the additional effect of significantly heightening the client's motivation. Other fluency shaping techniques include establishing fluency (characterized by slightly prolonged vowels, soft articulatory contacts on vowels and consonants, natural suprasegmental features) through modeling, choral speaking or reading, using mechanical devices (such as delayed auditory feedback machine, or metronome) or other externally driven methods, speaking loudly or in a whisper, using a dialect, or speaking to a rhythmic stimulus (such as movement of finger or head). For a client who demonstrates more severe symptoms, the clinician may first establish a fluent syllable and systematically shape it into increasingly longer and more complex units (using a progression—monosyllabic word, polysyllabic word, phrases, sentences). First using imitation, the clinician may move to delayed imitation, elicitation through pictures, and eventually more spontaneous forms. The clinician provides praise and other forms of positive reinforcement as a consequence of a fluent utterance.

Stuttering Modification

The clinician wants the client to discover that there are many different ways to stutter (e.g., hard or soft, long or short, loud or quiet, tense or relaxed, and so on). Modeling for the client, we want him to experiment with how he talks, thereby realizing that talking does not just happen; it is something that we do. Both fluency and disfluency are consequences of something we do differently with our speech apparatus. For many adults, this will be a new perspective. Telling an adult is not as effective as enabling him to discover for himself that he can modify his own speech. If it can be modified, that must mean that he has choices. Such an awareness (i.e., that I can change and thereby control the way I talk, that I have choices, and that fluency and disfluency represent the consequence of different choices), once discovered, is remarkably empowering and motivating. While self-discovery generally is the most effective teacher, adults, nevertheless, tend to be more disbelieving than children. Adults typically have longer histories of stuttering; fluency failure therefore has become more predictable. Many adults have been wounded by stuttering; they form inflexible impressions about themselves and the world; they doubt their abilities; they lose belief in themselves. Individualized fluency intervention seeks to work with them to create opportunities for fluency success, thus yielding an alternative set of data from which the adult must reconsider his beliefs about his communication skills, himself, and the world. A variety of stuttering modification techniques contribute to this self-discovery process. Several methods were discussed in Chapter 9, with which readers should be familiar. Several techniques will be listed now and elaborated within the treatment section.

- **Explain to the client that you will be putting his disfluencies into your own mouth.** You are not mocking him; rather, by internalizing what he does, you can better understand it. This conveys a powerful message to the client regarding the clinician's commitment and willingness to share the same bunker. The clinician is communicating, "Do as I do, not just as I say." Furthermore, once internalizing what the client does, the clinician is in a better position to model ways of stuttering differently.

- **Model slow, relaxed, prolonged speech.** Use gentle articulatory contacts and natural sounding suprasegmental features ("Yyou ssaid eearlier thhat yyou llike ssports. Wwhich ssport iis yyour ffavorite?").

- **Demonstrate easier versions of the client's stuttering.** Use a modeling and expansion format (*Client:* "I–I–I–I huh–huh–huh–had a huh–huh–hard t–ime fffffinding a–a–a–a puh–arking p–lace." *Clinician:* "II knnow. Ffinding a pparking pplace ccan bbe a rreal bbear aarround hhere.")

• **Demonstrate easy and eventually hard disfluencies in the clinician's speech.** Initially, the clinician will offer descriptive, emotionally neutral self-comments (such as, "Hey, that was a tough one") and later invite the client's comments and assessment (*Clinician:* "What did you think about that one?" *Client:* "That was pretty tough. You're starting to sound like me!")

• **Identify instances when the client uses gentle speech onset with light articulatory contact, describe what he did, and offer positive feedback.** These procedures heighten the client's awareness of how much and what type of fluent speech he already possesses, and model for the client eventually what he will do for himself (i.e., identify his fluency, describe what he did to produce fluent speech, and offer positive feedback).

• **Provide for the client one or two foci for positive assertions of behavior.** For example, the clinician will model slow and gentle speech (refer to Figure 9.2), pointing out that the two behavioral foci are "slow" and "gentle."

• **Explore and support the adult for expressions of feeling related to stuttering or himself as a communicator.**

• **Extend the discussion of where and with whom the client would expect his speech to be more and less fluent, and discuss his related feelings.** Hierarchies such as these help explore the client's feelings and perceptions, tailor treatment if recommended, and facilitate transfer from the outset of the clinical process.

POST-ASSESSMENT PROCEDURES

After engaging in conversation and more structured activities first with and then without communicative pressure and delineating preliminary impressions, the clinician then needs to analyze the results more thoroughly to accomplish the following:

- To quantify (numerically account using summary statistics) and qualify (narrowly describe) the nature of fluency and disfluency within and across speaking contexts

- To describe competence in other areas of communication (including language, articulation and phonology, and voice)

The clinician analyzes the data collected and makes statements of diagnosis, prognosis, and recommendations for intervention, in addition to statements of referral to other professionals if appropriate. These results, in preliminary form, are conveyed to the client and his family in a conference at the end of the evaluation and summarized subsequently in a more complete form within a written report. Frequently, the clinician and client meet again, either in person or on the phone, once the report has been received.

Speech Analysis

The actual analyses of conversational and structured speech samples from adults are similar to those from children. The procedures used for speech analysis are reviewed more thoroughly in Chapters 8 and 9. Assuming the word as the unit of measure, those analyses are summarized as follows:

Frequency of Speech Disfluency (i.e., Disfluency Frequency Index, DFI)

This is a general measure of the amount of disfluency, without consideration to the individual types or relative severity, that occurs in the client's speech. Reported as a percentage, the DFI is computed by dividing the total number of disfluent words by the total number of words spoken (disfluent and fluent), and then multiplying the resulting decimal by 100 to achieve the percentage. The frequency of speech disfluency typically is reported as a percentage of 100 words spoken, averaged over samples of 300 or 400 words.

Type of Speech Disfluency (i.e., Disfluency Type Index, DTI)

This measure identifies the individual proportions for each type of disfluency. It is computed by dividing the number of disfluencies of each individual type by the total number of disfluent words, and then multiplying by 100.

Molecular Description of Disfluency

This includes the duration and frequency (reported in terms of total, mean, and range) of the most prominent or otherwise significant forms (particularly within-word disfluencies).

Rate of Speech

This is a measure of the number of words spoken per minute. The more a person stutters, the more his rate of speech is reduced. As treatment decreases the degree and amount of disfluency, rate should steadily increase and approximate normal standards. Rate is computed by dividing the number of words the client has spoken by the client's talk time in minutes. For purposes of comparison, it is helpful to know what is considered to be an average or "normal" rate of speech for adults who do not stutter.

Those figures, expressed in words spoken per minute, range approximately from 116 to 164 for conversation (Andrews & Ingham, 1971), 114 to 173 for monologue (i.e., talking about one's job) (Williams et al., 1978), and 148 to 190 for reading (Williams et al., 1978).

Duchin and Mysak (1987) provided additional detail for speech rates, also expressed in words per minute, for adults (male only). Average (i.e., mean) rate of speech for adults aged 21 to 30 years was 182.7 in conversation (i.e., standard deviation, 17.2 words per minute), 151.4 in monologue (picture identification; standard deviation, 49.6), and 219.9 in reading (standard deviation, 37.1). For adults aged 45 to 54 years, average rate was 153.7 in conversation (standard deviation, 26.7), 133.7 in monologue (standard deviation, 27.4), and 182.1 in reading (standard deviation, 18.5). For those aged 55 to 64 years, the average rate was 168.7 in conversation (standard deviation, 37.6), 141.7 in monologue (standard deviation 30.7), and 190.1 in reading (standard deviation, 19.2). Adults aged 65 to 74 years revealed an average rate of 155.1 in conversation (standard deviation, 35.9), 131.0 in monologue (standard deviation, 21.7), and 182.5 in reading (standard deviation, 29.1). Finally, for adults aged 75 to 91 years, the average was 133.3 in conversation (standard deviation, 14.9), 117.8 in monologue (standard deviation, 16.8), and 167.9 in reading (standard deviation, 19.2).

Expressed in syllables spoken per minute, the average rate of speech ranges approximately from 162 to 230 for conversation and 210 to 265 in reading (Andrews & Ingham, 1971; Peters & Guitar, 1991).

Secondary Characteristics

The secondary or associated characteristics, both speech-related (such as audible inhalations or exhalations, pitch rises, and oral and neck tension) and nonspeech-related (such as facial, head, and eye movement or tension), are quantified and qualified. These may reflect the client's developing awareness of stuttering, coping mechanisms during stuttering, or attempts to prevent stuttering.

Severity Rating

This is an assessment of the client's relative degree of stuttering involvement considering a variety of speech and nonspeech factors. Use of the *Stuttering Severity Instrument–Third Edition* (SSI–3; see Figure 8.5), *Scale for Rating Severity of Stuttering* (see Figure 8.6), *Profile of Stuttering Severity* (see Figure 8.7), or other severity instruments helps standardize assessment of relative severity of a speaker's stuttering over time and across speakers. However, the information provided by such instruments proves to be confirmatory, if not redundant, with the other quantitative and qualitative information collected.

Adaptation and Consistency

This measures the degree to which an individual's disfluency resembles that of the overall group of people who stutter. Specifically, with repeated recitation of the same material, adaptation is the tendency for overall stuttering to decrease; consistency is the tendency for stuttering to occur on the same sounds or words.

Feelings and Attitudes

This assessment is pivotal to a clinician's understanding of a client's stuttering experience. It is an assessment of the degree to which a speaker is experiencing covert involvement related to the experience of stuttering. Haynes et al. (1992) reviewed 13 available protocols for assessing clients' feelings and attitudes. Nevertheless, just as Peters and Guitar (1991) noted that the most reliable measure of the client's feelings and attitudes is the clinician's judgment, Haynes et al. (1992) acknowledged that, "Ultimately, the most important diagnostic tool is the diagnostician" (p. 11).

Other

This is an open category that invites assessment of tempo, regularity, relative tension, smoothness of transitions, physical concomitants, in addition to any other overt or covert features not yet reported.

Diagnosis

The clinician analyzes and synthesizes all available information about the adult's communication skills and makes a statement of diagnosis. In doing so, the clinician determines if the client is demonstrating a communication exceptionality, namely stuttering or any other disorder of fluency. If an exceptionality is identified, the clinician determines if treatment is warranted and recommended and, if so, the nature and foci of treatment. The clinician also determines if there is a need to make a referral to other professionals and estimates the client's prognosis for improvement in the area of speech fluency.

Prognosis and Recommendations

The clinician estimates the client's prognosis for improvement based on a variety of sources. As noted previously, prognosis is a prediction of the outcome of a proposed course of treatment. This includes how effective treatment will be, how far the client will be expected to progress, and how long it will take (Haynes et al., 1992). We have noted also that estimating prognosis is an inexact science at best. Daly (1988) stated, "We cannot predict which clients will make significant improvements in their fluency and which will not" (p. 34). Stressing the importance of the clinician's attitude as a prognostic factor, Daly recommended that clinicians be positive and enthusiastic with every client who stutters. Indeed, "I would rather err in the direction of optimism than pessimism" (p. 34). Nevertheless, what we know about general predictors of successful treatment based on group trends will be reviewed first (Florance, 1986; Haynes et al., 1992; Prins, 1993), followed by a discussion of chronic perseverative stuttering syndrome (Cooper, 1987a, 1990a, 1990b, 1993a, 1993b, 1993c), a potential sub-category of stuttering that presents unique challenges to clients and clinicians.

Prognostic Musings

Nowhere is understanding the distinction between group trends and individual performance more important than in estimating prognosis. Group trends reflect general patterns that surface from the population of people under study, without regard to individual differences. Conture (1990b) noted that people who stutter enter our clinical facilities one at a time, not as a group. I want to caution clinicians to avoid ascribing greater predictive validity to the general prognostic indicators than they deserve. Too often, clinicians themselves are doubtful about a client's potential for improvement. Additionally, clinicians carry insecurity about their own professional skills with people who stutter and a negative preset about the efficacy of treatment with such persons (Conture, 1990b; Manning, 1996; Silverman, 1996). If we take seriously Daly's (1988) reminder, which I do, that the sincerity of the clinician's attitude regarding the client's ability to effect improvement is predictive of the change achieved, then we clinicians must be mindful of our attitudes.

In other words, too often clinicians inadvertently box our clients into our assumptions or predictions. Let us never become a burden or a handicap for people who stutter. Let us never put a lid on someone's potential for growth and change. Change is not time bound, and wonders never cease. Who is to say what one individual can and cannot achieve? Yes, I know that we must be realistic with our clients so that they do not form unrealistic performance expectations. I know that our Code of Ethics (ASHA, 1994a; see Appendix A.2) prohibits us from offering guarantees, and that issues of accountability and liability are real. However, clinicians must take seriously the importance of understanding both the visible and invisible aspects of each individual client's personal construct and his potential to dream. Just as clients learn about dreams and dreaming from clinicians, many clinicians can take a lesson from the great advances many clients make, some of which are unpredictable or come from clients who demonstrate clearly negative prognostic indicators. Never say never. Never even think never. An effective clinician will enable a client to imagine, work toward, and realize dreams, occasionally far beyond that imaginable to either participant. To say that "the sky is the limit" only conveys the limitations of our thinking and our inability to imagine the unimaginable. There should be no limits imposed on our clients who stutter. Stuttering may be viewed from one perspective as a limitation; from another as an opportunity for change, learning, and growth by the client, his family, and the clinician.

Discussing the advantages of early intervention, Peters and Guitar (1991) noted the following:

> Good treatment of mild and moderate stutterers in their preschool and early elementary school years may leave a child with little trace of stuttering, except perhaps during stress, fatigue, or illness. Most severe stutterers, or those who are treated after puberty, will make only a partial recovery. They will learn to speak more slowly or to stutter more easily, and to be less bothered by it. Some stutterers will not improve, despite our best efforts. For reasons we don't understand, a few stutterers just don't change significantly in treatment. (p. 4)

While some have found the nature and severity of stuttering behavior at the time of assessment to be unrelated to treatment outcome (Florance, 1986), others noted that a more severe stuttering pattern is predictive of more positive treatment outcome (Haynes et al., 1992). Predictors of prognosis are inexact in general, and particularly so with adolescents, adults, and senior adults who stutter. Guitar and Peters (1991) acknowledged that some people who stutter will not improve "for reasons we don't understand." Similarly, I might add that "for reasons we don't understand," some people who stutter severely, are older, and characterize a variety of other negative prognostic indicators achieve remarkable fluency, control over their lives, and advances as people and communicators that could not have been imagined. Van Riper (1974) noted that for many years he accepted onto his caseload one client who, for him as a clinician, held a "zero prognosis" (p. 105). Reflecting on such experiences, he indicated the following:

> With a few of them a most successful result ensued; with the others either some improvement or at least no harm occurred. They taught me much. Most important of their teachings was the revelation that I had more potential for growth than I had realized—and so had they. Over and over again I have found that they knew what they really needed to solve their problems or at least to make them more bearable and that if I could only understand their needs, I had something to give. Perhaps it was not enough, but it was something. Often out of many such moments of partial understanding and inadequate therapy came surprising changes for the better. (p. 105)

As clinicians, mindful of the value and limitations of prognostic indicators and what we know about stuttering and people who stutter, we owe it to our clients to assume that each can achieve great things.

Prognostic Indicators with Adolescents, Adults, and Senior Adults

Clinicians are advised to consider seriously the cautions presented above. Within this context, the following indicators tend to be associated with a more positive prognosis for clients in this group regarding improvement in the area of speech fluency (Bloodstein, 1995; Daly, 1988; Florance, 1986; Haynes et al., 1992; Prins, 1993):

• **No record of unsuccessful treatment.** An absence of treatment seems more conducive to treatment success than a history of therapeutic failure. However, I have worked with many adults (ages 18–70) who have had treatment on and off for most of their lives without permanent success, only to achieve their speech fluency goals later in life.

• **A cooperative and supportive family system.** Treatment outcome seems most promising when family members are willing to participate meaningfully in family counseling and the treatment process.

• **Cooperative interdisciplinary team members.** Similarly, the treatment effect is most potent when team members (teachers, allied educational and medical professionals, and associates) work together and communicate effectively.

• **More severe stuttering pattern.** Those with a more severe stuttering pattern tend to demonstrate greater motivation and therefore greater likelihood of improvement. Those with a less severe stuttering pattern tend to show less improvement.

• **No other significant, concomitant problems.** Additional problems that may hinder progress include other communication disorders; reading or learning disabilities independent of stuttering; intellectual, sensory, or motor limitations; and psychopathology.

• **Other available resources.** Those with various areas of interest or expertise (in areas such as outdoor interests, reading, or music) often are more well-rounded in their way of living—including behaviors, thoughts, attitudes—and tend to achieve greater fluency success.

• **Positive pretreatment motivation and attitude.** Not surprisingly, motivation (one's internal drive) to change is associated with greater improvement. Florance (1986) found that clients who self-referred were significantly more motivated and therefore achieved greater fluency success than those who were referred by parents or other family members. Therefore, she instituted a criterion stating that clients must independently choose to enroll; otherwise the client is given time after the evaluation to consider the benefits of treatment. She reported that most of the adults, particularly teenagers, who chose not to enroll immediately did so later with dramatically positive results. Similarly, Watson (1995) noted that, "Given the effort and time that therapy demands, it is important that a client has made the decision to address his problem and that such a decision was not made by a spouse, employer or other individual" (p. 149).

• **Significant timing and voluntary enrollment.** Clients' motivation for treatment often interacts with critical life experiences. People who have reached a point at which they feel blocked because of their stuttering (e.g., limitations in job advancement, education, employment, marriage, or family relations) and who voluntarily enroll in treatment often have a more positive prognosis. Many of the senior adults with whom I have worked acknowledged that previous decades of treatment had not been successful. But they wanted to try once more, particularly because they had the time to focus on their own communication needs. I have found intervention with such people to be remarkably successful. Success is always sweet, particularly when one has wished and worked for it for so long. The clinical portrait at the end of the chapter will profile one such client.

• **Commitment to a jointly determined treatment plan and schedule.** The client must share the process of determining a comprehensive treatment plan and appropriate schedule that must be followed with sincerity and internal motivation. Recommended plans and schedules vary with clinicians (e.g., no less than twice per week, Daly, 1988; daily treatment initially with subsequent reduction, Florance, 1986). However, I have found that the shared establishment and ownership of such factors (e.g., one weekly treatment session of between 1 to 2 hours in duration) combined with regular treatment-related activities that occur between scheduled sessions to be key in predicting prognosis.

• **Personality variables.** Tolerance for ambiguity, positive self-reinforcement, and internal locus of control contribute to a positive prognosis. Florance (1986) described a high tolerance for ambiguity as the ability to cope with uncertainty, often associated with creative people who like to be involved in different activities. In contrast, low tolerance for ambiguity often is associated with clients who fight to maintain status quo, prefer structure and order, and follow rules carefully. High self-reinforcers monitor and focus on increasing the positive aspects of one's speech fluency; low self-reinforcers focus on the disfluent behaviors and decreasing their frequency. Those with an internal locus of control see both disfluency and fluency as the consequence of something they actively do. Those with external locus of control feel that their speech behavior is controlled by their environment (believing that they are victims of fate) and blame people and external events for their stuttering and personal shortcomings they perceive to be associated with their stuttering.

Therefore, high pre-treatment tolerance for ambiguity, positive self-reinforcement, and an internal locus of control have been associated with greater readiness for change and successful treatment outcome. Significantly, however, I have found that previous unsuccessful treatment has left many clients with negative prognostic indicators in these areas—low tolerance for ambiguity, infrequent positive self-reinforcement, and external locus of control—at the time of reassessment. Nevertheless, effective management of initial treatment, in which the client experiences heightened awareness of existing fluency and increased production of fluency, alters early prognostic indicators to a more positive direction (such as increased degrees of tolerance for ambiguity, positive self-reinforcement, and internalized locus of control). I noted previously that the positive effects of early treatment experiences are seen in the clients' statements that reflect a shift from feeling unable ("I can't be fluent; I never could.") to able ("By golly, I did it. Did you hear the gentle *g* when I said girl? I love it!"), and from feeling controlled externally ("Why is this happening to me?") to being in control ("I used my controls seven times yesterday, and five the day before. I know I can do this. I know I can catch those blocks before they catch me.").

• **Positive yet realistic expectations regarding the commitment required for fluency intervention.** Necessary life adjustments accompany the process of addressing and resolving stuttering-related behaviors, feelings, and attitudes (Guitar, 1976; Guitar & Bass, 1978; Prins, 1993). Perkins (1979) underscored the importance of assessing the client's attitudinal readiness for change and targeting that change. He stated, "We have serious doubts about the long-term effectiveness of any behavioral program that is not systematically concerned with evaluating and effecting improvement in the stutterer's attitude" (p. 109). Indeed, as Daly (1988) pointed out, "Too many of our clients get fluent in their mouths but not in their heads. Despite success, they feel threatened and helpless when trying their new skills alone" (p. 35). Similarly, Perkins stated the following:

> So much of their lives has been built around stuttering that, suddenly freed of it, they realize the extensive role it has played for them. When fluent, they feel like unwelcome strangers to themselves. If stuttering has been used as a defense against an unrealistic self-concept, then its removal will arouse anxiety. . . . But for some it is more a matter of identity. They wish to feel like themselves, and stuttering is part of that self-image. (p. 121)

• **The clinician's attitudes and expectations.** The clinician's attitude and expectations toward the client are both prognostic indicators and critical elements of treatment. Daly (1988) indicated that "the clinician's attitudes toward stuttering and people who stutter have as much to do with the successful treatment of this disorder as the methods selected for therapy" (p. 34). In other words, the clinician must sincerely believe in the client and his potential for change, just as the client must believe in the clinician's ability to facilitate such change. Relating the efficacy literature on treatment of terminally ill cancer patients to those who stutter, Daly noted that a positive attitude toward treatment was a better predictor of treatment outcome than the severity of the disorder. Therefore, the attitude and expectations demonstrated by the clinician significantly impact that of the client, and thereby predict the outcome of treatment. Daly noted the following:

> Might our clients detect any insecurities or uncertainties in the clinician's attitudes or feelings about the treatment advocated? Clinical experience repeatedly demonstrates that intelligent persons will expend effort and energy in treatment only when they expect substantial results. When the clinician concentrates on negative behaviors or problems rather than positive objectives, clients are apt to get discouraged. Such incongruity between the clinician's expectations and the client's expectations may account for the high dropout rate among our stuttering clients. Roughly one-third of stuttering clients withdraw

from treatment prior to completion. . . . We have expended tremendous effort studying clients who stutter. Perhaps it is time we study ourselves. (pp. 34–35)

A Prognostic Caveat—Chronic Perseverative Stuttering Syndrome

We have already established that predicting reliably who will and who will not improve significantly in speech fluency is imprecise, if not impossible. Particularly poor in predicting treatment outcome are measures of pre-treatment stuttering frequency or severity (Cooper, 1987a, 1987b, 1993a, 1993b, 1993c; Daly, 1988; Florance, 1986). Cooper (1993a) noted, "I find no meaningful relationship between reports of the frequency with which adolescents and adults experience or experienced disfluencies and whether or not they are successful in obtaining an acceptable level of fluency" (p. 13). In the face of such imprecision of prognostic indicators and given the importance of both clinicians' and clients' attitudes within and about the intervention process, I have argued that clinicians owe every client the bias of optimism. In other words, clients need the benefit of a clinician's sincerely positive attitude about the potential benefits of treatment and the client's potential for change. Nevertheless, honesty demands that we own up to the fact that some people who stutter will not improve as they or we would like. They will learn specific speech motor (i.e., behavioral) strategies to stutter more easily and they will learn cognitive and affective strategies to cope with stuttering as a reality, all of which help the person who stutters feel more in control of himself and his communication. Making this point, Peters and Guitar (1991) noted, "Some stutterers will not improve, despite our best efforts. For reasons we don't understand, a few stutterers just don't change significantly in treatment" (p. 4). Similarly, Daly (1988) acknowledged the following in response to clients' questions regarding, "Can my stuttering be cured?":

> I point out that some people who stutter do indeed become fluent; others achieve higher levels of fluency control although they may still stutter periodically. Some clients continue to speak in a predominantly disfluent manner, but we strive to help them speak as effectively as possible. That is our goal—to help each client develop the best fluency possible. (p. 34)

Understanding subtypes of stuttering (the stuttering syndromes) may help in reliably predicting treatment outcome. Just such a focus has been undertaken recently. Cooper (1987a, 1987b, 1990a, 1990b, 1993a, 1993b, 1993c) and Cooper and Cooper (1993) distinguished between three distinct types of stuttering. Cooper (1993b) indicated, "Out of every five individuals who experience disfluencies of sufficient frequency to be labeled as 'stuttering,' two experience the developmental syndrome, two experience the remediable syndrome, and one experiences the chronic perseverative stuttering syndrome" (p. 22). Specifically, developmental stuttering is characterized by achievement of normal fluency control by 7 years without professional help but with knowledgeable and supportive parental assistance, no evidence of feeling loss of control when disfluent, little evidence that disfluency is problematic, and subsequent inability to recall earlier difficulty with fluency. Those with remedial stuttering typically make behavioral, affective, and cognitive adjustments to achieve normal fluency after age 7 years with professional assistance and a supportive home environment; experience a loss of control during moments of disfluency that, however, are episodic in nature, usually related to changes in one's physical, mental, and environmental situation; and recall their earlier difficulty with stuttering but do not think of themselves as still stuttering. Finally, chronic perseverative stuttering is known as "incurable stuttering." It is defined as follows (Cooper, 1987a):

> The chronic perseverative stuttering syndrome is an adolescent and adult disorder in the fluency of speech resulting from multiple coexisting physiological, psychological, and environmental factors, distinguished by (1) recurrence after periods of remission; (2) characteristic cognitive, affective, and behavioral response patterns; and (3) susceptibility to alleviation but, given the present state of the healing arts, not to eradication. (p. 386)

Cooper presented the characteristics of chronic perseverative stuttering (CPS) syndrome in an inventory (1987a), which he later revised and presented as a checklist (1993a). The elements of this checklist, represented in Table 10.1, must be taken seriously by clinicians.

The feeling of loss of control is a significant indicator that distinguishes remedial stuttering from chronic perseverative stuttering. Therefore, Cooper (1977, 1979, 1987a, 1987b, 1990a, 1990b, 1993a, 1993b, 1993c) has argued that the feeling of fluency control must be a major goal (indeed, the "end goal" or "ultimate goal") of fluency intervention. Cooper and Cooper (1985b, 1995) argued that speech fluency is a byproduct of the feeling of such fluency control. Cooper described attainment of speech fluency as a "fluency trap" (1993a, p. 14) because such an end goal of treatment is not realistic in many cases. Cooper acknowledged that the construct of CPS syndrome may be misinterpreted by some as "dream-shattering" (1993a, p. 14). He countered that it is a positive force, a construct that "relieves guilt and self-deprecation in those who, after in therapy or years of self-directed efforts to be fluent, remain abnormally disfluent" (p. 14). Cooper (1987a, 1993a) recommended that, at the end of the diagnostic interview with an individual who characterizes CPS syndrome, the clinician present both the "good news" and "bad news" to the client. Cooper (1987a) first presents, "The bad news is that you have the chronic perseverative stuttering syndrome which means that there is no cure for your stuttering" (p. 387). The "good news" is presented next, that the clinician can help the client add to the controls he presently is using and gain "the feeling of control over your speech" (p. 387). Cooper concludes as follows:

> When we finish, you most likely will still be disfluent, but you will be able to enter any situation knowing that no matter how tough it is, you have the skills to alter your speech and to communicate effectively. You will have the feeling of control. (1987a, p. 387)

Citing letters from clients and clinicians, Cooper (1993a) acknowledged that his notion of CPS syndrome is controversial. It is undeniable that for some people who stutter, speech fluency is an unrealistic treatment objective. It is undeniable also that many people who stutter are put to unnecessary and unfortunate feelings of frustration and failure. However, when and how such a determination (i.e., CPS syndrome) can be made remains debatable. I have seen

Table 10.1. CPS Syndrome Checklist

CPS Syndrome Checklist

- The individual's fluency disorder developed concomitantly with the development of language and speech.

- The individual's fluency disorder has persisted for 10 or more years.

- The individual's disfluencies are, or have been, accompanied by a fleeting but generalized feeling of loss of control.

- The individual has experienced periods of normal fluency accompanied by the feeling of control.

- The individual experiences a persistent fear of a catastrophic loss of fluency although, in fact, such occurrences occur rarely, if ever.

- The individual has identified one or more adjustments in speech production that generally, but not always, enhance fluency.

- Although capable of predicting the level of fluency to be experienced in most situations, the individual continues to experience unpredictable fluency failures.

- The individual has experienced fluent periods after a heightened and sustained period of psychic and physical concentration on attaining fluency, but has been unable to maintain that level of concentration or fluency.

- The individual's predominant self-perception is that of being a stutterer.

- The individual experiences periods of obsessive absorption in striving for normal fluency.

The factor most noticeably missing from this listing of identifying characteristics of the CPS syndrome is that of the frequency of disfluencies. I find no meaningful relationship between reports of the frequency with which adolescents and adults experience or experienced disfluencies and whether or not they are successful in obtaining an acceptable level of fluency.

Note. From "Chronic Perseverative Stuttering Syndrome: A Harmful or Helpful Construct?" by E. B. Cooper, 1993a, *American Journal of Speech–Language Pathology, 2* (3), p. 13. Copyright 1993 by the American Speech–Language–Hearing Association. Reprinted with permission.

too many senior adults achieve their lifelong fluency goals after so many years of previous, unsuccessful treatment to accept that such a determination can be made at the end of the initial diagnostic evaluation. I am convinced that prognosis is a dynamic, rather than static, entity. This means that one's prognosis fluctuates with different factors.

For example, timing is a critical factor impacting prognosis. Many young adults who are establishing marital relationships, raising children, building careers, or creating financial foundations, realistically do not have the opportunity to focus on their own individual needs including speech fluency. Once these and other factors no longer require primary attention (i.e., children are now adults and on their own, career is well established or completed, financial plans are in place, and so on), many such individuals then can focus on their own needs and achieve remarkable fluency progress. I would hate to discourage one's potential for speech fluency or any other aspect of human development. While I see a value for Cooper's construct, I am concerned about its potential overuse and misuse. After achieving her objectives for speech fluency and communication, one "chronic perseverative stutterer" or "incurable stutterer" I worked with told her discriminating employer where to put his company, and now is an extremely financially successful private practitioner in computer programming; another has become the chief psychiatrist at a Developmental Evaluation Center; another is enjoying his retirement, "going out fluent" as he says. All beat the odds against them and now feel in control and demonstrate spontaneous fluency or, occasionally, controlled fluency.

Another "incurable stutterer" comes to mind, the author of your book. While I make it a rule not to exploit my audiences (including clients, student clinicians, workshop participants, and readers) into hearing my story, I must confess that many well-intentioned clinicians who worked with me ultimately threw in the towel. In other words, they became frustrated with my progress and gave up. It is as though the checklist for CPS syndrome was written to describe me and my stuttering. Without treatment success, I stuttered severely for most of my first 25 years. Thankfully, for nearly 2 decades, I have enjoyed spontaneous fluency, although occasionally I resort to controlled fluency. *Never* throw in the towel. Too many well-meaning people become obstacles, inadvertently snuffing out the light of hope of someone else's dream. Within the limits of realism, which are individually defined, I am convinced that the most difficult challenges take the most time and energy, and those that seem impossible take even more. *Never* give up. People die not only when the pulse stops and brain waves cease. Too many people stop dreaming, which surely is an indication of premature death.

Recommendations

All of the information collected to this point, which led to the diagnosis and statement of prognosis, is integrated with intrafamily, extrafamily, and psychotherapeutic considerations in order to form treatment recommendations. As noted previously, intrafamily considerations focus on personal constructs (the way the adult views himself as a person and as a communicator, the extent to which he sees himself as successful or potentially successful as a more fluent or effective speaker), and aspects of the family system (the extent to which members of the family unit communicate openly, support each other, and sincerely participate in the clinical process). Extrafamily considerations address interdisciplinary teaming (the degree to which members of the interdisciplinary team communicate openly and contribute to an integrated fluency intervention program) and multicultural factors (the individual differences that might impact planning for, conducting, or interpreting the treatment experience). Psychotherapeutic considerations are those factors that help individualize the treatment plan based on the relative degree of involvement of overt and covert factors and seek to establish objectives that are appropriate to each individual (that is, fluency shaping and stuttering modification). When integrated, this pool of information yields informed treatment recommendations.

Post-Assessment Interview

The post-assessment conference, held immediately after the evaluation, is intended to summarize the results of assessment, provide recommendations, and discuss any remaining questions. It is supportive first to address the objectives, needs, and concerns expressed by the adult and his family, and to express positive observations about the adult's communication skills and the interactions among the family members. The positive tone in which the results are summarized and discussed establishes the style of interaction among all participants of the clinical process. Negativity generates a problem focus and one of repairing the adult's defective speech and the family's communication deficits. A more positive, albeit direct, realistic, yet optimistic, approach yields a solution and strategy focus directed toward achieving communication improvement and realizing fluency potential where all work together and support one another.

One of my student clinicians recently asked me if being so positive results in "sugar coating the truth." I don't believe so. Being positive yet realistic by nature provides a model for the clinical process as noted, but also helps the client and family be more receptive to the results being presented, the seriousness of the concern, and the recommendations for constructive change. As long as the truth is represented objectively and fairly, the clinical process can become a collaborative, positive endeavor in which all participants actively contribute, support each other, and share the outcome. The alternative that I do not find appealing is one in which the communication problem and clinical process are conceptualized in the light of misfortune or as gloom and doom. I guess I have always felt that everyone, even those who appear to be most successful, have unique limitations that require attention to offset their own strengths. For some, the limitations may not be as visible as for those who stutter. The clinician's personal construct about the clinical process and the respective roles of the participants within it significantly influence the nature of the process that results.

In the post-assessment conference, I summarize in understandable terms and with sufficient audible and visual illustration the nature of the adult's fluency and disfluency. I address the family's questions about causality by summarizing briefly what we know about predisposing factors and the importance of identifying and controlling for precipitating and perpetuating factors. I offer recommendations, remembering the importance of not just telling, but discussing, demonstrating, and directing/coaching the adult and family implementing the recommendations. Having discussed with the family the importance of making a joint decision and commitment to return to treatment (deciding they are ready to "open a can of worms"), I determine the relative confidence and consensus of the family's decision. If they are not fully decided, I encourage them to take their time deliberately, without offering any pressure or undue encouragement. Many of the adults I have worked with have pursued false promises and endured high pressure in the past. Perhaps I overcompensate, but I want to ensure that a decision to pursue treatment reflects a shared and confident decision without any external pressure.

Furthermore, I explain this premise as well as the nature of treatment. I explain that I have no magic and that I can offer no promises. Treatment is likely the hardest work one will ever do, requiring increasing degrees of vigilance. Treatment is a shared process that is tailored for each individual. I explain that I tend to be more directive toward the beginning of treatment and deliberately shift greater responsibility onto the client and family as the process progresses. I implore, however, that if the client ever does not fully understand what we are doing or why we are doing it, he should speak up. No instructions are to be followed blindly. Many clients have followed instructions without complete information in the past, and therefore may expect to do so again. I want all of the clients and their families to understand and participate in, and thereby own, all aspects of the treatment process. The client-related factors discussed to this point (i.e., making independent decisions to enter or reenter treatment, understanding and committing to the clinical process, demonstrating strong internal motivation, maintaining a positive yet realistic attitude regarding the treatment process and one's role within it, and contributing actively and independently to the treatment process) essentially screen or hand pick the clients who are likely to be successful. When possible, I prefer to stack the deck in favor of the client's potential for success. Some prospective clients may not have expected to be so involved in the process, or still may be in pursuit of the "quick fix." For others, the timing may be wrong. They may be viable candidates for intervention, but cannot commit to the time involved or degree of internalized vigilance and concentration required. For such individuals, I recommend that they consider seriously when might be a more appropriate time for them to enroll and I offer a welcome for whenever that time occurs.

Various resources may be discussed with and loaned to prospective clients. These include brochures ("Turning on to Therapy," "Using the Telephone: A Guide for People Who Stutter," and "Did You Know?"), booklets ("Do You Stutter: A Guide For Teens," "To the Stutterer: Self-Therapy for the Stutterer"), and videotapes (*Do You Stutter: Straight Talk for Teens*) distributed by the Stuttering Foundation of America; books containing personal accounts (*A Stutterer's Story: An Autobiography* [Murray & Edwards, 1980]; *Tangled Tongue: Living With a Stutter* [Carlisle, 1985]; *Stuttering: A Life Bound Up in Words* [Jezer, 1997]); and others. Additional information about these and other resources is found in Appendix B.

TREATMENT

In this present chapter, we have characterized adolescents, adults, and senior adults, reviewed a variety of assessment procedures, and addressed the imprecise practice of estimating one's prognosis for improvement in the area of speech fluency. Now we turn to integrating treatment procedures to address the behaviors, thoughts, and feelings of adolescents, adults, and senior adults who stutter.

Goals

Treatment goals for adolescents, adults, and senior adults who stutter are spontaneous or controlled fluency (i.e., acceptable stuttering if necessary) and the establishment or maintenance of a positive attitude (i.e., feelings and thoughts) toward communication and oneself as a communicator.

Objectives

Objectives for adolescents, adults, and senior adults who stutter are to establish or increase and transfer fluent speech, to develop resistance to potential fluency disrupters, to establish or maintain positive feelings about communication and oneself as a communicator, and to maintain the fluency-inducing effects of treatment on the communication-related behaviors, thoughts, and feelings.

Rationale

The goals and objectives for adolescents, adults, and senior adults appear similar to those for school-age children who stutter. Adolescence through senior adulthood is a time of transition that has been described variously as life after youth, an urge to merge, a solo flight, a predictable series of passages or adult crises, or otherwise a time of change (Sheehy, 1976). The conflict between the establishment of increasing independence and self-sufficiency and the loss of control experienced by people who stutter intensifies for adolescents, adults, and senior adults. While treatment approaches for people during this time of transition may appear similar on the surface, distinctions are seen in how the procedures are implemented, reflecting differences in intrafamily, extrafamily, and psychotherapeutic considerations.

Intrafamily Considerations

People who continue to stutter throughout their life span often develop an entire system of coping to accommodate the life and communication needs. Van Riper (1982) noted, "It is difficult for those who have not possessed or been possessed by the disorder to appreciate its impact on the stutterer's self-concepts, his roles, his way of living" (p. 1). Similarly, Peters and Guitar (1991) stated, "By adulthood, the fear of stuttering and the desire to avoid it create a whole lifestyle. An adult stutterer often copes with stuttering by limiting his work, friends, and fun to those that put fewer demands on his speech" (p. 4). What this means is that adults who stutter often have established a clearly defined personal construct (i.e., about oneself as a person and communicator) and a consistent lifestyle (involving educational and employment ambition, social dynamics, family relationships, and partner selection), both of which increase the individual's resistance to change. The nature of personal constructs was discussed in Chapter 5. Just as the stuttering behaviors have developed and become habituated over time, so have the thoughts, feelings, and attitudes of the person who stutters. Identifying and understanding the client's personal construct provides a major challenge to both clinicians and clients. Clients need to be able to envision how life as a communicator could be better by being fluent; they must develop the ability to imagine things that have never been.

It has been said that it is hard to imagine freedom until one has experienced it. That is why creating opportunities for clients to experience fluency success, and thereby fluency freedom, is so important. Clinicians must be able to observe objectively without judgment; to internalize another adult's reality; to consider alternative points of view (i.e., to distinguish between an event and its multiple interpretations); and to strive toward understanding, insight, and acceptance. These and other clinician competencies are discussed in Chapter 11. Such competencies and component tasks present a particular challenge to clinicians when working with clients whose life passages they have not experienced. For example, although many clinicians have not yet experienced later or senior adulthood, they nevertheless must be able to learn from and thereby relate to their clients in order to meet their clients' diverse needs. Whereas the personal constructs of younger people who stutter are in evolution, that of older people tend to be more firmly established. While personal constructs are not impenetrable, the attitudes, thoughts, and feelings generally that have a longer history and buttress surface behaviors make intervention and the process of change uniquely challenging for clinicians and clients. As will be discussed, the treatment events around which older clients experience fluency success must be salient enough to create a critical incident that compels them to reconsider the way they have viewed themselves and their communicative futures.

Also potentially impacting the intervention process are the communication dynamics within the family system. A change experienced by one member of a family unit affects all other members in some way. For this reason, all family members must be considered, if not involved directly, in treatment. As discussed in Chapter 5, the communication dynamics are affected by the diversity, characteristics, interactions, functions, and life cycle of the family. As the person who stutters and his family grows and matures, certain aspects of the interpersonal dynamics tend to become patternized or ritualized (in terms of who speaks to whom, who orders for whom in restaurants, who seeks whom for advice, who is responsible for providing discipline, and so forth). Clinicians must be aware of and sensitive to such dynamics in order to design, with the family, treatment procedures that are most effective for achieving the changes desired. The family members are absolutely critical participants on the intervention team. The clinician must understand the family system and the feelings, thoughts, and needs of each member. The changing needs of the person who stutters and that of all other family members must be met simultaneously. Doing so creates unique challenges for clinicians, yet is a key to effective intervention. The importance of forming a "therapeutic alliance" with older clients is evident in the following advice, "If you want to help me, help my family" (Hooper, 1996, p. 43).

Extrafamily Considerations

In Chapter 6, we discussed the importance of working collaboratively with members of interdisciplinary teams, as well as with an awareness of the client's unique system of beliefs and traditions. We noted earlier that for adolescents who stutter and are receiving treatment in the schools, clinicians have the luxury of relatively easy access, as needed, to other allied educational, medical, and health professionals—learning disability and other special education specialists, psychometrists, psychologists, principals, counselors, psychotherapists, physicians, nurses, physical therapists, occupational therapists, nutritionists, and dietitians. While access to allied professionals may not be as easy or affordable for people being treated in clinical settings outside of the schools, such collaborative opportunities are available and should be explored as needed. The adult's educational, vocational, and multicultural experiences impact the content and process of treatment. These experiences reflect the client's diversity, which the clinician must understand and relate to within the treatment process. In addition to unique ethnic or cultural beliefs or traditions, clinicians also must understand the client's stage within and individual interpretation of the life cycle. These domains overlap with the client's personal construct and family system. Furthermore, the clinician must understand each individual client's experience as an adolescent, adult, or senior adult, realizing that such life experiences are dynamic. In other words, each individual experiences and is affected by life differently. This means that while generalizations of any group may be tempting, clinicians must be cautious to recognize and address the uniqueness of each person who stutters. Haynes et al. (1992) aptly stated, "Although there are certain generalizations that are useful for planning and conducting evaluations, elderly people are not any more 'all alike' than children or adolescents" (p. 20).

Psychotherapeutic Considerations

Just as the behaviors, thoughts, feelings, and attitudes of people who stutter typically evolve across the life span, so does the distinction between stuttering modification and fluency shaping procedures. As noted in Chapter 7, the relative severity of stuttering behavior has little directly to do with the design of treatment slanted more in one direction of the continuum than the other. Rather, a stuttering modification emphasis is indicated when the client avoids or attempts to conceal his stuttering, demonstrates upset or embarrassment because of the stuttering, feels negative about communicating or himself as a communicator, experiences intentional or inadvertent punishment in any settings because he stutters, and demonstrates a positive response to stuttering modification techniques during trial management. A fluency shaping emphasis is indicated when the client stutters openly without trying to hide or conceal it, does not avoid speaking, exhibits relative emotional neutrality about himself as a communicator, and demonstrates a positive response to fluency shaping techniques during trial management. The severity of stuttering has little directly to do with the relative emphasis of treatment design. The severity of stuttering behavior, however, impacts and is impacted by the thoughts, feelings, and attitudes of the person who stutters. Therefore, stuttering severity may indirectly impact the design of treatment. As discussed in Chapter 7, when fluency shaping and stuttering modification techniques are compared, fluency shaping tends to be more efficient in changing speech behaviors, while stuttering modification tends to be more efficient in reducing fears, changing attitudes, and strengthening generalization.

Procedures

A discussion of the integration of treatment procedures with respect to each objective noted earlier follows. The order in which the objectives are presented reflects a logical sequence that facilitates instruction. In reality, however, the objectives and procedures are multidimensional and overlapping. Readers will notice similarity between procedures discussed here with those discussed for school-age children. Major distinctions are seen more in how the procedures are implemented than in what the procedures are; how the intrafamily, extrafamily, and psychotherapeutic considerations impact the design of treatment; and how thoughts, feelings, and attitudes are addressed. To minimize redundancy, the procedures will be summarized herein with distinctions highlighted as they relate to adolescents, adults, and senior adults. The discussion of treatment procedures in this chapter assumes an understanding of those presented in the last chapter. Readers may want to review the treatment procedures discussed in Chapter 9 now.

Increase and Transfer Fluent Speech

Adolescents, adults, and senior adults who stutter first need to increase the absolute and relative amount of fluent speech—the degree and frequency of fluency compared to itself and that of disfluency over time—and to transfer the fluency facilitating techniques that are learned in treatment to extraclinical settings. To do so, the behaviors, thoughts, and feelings are addressed directly, as follows:

Establish the treatment setting as a "safe house" where clients and clinicians learn with and from each other and, as a consequence, grow together. A safe house is a retreat, a refuge or shelter, where people feel accepted, nurtured, and secure. People of all ages, not just children, need to feel safe. How do we help our client feel safe? We express our sincere interest in him as a person, in his family, his work, his interests. We focus on his communication abilities, what he already is doing well, and only within that positive context do we provide constructive strategies to increase his ability to be and feel fluent. By learning that he is fluent most of the time, that both fluency and disfluency are consequences of what he does, and that he already possesses the ability to be fluent even more often, the client feels empowered and motivated. We help the client maintain such feelings by designing treatment activities in which he will succeed, and we nurture him for his effort and success. Within such an environment, dreams are born. Clients begin to consider how they have viewed communication and themselves as communicators, reconsider the appropriateness of such constructs, and thereby ultimately believe in themselves and their communicative potential.

We noted that within a "safe" environment, clients often express themselves freely, whether fluent or disfluent. In fact, the degree of expression and self-disclosure occasionally takes the unexpecting clinician by surprise. Two former clients, both in their 40s, come to mind. One was a successful attorney who presented the picture of poise and confidence. Handsomely dressed in the finest clothing, sporting a winning smile at best (most frequently) or a poker face at worst, my student clinicians concluded that he felt positive about himself as a person and as a communicator. When I provided him an opportunity to receive positive feedback about his fluent speech and to consider what he wanted to achieve from the treatment experience (a procedure discussed in the next section), my student clinicians were astonished when his eyes began to water and he emotionally described his "impossible dream," a dream that he could be as confident about himself inside as he knew he projected on the outside. He discussed his success as an attorney, noting that he can act, or adopt another persona, all the while continuing to feel insecure about himself as a communicator and continuing to expect impending doom. Another client was a social worker. She ably masked her inner feelings about herself, projecting the picture of confidence and communicative assertiveness. When nurtured regarding her present level of fluency and when asked about her family and work, she described herself as an "impostor," always trying to be something she is not. She also described ongoing turbulence in her marriage and in her work. Both clients, through speech intervention and professional counseling services, ultimately were successful in achieving, transferring, and maintaining more positive feelings and thoughts about themselves in addition to improved speech fluency. The point is that people of all ages flourish within a safe house and that clinicians should not be fooled by deceptive appearances. Recall earlier discussions about the "interiorized stutterer" (Douglass & Quarrington, 1952) and the importance of understanding the client's personal construct and approaching treatment from an interdisciplinary perspective.

Invite treatment objectives from the client. I discuss with my clients what they want and hope to achieve as a result of treatment. Some clients express astonishment at having a professional invite their input. Such clients report being accustomed to being told what will be accomplished and how it will be done. I explain that surely I have ideas about how I would like to see treatment designed. Before sharing those ideas, however, I must understand how the client envisions the treatment experience and what he hopes to accomplish. Some clients know specifically what they want to accomplish (e.g., I want to be able to speak freely without having to scan my words; I want to be able to present psychiatric depositions in court; I want to be able to introduce myself on the golf course without waiting to be introduced.). Others are less specific. Recall the man who could not even imagine what it would be like to be more fluent "because stuttering is all I have ever known." Dialogue of this sort provides the clinician an understanding of the client's previous communication and clinical experiences and attitudes about himself as a communicator. Furthermore, the client begins to understand that his active participation is critical to the process of treatment and its outcome, and that treatment is a joint, collaborative venture.

Discussing what the client hopes to achieve in treatment often leads into designing communication hierarchies, which are lists of speaking situations in order of perceived difficulty. These lists help individualize the treatment experience, facilitate transfer of treatment gains to outside settings, and help the client discuss and thereby understand objectives and related thoughts, feelings, and attitudes. Such hierarchies address a variety of different speaking contexts including individual conversational partners (e.g., family, friends, superiors, strangers), audience size (few to many people), location (home, school, work, stores, restaurants), content (casual conversation about family scheduling, i.e., who will do what and when; versus talking with a professor about a grade or an employer about a promotion or a pay raise), and other contexts. Hierarchies, preliminary estimates of anticipated communication difficulty, are designed initially with the clinician and are expanded by client and family between scheduled treatment meetings. As a working plan, hierarchies are discussed regularly between the clinician and client and revised as necessary. Importantly, hierarchies individualize the treatment experience, reinforce the importance of the client's active participation in treatment, and facilitate generalization of treatment gains to outside settings from the outset of treatment.

Create opportunities for the client to experience fluency success. Nothing stimulates motivation to achieve speech fluency more than fluency success itself. For this reason, I begin with a fluency shaping exercise to enable the client to experience speech fluency, thus helping the client to visualize, internalize, and personalize the goals to which he is striving. Some clients may be unable to project treatment objectives or to visualize themselves as more fluent speakers. I remember one such client in his 50s, whose wife was responsible for him pursuing assessment and treatment. During the evaluation experience, he was skeptical at best about the possible benefits of treatment. I recall vividly his disbelieving glances at his wife as if to say, "Look what you got me into now," and his disparaging comments suggesting, "What does this young whipper-snapper think he has that I might be interested in?" (i.e., emphasis more on "whipper-snapper" than "young"). When engaged in a choral reading experience, his stuttering dramatically (predictably) disappeared resulting in the client's stunned, awestruck expression. He began to laugh, then cry, exclaiming, "What is going on? I've never been able to speak like this." I use a fluency shaping experience deliberately to confirm the presence of stuttering (through differential diagnosis) and to provide the client an experience, sometimes his first, to feel or own fluency directly. Clinicians must heed Manning's (1996) warning, however, not to mislead clients with such procedures yielding dramatic and predictable results. These results are temporary at best and do not by themselves generalize. Clinicians must be mindful not to generate false hopes in clients. Specific procedures, including how the clinician establishes an appropriate model, varies and fades her volume, and returns so as to prevent the client's disfluency, among others, were reviewed in the last chapter.

Many adolescents, adults, and senior adults who stutter expect, based upon previous experiences, that they will stutter. This is part of their personal construct. By creating a foundation of successful speaking experiences as salient as that of stuttering, the client will need to reconsider how he anticipates communication and himself as a communicator. Regular fluency failure has led the client to predict that he will stutter. Deliberately helping the client to amass successful fluency experiences, he will begin to expect speech fluency over stuttering. Therefore, we design treatment so as to create opportunities for speech fluency. The fluency shaping exercise, development of speaking hierarchies, focus on fluency before disfluency, advancing in treatment by small steps, and other aspects of treatment, all are intended to contribute to such an alternative (i.e., fluent) foundation. Data collected on self-comments and speech fluency often result in predictable covariance. Increases in speech fluency often coincide with significant increases in the positive statements about one's communication ability and control over fluency; decreases in speech disfluency coincide with decreases in negative statements about one's communication ability and control over fluency. These data provide a valuable record of treatment efficacy and visual representation to maintain the client's motivation (Gouge & Shapiro, 1989–1990).

The main point, however, is that clinicians must design treatment activities so as to ensure the client's fluency success. The experiences must be dramatic in their effect on the client and facilitate an internalized feeling of control, from which the client will be compelled to reconsider his view of himself as a communicator and how these views have developed, and to begin to entertain adjustments to such views (his personal construct) for the future. Indeed, seeing is believing. This is particularly true for older clients who have longer histories of stuttering, thus requiring more and indisputable data (i.e., successful fluency experiences) from which to consider revisions or alternatives to present personal constructs. Creating such opportunities both within and outside of the treatment setting indeed is within the domain of the speech–language pathologist.

Heighten the client's awareness of his speech fluency. Make the client's speech fluency (i.e., and only then, disfluency) the object of study. After creating initial opportunities for the client to experience fluency success, the client and clinician analyze and discuss the behaviors, thoughts, and feelings that characterize "speech fluency." At first, the clinician assumes greater responsibility by identifying when the client uses gentle speech (e.g., "Right there! You just did it!"), modeling what the client did (e.g., "You said, 'Sshe.'"), and describing (i.e., using slow, gentle, natural sounding speech) what the client did and encouraging its continuation (e.g., "Ffantastic! Yyou wwere rreally ggentle on Sssshe. Keep it up!"). The clinician and client discuss articulator placement, proprioceptive feedback, and the client's thoughts and feelings about his speech and himself as a communicator. As detailed and discussed in Chapter 9, responsibility deliberately shifts to the client who ultimately identifies instances of speech fluency, describing what he did while demonstrating an appropriate speech model, and offering description of proprioceptive feedback and affective reactions, to all of which the clinician offers support and encouragement. Treatment activities of this nature heighten the client's awareness of his fluent speech, convey that he already is doing much of what he needs to do more often, and enable the client to gain a feeling of control by becoming aware of what he is doing right in addition to proprioceptive feedback and his affective reactions.

Recognizing that time in treatment is an important predictor of treatment success (Andrews et al., 1983), specific treatment activities (i.e., extraclinical assignments) conducted regularly between scheduled treatment sessions are critical. Jointly designed between the clinician and client, these assignments must be clear and specific so as to ensure success. Typically, assignments are mastered with the clinician before they are conducted by the client outside of the treatment setting (i.e., recall the three Ds; *d*iscuss, *d*emonstrate, *d*irect/ coach). To heighten the awareness of his own speech fluency, the client may describe initially in a pocket notebook one word per day spoken fluently. These assignments may increase in frequency or focus. For example, assignments may increase the frequency and/or duration of the client's attention to his fluent productions. As noted previously, such fluency focus ultimately is associated with frequently occurring events (e.g., when around anything edible, when using the phone, when asking questions, when engaged in social small talk).

Another common assignment is to have clients attend to the speech of others, particularly those whom they consider to be exemplars of superior or inferior speaking effectiveness. Such assignments help the client discover that much of the speech of people who stutter is fluent; much of the speech of people who do not stutter is disfluent. Watson (1995) noted that, "As a group, adults who stutter may have unrealistic expectations about their speaking capabilities as they view the speech of others as unrealistically excellent" (p. 154). Other assignments change as treatment progresses, reflecting and supporting treatment progress. In this way, while assignments have commonalities across people who stutter, there are unique features reflecting the individual treatment of each client. Daly et al. (1995) underscored the importance of having clients keep "success journals," which help maintain motivation. Furthermore, actually documenting assignments ensures completion (i.e., "no notebook, no change," Lazarus & Fay, 1975; cited in Daly et al., 1995).

Occasionally, clients complain that there is not enough time to do speech assignments outside of treatment. At this, I acknowledge and offer my respect for their busy schedules, restate the importance of treatment conducted between scheduled sessions, and emphasize that the assignments are to be done as much as possible during one's regular activities. Clinicians must be familiar with the client's daily routine and obligations in order to help design assignments that will not interfere with these activities. Assignments require that the client attend to speech fluency during his regular activities in ways that he otherwise would not. Regularly attending to speech fluency is absolutely critical for identifying and replacing habituated speech patterns. Too often, clinicians and clients assume that speech-related assignments are done apart from one's daily speaking interactions. Rather, the assignments need to be viewed as an extension of treatment, both of which are hierarchically based and conducted during one's regular activities. Often the client may be the only one aware that an assignment is being implemented (his conversational partner may not be aware). He may internalize his focus, thus gaining a feeling of fluency control, recording in the speech notebook what has been designed and agreed to when he feels appropriate. This means that the client need not report completion of his assignment in front of his unsuspecting conversational partner. Clients indicate that they want their assignments to be "their business," not drawing additional attention to themselves. I respect and support this need, as long as the client reports his progress regularly and as soon after completion of the assignment as appropriate and possible.

Develop or improve use of fluency facilitating techniques during instances of stuttering. Before working to improve fluency control, the clinician must establish a safe clinical environment, design and plan objectives with the client, immerse the client in speaking experiences that highlight fluency success, and help the client become aware of the nature of his speech fluency and that of other speakers. Once the client understands that speech fluency and disfluency are consequences of things he is doing, then he can both increase the frequency and consistency of the behaviors that result in fluency (i.e., slow, gentle, soft articulatory contact, natural prosody) and vary the forms of disfluency in order to stutter with less abnormality. The knowledge of and the ability to vary what he does enable the client to break the habit strength of stereotyped behaviors and to realize that he has choices. Entertaining and exercising choices is the essence of the feeling of fluency control, a significant factor leading to the behaviors, thoughts, and feelings of speech fluency (Cooper, 1993c; Cooper & Cooper, 1995).

We decide with the client one or two behaviors that he can do that will have a pervasive and positive effect on his speech fluency. Important procedures were reviewed in the last chapter, specifically how to discuss, demonstrate, and direct/coach the characteristics of slow and gentle speech (see Figure 9.2); to discuss the importance of advising clients about dramatic, albeit temporary, increases or decreases in speech fluency during the early stages of treatment; and to help clients become more aware of and in control of their articulatory postures. Furthermore, intervention typically occurs within the context of conversation, resulting in more fluent speech with slightly reduced and more regular rate, softened articulatory contacts, gentle onsets, and continual, gentle airflow. Other procedures reviewed include *dos* and *don'ts* for clinicians and clients learning to establish slow, gentle, normal-sounding speech; useful fluency modification techniques (such as cancellations, pull-outs, and preparatory sets; Van Riper, 1973; see Figure 7.1); and how to combine different forms of treatment including airflow therapy, relaxation, and cognitive restructuring and visualization. Readers are encouraged to review the section in Chapter 9 titled, "Develop or improve use of fluency facilitating techniques during instances of stuttering."

Address thoughts, feelings, and attitudes directly. One distinction in working with adolescents, adults, and senior adults compared to working with school-age children is how thoughts, feelings, and attitudes are addressed. Generally, such discussions, including positive and negative expressions of feeling, are more direct. We may ask the following: "About that slow, gentle fluency we just heard coming out of your mouth, what does it make you think or feel about yourself?" "How did you feel when you asked Amy to go out with you and she did not maintain eye contact when you stuttered?" "What do you feel when you go to discipline your children and you find yourself stuttering?" "What is it like ordering for your wife in a restaurant for the first time in your 35-year marriage?" Such questions and resulting dialogue assume a maturity of expression within the affective domain, for both a client and a clinician.

Clients vary with respect to their comfort and willingness to interact affectively. Some are not comfortable because of lack of experience; others because of negative experience. For example, listeners may have minimized or negated sincere expressions of feeling by responding, "Don't sweat the small stuff" or "Don't let it bother you. Just remember, 'Sticks and stones may break my bones but names will never harm me.'" Some people, particularly older adults, are unwilling to share feelings because, in the words of a former client, "that is something grown men just don't do." Similarly, clinicians vary in their ability and willingness to engage affectively. I have had a number of student clinicians and practicing speech–language pathologists in workshops acknowledge the importance of addressing the thoughts and feelings of a client and his family, but confess discomfort, feeling unprepared actually to do so. Watson (1995) noted the following:

> Despite the clinical and empirical support that attitudes are an important consideration in the therapy process, many clinicians seem to be reluctant to address these more covert aspects or express a low comfort level in dealing with attitudes related to the complex problem of stuttering. This reluctance or discomfort may be due in part to an overall lack of confidence in working with people who stutter. . . . Moreover, many clinicians have little to no formal training in counseling and, hence, feel ill prepared to deal with attitudinal issues. And finally, recent efforts in our field to document treatment efficacy have resulted in a focus on outcomes that can be reliably and validly measured, such as stuttering frequency. Although we are making gains in assessing the more covert aspects of stuttering, we continue to struggle with quantifying these constructs. This struggle is highlighted by clinicians' reluctance to provide services to individuals who report fears, avoidances and severe speech anxiety but exhibit overt behaviors characteristic of stuttering. (p. 144)

Interacting affectively is one of the areas of a clinician's preparation and competence that will be discussed in the next chapter. Not only must clinicians be able to interact affectively, they must see how a client's expressed or unexpressed feelings relate to his personal construct, as well as how his personal construct reflects what he thinks and knows about himself and the world.

Transfer fluency facilitating techniques to extraclinical settings. All aspects of treatment discussed to this point emphasize transfer of speech fluency to extraclinical settings. This is accomplished by (a) emphasizing the active role of the client and his family throughout the treatment experience, (b) individualizing activities for each client, and (c) helping the client gain the feeling and experience of fluency control reflected in behaviors, thoughts, and feelings. For example, specific strategies help construct a foundation on which the client may begin to address developing or improving his use of fluency facilitating techniques during stuttering and understanding and adjusting, as necessary, his thoughts, feelings, and attitudes about himself as a communicator. These strategies include: building an environment within which the client feels safe to take risks with the ongoing and unconditional support of the clinician, inviting objectives from the client, creating opportunities for fluency success, and heightening the client's awareness of his speech fluency and that of other speakers. The fluency facilitating techniques themselves are built upon our knowledge of communication and one's role as a communicator, help internalize the motor sequence and proprioceptive feedback, and address the client's thoughts, feelings, and attitudes. Furthermore, the extraclinical assignments deliberately extend the treatment experience beyond the treatment room; the hierarchies tailor the treatment process for each individual client; and the conversational context within which most treatment is conducted creates a medium that is portable and transferable to any extraclinical setting.

As noted in the last chapter, other aspects that facilitate transfer of increased fluency and fluency facilitating control include (a) emphasizing what the client already is doing that is facilitative of speech fluency, (b) encouraging an increase of the speech fluency already demonstrated, (c) providing strategies for the client to do (rather than focusing on what not to do), (d) building social and situational hierarchies, (e) careful and regular monitoring by the clinician and client, (f) encouraging regular assignments and monitoring by the client and family outside of treatment, (g) designing specific objectives to ensure success, (h) modeling consistently to encourage self-monitoring, (i) shifting responsibility from the clinician to the client, and (j) engaging family and friends in all treatment phases. As before, one major factor emphasizing transfer is the client's active involvement in and ownership of the treatment process from the very beginning.

Develop Resistance to Potential Fluency Disrupters

While clients are engaged in increasing and transferring behaviors, thoughts, and feelings consistent with fluent speech, they need also to develop resistance to the potential effects of fluency disrupters. Several techniques reviewed earlier for transferring fluency facilitating controls to outside settings build the client's resistance to fluency disruption. Other techniques for establishing resistance to behavioral interference will be reviewed here. Those for establishing resistance to affective and cognitive interference will be addressed in the next section.

Introduce direct fluency challenge. Behaviors cannot be considered to be established until they withstand direct, varied, and repeated challenge over time. Therefore, those stimuli that have been eliminated in order to prevent the client from stuttering need to be reintroduced gradually within the treatment setting. These stimuli vary with each client. For example, we may gradually begin to deliberately compete with the client, talk too fast, interrupt, ask a question and then ask another before the client has finished responding to the first, shift topics abruptly, contradict ourselves or our clients, or overestimate the client's familiarity with the topic being discussed. This stage of treatment provides a challenge for the client and clinician but should be entertained in good nature and within a context of fun. Challenge should be varied so that the client successfully maintains his fluency, in terms of both ease and effort. While challenge needs to systematically vary and increase, no constructive purpose is achieved by enabling the client to experience persistent failure. Success begets success; success enhances motivation to achieve increasing levels of challenge. Failure begets failure; failure when sustained causes clients to recoil, solidifying old constructs of being unable and out of control. Clinicians, and ultimately clients, need to regulate the degree of challenge presented to ensure internalized feelings of control and resulting fluency success.

Revisit and advance toward the top rung of communication hierarchies. The hierarchies designed with the clients individualize the treatment process, actively engage clients into that process, and organize extraclinical speaking activities and assignments. Throughout treatment, the client and clinician have reassessed and revised the hierarchies as necessary. In other words, hierarchies were established on the basis of the client's perceptions of how, where, and with whom speech fluency would be increasingly challenged. Experience reveals errors; some contexts prove more difficult, while others prove less difficult, than expected. At this advanced stage of treatment, adolescent, adult, and senior adult clients should be conversing fluently with partners, about topics, and under circumstances listed in the hierarchies as representing the most difficult level of challenge. This might involve asking or responding with a question in class, asking someone out for a social engagement, making phone calls, ordering for one's family in a restaurant, introducing oneself on the golf course, or negotiating with the social security office about funds to be received. Whatever the specific experiences of each client are, he should feel accomplished about his increasing ability to remain fluent and to use fluency facilitating controls in the face of persistent and varied communication disruption.

Prepare for relapse: Relapse happens! Indeed, relapse is more likely among adults than children who stutter (Manning, 1996; Peters & Guitar, 1991; Starkweather et al., 1990). Van Riper (1973) described relapse as more the rule than the exception among adults who stutter. Clients need to be prepared for this likelihood in order to deal constructively with its occurrence. The course of relapse has been described in different ways. Starkweather (1993) noted the following:

With adults the typical scenario is that the controls are given up slowly, behavioral piece by behavioral piece, as the stutterer says to himself, "Oh that was just a little one, hardly anyone could notice; I won't be bothered with it." From this point on, "little ones" are not worried about. Then pretty soon, a behavior that is a little "bigger" is let go without control, and the level of uncontrolled behavior is recalibrated to a higher level of acceptance. Slowly, the old behaviors return, until suddenly the client realizes that he has begun to stutter again. . . . Occasionally, the relapse does occur suddenly, when the stutterer makes a kind of decision that he just cannot stand the burden of using controls any longer—he would rather stutter. Then there is a sudden crash. (p. 164)

Describing and predicting relapse, Manning (1996) noted the following:

The frequency of overt stuttering events is one indicator [predictor], but usually it is far from the only and typically not the initial indicator of regression. . . . The attitude and cognitive aspects of the problem, often in the form of negative self-talk, are likely to take the lead in the progression of relapse. As elements of avoidance and fear begin to multiply and increasingly influence the speaker's decision making, overt stuttering will not be far behind. (p. 241)

Despite our best efforts at prevention, relapse may be unavoidable. Nevertheless, we must help clients and their families understand the nature of relapse and prepare them for the likelihood of its occurrence. If knowledge is power, then talking with the client about relapse is the first step in preparation. It has been said that "forewarned is forearmed." Once informed (i.e., forewarned), the client can develop behavioral, affective, and cognitive strategies in advance in order to respond constructively should relapse happen (i.e., forearmed), and to view the experience as a developmental opportunity within the progression of fluency establishment, transfer, and maintenance. Left unprepared, the emotional consequences resulting from the client's communicative defenselessness and helplessness can be deleterious to the process and progress of treatment.

I remember an experience vividly that reflects a critical moment in my growth as a communicator. It also indicates the benefits of being prepared for relapse and developing constructive strategies for dealing with its recurrence. For more than 20 years, I experienced severe stuttering behavior and feelings of incompetence as a person and as a communicator. Over the years, however, I have achieved a level of spontaneous fluency and positive feelings and thoughts about myself, reverting infrequently to controlled fluency during times of extreme fatigue or stress. A university meeting several years ago was a doozy! Meeting in the Chancellor's Conference Room, the chairperson suggested that we go around the boardroom table and introduce ourselves. "No, don't do it! Not today! We all know each other," I thought to myself. I had been up at 4:00 a.m. grading papers, and the meeting was at 4:30 p.m. The participants were all senior faculty members and high-ranking administrators within our university. In other words, I was exhausted and these were to me very important people, a sure formula for disaster! To make matters worse, the first to introduce himself established a quick, crisp, staccato pattern of introduction. It went something like, *Bum-Bum,* (pause) *Bum!* I could tell we were each allowed two (i.e., and only two) bursts of sound. Each member followed the same pattern—Alvin

Jerkface, Psychology; Rita Repulsa, Criminal Justice; and so on. Great way to get up close and personal. On with the sweaty palms, the beating heart, the red face. No way out!

As it came to my turn, I was rehearsing internally, telling myself, "You can do it. Just sound as pitiful as everyone else." As I began to introduce myself, I felt my articulators tensing slightly, but not locking. I knew I could do it. I indulged in the slightest delay, the most minute deviation, before beginning, poised and relatively relaxed given the circumstances. Just as I was shaping the *d* in David, I heard—to my horror—the person who was to follow me say, "David Shapiro, Human Services. Come on. Say it!" Could this really be happening? While seemingly the entire boardroom started to laugh, I reflected—for one humiliated moment—on many things timeless, placeless, nameless. As the laughter subsided, I regrouped and said, "David Shapiro, Human Services." After a momentary, tensionless pause, I did my *Bum-Bum,* (pause) *Bum*. As the introductions continued, I heard very little. While I was tempted to indulge in feelings of self-pity and worthlessness (wondering, "How could I have been so stupid? How could they have ever hired me *and* tenured me *and* promoted me to full professor?"), I stopped and realized that this experience was not about me at all. It did not reflect on me in the least. Instead, it reflected on the person who interrupted me and demonstrated his professional immaturity, intolerance, and impertinence. Acknowledging his unprofessionalism only to myself, I felt so glad to be me. We all have to live with ourselves. Feeling proud despite my faults, I smiled so big inside. What is the story about the last laugh? It has to do with coping strategies and continuing to feel successful and maintaining integrity in the face of potential adversity. At least, that's how I remember it.

Blood (1995a, 1995b) addressed directly the issue of relapse and its management. He designed a relapse management program for adolescents and adults who stutter. Taking the form of a cognitive–behavioral board game, the program includes "training techniques in problem solving, general communication skills, and assertiveness, as well as coping responses for stuttering episodes and realistic expectations for fluency and relapse" (1995b, p. 169). The program's name, POWER[2], is an acronym for *P*ermission, *O*wnership, *W*ell-Being, *E*steem of One's Self, *R*esilience, and *R*esponsibility. Each step addresses different topics and related activities including stuttering, the impact of stuttering on client's lives, ways to deal and cope with the challenges of stuttering, and the concept of resilience or hardiness. According to Blood, the program provides an opportunity to teach and discuss awareness of the problem, problem-solving techniques, negotiating and owning short- and long-term goals (for speaking, feeling, and thinking), facilitators and inhibitors of carryover, self-esteem issues related to relapse (e.g., speaking assertiveness, self-talk, enhancing feelings and thoughts about stuttering and oneself), perceived control issues (e.g., control over and reactions to relapse, realistic objectives, mental and physical persistence), social support factors in maintaining fluency, and assumption of responsibility (i.e., change and functional use of motor and cognitive skills, identity change, and different types of coping).

Establish or Maintain Positive Thoughts and Feelings About Communication and Oneself as a Communicator

We have noted repeatedly that one's behaviors, thoughts, and feelings are intricately and dynamically interrelated. In other words, one's attitudes (i.e., thoughts and feelings) affect one's behavior (i.e., speech fluency); one's behavior affects one's attitudes. The connection between attitudes and behavior is not a novel idea. Blood (1995b) noted that, "The fact remains that the motor changes of reduced rate, prolongation, airflow changes, or continuous phonation are necessary. However, these changes may be maintained and enhanced with the aid of counseling techniques and self-monitoring skills for cognitive change" (p. 172). Daly et al. (1995) indicated that, "A combination of both behavioral and cognitive treatment strategies . . . is necessary for successful treatment outcome" (p. 167). Cooper and Cooper (1995) noted that, "From the beginning of therapy, the focus should be on the development of feelings, attitudes, and motor skills that enhance the feeling of control. Behaviorally focused fluency programs not addressing the attitudinal and cognitive features of oral language fluency control may be the single major factor leading to the needless guilt and shame experienced by individuals with chronic perseverative stuttering syndrome" (p. 130). Therefore, the client's attitudinal and cognitive strategies for developing and maintaining a positive attitude about himself as a communicator are at least as important as the behavioral strategies for maintaining the motor skills associated with speech fluency. The attitudinal and cognitive strategies are addressed in this section.

Treat teasing and relapse as probabilities rather than possibilities. Empower clients with constructive strategies to withstand the potential ill effects of teasing and relapse. Clients need to be prepared with strategies to remain positive about communication and themselves as communicators in the face of teasing or relapse. Teasing tends to occur less frequently among older clients than among children. However, the relative infrequency of occurrence may exacerbate the potential ill effects. As with children, negative thinking inhibits fluency facilitating control and increases the likelihood of relapse. The treatment as described helps clients maintain positive thinking. By focusing on, understanding, and increasing the client's fluent speech; by creating opportunities for the client to succeed; by involving the client and his family in all aspects of the treatment process; and by attending to and supporting the client's feelings and thoughts related to speech fluency, the client moves from feeling unable and out of control to able and in control. Other strategies, however, often are necessary to combat negative thinking and learned helplessness in order to achieve positive thinking, self-assurance, and fluency success.

A variety of cognitive coping strategies is useful to help clients adjust to their improved speech fluency and to react constructively to teasing and relapse. Recall Daly (1988) noting that, "Too many of our clients get fluent in their mouths but not in their heads" (p. 34). Before a person can change, he must understand and adjust how he views himself. Relaxation, mental imagery, visualization, and positive self-talk may be used as discrete elements for cognitive intervention or may be used in combination (Daly et al., 1995). Relaxation is the refreshment of body and mind resulting from being aware of and voluntarily adjusting the relative tension perceived in specific or general body locations. This is done with or without external stimuli (e.g., auditory, visual, proprioceptive, and so on). Mental imagery is picturing or mentally rehearsing an event before it occurs. Just as anticipation of fluency failure can contribute to its occurrence (as in a self-fulfilling prophesy), rehearsing, visualizing, and internalizing fluency success (i.e., specific to the task or stage in treatment) contributes to its occurrence. During the recent Olympic Games, several athletes interviewed after their successful events reported having mentally imagined their entire performance before it actually occurred. Much has been written about and by persons in athletics, science, and business who use or recommend mental imagery.

Visualization is creating soothing pictures in one's mind that contribute to a more relaxed state, positive self-image, and behavioral adjustment. We discussed earlier visualization and relaxation exercises in which initially the clinician led the client through a description of a leaf moving gently on a flowing stream; eventually the client led the clinician through the exercise; and ultimately the client internalized the experience completely with no verbalization. Positive self-talk, also referred to as "affirmation training" (Daly et al., 1995), is making statements about oneself in positive and first person language. These statements may reflect truth, or what the client wishes to be true in the future. Daly et al. (1995) noted that, "Repeating positive, success-oriented statements increases positive expectations of future improvement and strengthens the students' belief in their own abilities" (p. 166). In the example earlier in this chapter, as I was sitting around the boardroom anticipating introducing myself, I deliberately relaxed my articulators, mentally rehearsed what I was about to say with both fluency and confidence, and engaged in positive self-talk (e.g., "You can do it. You are fluent. Picture yourself relaxed. Now just do it slowly, gently, and natural sounding, and with confidence."). These cognitive coping procedures are related to many others referred to earlier. For example, we have emphasized the importance of identifying and rewarding clients for their speech fluency initially and throughout treatment, and of having clients maintain a record of fluency success in their speech notebooks. Daly et al. (1995) noted the following:

> When practicing speech techniques and cognitive strategies, students are encouraged to strive to do their best, rather than trying to be perfect or the best. . . . The speech–language pathologist's commitment to being positive, patient, and persistent with adolescent students with fluency disorders is critical for maintaining therapeutic trust. (p. 166)

Help clients maintain positive thinking about communication and themselves as communicators. The treatment procedures and cognitive coping strategies that were reviewed for helping clients withstand the potential ill effects of teasing and relapse also help clients maintain positive thinking about themselves as communicators. Additionally, there are specific treatment procedures that may help clients remain focused on their successes and, as a result, positive and optimistic in nature. For example, such techniques as reframing, confronting, encouraging, empathic listening, and using humor (Blood, 1995a; Manning, 1996) may be used singly or in combination. For example, let's consider those who "get fluent in their mouths but not in their heads." These are the clients who, despite remarkable improvement in the fluency of their speech behavior, continue to view themselves as communicatively ineffective, unable, and out of control.

Reframing means shifting perspective to consider another point of view. When the client says, "I always stutter," or "I never will be able to talk right," the clinician can help the client realize that a such a global assessment is not based in fact. In fact, the data collected by both clinician and client suggest that the client is steadily improving, although there seems to be a mismatch between what the client does and how he thinks and feels about himself. Confrontation is a direct form of bringing something to someone's attention for identification or confirmation. For example, when the client demonstrates slow, gentle, natural sounding speech, the clinician might say, "That's it! Did you catch it? You just said the *b* in boy really gently." I noted previously that ultimately we want the client to identify, describe, and praise himself when he hears himself using speech fluency or successfully completing any other treatment procedure or assignment. Encouragement is another clinical technique. It helps the client build on what he has just said or done. For example, when the client begins to identify his own disfluency and says, "I just did it," the clinician might say, "That's right, you surely did. Tell me more about what you just did and how it felt." Empathic or active listening is yet another technique, although somewhat less direct, of seeking clarification or confirmation of what the client just said. It reinforces that the clinician is interested, engaged, and understands what the client is sharing, and that she is sensitive to the needs and emotions being expressed. It confirms to the client that he is operating within a safe house. The clinician might say, "So you're saying that you feel you were denied the promotion because of your stuttering," or "It sounds like you feel excited about the successes you just shared."

A final method of helping clients maintain a positive outlook on communication and themselves as communicators is the use of therapeutic humor. Manning (1996) discussed the clinical implications of humor by indicating its positive correlation with personality characteristics including enthusiasm, playfulness, hopefulness, excitement, and vigorousness, and its negative correlation with fear, depression, anger, indifference, and aloofness. Furthermore, humor invites a natural expression of amusement (laughter) in response to an immediate conceptual shift using contradiction, incongruity, or integration of contradictory ideas. Manning noted that humor reflects the spontaneity in timing within a therapeutic relationship that has achieved some level of intimacy, and that humor and laughter frequently occur during successful treatment sessions. Clinicians need to be able to model the ability to see humor in life, to value humor as a tonic, and to laugh at oneself. The ability to laugh at oneself and life's ironies enables a client (i.e., and the clinician) to remain positive for the long haul.

I still remember fretting with two of my colleagues years ago in a hotel room the night before our first presentations at a national conference. While each of us had a personal background of severe stuttering, we achieved different levels of fluency success. Discussing our concern about being able to control our fluency the following day, one of us began to stutter deliberately, the next outstuttered the first, and before long we were convulsively stuttering and laughing at ourselves. Does this mean that we are insensitive to the problem of stuttering? I don't think so. We were among friends and we felt safe. Being able to laugh at ourselves and each other enabled us to reframe our concern (i.e., to realize that our global concern was unfounded), to shift perspective (i.e., to realize that we were all well prepared and that we should derive confidence in that), and to enjoy the therapeutic catharsis resulting from contradiction and incongruity (i.e., three academics demonstrating their worst nightmare in Technicolor).

Ultimately, this experience enabled us to succeed the following day, knowing that we had the necessary fluency facilitating controls, knowledge, confidence, and strength of friendship.

Talk with clients in positive ways. Help clients understand how they speak, think, and feel about themselves. Clinicians must be aware of and both sensitive and responsive to a client's personal construct. Clinicians ask, "How do we assess and influence the degree to which a client's thoughts about himself are positive, while at the same time trying to increase the client's fluency?" Similarly as with our school-age clients, this is influenced by how we talk with clients and what we say, and the opportunities we provide for clients to experience successful control over their speech and to believe in themselves. Enlightenment awaits both clinicians and clients who videotape-record and analyze their own talking. Clinicians should listen to what they say to their clients, as well as how they say it. Does the clinician convey sincere enthusiasm about the client's potential, focus on what the client can rather than cannot do, address fluency at least as often as disfluency, use positive terminology even when offering corrections, invite the client's input for treatment-related decisions, reflect on what the client has shared, involve the client actively in the treatment process, and demonstrate both patience and persistence regarding the client's self-discoveries? Clients should listen to how they speak about themselves. Does he emphasize what he can do and has done successfully? Does he reflect an awareness that both fluency and disfluency reflect the consequences of things he is doing, albeit differently? Does he take charge, remaining active in his role within the treatment process, or does he defer passively to the clinician? A variety of interaction analysis systems, discussed in Chapter 12, is available for the clinician and client to facilitate observation of the clinical process and changes as appropriate (Anderson, 1988; Boone & Prescott, 1972; Casey, Smith, & Ulrich, 1988; Schubert, Miner, & Till, 1973; Shapiro, 1994a).

Maintain the Fluency-Inducing Effects of Treatment

We discussed in the last chapter that of all the treatment objectives, maintenance of speech fluency after the completion of treatment proves to be the most vexing. As the client improves throughout treatment, his remaining speech disfluency comes to be less handicapping. The communicative need, which has been the source of great motivation, wanes. Therefore, safeguards for maintenance of speech fluency must be addressed early, directly, and throughout treatment. Some specific suggestions follow:

Help the client become his own clinician. Both transfer and maintenance of speech fluency originate at the beginning, rather than the end, of formal treatment. In word and deed, the client must assume increasing degrees of responsibility for monitoring and regulating his speech behavior. Both the client and clinician must understand and be committed to this basic objective and must be able to relinquish and assume different responsibilities as appropriate. The clinical process is dynamic. The feedback loop (i.e., the process by which a client receives feedback and adjusts his behaviors, thoughts, and feelings thereto) must move from being externally controlled (by the clinician) to internally controlled (by the client). Clients must resist the temptation to become dependent upon the clinician. Clinicians must be aware of and address their own need to be needed, so as to serve, rather than exploit, their client. Maintenance of speech fluency is accomplished by discussing the roles and responsibilities of each participant and jointly establishing objectives, designing procedures and assignments, providing feedback, and monitoring speech production and progress. Initially, the clinician is more assertive. However, as the client comes to understand the process and share in its ownership, he assumes increasing responsibilities for these and other responsibilities related to clinical decision making. The more the client participates actively in treatment and both internalizes and habituates the key elements of the process, the more he will maintain the behaviors, thoughts, and feelings conducive to speech fluency.

Decrease the frequency of scheduled treatment. Once the treatment goals addressing behaviors, thoughts, and feelings related to speech fluency have been met and are being maintained—and the client is using his fluency facilitating controls independently, assuming responsibility for self-evaluation and self-monitoring, as well as feeling positive and in control—then the frequency of scheduled direct treatment is decreased. Doing so reflects the client's success and increasing responsibility for managing his communication and himself as a communicator. The scheduled meetings of decreasing frequency become maintenance checks, wherein the clinician actively listens while the client summarizes, evaluates, and projects his ability to internalize communication responsibility.

During several recent monthly meetings of this nature, one client who was 22 years old discussed how excited and proud she was to have self-monitored and adjusted her fluency during a series of oral reports and other presentations in college classes. As she reviewed and shared the notes she had collected about these experiences, she indicated, "I knew I could do it. It felt so good to be in control and I am so happy inside." Another client who was 55 recalled from his notes how he had remembered to focus on his fluency facilitating controls during visits to the barber shop, auto parts store, physical therapist, and physician. He shared that the experience at the barber shop was particularly noteworthy because he elected to speak knowing that he did not need to, and because his audience grew from only the barber initially to eight others who entered consecutively. He shared, "The fluency was good and I was in control. I am so pleased about that." These experiences are no small victories. Furthermore, they reflect the importance of enabling the client to become his own clinician and, in so doing, of decreasing the frequency of scheduled treatment.

Maintain regular maintenance checks of decreasing frequency for at least 2 years post-treatment. As noted, the client becomes increasingly responsible for reporting, evaluating, monitoring, and adjusting his behaviors, thoughts, and feelings. Initially, the maintenance checks with the clinician may be once monthly, moving to bimonthly, every 4 months, 6 months, 1 year, then 2 years. The importance of the client internalizing the role of the clinician and assuming responsibility for his communication skills must be underscored. We noted earlier that the risk of relapse typically is greater for adolescents, adults, and senior adults than for children and for those whose pretreatment level of fluency is less severe (Manning, 1996; Peters & Guitar, 1991). Most clients experience the need for some type of follow-up. Therefore, they should be prepared for this fact and should feel welcome and encouraged to return for as long as they need it. Needing to return for some type of refresher should not be seen as failure; rather, it should be seen as a necessary component of long-term change. Individual follow-up, group treatment sessions, or support or self-help group meetings generally will enable clients to continue making progress.

Institute regular, client-initiated benchmarking. In the last chapter, we discussed the concept of benchmarking as a means to facilitate maintenance of speech fluency. Benchmarking means reassessing where one is, where one wants to be, and addressing any discrepancy. The client benchmarks by reassessing his progress regularly with respect to each long-term goal and makes adjustments as necessary. Once maintenance of fluency is receiving the client's primary attention, he benchmarks his present level of fluency-related behaviors, thoughts, and feelings on the basis of pre- and post-treatment levels and projections. If the client's present level of functioning is consistent with earlier projections, then he internalizes the reward for maintaining progress. If not, the client interprets the discrepancy with respect to relevant circumstances and designs a realistic, specific strategy for change. Occasionally, when a client feels he has dipped with respect to expectations, a follow-up visit with the clinician in a supportive, nurturing environment proves beneficial. Similarly, ongoing support from other members within the communication system proves invaluable for maintaining the long-term benefits of treatment.

For example, I met recently with a 44-year-old client whom I dismissed from formal treatment over a year ago. She is a mother, wife, and successful professional and had been benchmarking successfully with respect to behaviors, thoughts, and feelings. However, recently she noticed an increase in her disfluency, which had generated old feelings of being out of control. She described her feelings as follows: "It's like I am falling from a building not knowing how far I will fall, what's at the bottom, or whether or not someone is there to catch me." When we met, she brought a friend who also is a professional colleague. It became evident that the client was using fluency facilitating controls successfully, but was internalizing an unfounded fear that her controls would fail her. It also became evident that she was experiencing stress within her family because her husband became unemployed several months prior to our meeting. She decided to increase the frequency of her benchmarking from biweekly to weekly, during which she reviewed her daily log of use of fluency controls and resulting positive feelings and thoughts about herself as a communicator. During the meeting, she discovered that she had been triangulating her financial and emotional concerns resulting from her husband's unemployment onto her speech which she perceived as a loss of control. She decided to explore the family counseling that she and her husband had already discussed. She wrote to me later that her speech fluency gains were being maintained, as was her positive attitude about herself as a communicator. She also shared that the family counseling sessions were successful, that she and her husband were talking openly, and that his employment options appeared bright. This example illustrates the importance of fluency-related benchmarking, supportive follow-up visits with the clinician, and monitoring personal constructs and family systems.

Deliberately revisit the past. Clients are prepared to view a videotape of pre-treatment communication for the two purposes previously reviewed (i.e., to celebrate the client's accomplishments and to maintain the post-treatment level of speech fluency). The preparation helps the client focus on the forms of disfluency that he has left behind and the fluency that has resulted. When viewing the videotape, the client is encouraged to discuss his previous thoughts and feelings about himself as a communicator, and how these have evolved and changed in a more positive direction as a result of treatment success. It is particularly important for clinicians to be sensitive and supportive at this time. While the clinician intends to maintain a positive focus, viewing the videotape is disturbing for some clients. It is hard to return to times past and see oneself struggle and contort. Even within the context of, "Look at all you have left behind," some clients nevertheless experience such feelings as, "How could I have been so dreadful for so many years?" Clinicians are challenged to maintain a delicate balance between remaining focused on the positive aspects of change while presenting a disturbing, albeit past, reality, the combination of which rewards progress, yet prevents a return to pretreatment levels.

It is not uncommon for clinicians to follow-up with clients by phone after such a visit to times past to ensure the maintenance of a positive attitude. Sometimes, clients feel positive and accomplished when reviewing the videotape with the clinician, but find that reality strikes after they leave the security and support provided by the clinician. Some clients reflect on the videotape and center on the bizarre or grotesque nature of their earlier disfluency. Older clients occasionally confront feelings of how things could have been different had they accomplished fluency success earlier in their life. Some wonder about career choices, financial status, family issues, even selection of partners. We discussed earlier that intervention with adolescents, adults, and senior adults in ways might be like opening a can of worms. Every person has his own Pandora's Box. Nowhere is ongoing support and understanding of the client and his family more important than now. And nowhere is an appreciation of the dynamics of one's personal construct and the uniqueness of one's family system more important than here. Memories are dear and exist in the soul of a person. Clinicians must be aware of the territory they are exploring.

Reexamine the client's personal construct. Be sure the changes are integrated into the client's personal construct. In order for affective, behavioral, and cognitive changes to be maintained after the conclusion of treatment, the changes must be integrated into one's personal construct. Unless the client feels that the changes "fit," they will not last. We have discussed the importance of helping the client shift from feeling unable and externally controlled to feeling able and internally in control. We have done this by helping the client understand the nature of his fluency and that he already possessed a great deal of fluency and the skills necessary to be fluent even more often. We deliberately designed opportunities for the client to experience fluency success, and we involved him and his family actively in the treatment process and related decisions. From amassing a foundation of fluency success, the client had to take, with our support, a closer look at how he has viewed himself as a communicator. We have helped him to know what to say and how to speak within social constraints (i.e., to develop pragmatic fluency), now that he can predict speech fluency. We have helped the client in all ways to think of himself as something other than a person who stutters and to make changes in his lifestyle throughout the treatment process that support the evolving view of himself. Despite our best efforts to enable the client to change and to feel comfortable with the changes, some report not feeling like themselves. They feel that they have deceived everyone but themselves. How we integrate such changes into one's personal construct represents a major difference in our work with adolescents, adults, and senior adults.

It is true that behaviors, thoughts, and feelings about which clients or any of us remain unaware perpetuate. It is also true that older clients tend to develop more firmly held opinions about communication and themselves as communicators, yet possess relative emotional and cognitive maturity to be able to analyze directly, with our assistance, such opinions and constructs. These opinions form the core of one's personal construct, the cumulative and integrative filters through which one views his world and predicts his future. The combination of opinions and potential for insight and change can be used to the client's communication advantage by a knowledgeable clinician. I have emphasized the importance of identifying and understanding the client's personal construct, which provides a window into one's affective self. In order to help clients establish and maintain positive feelings about communication and themselves as communicators, the client and clinician need to identify the client's feelings, assess the extent to which such perspectives are justified in fact, and determine whether a reconsideration is warranted. This process must be systematic, as it addresses sensitive issues including thoughts, feelings, and behaviors, essentially the heart of our client.

In earlier publications (Moses & Shapiro, 1996; Shapiro & Moses, 1989), my colleague and I presented a model of problem solving based on cognitive learning theory that has applications when a client encounters a novel situation, thus presenting a clinical problem. Adjusting one's personal construct to changes experienced in communication competence is one such situation. The model contains a series of component operations that generates a variety of procedures, enabling the clinician and client initially to identify their own perspective and ultimately to shift perspective so as to consider, if not to construct, alternative points of view. The model will be applied briefly to a client who is adjusting his personal construct to accommodate a communicative change (i.e., improved speech fluency and communicative independence). This discussion assumes that the client understands how his thoughts, feelings, and behaviors are interrelated and represented within his personal construct.

The client may be asked to write or present an autobiographical account of himself as a communicator, focusing particularly on behaviors, thoughts, and feelings. As noted previously, earlier accounts typically reveal that thoughts and feelings expressing inability (e.g., "I can't be fluent. I never could talk well.") and being externally controlled (e.g., "Why does this stuttering have to happen to me?") are often paired with observed speech disfluency. As the client succeeds in the treatment activities described earlier, thereby demonstrating increases in speech fluency, his comments should reflect a shift to thoughts and feelings of ability (e.g., "I can do this!") and control (e.g., "I know I can be fluent by remembering to speak slowly, gently, and naturally more often."). This positive shift in thoughts and feelings, when paired with improved behavior, should be discussed explicitly with the client so as to facilitate the adjustment in how the client views himself as a communicator. If the client continues to feel unable and out of control (i.e., externally controlled) despite observable evidence to the contrary, then this mismatch between his thoughts and feelings compared to his speech behavior represents a significant clinical problem and must be addressed directly. In doing so, it is useful to understand a series of component operations of problem solving (Shapiro & Moses, 1989) from the client's perspective, as follows:

1. *Identification*—identifying a problem from one's own perspective

2. *Disequilibrium*—feeling uncomfortable or anxious as a result of identifying a problem

3. *Reflection*—thinking about and initiating causal interpretations

4. *Exploration*—discovering and differentiating one's own from another's perspective

5. *Solidification of conflicting perspectives*—believing even more strongly in one's own perspective. Typically, within the operation of solidification, disequilibrium intensifies

6. *Negotiation*—internal distancing and abstraction from one's own perspective

7. *Modification of perspective*—generating problem-solving procedures. Within this operation, resolution of conflict entails applying or constructing knowledge, thereby reducing disequilibrium

8. *Evaluation*—evaluating the efficacy of procedures and solutions in terms of the resolution of the problem

9. *Construction or modification of causal theories*—the end goal of problem solving. In this final operation, causal theories are constructed, or at least modified, by reflecting on and interpreting events with reference to causality

These component operations generate a variety of possible procedures for the client who is adjusting his personal construct to accommodate observed changes. These procedures will be discussed briefly and applied to the experiences of one former client. Specifically, the client's feelings about himself as a communicator were resistant to change, despite his improved speech fluency.

First, the client must identify that a problem exists (recognizing the mismatch in thoughts and feelings compared to behaviors) and be able to describe the problem from his own perspective (e.g., "I feel like an impostor," "I don't feel fluent even though I behave fluently.").

Second, the client identifies and reflects upon his assumptions about the problem situation and about learning and change. The client reflects on the mismatch, causal elements (i.e., the three Ps), and similarities and differences to other life events. The client may become anxious because the feeling "just doesn't make sense" and is inconsistent with the observed behavior. Interestingly, the client's increase in disequilibrium occasionally may lead to increased disfluency. This turn of events may be circular, leading the client to feel, "You see, I don't feel fluent inside because I just stuttered again," which may reduce disequilibrium temporarily. The client needs to be reminded that he is and has been fluent, and specifically that is the observation that must agree with the way he feels.

Third, the client evaluates the problem situation from the perspectives of all participants involved or affected. Those affected might include the clinician, family members, friends, and co-workers, among others. The client reflected, "Everybody is telling me that I sound so good. I have improved. I know I have. Why can't I believe it? Why can't I feel as fluent as I sound?"

Fourth, the client and clinician specify and define the desired change. Once the client is aware of his own perception and assumptions and those of others, the desired change is discussed. Specifically, the client wanted to integrate his improved speech behavior into his thoughts and feelings (i.e., he wanted to feel fluent, internally in control of his communication abilities, and thereby to think of himself as a relatively fluent speaker).

Fifth, the client and clinician plan a strategy for provoking change with respect to the problem situation that has been identified and evaluated. Specifically, the client agreed to do three things—to engage in visualization and cognitive imagery one time per day of himself as a fluent speaker (i.e., to mentally rehearse the behavioral synchrony and proprioceptive feedback, thoughts, and feelings of fluency, like the gymnast visualizing the perfect routine); to engage in one additional speaking interaction per day that would not otherwise occur (i.e., deliberately flooding himself with successful speaking opportunities); and to evaluate and benchmark his progress every weekend. The client and clinician met to discuss and evaluate the strategy implemented.

Sixth, the client and clinician implement the strategy for provoking the change that has been described. The plan was implemented as described.

Seventh, the client and clinician evaluate the strategy implemented regarding the change achieved. The client and clinician met as described, agreeing that the data collected were indicative of a successful strategy. The client reported that the strategy enabled him to focus more on his thoughts and feelings, and that the flood of additional successful speaking experiences resulted in greater confidence as he approached unplanned and more challenging speaking encounters.

Eighth, the client and clinician reflect on their assumptions about the problem situation, learning, and change in light of the change achieved. This opportunity to reflect enabled the client and clinician to clarify their own assumptions, agreeing that behavior (i.e., affective, behavioral, or cognitive domain) about which we become aware can be changed; that about which we remain unaware perpetuates. The client noted that, "I really feel in control now, knowing that I can feel as fluent as I sound. I guess you can teach an old dog new tricks."

Finally, the client and clinician, individually or jointly, approach new problem situations with clarified assumptions and the wisdom gained from focused and shared experience.

These nine procedures reviewed here originated from the component operations noted earlier and can be applied to the resolution of novel or problem situations through a systematic, nonjudgmental, objective strategy. Systematic problem solving contributes to the client's and clinician's growth as people, communicators, and clinical colleagues (i.e., "comrades in a common struggle"), and particularly to the client's communicative skills.

Integrate treatment changes within the communication system. It is not only clients who need to adjust to the affective, behavioral, and cognitive changes resulting from increased fluency and communication independence. Conversational partners within the client's communication system (including family, friends, and co-workers) need to adjust to the "new" speaker as well. With increased communication skills, the client will participate more and will take increased communicative risks and conversational partners must adjust their expectations. Clinicians can help the conversational partners understand the nature of the changes that are occurring, how to react in ways that are supportive of such changes, and ultimately, how to continue to feel needed in different ways. Family members who have become accustomed to speaking for another who stutters will need direction in when and how to let him speak for himself (e.g., in restaurants, on the phone, and at family gatherings). Teachers and employers who have become accustomed to altering tasks so as not to penalize the person who stutters will need guidance in how to include the client and what to expect of him. I have found that spouses need to get used to their partners talking so much more. Grandchildren are not accustomed to grandpa talking so much, or vice versa. There are new rules, and all must continue to be supported along the change process.

In most cases, people within the communication system are more than willing to change with the person who stutters and appreciate the guidance and support along the way. Parents are happy to see their adolescent children become more independent on the phone, in social settings, and in school or work activities. Spouses or significant others are more than happy to be introduced, rather than always scanning the social situation to determine whether to introduce the person who stutters so as to prevent him embarrassment or wait to be introduced. In most cases, change is welcomed by those who care for and communicate with people who stutter. However, there are situations in which conversational partners are resistant to change, particularly when the relationship is based more on need than mutual support. In such relationships, a partner who has felt needed and important as a ready spokesperson may feel threatened by the increasing communicative independence of the person who stutters. Recall from Chapter 1 the woman who conveyed that while she would do anything to support her husband's fluency goals, she was concerned that he would find her "less attractive" when he achieved fluency independence.

I always will remember with regret a family for whom the changes created by one member's improved fluency could not be integrated into the interpersonal dynamics. A 35-year-old man referred himself to me after a 15-year hiatus from fluency shaping treatment. Interestingly, his earlier clinical reports indicated that he was dismissed because all of his fluency goals had been met; however, his prognosis was "guarded." He and his wife had two sons. He explained that his continuing stuttering was interfering with his parenting and his work. In an individualized program that combined stuttering modification and fluency shaping, his progress was steady. I met with both of his sons during the first several months, yet was unable to meet with his wife. While I made several appointments at times that were intended to accommodate her work schedule, she ultimately canceled each one. When I initiated phone contacts, she seemed rushed and I always felt that my calls were at times that were inconvenient for her. I expressed early that everyone within a communication system affects and is affected by everyone else. I believed that his improvement would continue and that the changes caused by it would need to be integrated into the family system.

Ultimately, I never met with the man's wife. At my suggestion, he pursued family counseling; however, they were divorced within 1 year. Did the improvement in his speech cause the divorce? Probably not, but the changes imposed by his increasing communication independence only contributed to and revealed an unstable marriage. In other words, the changes created demands that exceeded the family's capacity to remain integrated as a family unit. Perhaps the communication changes presented the proverbial "last straw." In most cases, one's gain contributes to the gain of all (creating a win–win situation). In this case, one's gain was seen as another's loss (yielding a win–lose, or zero sum situation). According to my client, his wife felt no longer useful because she was not needed as his spokesperson. If I had not actively pursued involvement of his wife and integration of the communication changes within the family system, I would have felt directly responsible for the dissolution of the family. The moral here is to be mindful of the impact of communication changes within the family system, and to do all possible to facilitate those changes, while being sensitive to the unique roles and contributions of each member.

Respect the primary role of the conversational partners and help support their needs. In the last chapter, I cautioned clinicians to remember the primary role of those within the communication system who are helping the person who stutters to transfer and maintain his fluency. Too often, clinicians and clients assume these people to be "clinicians in absentia," expecting them to provide correction and other forms of feedback as would the clinician. They may say, "Wait a minute. What about your gentle speech?" or "You forgot to correct that one." A situation such as this ultimately inhibits communication because the person who stutters becomes reluctant to talk, knowing that he is facing certain correction. In fact, emotional upset may result. Clients find themselves feeling or saying, "You're my [*mother/father, girlfriend/boyfriend, wife/husband*], not my clinician!" Indeed, the role of clinician in absentia may interfere with the interpersonal dynamics within the family. Inadvertently, a dependence on the clinician shifts to a dependence on the conversational partner, rather than fostering a communication independence by the person who stutters. I have had spouses express feelings that they are letting their partners down if they do not correct them. I have found also that clients will enable their partners to assume this role because it is easier than internalizing responsibility for self-corrections.

Clinicians need to talk with the clients and their families to help them understand that the client must become his own clinician. Family members should be advised to offer supportive comments for all they see the client is doing right (e.g., "Hey, you're doing great today! You really are remembering your controls. I am so proud of you!"). Surely, they may offer correction occasionally, but they should not feel compelled to do so. We have noted before that all of us are inclined to do more of what we feel we are doing right; constant corrections close one down as a communicator and encourage conversational passivity. In fact, the client's occasional disfluency may serve to remind the supportive family members to comment on the fluency when it is observed, and to model and expand slow, gentle, natural sounding speech with even more deliberateness and frequency. Clients should be reminded that they, not their supportive partners, should internalize the responsibility to monitor and control their speech fluency. While it is tempting and understandable for the client to want his partner to take the monitoring and correction load off his shoulders, this must not happen. This is the client's job as his own clinician.

Another related reminder is that we must recognize and support the ongoing and dynamic needs of the conversational partners within the communication system. It would be easy to address only the communication needs of the adolescent, adult, or senior adult who stutters. The significant others have behavioral, affective, and cognitive needs as well. We have addressed the importance of clinicians helping the significant others know how best to contribute to the client's establishment, transfer, and maintenance of speech fluency. What to *do,* however, often is the least puzzling to those interacting closely with people who stutter. Addressing the affective and cognitive needs of significant others tends to be more challenging for clinicians. Many parents, siblings, spouses, and others have intense, albeit initially inarticulate, feelings about the client's stuttering. We noted before that some feel responsible, some feel helpless, some even feel resentment. Some are not precisely aware of what they feel. Again, asking general but leading questions, combined with active listening and reflective speech, enables the significant others to see that we care about them. Caring about significant others invites them to tell their story, thus clarifying and communicating their thoughts and feelings both to themselves and the clinician. Occasional constructive silences encourage them to share their feelings, forming insights about themselves, their family member who stutters, and the family system. Clinicians need to alleviate feelings of guilt by inviting, accepting, and supporting expressions of feeling and insight, yet providing information and alternative suggestions where appropriate.

Related to the significant others' affective need is a cognitive need, or need for knowledge. What people do or say to help the person who stutters generally reflects what they think or know about communication and stuttering. Again, clinicians need to determine the beliefs and assumptions of significant others, offering support, information, and alternatives. Regularly, I meet with the significant others, both with and without the client present, to ensure that I understand their experiences related to the change process, their unfolding needs, and that their needs are being met. I might ask any of the following:

- "So, how do you think things are going?"

- "How do you feel about your role in the change process both inside and outside of treatment?"

- "How are you all adjusting to the changes in Paul's speech fluency?"

- "Are there any things that you feel we need to talk about regarding the communication environment at home?"

In other words, we need to check in occasionally, yet deliberately, with the significant others to ensure that their needs are being met (one of which is their need to be needed), that they are contributing meaningfully to the treatment process and perceive themselves in this way, and that the family system is adjusting to and supportive of the changes resulting from the client's improved communication skills.

Clinical Portrait: Bill Rice

Selected Background Information

Bill* was 55 years old when he was referred by his family physician for a communication assessment because of "severe disruption of speech fluency." An informal preassessment meeting was held with Bill and his wife, Francis, to address initial questions and discuss general intervention options and implications. After deciding to pursue a diagnostic evaluation, Bill and Francis attended the scheduled evaluation. Bill described his stuttering as "aggravating." Francis described Bill as a "severe stutterer" who never let his disfluency hold him back and who persisted until his listeners understood what he had to say. Bill's disfluency reportedly began early in childhood and remained constant in degree and type as long as both Bill and Francis could recall. While Bill received no treatment over the last 30 years, he did experience brief periods of treatment before that time involving oral elocution (i.e., exercises requiring him to practice consonant and vowel combinations, and squeeze his abdomen and contract his neck muscles while speaking, among others), neuropharmacology (i.e., medication by prescription), and psychiatric intervention. Reportedly, Bill was told by numerous physicians that he would in time outgrow his stuttering. While typically severely disfluent, Bill could only predict fluency when talking alone or to the family dog. When asked how improvement of communication skills would affect his life, Bill indicated that he could not respond because he has always stuttered and could not imagine what it would be like not to stutter, saying, "This is all that I've ever had." Bill had no causal explanation, but acknowledged that his parents associated its onset with a car accident in which he was involved as a child. No hospitalization or loss of consciousness was reported, however. Bill's sister reportedly demonstrated mild stuttering behavior when she was young, and his father demonstrated imprecise articulation of speech sounds. Both Bill and Francis reported that his disfluency at the time of the evaluation was representative of his regular communication skills. Bill shared that his pursuit of the evaluation and related intervention options resulted from the ongoing support and encouragement received from his wife. Bill was a long time factory employee; Francis was an educator in a local public school. Bill and Francis' one adult son was employed and lived in their home.

Abbreviated Speech–Language Analysis

Bill's communication was analyzed from conversation, reading, and word and sentence repetition.

Conversation

Bill's conversational speech revealed an average of 41 fluent words per minute (163 in 4 minutes), significantly below the normal average of 115–165, reflecting the severity of Bill's disfluency. His disfluencies included the following:

- initial (e.g., tuhtuhtuhtuhtuhto; i.e., *t* + *uh* vowel = *tuh*) and medial (e.g., remuhmuhmuhmuhmember; i.e., *m* + *uh* vowel = *muh*) syllable repetitions (i.e., units rapidly repeated from 1 to 16 seconds),

- word repetition (e.g., I–I–I–I would say; 1 to 9 units repeated) and part word repetition (e.g., under–under–understand; 1 to 6 units repeated),

- phrase repetitions (e.g., It is–it is–it is–it is a rhythm; 1 to 7 units repeated),

- syllable interjections (e.g., uh–uh–uh socially; 1 to 9 units interjected/repeated),

*All clinical portrait names have been changed to protect confidentiality.

- word and phrase interjection (e.g., Well, I a–a–a–a–a usually, 1 to 10 units interjected/repeated; That well–a–well–a–well–a–well–a gets people, 1 to 6 units interjected/repeated). Occasionally, words were interjected within word boundaries (e.g., under–well—stand; 1 unit interjected).

- combinations of disfluency types noted above (i.e., up to 50 distinct units chained together for a sentence of 13 words that lasted 55 seconds, e.g., Well socially I'd say well that it a that it uh uh uh that it a a a well that it it it it a a a it you know a a a well well a a a chose well a social that well luhluhluhluhluh well a well a well luhluhluh well luhluhluhluh . . . life. I don't know).

Bill's disfluency was associated with tight eye closure, pitch increases indicative of laryngeal tension and rapid vertical jaw movements during syllable repetitions, and visible facial tension. The disfluency reduced Bill's rate of speech, general communication output, and overall speech intelligibility. Within Bill's conversational speech, there were islands of fluency of up to 16 words (e.g., "That's what they say but I don't know whether that had anything to do with it."). This fluent speech was characterized as gentle with good (i.e., normal) intonation, inflection, phrasing, and juncture.

Reading

Bill read the initial part of a phonetically balanced passage (i.e., "My Grandfather," also used to evaluate sound production skills). His rate of speech in this context was 12 fluent words per minute (37 words/3 minutes). Forms of disfluency were consistent with those noted above. However, the severity and intensity of the forms were more pronounced. For example, syllable repetition (e.g., guhguhguhguh . . . grandfather, nuhnuhnuhnuh . . . nearly) was extremely rapid and lasted up to 90 seconds in duration. After a 90-second repetition of the *g* + *uh* vowel targeting the *g* in grandfather, Bill stopped without having stated the complete word and remarked, "I can't say that word" with absolute fluency. Word interjection (e.g., a–a–a–a–a–a–a–a to know) lasted for up to 20 seconds per instance. The reading exercise was terminated due to Bill's difficulty with this context.

Word/Sentence Repetition

Bill repeated 6 of the 10 monosyllable words (e.g., *to, you, hat*) without disfluency and 1 of the 10 multisyllabic words (e.g., *statistics*) without disfluency. All of the sentences of increasing length and complexity contained disfluency (i.e., from 1 to 3 disfluent words in sentences of up to 8 words in length). The form of disfluency was consistent with those noted above. The difference in overall fluency within this context (i.e., greater disfluency on longer, more complex words and sentences) was consistent with stuttering behavior.

Other

All other aspects of assessment revealed appropriate speech (articulation and phonology) and language (semantics, syntax, and pragmatics) consistent with regional dialectical patterns. All parameters of voice, except during instances of laryngeal tension noted, and hearing were within normal limits.

Trial Management

Several trial management techniques including both fluency shaping and stuttering modification were used during the evaluation. These techniques focused on helping Bill experience more fluent speech and gain a better understanding of the nature of his fluent, as compared to his disfluent, speech. A particular objective of the trial management was to provide Bill an opportunity to experience speech fluency (i.e., to get a glimpse of "fluency freedom"), an experience he reported having never had previously. No disfluency was observed during song or choral speaking or choral reading. Bill was successful at discussing the nature of his fluency and disfluency and related feelings. It was emphasized that disfluency is much less likely to occur in the context of slow, gentle speech, and that both fluency and disfluency are the consequences of something we actively do. Results indicated that Bill's disfluency indeed was stuttering behavior and that a combined fluency shaping (direct manipulation of symptoms) and stuttering modification (analysis of fluency, disfluency, and related feelings) approach would prove successful in reducing his disfluency.

To indicate the improvement resulting from the trial management, another sample of Bill's conversation and reading after the trial management was transcribed and analyzed. The conversational sample revealed an average rate of 120 words per minute (120 words in 1 minute), containing a total of 6 disfluent words. A reading of the complete "My Grandfather" passage revealed a speech rate of 89 words per minute (133 words in 1.5 minutes), containing a total of 3 disfluent words. All of the disfluent words were characterized by silent articulatory fixations or syllable repetitions, however, with significantly reduced struggle and tension behavior. Bill and Francis both acknowledged that they have never observed this degree of fluency in Bill's speech. These data revealed a marked improvement as a result of trial management and suggested that Bill possessed the ability to speak with greater fluency and communication independence. Also discussed in the evaluation and trial management was the importance of making a joint, family decision regarding initiating the treatment process. Bill and Francis indicated that they intended to pursue scheduled treatment. The significance of the family communication system was addressed, as all members of this unit would be directly or indirectly affected by Bill's fluency focus and projected improvement.

Recommendations, Goals, and Objectives

Recommendations

Based on the results of the evaluation, the positive influence of trial management procedures, the internal motivation demonstrated, and the ready support of his family (his wife and his son with whom I spoke separately), Bill was recommended to receive direct fluency intervention for 1 hour per week.

Goals

The goals for Bill to accomplish by the end of scheduled direct treatment, tentatively projected for 1 to 2 years from the beginning of treatment, were as follows:

- Bill will develop and use specific fluency facilitating controls and self-monitoring skills.

- Bill will replace the present forms of disfluency with the fluency facilitating controls of pull-outs and preparatory sets (Van Riper, 1973). This means that he will replace an instance of stuttering while it is occurring within a word (pull-out), and eventually before it occurs (preparatory set).

- Bill will transfer fluency facilitating controls to outside settings.

- Bill will understand and discuss his communication-related feelings.

- Bill will participate actively in all aspects of treatment planning, execution, follow-up, and evaluation.

These goals were considered appropriate for Bill on the bases of baseline data, status of fluency at the time the goals were designed, success in trial management during and subsequent to the diagnostic evaluation, and the dialogue with Bill and his family members. Furthermore, the goals resulted from an understanding of Bill's views toward himself as a person and a communicator within a social world and the cognitive, behavioral/sensorimotor, and emotional/psychosocial dynamics (Klein & Moses, in press; Shapiro, in press) that operate within Bill's family.

Rationale and Procedural Approach to Goals

The procedural approach to achieving Bill's goals took the form of a combined stuttering modification and fluency shaping approach within a family systems context. The combined intervention approach provided an opportunity to help Bill experience more fluent speech and gain a better understanding of the nature of his fluent, as compared to his disfluent, speech. Furthermore, this approach provided an opportunity for Bill to experience controlled, volitional fluency—thereby getting a glimpse of "fluency freedom"—an important experience he reported having never had previously. The approach also allowed Bill to identify, discuss, understand, and gain control of his communication-related feelings and attitudes; and all members of Bill's family, particularly his wife Francis, to participate actively and regularly in all aspects of the intervention process. The approach was interactive and collaborative.

The design of treatment resulted from an awareness of cognitive, behavioral, and emotional dynamics that tended to perpetuate Bill's stuttering. These will be reviewed briefly now. Additionally, intrafamily, extrafamily, and psychotherapeutic considerations guided the design of treatment, and will be reviewed later. Of significance and related to cognitive factors, Bill indicated that he could not imagine how improvement in communication skills would affect his life because he had always stuttered and knew nothing else. Providing Bill an opportunity to experience fluency success was essential in enabling him to begin to visualize, internalize, and personalize the goals that he helped design and was striving to accomplish. Behaviorally, Bill reported being unable to control his disfluency, and being unaware that his articulatory postures during fixations were frequently inappropriate compared his target sound. Providing Bill an opportunity to heighten his understanding of his fluency and disfluency in addition to gaining control was essential in order to break the habit strength that had persisted for so many years. Emotionally, Bill's family, particularly his wife, shared Bill's commitment toward a brighter fluency future and expressed a willingness to do all they could in active pursuit of shared goals. However, life was so busy and chaotic that there was at best minimal time for real communicative dialogue, and what did exist was rushed and fractured. As will be seen, this maintaining or perpetuating factor not only contributed to the design of goals, but to the objectives and procedures as well.

Objectives

The objectives for Bill to accomplish approximately within a 2-month period included the following:

- Bill will heighten his awareness of the nature of his fluent speech.

- Bill will discuss specifically what he does when he is fluent, and compare that to what he does differently when he stutters.

- Bill will compare the feelings associated with fluency and those associated with stuttering.

- Bill will reduce the severity of his stuttering by varying and experimenting with the form and degree of disfluency.

- Bill will begin to "cancel" (Van Riper, 1973) instances of disfluency. This means that he will finish uttering the word that contains an instance of stuttering. Before going on, he will return to the beginning of that word and not before to institute a slow, gentle, yet natural sounding posture to replace the instance of stuttering. In this way, Bill will begin to gain control over the speech after an instance of stuttering has occurred.

- Bill will determine with his family a regular, predictable time for uninterrupted, quality family interaction.

The objectives were determined from an awareness that they are elemental to the goals described earlier. Bill needed to gain an understanding of the nature of his fluent speech. In the speech of most people who stutter, even among those who stutter severely, fluency is observed more often than disfluency. However, disfluency tends to draw more attention to itself and therefore is often not as noticeable as the stuttered speech. Bill needed to understand and be able to describe specifically what he does when he is fluent in order to be able to do it even more often. This is highly motivating and a necessary step before beginning to control his stuttered speech, and ultimately replacing it with fluency facilitating controls. Also, Bill and his family needed to find time to communicate, discuss the intervention process, and share responsibility for it. For these reasons, intervention helped Bill and his family develop a communication context that was more conducive to meaningful, less frenetic interaction. This could only happen through involvement with and an understanding of the family leading to communicative restructuring.

Rationale and Procedural Approach to Objectives

Although working within the client's home may have provided a more ecologically valid setting for conversational interaction, the university Speech and Hearing Center was used for practical reasons. The room itself was arranged to encourage informal dialogue and sharing of ideas. This was achieved by the clinician's supportive, professional manner of encouragement, active listening, positive facial expressions and eye contact, and unconditional positive regard. I recently stated the following:

> While appropriate furniture for casual, focused interaction combined with appropriate lighting is important, all the furniture in the world cannot replace the significance of the clinician's manner, sincerity, and attitude toward the family and the client's potential for fluency success. In fact, I have become convinced that the clinician's attitude is one of the key elements related directly to and predictive of the client's and family's communication success. (Shapiro, in press)

The objectives and procedures were designed in order to provide Bill with experiences that would enable him to consider alternative and expanded perceptions of himself. They allowed him to move from, "I cannot succeed. I am a stutterer," to "I am able, and since I know I have achieved some fluency success, I know I can achieve more." I noted previously the significance of tracking the client's comments about himself over time (Gouge & Shapiro, 1989–1990). Typically, such comments move from expressions of inability ("I can't speak fluently. I never could do that.") to ability ("I just used a gentle slide. I know I can do this."), and from being out of control or externally controlled ("Why is this happening to me?") to being in control or internally controlled ("I just self-corrected. I know I can blast those blocks before they get me."). These experiences had direct cognitive implications, enabling Bill to study and revise his personal construct of himself as a communicator. Furthermore, recall that Bill initially demonstrated a lack of fluency control and inappropriate articulatory postures. Related to behavioral factors, the setting, objectives, and procedures provided a supportive context encouraging Bill's active participation, systematic approximations for success, and heightened auditory, visual, and proprioceptive feedback, all of which are prerequisites to fluency control. The ongoing involvement of Francis and other family members in Bill's fluency treatment provided both the opportunity for and model of meaningful conversational interaction that was carried over into the home and other settings outside of the clinic.

Treatment Snapshot

The previous section that addressed recommendations, goals, and objectives also covered the rationale for the procedural approach taken with Bill and his family during intervention. This section will provide a few additional highlights about the treatment process and its outcome.

Two days after Bill's evaluation, I received an audiotape-recorded letter from him containing spontaneous speech and a reading sample. Both samples revealed appropriate use of the fluency facilitating controls we had discussed in the evaluation, including reduced rate, soft articulatory contacts, and slight prolongation on initial sounds in words. He explained that he had never sent a tape-recorded letter before, and wondered, "Why can I be completely free of stuttering when I am alone, yet when I am with people, stuttering shows its ugly head?" I called Bill immediately and pointed out to him that while he stated that he was "alone," he actually was speaking to an audience once removed (i.e., the clinician). I explained that the fluency he demonstrated in addition to his ability to integrate the suggestions discussed during the initial evaluation were indicative of his ability to speak more fluently and his motivation to improve his speech. I also reminded him of our discussions regarding the predictable yet temporary effects he might expect (such as a significant increase or decrease in fluency) that represent his increasing communication awareness. Bill expressed his interest to "get started in treatment," and followed-up with a postcard in which he stated, "Thanks again for your time that you gave me yesterday. I am looking forward to being involved in your program and working with you in any way that I can."

In the preassessment and assessment conferences, Bill, Francis, and I talked about the dynamic nature of the family system and how all members affect and are affected by each other. We discussed treatment as an exciting multidimensional process that takes a lot of work and commitment for all involved. Furthermore, I encouraged Bill to consider his family members when entertaining intervention decisions and to know that I would be doing just that. I explained that making a decision to return to treatment is a major decision for all involved, often not unlike "opening a can of worms." "In other words," I explained, "sometimes you just don't know exactly what you are getting into. Others will be expected to change along with you and typically need support to know how to change and to feel good about it. Furthermore, sometimes change triggers thoughts and feelings that you may not have known you even had." Bill's one son was less directly involved in treatment meetings because of the travel distance involved and resultant schedule conflicts. However, the following was taken from one of his letters:

> I enjoyed talking with you this morning and especially appreciate your generosity of time, knowledge, and personal experiences. Your concerns about the effect such changes would have on the family, as well as Dad as an individual, are probably well founded. In my own therapy, I have learned how closely I've identified with Mom in temperament as well as personality. I have a hunch that Mom will be giving up a great deal as Dad improves. I believe if there's any way to include her in your intervention, it would make it much easier for Dad to develop more fully.

Treatment began by establishing social, human connections between Bill, Francis, and the clinician. The clinician learned that Bill maintained a farm in addition to his other work, was highly skilled at carpentry, enjoyed travel, loved to cook and eat out, and had a remarkably dry sense of humor. The procedures, as discussed earlier in this chapter, were used to increase, establish, and subsequently transfer Bill's fluent speech, to develop resistance to potential fluency disrupters, to establish and maintain positive feelings about communication and himself as a communicator, and to maintain the fluency-inducing effects of treatment including behaviors, thoughts, and feelings. The initial sessions enabled Bill to explore and better understand the nature of his communication behaviors and related thoughts and feelings. Bill was provided a variety of opportunities to experience speech fluency and control of his communication.

Within related assignments, Bill described once per day in a speech notebook a word he spoke fluently. He made this notation as soon as he could after the event as appropriate, recording the specific word, with whom he was talking, the topic of conversation, and related thoughts and feelings about himself and the experience of control. After a social update, sessions began by having Bill summarize and describe the nature of his assignments since the previous session. In so doing, Bill discussed, and thereby internalized, the nature of fluency. Not long afterward, Bill shared in treatment that, "I want to be able to carry on a conversation. Then I wouldn't have to depend on anyone else." This statement was discussed as particularly significant because having experienced fluency success and some initial sense of control, he was beginning to imagine for himself what might become possible. Subsequent assignments enabled Bill to focus on his fluency (and later, the establishment, transfer, and maintenance of fluency facilitating control) even more often, thus providing a source of internalized and positive feedback, solidifying previous gains, and nurturing future improvements.

Experiencing success in treatment, Bill began to consider alternatives to the way he pictured himself as a person and as a communicator. Other assignments included completing hierarchies begun in treatment. He determined that the challenge of speaking fluently increased in the following order of contexts—alone, with his dog, with his wife, and with close friends. Among the most difficult were speaking to larger groups of people and on the phone.

Within 2 months, Bill's conversational rate of speech nearly doubled, from 41 to 75 fluent words per minute. Reading went from 12 to 90 fluent words per minute. Within 3 months, his use of cancellations as a fluency facilitating control increased from nonexistence to an average of 80%. The length of his longest disfluency in conversation decreased from 55 seconds to less than 5 seconds; in reading from 90 seconds to 14 seconds. Secondary features decreased noticeably as well. Within 1 year, his rate of speech in conversation and reading reached 100 fluent words per minute. About his regular assignments in which he recorded evidence of speech fluency, fluency facilitating control, and fluency-related thoughts and feelings, Bill commented, "I've got so much fluency now. I don't have time to write it all down!" Of significance, Bill was observed in treatment to subvocalize when the clinician offered models and expansions as a form of fluency correction. This means that Bill demonstrated without vocalization the motor sequences being modeled, thus indicating that he was internalizing and processing the necessary adjustments. Francis noted that she had been receiving positive comments from family and friends about Bill's improved communication skills. Comments from those who did not know that Bill was involved in fluency intervention were particularly appreciated. Francis also noted that she had begun to have difficulty distinguishing between Bill's voice and that of their son when she made phone calls to the house. Bill and Francis both reported feeling pleased with the process and products of intervention.

Treatment continued for nearly 2 years. After 14 weekly meetings, frequency of direct treatment reduced steadily (biweekly, then every 3 weeks, then monthly), thus requiring increased responsibility for Bill to transfer and maintain his fluency facilitating controls. These techniques were challenged deliberately by the clinician in the treatment setting, and by Bill and others in home, work, social, and other interpersonal settings. Bill was dismissed with an explicit welcome to return anytime.

Follow-Up and Epilogue

Follow-up continued for 2 years. Bill's rate of speech in conversation and reading stabilized between 150 and 160 fluent words per minute. His frequency of disfluency remained no greater than 2% (i.e., 2 disfluent words per 100 words spoken). Bill reliably adjusted his oral postures in advance of the anticipated block (i.e., preparatory sets), although occasionally needed to perform an adjustment while the block was occurring (i.e., pull-out). Fixations were silent, gentle, and with eyes open, lasting less than 1 second. Bill reported that he continued to ask himself the two "golden questions"—Are my articulators in the right position? If *yes,* go gentle. If *no,* what do I need to do to get there? The only remaining disfluency, therefore, was gentle prolongation of a fleeting nature. These behavioral data, combined with self-reports indicating positive feelings and thoughts about himself as a person and as a communicator and reports from Francis, other family members, and friends of maintained fluency success, all revealed significant fluency progress that was being maintained. In the later stages of treatment, Bill shared the following:

> There is no magic. You make your own magic. When I began, I had no idea I'd be where I am today. I just didn't believe it was possible. I didn't think it would be quite

that hard, but it can be overcome. Take it slow and easy. And if you have to, use stretches.

A cousin who was 85 years old with whom Bill and Francis visited regularly sent me a letter after a clinical meeting in which she shared the following:

> You certainly are not the typical college professor (of course they may have changed in the last 65 years). You are easy to talk to, you have a lot of personal charm, and I might add you are handsome. I think you have found friends for life in the Rices. Francis is pleased with the improvement in Bill's personality and in life in general. There was a time he was bound up in himself by a speech impediment. He now orders his meals in the restaurant and also answers the phone. I am excited over his progress.

Central and Guiding Intervention Assumptions

We return briefly to the assumptions that are central to and guide our design of intervention and its evaluation. These assumptions are the intrafamily (personal constructs and family systems), extrafamily (interdisciplinary teaming and multicultural awareness), and psychotherapeutic (fluency shaping and stuttering modification) considerations.

Intrafamily Considerations

Bill viewed himself as a "stutterer." This was his personal construct. Stuttering was his past, and the basis on which he anticipated his future. He could not imagine any other alternative interpretation. Providing him those alternatives, not by word, but by systematic intervention planning, was the clinician's responsibility. In other words, the clinician could not convince Bill to believe differently. However, it was incumbent upon the clinician to create the necessary opportunities for him to experience success from which Bill would draw alternative conclusions. Bill's family, and particularly an understanding of his family system, played an important role in the success of Bill's intervention. Bill and Francis had been married a long time. His development of fluency control was a change that potentially would alter the communication dynamics that had existed for a long time. Just because he changed through improved speech fluency and communication independence did not mean that his wife or other family members necessarily would know how to change with him. Without attending to the needs, thoughts, and feelings of the other family members, it would have been unfortunate, yet understandable, for them to feel less needed as Bill spoke more for himself. Francis and the other family members were involved regularly both inside and outside of the clinical setting to help Bill transfer and maintain his fluency, and to help them adjust to the altered communication dynamics as Bill achieved increased fluency control.

Extrafamily Considerations

While no allied professionals participated directly in Bill's intervention program, others within Bill's communication system including work colleagues, friends, and personal and professional associates were involved in transfer and maintenance activities. Also, there were several significant multicultural considerations that influenced the intervention process. Examples of these included level of education and type of professional employment, place of origin, chronological age, and religion. What could have been potential barriers to communication proved to be facilitators, creating opportunities for the clinician and client to learn from each other and, occasionally, for both to laugh at the unlikely, albeit sincere, union between people so different. Bill was a skilled factory employee who also maintained a farm; the clinician held a PhD and knew only that "hay is for horses." The client was from the south; the clinician was from the north and never even heard of butter beans. The client was significantly older than the clinician, providing an opportunity to learn about passages related to Bill's health, family, and approaching retirement. The client was Christian; the clinician was Jewish and never heard of progressive dinners. In fact, the clinician thought that a progressive dinner was a liberal church function. Indeed the client and clinician learned from each other and never ran out of things to talk about. Differences and similarities became shared topics of interest. Conversation and sincere dialogue were the mediums of intervention, presenting a context within which the participants contributed willingly to the process and learned from and with each other.

Psychotherapeutic Considerations

Bill's treatment initially emphasized fluency shaping in order to develop a measure of functional, albeit controlled if not artificial, fluency and heightened motivation. Bill was given opportunities to gain control over his fluency and thereby generalize these methods to instances of disfluency. Thereafter, a combined approach favored stuttering modification for the purpose of reducing the severity of Bill's stuttering and developing increased communication independence while providing him an opportunity to identify and understand his thoughts and feelings about himself as a communicator. Treatment emphasized the fluency already contained within Bill's speech and the importance of transfer activities conducted on a daily basis between scheduled sessions to facilitate control and self-monitoring skills. All procedures encouraged Bill's active role in achievement of fluency success, heightening his understanding and thereby acceptance of himself as an effective communicator, and transfer of fluency facilitating control and self-monitoring skills to outside settings. The people within Bill's family system participated in planning, implementing, and evaluating the treatment process, all with Bill's communication-related behaviors, thoughts, and feelings in mind. Similarly, Bill was reminded regularly of the importance of supporting the needs and feelings of his family members as he received their support. Bill came to realize that fluency and disfluency each represent active and deliberate choices available to him. He set out to achieve as much control over his communication skills as he was capable of, rather than striving toward perfect fluency. The intervention context was a positive one in which Bill actively constructed a revision of how he viewed himself and lived his life as a communicator. This context enabled Bill to achieve and maintain significant gains, providing his family with the opportunity to learn and grow together and celebrate in shared accomplishment.

CHAPTER SUMMARY

This chapter presented specific strategies for assessing and treating adolescents, adults, and senior adults who stutter. In so doing, we emphasized several major points. First, clients from these three groups must understand, be in control of, and thereby increase their speech fluency before effecting reduction in their disfluency. Second, clinicians must help clients who stutter manage not only the behavioral aspects of stuttering, but the more central thoughts and feelings about communication and themselves as communicators as well. Third, effective intervention must consider and be responsive to intrafamily (personal constructs and family systems), extrafamily (interdisciplinary teaming and multicultural awareness), and psychotherapeutic (fluency shaping and stuttering modification) factors. Finally, intervention with senior adults who stutter is a positive, inviting, and enlightening opportunity. Indeed, change is realistic, desirable, and possible at any age across the life span.

We noted that adolescents, adults, and senior adults who stutter typically have been stuttering for a number of years; often have increasingly complex behaviors, thoughts, and feelings related to the longer duration of stuttering;

may have a prognosis more related to the age of their stuttering than chronological age; and have stories to tell. Adolescence is an often confusing period of transition between childhood and adulthood. Adolescents often demonstrate a strong desire to be like others and to be liked by others and are remarkably vulnerable even when they may appear stalwart and confident. Adulthood is operationally defined as the working years, generally beginning between 18 and 21 years of age and ending between 55 and 65 years of age. Stuttering may become more or less severe during adulthood. Senior adulthood begins between 55 and 65 years of age, when an adult has completed his or her career and when his or her children are independent. Senior adults represent a growing and increasingly diverse population. While persons who do not stutter typically become more disfluent as they age, persons who stutter typically become less disfluent with age.

Preassessment procedures for adolescents, adults, and senior adults include completion of a case history form, review of an audio- or videotape recording of the client while engaged in family interaction, a preliminary phone call, and occasionally a preassessment conference. Assessment of adolescents, adults, and senior adults should occur within a supportive, nurturing, conversational context and includes a client and family interview, speech–language sampling and structured activities with and without communicative pressure, and trial management. The client and family interview begins with a social greeting and continues in an informal, conversational tone. Various topics are addressed including the client's and family's assumptions about the assessment process and about their past, present, and future with respect to communication and the communication impairment. The speech–language sample without communicative pressure may include or be a continuation of the questions and dialogue in the client and family interview. It should be no less than 300 words or 5 minutes of the client's talking. Structured activities without communicative pressure may include reading at different levels of complexity, recalling and describing both simple and concrete as well as complex and abstract events or things, repeating words and sentences of differing lengths and complexity, and responding to questions requiring answers of differing lengths and complexity. The speech–language sample and structured activities with communicative pressure may include activities involving time pressure, linguistic ambiguity, or violation of conversational rules. Trial management includes fluency shaping and stuttering modification techniques and enables the clinician to (a) help the client by adjusting and exploring his behaviors, thoughts, and feelings; (b) determine the relative effectiveness of different techniques with a particular client; and (c) design specific treatment recommendations.

Post-assessment procedures include a thorough analysis of speech and language leading to a determination of diagnosis, prognosis, and specific recommendations. Speech analyses address the frequency, types, molecular description, rate, secondary characteristics, severity, and adaptation and consistency of the speech disfluency. The diagnosis integrates all of the information available to determine the nature of the client's speech fluency and disfluency and whether or not treatment is warranted and recommended. If intervention is indicated, the clinician estimates the client's prognosis for improvement within a proposed course of treatment. Treatment recommendations vary with each individual, particularly with respect to intrafamily, extrafamily, and psychotherapeutic considerations, and are discussed with all parties involved.

Treatment goals for adolescents, adults, and senior adults who stutter are spontaneous or controlled fluency and establishment or maintenance of a positive attitude toward communication and oneself as a communicator. Specific and comprehensive treatment recommendations were presented, discussed, and applied for the purpose of achieving the following objectives: establishing or increasing and transferring fluent speech, developing resistance to potential disrupters, establishing or maintaining positive feelings about communication and oneself as a communicator, and maintaining the fluency-inducing effects of treatment (i.e., on communication-related behaviors, thoughts, feelings, and attitudes). Increasing and transferring fluent speech involves establishing a "safe house," inviting treatment objectives from the client, creating opportunities for the client to experience fluency success, heightening the client's awareness of his fluent speech, developing or improving the client's use of fluency facilitating techniques during instances of stuttering, addressing the client's thoughts and feelings directly, and transferring fluency facilitating techniques to extraclinical settings. Developing resistance to potential fluency disrupters involves introducing direct fluency challenge, revisiting and advancing toward the top rung of the client's communication hierarchies, and preparing for relapse.

Establishing or maintaining positive thoughts and feelings about communication or oneself as a communicator involves addressing teasing and relapse as probabilities rather than possibilities, empowering clients with constructive strategies to withstand teasing and relapse, helping clients maintain positive thinking about communication and oneself as a communicator, and talking with clients in positive ways. Finally, maintaining the fluency-inducing effects of treatment involves helping the client to become his own clinician, decreasing the frequency of scheduled treatment, implementing regular maintenance checks of decreasing frequency for at least 2 years post-treatment, instituting regular client-initiated benchmarking, deliberately revisiting the past, and integrating treatment changes within the communication system.

The chapter ended with a clinical portrait of Bill Rice, a 55-year-old man, in order to apply and discuss the assessment and treatment suggestions in addition to intrafamily, extrafamily, and psychotherapeutic intervention considerations. In doing so, we discussed selected background information, an abbreviated speech–language analysis, recommendations, goals and objectives, rationale and procedural approaches to goals and objectives, a snapshot of treatment, and a follow-up and epilogue.

Chapter 10 Study Questions

1. We reviewed a variety of prognostic factors and their implications for adolescents, adults, and senior adults who stutter. We stated that predicting treatment outcome is an inexact science at best. Given the concerns about the predictive validity of such factors, why do we continue to make statements of prognosis for our clients? How might the clinician's statement of prognosis affect the treatment process and its outcome? How might such statements impact all parties involved—the client, family, and clinician? Could one clinician's statement of prognosis affect that of another? How might a previous clinician's statement of prognosis impact your estimation of the client's potential? How might your estimation affect that of a subsequent clinician? What do you feel are the advantages and limitations of Van Riper's policy to accept at least one client who holds a "zero prognosis"? What do you feel are the advantages and limitations of Cooper's designation of "Chronic Perseverative Stuttering Syndrome"? Could you diagnose this syndrome within the scheduled evaluation session? What factors will you use to estimate one's prognosis? What are the implications of such factors?

2. Part of the assessment process includes assessing speech fluency under conditions of communicative pressure. How can clinicians provide communicative pressure without jeopardizing the supportive, nurturing environment that is so necessary for clinical intervention, both assessment and treatment?

3. One goal of fluency intervention is establishing and maintaining positive thoughts and feelings about communication and oneself as a communicator. When discussing stuttering modification approaches, we indicated that such procedures require more advanced interpersonal and counseling skills on the part of the clinician. How are such skills acquired? When using such skills and interacting with your adult clients about a variety of topics, how will you ensure that you remain within the boundaries of your professional training? When might interacting with your client about sensitive topics (e.g., client's marriage, client's thoughts about his partner, interpersonal dynamics, or family and social relationships) be *within* versus *beyond* the limits of your training? How will you remain sensitive to and detect the difference? What would you do if you found that you were approaching the limits of and extending beyond your training?

4. We discussed different aspects of adolescence, adulthood, and senior adulthood. What particular strengths might each of the groups bring with them to the treatment setting that would positively influence the treatment outcome? What special challenges might each group provide? What factors would likely motivate a person in each group to seek treatment? How might what we know about these three phases of life impact our intervention with members of the different groups? What are the dangers of stereotyping members of any group? What type of "radar" or other detection device would you have operating to prevent the inadvertent, yet frequent, experience of stereotyping?

Unit IV

◆ ◆ ◆ ◆ ◆ ◆ ◆ ◆ ◆ ◆ ◆ ◆ ◆ ◆ ◆ ◆ ◆ ◆ ◆

The Clinician: A Paragon of Change

Chapter 11
The Clinician and the Client–Clinician Relationship

Chapter 12
Professional Preparation and Lifelong Learning:
The Making of a Clinician

Chapter 11

The Clinician and the Client–Clinician Relationship

◆ ◆ ◆ ◆ ◆ ◆ ◆ ◆ ◆ ◆ ◆ ◆ ◆ ◆ ◆ ◆

Importance of Clinicians to the Change Process   450

Interpersonal Factors of Effective Clinicians   452

    Clinician Behaviors   452

    Clinician Attributes and Manner of Interaction   452

        Empathy   453

        Warmth   454

        Genuineness   455

        Personal Magnetism   457

        Compatible Friction   458

        Realistic, Focused Optimism   458

    Clinician Language   460

Intrapersonal Factors of Effective Clinicians   460

    Clinician Thoughts, Feelings, and Beliefs   460

        Significance of Clinicians' Personal Constructs   460

        Persistence of Clinicians' Negative Attitudes   461

        Interaction of Attitudes and Professional Preparation   462

        Interaction of Attitudes and Understanding of Stuttering   463

        Interaction of Attitudes and Positive Observation and/or Treatment Experience   463

    Clinician Needs   464

    Clinician Satisfaction and Rewards   466

The Clinician as Guardian Angel   468

Chapter Summary   470

Chapter 11 Study Questions   472

There seems to be an element of magic in stuttering therapy, an elusive, ephemeral, and yet powerful force which most clinicians acknowledge but few can precisely identify. The catalytic agent of this force appears to be the interpersonal relationship between the clinician and his client, for regardless of the particular procedures or techniques involved, changes in the stutterer's behavior are mediated by person-to-person interaction.

(EMERICK, 1974B, P. 92)

The clinical magic (Emerick, 1974b) embodied in the interaction between a clinician and client is the focus of the present chapter. It seems that this magic is recognizable and powerful when it occurs. Like any other aesthetic experience, effective clinical interaction is hard to describe and harder to recreate in identical form. Clinical artistry reminds me of good cooking. Just as a cook reveals the recipe as "a little of this and a little of that," our attempts to recreate the prescribed steps never result in a meal that tastes the same. There is something intangible, yet essential and absolutely unique, to each master clinician. We can and will describe the inter- and intrapersonal factors revealed by the best clinicians. Nevertheless, attempts to create clinical effectiveness or those quintessential moments of clinical magic by demonstrating its component elements are doomed to disappointment. Clinical effectiveness is that connection of mind, body, and soul between caring clinicians and clients—those moments of ultimate communication and shared growth that are focused, yet timeless and placeless. Knowing that any attempt to capture that magical experience can be an approximation at best, let us begin.

In Unit I, we established that planning and conducting intervention with people who stutter require a solid understanding of stuttering including its onset, development, nature, and etiology and treatment from past and present perspectives. Furthermore, we established the importance of clinicians being able to distinguish and differentially diagnose stuttering from other disorders of fluency. In Unit II, we developed a model of intervention consisting of central and guiding assumptions including intrafamily, extrafamily, and psychotherapeutic considerations. In Unit III, we applied the material presented in the previous two units to address comprehensively the processes of assessment and treatment with preschool children and school-age children, adolescents, adults, and senior adults who stutter. Now, in this last unit, we will discuss the clinician and the client–clinician relationship (in Chapter 11) and the processes involved in professional preparation and lifelong learning (in Chapter 12). Specifically, Chapter 11 will address the importance of the clinician and the client–clinician relationship to the change process, and the interpersonal and intrapersonal competencies that are necessary for clinicians to work effectively with people who stutter and their families. In Chapter 12, we will address the academic, clinical, and supervisory processes by which such competencies are developed, and then we will end with a discussion of three elements that are critical for maintaining and upgrading a clinician's competence across her professional career.

In this chapter, we will emphasize the following major points:

- The clinician is the single most critical variable in the process of change. Clients neither communicate nor improve communication in a vacuum. The clinician enables the client to imagine, work toward, and achieve communicative dreams.

- There are certain interpersonal factors that characterize effective clinicians who work with people who stutter. These include clinician behaviors, affective attributes (i.e., manner of interaction), and language factors.

- Additionally, there are intrapersonal factors about which effective clinicians are aware and of which they are in control. These include thoughts, feelings, and beliefs; personal needs; and enduring satisfaction and internal rewards.

- Once personally and professionally self-aware (i.e., aware of and in control of interpersonal and intrapersonal factors), clinicians can develop or improve their professional skills.

IMPORTANCE OF CLINICIANS TO THE CHANGE PROCESS

The clinician and the interpersonal clinical relationship are among the most significant factors that influence, if not foretell, the outcome of treatment. Indeed, as Murphy and FitzSimons (1960) noted, "The most important single variable affecting success in the treatment of stutterers is—the clinician" (p. 27). Van Riper (1975) stated, "No matter what kind of treatment is used and no matter what its rationale may be, the clinician is always a significant part of the therapeutic dyad" (p. 455). Nevertheless, compared to the numerous investigations of children and adults who stutter, the clinician has been relatively unstudied. Van Riper (1975) observed further that, "Millions of words have been written about stutterers, but only a few about the clinicians who have treated them. Surely it is time to examine stuttering therapy from this other perspective" (p. 455).

It is no secret that clinicians vary in professional effectiveness. This conclusion is based on the clinical literature (ASHA, 1995; Argeropoulos, 1974; Brutten, 1993; Carkhuff, 1969a, 1969b; Cooper & Cooper, 1985b; Manning, 1996) and more than 20 years of working directly with and observing clients and clinicians and discussing with both what they find to be most and least effective about the clinical experience. Nevertheless, there are certain qualities that tend to characterize clinicians who are considered most effective. Manning (1996) noted that there is no exclusive set of attributes that characterize an expert clinician. Indeed, clinicians' professional and personal attributes vary as do clients' behaviors, thoughts, and feelings, thus creating a dynamic and unique clinical interaction. Manning (1996) added the following:

> It is clear that some clinicians are considerably better than others at motivating and guiding their clients. The attitudes and abilities these clinicians possess distinguish them from the clinicians who are less effective. It is the effec-

tive clinicians who are able to discover appropriate therapeutic strategies and design associated techniques. Perhaps more than any other quality, the best clinicians are uncommonly effective in motivating and supporting their clients along the often arduous path of treatment. (p. 2)

Some might argue that the clinician tends to be more significant to the clinical process when treatment takes on more of a stuttering modification, or counseling, focus compared to a fluency shaping, or behavior-driven, focus. Others (Cooper & Cooper, 1985b; Hood, 1974; Manning, 1996; Van Riper, 1975) countered that independent of the form of treatment, the clinician remains a key ingredient to its effectiveness. The following citations represent the importance of the clinician in the process of change:

- Workers in every phase of the helping professions recognize that the client-clinician relationship is a, if not the, crucial variable in the treatment process. (Emerick & Hood, 1974, p. vii)

- The enthusiast may be influencing his patient more by his personality than by his method. The method becomes only the vehicle for this transmission. It may be that what makes a therapist an expert is an increase in his self-expressive ability through the selection and alteration of a chosen system. (Walle, 1974, p. 6)

- Methods and materials used in therapy remain insignificant until touched by a spark, the individual clinician's uniqueness, which elevates them beyond the commonplace. Regardless of approach, his personal conception of the clinical interface, his attitude concerning the personal dimensions of the encounter called therapy, his blend of thinking, feeling and doing, and his way of life deeply affect both the nature of the interaction and its degree of success, be it objectively or subjectively defined. Such behavior can constitute the advocacy of a certain clinical orientation or mood, a form of attitude toward action appropriate with humans who stutter. (Murphy, 1974, p. 30)

To emphasize the importance of the clinician and the interaction within the clinical process does not negate or even challenge the importance of other aspects of the clinical process, such as understanding, planning, observing, analyzing, and integrating. Indeed, we will highlight the behavior of effective clinicians, including goals, processes, and competencies related to assessment, management, and transfer and maintenance of fluency (ASHA, 1995). Many disparate kinds of treatment have resulted in communicative improvement of different kinds and degrees of durability (Andrews et al., 1983; Brutten, 1993; Emerick, 1974a, 1974b; Luper, 1968; Van Riper, 1974). We know that the affective or interpersonal dimension contributes significantly to the overall clinical experience and its outcome. However, to estimate in concrete terms the relative contribution of this dimension is conjecture. About the relative import of the interpersonal element, Emerick (1974b) noted the following:

How large a segment this interpersonal dimension occupies within the therapeutic process I do not know; some experienced clinicians suggest that at least half of what occurs in therapy is simply inspirational and elicits the release of healing processes within the individual. . . . After laboring with stutterers for over a decade, I am convinced that it is not only what I do that helps the person get better but also how I do it and who I am. (pp. 92–93)

While attempts to quantify the influence of the clinician may fail, the point remains that the clinician is at least a critical element in the client–clinician relationship. We will attempt to describe elements of that relationship and particularly interpersonal and intrapersonal factors of effective clinicians who succeed in creating clinical magic.

INTERPERSONAL FACTORS OF EFFECTIVE CLINICIANS

Clinician Behaviors

Analyzing and describing the behaviors of effective clinicians, as will be seen, present the least degree of difficulty. The Special Interest Division on Fluency and Fluency Disorders recently presented a cogent set of "Guidelines for Practice in Stuttering Treatment" (ASHA, 1995). This document (see Appendix A.3) addressed such issues as:

- *General guidelines for practice*—timing and duration of treatment sessions; setting, duration, complexity, and cost of treatment;

- *Personal attributes of clinicians*—interest and commitment, willingness to develop knowledge and skill, problem-solving skills, and flexibility;

- *Learned attributes of clinicians*—an understanding of the literature, knowledge of phenomenology, a focused yet broad perspective, an understanding of the clinical process, good communication skills; and

- *Specific guidelines for practice*—goals, processes, and competencies for assessment, management, and transfer and maintenance.

The specific guidelines represent the most comprehensive delineation to date of "all goals that are considered appropriate by all philosophies of treatment currently held by speech-language pathologists who treat people who stutter" (p. 28), processes that are useful for achieving specific goals, and competencies (including skills and knowledge) that clinicians can use to engage in the processes identified. Notwithstanding, the guidelines understandably are stated in behavioral terms, thus emphasizing the behavioral domain. What remains to be addressed are the less tangible, albeit critical, manifestations of the clinician's affective and cognitive dimensions.

Clinician Attributes and Manner of Interaction

We have long known the importance of the clinician's affective characteristics. In an earlier publication (Shapiro, 1994a), I discussed the work of Carkhuff (1969a, 1969b), Gazda, Asbury, Balzer, Childers, and Walters (1977), and Rogers (1957) and applied this work to interaction analysis and self-study. The integrative premise across these works is that, if certain facilitative conditions are present within the clinical interaction and if they are perceived by the client, then the client will experience positive changes. Various master clinicians have described the elements of this affective dimension, which are recognizable, yet hard to measure. Van Riper (1975) described such essential clinician characteristics as empathy, warmth, genuineness, and charisma. Emerick (1974b) described the critical dimensions of interpersonal sensitivity as compatible friction, focused optimism, and personal magnetism. Because of their relevance to the importance of the interpersonal process in the treatment of people who stutter, these elements, which do overlap with one another, will be described briefly.

Empathy

Empathy is an "authentic sensitivity for the client" (Manning, 1996, p. 6), "the ability to imagine how it feels to be inside another person's skin" (Van Riper, 1975, p. 461). Van Riper (1975) compared the empathic perceptiveness between an effective clinician and client to that in a long and successful marriage in which each partner knows what the other is thinking and feeling. Empathy requires objective observations that are distinct from hypotheses or inferences. Furthermore, since all observation is selective (i.e., no clinician can observe all behaviors of people who stutter; inherent selectivity may distort the picture), clinicians deliberately must open their field of view and consider alternative points of view. Empathy also requires sensitivity to clients' internal thoughts and feelings, which may or may not be revealed by what the client does or does not say. Empathy requires the clinician's self-awareness and the ability to observe herself while she is observing the client. Van Riper (1975) cautioned against overidentification or overinvolvement, noting that clinicians' and clients' circles should intersect but never be concentric. There must always be a clear area outside the intersection to be able to help people who stutter. In other words, in our attempt to feel the way the client feels, we must not become so close that we take on all of these feelings or lose perspective or objectivity. Similarly, Rogers (1961) advised clinicians to retain the "as if" quality; that is, to understand the client's angers, fears, and confusions *as if* it were our own, without letting our own angers, fears, and confusions become bound up. This is empathy.

I am doubtful that empathy can be learned; rather, I believe it is discovered. Sometimes discovering one's own capacity for empathy is challenging, if not unsettling. Student and other novice clinicians often have expressed concern that they will become emotional in the presence of a client. "What if I cry, or totally lose it?" they say to me. I explain that our ability to relate to another person and his life is one of the reasons we decided to enter this profession. To relate to, to internalize, and even to make "as if" one's own the reality of another person; this is healthy, sound, and professional. We should not be reluctant to build our understanding of another person upon our own solid emotional foundation. This may mean that occasionally we share both a tear and a smile with someone we care for deeply. However, for us to superimpose another person's reality upon ourselves leading to a loss of our emotional composure (including crying uncontrollably, becoming visibly angry, or becoming internally fearful) is professionally unacceptable. Doing so inappropriately shifts the clinical focus from the client onto the clinician. Typically clinicians become more comfortable with their own empathic side as they become familiar with it. Rarely have I seen a clinician who cannot develop and maintain the "as if" quality. In such few instances, I have seen clinicians sob uncontrollably in class when learning about one's pain from a guest presentation or an interview replayed from videotape. In only one instance that I can recall was a student counseled out of the program because of chronic overidentification with clients, despite exhaustive instructional intervention efforts.

Warmth

Warmth is no more concrete a term than is empathy. Warmth is a composite of behaviors including understanding, sincerity, friendliness, and respect (i.e., "unconditional positive regard;" Rogers, 1957) that, when offered, typically receives a similar response in return. I often hear warmth discussed as a tag to other affective qualities (e.g., warm and friendly, warmth and hospitality). Over the years, I have seen warmth blossom in countless clinicians. I do not believe that they had to "learn" warmth. I believe that they needed to address their own needs (e.g., anxiety, confidence, feelings of competence) before they could focus without distraction on their clients. It is that connection, that shared commitment in focused communication, that is timeless and placeless, enabling warmth to surface. I have seen so often clinicians' early interviews look like interrogations (i.e., series of staccato questions without reflection or any shared affective interaction), only to move to conversational, inviting, reflective, problem-solving dialogues. Murphy (1974) spoke of "two monologues in search of a dialogue" (p. 29). The conversational dialogue emanating from and connecting with the head and heart; this is warmth.

Van Riper (1975) noted that clients "must feel vividly that we like, respect, and care for them as persons. . . . When we could not really like a stutterer we always failed" (p. 466). Given the significant impact of clinicians' attitudes on clients' improvement (Daly, 1988), it is not surprising that the warmth conveyed by the clinician influences the client's potential communication improvement. Murphy and FitzSimons (1960) noted, "The successful clinician is the worker who is able to establish the warm relationship on which new learning is dependent" (p. 28). In most cases, clinicians have no problem relating to and liking their clients. However, what happens when clinicians are faced with a client they find unpleasant, unappealing, or otherwise unlikable as a person?

I remember one such client. He was a senior adult with a litany of medical woes. He was being treated psychiatrically for clinical depression, negativity, paranoia, and passive dependency syndrome. We were working collaboratively with other family members, psychiatric services, and other allied medical and human service professionals. I remember several male and female clinicians who were well-meaning, positive, perky, and young-spirited when they prepared for and began this man's treatment, but who later demonstrated visibly a slow emotional crumble that ended with two broken souls leaving the treatment room. "Wait a minute," I admonished one clinician, "You are to help and support your client but not to become him." She replied, "But I don't like him. He's horrible. I think I hate him." Impressed with the student clinician's degree of self-disclosure, at once I needed figuratively to scrape her off the floor while impressing upon her the importance of empathic understanding and warmth.

The question remained, however, how do you express warmth, which must be sincere, to a person you don't like or respect? Fortunately, in most cases, clients and clinicians develop a sincere and positive regard for each other as the therapeutic relationship develops and progresses and as they relate to each other as people. Granted, in any relationship there are times when we may not like all of what we see in others or in ourselves. Again, I am reminded that when we point an accusing finger at another person, at least three are pointed at ourselves. Go ahead, try it! As the clinical relationship develops, its participants often become increasingly candid. Usually this candor contributes in positive ways to the development of the clinical interaction.

However, I have worked with clients who, in my presence, expressed thoughts and beliefs reflecting bigotry, racism, sexism, anti-Semitism, ego- and ethnocentrism, and other woeful constructs. I must confess that on such thankfully few occasions, my attempts to interact on the basis of our shared interests were indeed challenging and atypically deliberate. Furthermore, my manner of conveying empathy and warmth was affected by my attempts to accept a person whose views I found unacceptable. In such instances, I repeated the words I learned from a clinician whose clinical fellowship I supervised ("I know you feel that way. However, I see things differently.") (B. Baxley, personal communication, 1985). By attending to communication objectives and by redirecting conversation that does not have at its heart the client as a communicator or the client's communication system, I never have referred a client to another clinician because of "personality conflicts" or "irreconcilable differences." Theoretically, however, I see this as possible and occasionally a wise professional choice. People are different. Indeed we do not need to like everything we see in or hear from our clients. But we do need to remember the value of empathy and warmth in creating a clinical climate that is conducive to meaningful change.

Genuineness

Genuineness is the ability to be one's true self as a person with a client while conveying professional competence and personal confidence. Rogers (1957, 1961) noted that the clinician's "congruence" is critical to her influence on the client. This refers to being aware, accepting, and honest about oneself and how one presents herself to each client. In addition to personal honesty, competence is another aspect of genuineness. Clinicians must be and feel competent and be able to demonstrate this competence. Clients need to know that their clinicians are competent in order to begin to trust their clinician and believe that the clinical process really will result in meaningful change. Usually, the client's need to believe that the clinician is competent is implicit, although rarely expressed. On one occasion, however, I was intrigued by how much one adult client knew about me at the time of her diagnostic evaluation. It came out that before scheduling the appointment, she visited our university, which was 150 miles from her home, to review my professional vita, publications, and videotape recordings of television spots I have done for the university about my work with people who stutter. When she expressed concern that I might feel offended at the thoroughness of her investigation, I shared that I wish all prospective clients would be equally responsible and as informed as consumers. Indeed she knew my record as she should. We were about to enter into an agreement, a clinical commitment that Van Riper (1975) referred to as "an invisible contract." Before "signing," she should know about the person with whom she is making a major decision.

All clients must be comfortable with their clinicians as people and as competent professionals. About clients' need for competent clinicians, Van Riper (1975) noted the following:

> No matter how warm and understanding and genuine we may be, they [clients] also want something more in their clinicians. They want competence. Too many amateurs have had their dirty fingers in the stutterer's pie. Stutterers demand guides who know the terrain, who know where the stutterers are in the swamp and which way they must go to get out of it. They want guides who will not abandon them, who are strong, warm, and understanding; but above all, they want their guides to be experienced and skillful and to have some kind of map. (p. 470)

Van Riper (1975) indicated that in order to gain such competence, clinicians must acquire a solid foundation of information about the nature of stuttering; know a large number of people who stutter personally; and "assume the role of a severe stutterer long enough, and in enough situations, to enable them to experience the frustrations, anxiety, shame, and other negative emotions that constitute the context of the stutterer's daily life" (p. 470). The importance of these suggestions cannot be overstated. Students in classes on fluency disorders typically are assigned to "stutter" in public in order to heighten their awareness of that reality. It is interesting to note that students typically learn as much about themselves (i.e., thoughts, feelings, attitudes) as they do about the stuttering experience. A few remain unwilling to participate in the assignment. Some explain that they feel they are mocking people who stutter; others display utter discomfort even in the anticipation of temporary deviance. How can one begin to understand the reality of another if she remains unwilling or unable to see it, to touch it, to feel it, to experience it?

I remember how significant the experience of stuttering deliberately in public was for me. The professor of my Seminar on Stuttering in graduate school was Dr. Barry Guitar, for whom I hold the highest respect and lasting appreciation. He and I spoke occasionally outside of class about our personal experiences as people who stutter. When the students were to report in class on an experience of stuttering in public, I had not given the assignment much attention. I figured that I had a broad enough experiential basis from which to report on a single episode. Furthermore, I figured this assignment was intended for those who had not any personal experience of stuttering. Shortly after I began sharing my experience in class, Barry challenged with, "David, did you do the assignment?" I began my explanation something like, "Well, Barry, actually I did stutter in public but not for this assignment," all the while masking my avoidance only to myself. Seeing right through my sorry excuse and being committed to the instructional value of stuttering deliberately in public, Barry directed me, "David, leave the class and don't return until you have done the assignment." "That was direct!" I thought. Somewhat shaken and not understanding the importance of the assignment, I left reluctantly to follow his instructions. Not until completing the assignment did I realize how much I still was avoiding stuttering and how much I was permitting stuttering to impact my thoughts, feelings, and attitudes about communication and myself as a communicator. That one experience for me was a turning point in my life and in my development as a clinician. I share this experience with my students to help them see that I might understand their degree of reluctance and how fear may impact our behavior.

Personal Magnetism

There are certain additional personal qualities of the clinician that naturally are attractive and arouse hope in a client. Such qualities, again easier to recognize than define, have been called personal magnetism (Emerick, 1974b; West, 1958) and charisma (Van Riper, 1975). The enchantment, sincere if not innate, that begets hope is perhaps the most critical gift of an effective clinician. It is born of the clinician's internal peace, professional knowledge, faith in the client's potential for change, and confidence in the clinical process. West (1958) described such seemingly intangible qualities in the clinician that generate the client's hope as:

> that subtle, difficult-to-define thing called personal magnetism. This is a complex of impressions made upon the patient. The therapist possessed of this ability to impress the patient seems to be frank but tactful; penetrating but understanding; professional but kind; confident but humble. (p. 220)

Similarly, Emerick (1974b) described personal magnetism or charisma as a form of electromagnetic energy from the clinician to the client, a high energy output that leaves the client exhilarated and the clinician drained and exhausted. He described such magnetism as follows:

> This therapeutic approach flows from a philosophy of life that encompasses a commitment to the principles of performing everything I do at the limit of my capacity. I decided long ago that I would rather wear out than rust out. . . . Most speech clinicians I have encountered in my travels are turned-on people; they are enthusiastic about the work they do, and it shows in the way they talk about their profession. . . . Charisma or personal magnetism comes in many forms and styles but it seems essential to therapy. Without this individualized spark, the treatment process would indeed be a rather somber transaction. (pp. 99–100)

In whatever form, personal magnetism is part of what helps a client believe in himself and begin to hope for a better fluency future. Van Riper (1973) expressed the essential nature and critical interaction between a clinician's faith and a client's hope:

> Recognizing that hope is the very essence of motivation, the therapist must either create it or at least blow upon its faint embers until they glow. To do so, the therapist must himself have some confidence in his own abilities to help his client. If molehills or mountains are to be moved, some of the energy necessary to move them will be found in the therapist's faith in himself. This is not to say that one can always be certain of the outcome, but any therapist knows in his bones that he can do much to ease the client's suffering. Like fishermen, good therapists are optimists. Most of them have come to have a profound respect for the latent potential for self-healing that exists in all troubled souls. They resemble Michelangelo who, when asked by a bystander how he could carve

such glorious angels from just a slab of stone, replied, "Oh they're already in there. I just have to chip away the stone that surrounds them." Out of the therapist's faith can come the stutterer's hope. (p. 230)

Compatible Friction

Compatible friction is another critical dimension of interpersonal sensitivity. Emerick (1974b) noted that this concept combines a philosophy of living and teaching with "an inextricable union of love and confrontation," or "a judicious wedding of positive regard and frustration" (p. 94). First, a positive tone or compatible interpersonal context is established between clinician and client, communicating that she is committed to the client's communication welfare. Then, since the clinician intends the client to change, the clinician must disturb the equilibrium or homeostasis, introducing friction or confrontation. How is compatible friction established? Compatibility is born of empathy, warmth, and genuineness, reviewed earlier. The clinician conveys her understanding of the client's situation, from the client's own perspective, as if it were her own. The clinician expresses and demonstrates her commitment to the client and his communication needs, from which a commonality or feeling of shared identification is established. Such commitment and commonality yield essential honesty, candor, and genuineness that transform a potentially contrived interaction into sincere human discourse of hearts and minds.

Compatibility, however, while essential, is not enough to achieve the objective of change. Change is stimulated by friction caused by some type of imbalance, challenge, or constructive disequilibrium (Moses & Shapiro, 1996; Shapiro & Moses, 1989). Emerick (1974b) noted that, "Man seeks imbalance as well as balance—if he is appropriately supported (compatible) during the period of disequilibrium. But it takes friction to get the gears moving in new cycles and unfamiliar patterns" (p. 96). In other words, unless challenged causing discomfort, old patterns perpetuate. Change requires a willingness to approach and engage in risk, knowing that a comrade is there with confidence holding a safety net should it be necessary. Challenge or friction is calibrated to the individual client (Emerick, 1974b; Manning, 1996). We discussed in Chapters 8, 9, and 10 how to introduce increasing degrees of challenge within a positive context, all the while helping clients imagine and achieve communication goals otherwise considered impossible.

Realistic, Focused Optimism

Apparently, I am a positive, optimistic person (Shapiro, 1994b). At least this is what I hear from my clients and students. One client who was a physician called me "the rah rah man." He did not mean that I was a "sis boom bah" type of cheerleader. Rather, I believe he saw me as identifying his strengths and abilities, particularly when he could not, thus creating in him a positive expectation set. In so doing, he came to expect that he would improve in his communication, and even more importantly, that he possessed the ability to succeed. This sharing of realistic, focused optimism inspires the client and creates in him faith or hope. Emerick (1974b) noted that, "The concept of focused optimism involves the creation of hope or faith centered upon one or two potentials I witness in the stutterer; these serve as rallying points for the development of the achievement motive" (p. 98). Furthermore, since each client acts according to the expectations and assumptions (or personal construct) he holds about himself, clinicians must enable the client to create an alternative perspective. From structured, individually designed clinical activities, the client experiences fluency success and the feeling of communication control, ones from which he begins to visualize himself as a more competent, fluent communicator. Methodologies for achieving focused optimism and adjustments to one's personal construct were reviewed in the last unit. Emerick (1974b) discussed several other valuable attitudinal considerations (pp. 98–99), including the following:

- *General Capacity for Transcendence:* Suitably invited, supported, and challenged, a person can overcome seemingly overwhelming odds. People possess an inner urge to become something better or greater. The clinician's role is to facilitate that process of becoming.

- *The Clinician's Attitude:* The clinician's attitude about the client's potential for change and confidence in herself as a facilitative agent for change are critical to the outcome of treatment. Emerick (1974b) noted, "The clinician's prognostic expectations have profound influence on the outcome of therapy. . . . Hope makes even an elusive goal look possible" (p. 98). Van Riper (1975) noted similarly:

> Whenever I see a new stutterer, I find in him so much more strength and potential than I remember having at that age that I immediately expect a favorable outcome. The feeling is this: "Lord, if that weak, miserable mess that once inhabited my skin could solve his problems and become reasonably fluent, then surely this potential client can!" Moreover, I have known other stutterers for whom the prognosis looked pretty poor but who were also able to master their tangled tongues and selves with my help. Perhaps other clinicians who create hope in their clients have similar perceptions. (p. 476)

- *Treatment as Work:* An effective clinician, at times, must be bold. Emerick noted that more clincians have failed because they were timid and temporizing than because they boldly set forth a treatment plan. Similarly, Manning (1996) noted, "If clinicians, including myself, are to be faulted for any one thing, we are most likely guilty of not pushing our adult clients hard enough" (p. 13). He added that clients want and expect to be pushed hard, but that clinicians are reluctant in fear of eliciting a negative reaction. I add, however, that as we push, clients must increasingly assume greater responsibility for the process and products of treatment.

- *Dyadic, Dynamic Interaction:* One person's behavior in a clinical interaction influences that of the other. Emerick noted that maternal behavior on the part of the clinician will tend to elicit immaturity in the client and dependence on the clinician. Consequently, he recommended that clinicians reflect vivid expectations for improvement.

- *Resilience and Error:* The treatment interaction can withstand and adjust to error. Emerick spoke of a homeostatic mechanism whereby stress and resistance created in one session may be followed by relative quiescence in the next. Furthermore, Van Riper (1975) discussed the inevitability of error and the clinician's responsibility to identify and correct it, as follows:

The clinician's errors in judgment show their effects very quickly in the stutterer's behavior and thus revision and correction take place. No one does any therapy without making mistakes. Competent clinicians are those who know they will make errors in judgment and are alert to their occurrence, so they can make the necessary changes in their approach to the problems encountered. Passivity, resistance, and emotional upheavals of many kinds are the signals that tell clinicians they must reassess the stutterers' needs. (pp. 476–477)

Clinician Language

Ours is an interactive, human service profession. Indeed, much of what we do and accomplish in speech–language pathology depends upon the language we use. It is incumbent upon clinicians to know how we talk while engaged in treatment with clients who stutter and their families. Language, therefore, is a critical interpersonal variable within the client–clinician relationship.

How do we become aware of our verbal and nonverbal language? That is the domain of self-study, a process by which we collect, analyze, and evaluate objective data from systematic observation of the clinical interaction. These data, or feedback, help us become aware of what we do in order to consider desired alternatives and to design and implement strategies for change (Shapiro, 1994a). Like communication behaviors among clients, our clinical behaviors can only be changed once we are aware of what is occurring. Behaviors about which we are unaware perpetuate. There are many methods available for collecting objective data, including verbatim recording, selected verbatim recording, rating, tally, interaction analysis, nonverbal analysis, and a variety of individually designed methods (Anderson, 1988; Casey et al., 1988; Shapiro, 1985, 1987, 1994a).

Having used most of the methods listed, I have found the use of interaction analysis systems to be the most instructive (Shapiro, 1994a). In the next chapter, I will introduce such systems and discuss their use and application in professional preparation, specifically in the clinical and supervisory processes. Suffice it here to say that our best efforts to implement change are only as effective as the language we use. Heightened awareness of our verbal and nonverbal behaviors contributes significantly to the effectiveness of the change process and to our own professional growth.

INTRAPERSONAL FACTORS OF EFFECTIVE CLINICIANS

Clinician Thoughts, Feelings, and Beliefs

Significance of Clinicians' Personal Constructs

We have emphasized the importance of clinicians understanding clients' personal constructs about communication and themselves as communicators. The thoughts and feelings that embody the client's personal construct influence how he perceives, predicts, and interacts within his world. Of no less importance, the clinician must understand her own personal construct about communication, stuttering, people who stutter, and the processes of learning, intervention, and change. Similarly, the clinician's behavior is most influenced by her concepts about the nature of the disorder and her role within the change process (Manning, 1996; Van Riper, 1975). In other words, there is a reciprocal relationship between what clinicians think and know and what they do with people who stutter. The diversity in beliefs and attitudes, in part, accounts for the variety of intervention procedures. Discussing such variety, Van Riper (1975) noted the following:

> For some, the preferred cloak is that of authoritarian controller, the omniscient dispenser of punishment and reward. For others, the role of priest in the confessional may be favored. For other clinicians, the cap and gown of information giver seem to be worn most frequently. Indeed, it is possible that not only our roles as clinicians but our basic beliefs concerning the nature of stuttering as well as its treatment may be determined largely by the sort of roles we prefer or have been conditioned to accept. (p. 456)

If we take seriously that the clinicians' beliefs and attitudes influence her perceptions and how she works with people who stutter, then clinicians must become explicitly aware of such internal preconceptions before planning and implementing an intervention program. Such preconceptions contribute to the success or detriment of the clinical process and, in fact, whether a clinician even chooses to work with people who stutter.

Persistence of Clinicians' Negative Attitudes

That clinicians' attitudes have a significant impact on the change process is not debatable. What we need to monitor both individually and collectively, however, is the nature of that impact. We have noted that the attitudes and expectations of the clinician are highly predictive of the client's progress, and that more effective clinicians typically believe sincerely that their clients are able to succeed as a result of treatment (Daly, 1988; Emerick, 1974a, 1974b; Van Riper, 1975). Despite such convincing arguments, the profession continues to battle negative attitudes toward stuttering and people who stutter from student and professional speech–language pathologists as well (Cooper & Cooper, 1985a, 1996; Cooper & Rustin, 1985; Lass, Ruscello, Pannbacker, Schmitt, & Everly-Myers, 1989; Mallard et al., 1988; Ragsdale & Ashby, 1982; St. Louis & Lass, 1981; Turnbaugh et al., 1979; Woods & Williams, 1971, 1976; Yairi & Williams, 1970). Apparently making matters worse, university training program directors and school supervisors have reported that clinical practicum experiences for student clinicians and in-service training opportunities for professional speech–language pathologists are lacking in the area of fluency disorders (Sommers & Caruso, 1995). Similarly, professional clinicians themselves report feeling less competent when working with people who have fluency disorders than those with other communication disorders (Cooper & Cooper, 1985a, 1996; St. Louis & Durrenberger, 1993). The most recent review of clinicians' attitudes was conducted by Cooper and Cooper (1996), who studied the attitudes of 1,198 speech–language pathologists toward stuttering, people who stutter, and their parents, treatment, and related issues. The results of this study conducted between 1983 and 1991 were compared with those of an identical study conducted between 1973 and 1983 of 674 speech–language pathologists (Cooper & Cooper, 1985a). Positive changes in attitudes over the 18-year period included rejection of concepts suggesting parental causality in fluency disorders, dangers in early intervention, and the perception that individuals who stutter possess characteristic personality traits. However, a significant number of clinicians continued to hold unsubstantiated beliefs regarding the personality characteristics of people who stutter, their parents, and the efficacy of early intervention with preschool children who stutter. Furthermore, a significant number of clinicians continued to feel less competent in the area of fluency disorders and believed that this feeling is shared by most clinicians working with people who stutter. Cooper and Cooper (1996) noted the following concern:

> While it is comforting to note that a shift away from viewing individuals who stutter as having psychological problems and distorted perceptions has occurred, it remains disturbing to note that 36% of the clinicians persist in their beliefs that most people who stutter have psychological problems, that 58% believe individuals who stutter possess characteristic personality traits, and that over 63% believe those who stutter have feelings of inferiority. Where and how clinicians develop these perceptions continues to be a mystery. (p. 132)

Interaction of Attitudes and Professional Preparation

Clinicians' attitudes toward stuttering and people who stutter are influenced by the professional preparation received during their undergraduate and graduate degree programs. I expressed previously my concern regarding the relative effectiveness of professional preparation to impact student clinicians' affective processes compared to behavioral and cognitive processes. Manning (1996) noted the following:

> Our attitude about those who come to us for help and our understanding of their communication problems have a fundamental influence on how we approach them as people during both assessment and treatment. What the clinician has been told and what she has been able to observe about stuttering and the people who stutter will determine whether she will even have the desire to work with such clients. (pp. 2–3)

There are clinicians who complete programs of professional preparation and wish to avoid working with people who stutter (Conture, 1990b; Manning, 1996; Silverman, 1996; St. Louis & Durrenberger, 1993; Van Riper, 1991). Unfortunately, as noted previously, student and professional clinicians occasionally report past instructors who have "taught" that "treatment for fluency disorders was rarely successful and that the student would be well advised to concentrate on those clients who were more likely to make progress" (Manning, 1996, p. 142). What concerns me most are the clinicians who wish not to work with people who stutter and feel less than fully competent in this area, yet for a variety reasons continue to take on clients who stutter. This clinical arrangement is doomed to failure before it begins.

The situation just described would be less likely to exist if programs of professional preparation committed to curricula containing both depth and breadth in the area of fluency disorders. However, as of this writing, the American Speech–Language–Hearing Association does not mandate a minimum number of hours in the assessment or treatment of children or adults with fluency disorders, or that a student take even one course in fluency disorders. Therefore the degree of preparedness of clinicians in the area of fluency disorders is dictated by the mission of the individual program, scheduling or other practical concerns, or preferences expressed by faculty and students. Unfortunately, I know of professional speech–language pathologists who had no clinical or academic preparation in the area of fluency disorders during their undergraduate and graduate programs. Such anecdotal reports and comprehensive analyses identifying critical areas of education that are lacking in professional preparation contribute to the movement toward upgrading current professional education of the general practitioners and designing programs to educate specialists in the area of fluency disorders (ASHA, 1995, 1996a, 1996b; Cooper & Cooper, 1996; Starkweather & Givens-Ackerman, 1997).

Interaction of Attitudes and Understanding of Stuttering

A clinician's attitude toward fluency, fluency disorders, and people who stutter is profoundly influenced by her understanding of its nature. Manning (1996) noted that if stuttering is viewed as a mysterious disorder, clinicians understandably will be wary about treating these clients. However, if stuttering is viewed as complex, multidimensional, yet fairly rule governed, the challenge tends to be more inviting. Indeed, while we do not fully understand the nature of stuttering, we do know a lot. We do understand the importance of identifying and controlling for precipitating and perpetuating factors. We know the importance of understanding and involving clients and their families in the treatment process. We know the importance of understanding clients from their own point of view and providing opportunities for success and graduated challenge. We know that many children and adults who stutter achieve great progress. Van Riper (1975) expanded as follows:

> Indeed we know a lot about the nature of stuttering even though we may not know all. We know, for example, that many of the behaviors shown by stutterers are learned responses to the expectancy or the experience of fractured fluency. We know that stutterers have fears—reasonable fears, not phobias—and a good many other negative emotions that contribute to the frequency and abnormality of the disorder. We know that there is evidence of mistiming of the sequencing of motor speech. We recognize that stutterers' self-concepts have been affected by their stuttering. We see the impact of the disorder on their language, perception, thinking, and social relationships. We have clear evidence that the frequency, duration, and kinds of their stuttering behaviors are not only variable but that they can be decreased by a variety of clinical techniques. Certainly, then, no clinician need despair of ever having a dearth of available knowledge on which to base his beliefs or therapeutic regime. What is necessary, however, is that he acquire that knowledge and then evaluate it. (pp. 457–458)

Interaction of Attitudes and Positive Observation and/or Treatment Experience

Finally, clinicians' attitudes are influenced by the treatment they have experienced or observed. Manning (1996) noted that the more students observe clinicians who are not afraid of stuttering and have had success with people who stutter, the more clinicians will be enthusiastic about intervention with people who stutter. He also noted that one of the strengths of clinical preparation (i.e., working with clients who demonstrate a wide range of communication disorders) may also be one of its limitations (i.e., clinicians rarely experience the long view of progress). In other words, student clinicians rarely follow clients throughout the continuum of change. Manning (1996) added, "The window available to student clinicians in graduate programs is a small one" (p. 5). This limitation is not experienced by student clinicians alone. Professional speech–language pathologists rarely follow clients beyond a few months or years after dismissal from formal treatment. Therefore, student clinicians and professional speech–language pathologists should explore opportunities to observe successful treatment and to follow the process and progress of change across the long haul.

Clinician Needs

When approaching and planning intervention, clinicians generally think about clients' needs, but rarely about their own. Surely more has been written about clients' needs. Clinicians, however, have needs too. Because clinicians' needs act like a filter through which clinical interactions are processed and interpreted, clinicians must identify, acknowledge, and address their own needs. Unless clinicians are aware of and control for their own needs, which may change over time, they run the risk of inadvertently exploiting, rather than serving, their clients. Indeed, clinicians would not exploit clients knowingly. Van Riper (1975) aptly noted the following:

> We have trained many clinicians in the course of a lifetime, and it is our impression that those who became the most successful were able to undergo this self-scrutiny. All of us have suffered deprivations of one sort or another in our youth and childhood, and few of us are without currently unsatisfied hungers. Perhaps we were status-deprived; if so, we should beware of our tendency toward assuming the role of authority. Perhaps we were overcontrolled in our childhood; if so, we must guard against an excessive need to control others or its opposite, the compulsion to delegate all responsibility to the client. Certainly, few of us ever got enough love, for the need to be loved seems insatiable; we must therefore be alert to the problems presented by transference. (p. 459)

I remember clearly a nontraditional (i.e., somewhat older) undergraduate student whom I interviewed before she declared her major in communication disorders. I asked her why she decided on communication disorders as an academic concentration and professional ambition. She explained that because of being physically challenged and having experienced inconvenience and ridicule as a result of using a wheelchair, she felt particularly suited to work with others who live with a handicap (i.e., communication disorder). "I can relate to them better than others who have nothing wrong with them at all," she explained. I asked her to elaborate how she felt her personal experiences might both facilitate and inhibit her prospective functioning as a human service professional. She reiterated her sensitivity and empathic inclination for others who have a handicap, but could not conceptualize or foresee any possible limitation. I talked about how we who have or have had an exceptionality indeed experience heightened sensitivities for the human condition, and that this may serve as a professional advantage. However, a potential advantage such as this is balanced by the risk of superimposing our experiences onto another person or losing our objectivity. Doing so would assume that someone else's experiences are the same as our own, thus interpreting one's experience from our, rather than his, assumptions and constructs. In other words, when we are unaware of and without control over our own experiences and needs, we risk treating another person as we were treated or wish we had been treated, rather than acting according to the client's strengths and needs. After discussing these issues, the student and I then had an enlightening conversation about needs and competencies for effective intervention (ASHA, 1995; see Appendix A.3), about the nature of a clinician's personal construct (see Chapter 5), and about the importance of a clinician being aware of and in control of her personal needs. These factors and others are critical for ensuring our objective understanding of the clients we serve and for delivering individualized intervention services of the highest quality.

I frequently encounter any of a series of questions that result in a similar line of dialogue. These questions are:

- "Should one person who stutters treat another?"

- "Do you think that people who have not stuttered can be as effective as those who have in treating people who stutter?"

- "Aren't you more suited to treat people who stutter because you yourself have stuttered and achieved significant fluency success?"

I remain reluctant to give a blanket answer to any of these questions. Again, I view previous personal experiences as a potential advantage (i.e., sensitivity, empathy) balanced with a potential disadvantage (i.e., bias, loss of objectivity). A client who stutters would be unlikely to accuse a clinician who has stuttered or does stutter that she cannot comprehend the difficulty imposed in one's life by stuttering. This may be seen as an advantage, compared to clinicians who do not stutter being criticized that they cannot know what it is like. Furthermore, clinicians who stutter typically do not approach clients who stutter with trepidation, as might clinicians who do not stutter. In fact, as Van Riper (1975) indicated,

> Stuttering clinicians, at least, are not afraid of stutterers. They know from their personal experience that they are tough animals, that they have endured and survived, and moreover that most stutterers respect a clinician who will not handle them gingerly" (p. 460).

However, a clinician's own experience with stuttering may be a disadvantage, particularly if the clinician stutters noticeably, for clients who feel directed by clinicians to, "Do as I say, not as I do." In other words, clients may question the clinical effectiveness of clinicians who are yet to gain control over their own fluency. I know several professional colleagues at universities who have not experienced successful fluency control, and therefore voluntarily ceased to teach courses in fluency disorders or to see clients who stutter. One colleague (personal communication, November, 1994) explained to me the following:

> I feel like the blind leading the blind. How can I convey, "Do as I say, not as I do"? That's just not right. The field is large enough now to acknowledge that

certain clinicians are more suited to work with certain clients. Knowing my limitations is a professional strength.

I have found that among student and professional clinicians, whether people who stutter without fluency control are suited to work with others who stutter is debatable and controversial (Shapiro, Brotherton, & Ogletree, 1995). Relatively recent federal legislation has been enacted to help interpret such thorny issues (e.g., Federal Rehabilitation Act of 1973, Section 504; Americans with Disabilities Act of 1990, P.L. 101-336). Notwithstanding their limitations, many people who stutter have made significant and lasting contributions to our profession. Discussing earlier days when training programs routinely rejected, discouraged, if not discriminated against, any person who stuttered from entering professional preparation in communication disorders, Van Riper (1975) noted, "Had such a practice been universal in the early days of our profession, its development would have been markedly retarded, for stutterers have made major contributions" (p. 459).

Returning to clinicians' needs, clinicians must know themselves well before they work with clients. Clinicians prepare for, enter, and remain in the profession for different reasons. Most, however, want to make a difference in some meaningful way in the life of another person, enjoy the feeling of having the ability to relieve pain and suffering, and experience rewards when a client noticeably shows improvement. Nevertheless, clinicians have individual needs. Clinicians filter clinical interaction, in addition to all other experiences, through these needs and other components of their personal construct. Being aware of their needs, thoughts, feelings, and attitudes enables clinicians to control for them, thereby recognizing and addressing the uniqueness of the client's experience. Initially, novice clinicians often justify their professional commitment by expressing a motivation of altruism (i.e., selflessly serving others). Career speech–language pathologists know that helping others is both a motivation and a source of personal reward. To be motivated and personally rewarded are needs of all people, including clinicians. Walle (1974) discussed the reciprocal relationship between clients' and clinicians' needs and behaviors, as follows:

> The therapist must achieve satisfaction from the interpersonal exchange, or his dissatisfaction may defeat the patient. . . . Who needs therapy? The therapist needs the therapy! If experiences are not therapeutic, they can be disruptive and even painful. When we choose the kinds of patients we think we can help, we are also attempting to choose those who can satisfy us. The therapeutic approach must suit the therapist; the therapist must suit the patient." (pp. 8–9)

Clinician Satisfaction and Rewards

We have already discussed the clinician's thoughts, feelings, beliefs, and needs as critical intrapersonal factors about which effective clinicians must remain aware. Other intrapersonal factors are the satisfaction and rewards experienced by clinicians. Just as some clinicians are loath to consider their own needs, erroneously fearing that so doing inhibits rather than facilitates addressing the client's needs, similar reluctance is found among clinicians to identify their sources of internal satisfaction and personal reward. I argue that clinicians must keep a finger on their own pulse of satisfaction and reward, both of which provide a sense of inherent meaning, in order to remain effective over the long run. Life must have meaning. Reminding us of our sense of inherent meaning, our satisfaction and rewards are what keep us excited, committed, and passionate about what we do professionally with people who stutter.

Van Riper (1974) eloquently described his sense of inherent meaning found in having intimate and ultimate "impact" on another human being. Furthermore, he (1975) expressed satisfaction in being challenged to use professional competence, learning and growing, participating in the human capacity for triumph over significant obstacles, engaging intricately in the craftsmanship of intervention, and knowing the awareness of meaningfulness. Emerick (1974a, 1974b) captured his sense of satisfaction in promoting growth in his clients, and thereby in himself, by means of continual self-confrontation. Walle (1974) discussed his satisfaction from setting in motion factors that engender hope, thereby bringing about positive changes in both the client's and clinician's life. Significantly, these and other master clinicians discuss their satisfaction and rewards as internal, or intrapersonal, factors that renew and energize. Clinicians' satisfaction and rewards differ, but clinicians must feel satisfied and rewarded in order to remain in the profession and to contribute meaningfully over their professional lifetime.

I have been a speech–language pathologist for more than 20 years. Honestly, not a single day has passed when I have not felt thankful for the privilege of working with people who stutter and their families. I sincerely enjoy my work and believe that it is important. I appreciate the opportunity to learn and grow, on a daily basis, with and from my client, student, faculty, and administrative colleagues (Shapiro, 1994b). At one time in my life, I hoped that I could change the world. Knowing better now, optimistically rather than in defeat, I feel fortunate to be a part of helping our clients and their families change their own communicative world. As a result, I feel a connection with the human condition that transcends any conceivable limitation, and a satisfaction in being constantly challenged to recall, apply, create, and thereby advance our knowledge of communication and its disorders. What keeps me fresh is the internal satisfaction in believing in what I do, with whom I do it, and the ultimate importance of the process and products of communication.

Discussing such aspects of communication, Gardner (1983) developed the concept of personal intelligence, including both intrapersonal and interpersonal elements. Intrapersonal intelligence was expressed in this way:

> On the one side, there is the development of the internal aspects of a person. The core capacity at work here is access to one's own feeling life—one's range of affects or emotions: the capacity instantly to effect discriminations among these feelings and, eventually, to label them, to enmesh them in symbolic codes, to draw upon them as a means of understanding and guiding one's behavior. (p. 239)

Intrapersonal knowledge is what enables clinicians and clients to understand their own feelings and those of each other. It is from this knowledge base that we think and talk introspectively about feelings, and from which we become aware of and thereby control our feelings in order to address our clients' needs.

Our intrapersonal knowledge is what enables us to come to understand our client's personal construct, and that of ourselves.

Another aspect of personal intelligence, interpersonal knowledge, was expressed by Gardner (1983) in this way:

> The other personal intelligence turns outward, to other individuals. The core capacity here is the ability to notice and make distinctions among other individuals and, in particular, among their moods, temperaments, motivations, and intentions. (p. 239)

This type of knowledge is what enables clinicians to understand the intentions and desires of our clients and their families and to act upon that knowledge. We discussed in Unit III the importance of creating opportunities for clients to discuss, and thereby understand, their own objectives, thus becoming centrally involved in (i.e., "owning") the clinical process. Development of personal intelligence in clients and clinicians has at its core an emerging sense of self, an interaction between intrapersonal (i.e., inner feelings) and interpersonal (i.e., other person) knowledge.

Within this chapter, we have considered intra- and interpersonal factors of effective clinicians. Such a development of self, in this case one's professional self, is what Gardner (1983) refers to as "the highest achievement of human beings, . . . that capacity about which individuals have the strongest and most intimate views; thus it becomes a sensitive (as well as an elusive) target to examine" (pp. 242–243). It is that opportunity to develop my intra- and interpersonal knowledge as a clinician and that of the clients and their families we serve about which I am most grateful and from which I accrue lasting satisfaction and internal reward.

THE CLINICIAN AS GUARDIAN ANGEL

Perhaps one indicator of an effective clinician is the ability to develop a sense of self including the interpersonal and intrapersonal factors discussed in this chapter. As noted, the clinician's behaviors (ASHA, 1995) present only one aspect of the dynamic amalgam that is the clinician. Of continuing challenge for the novice and seasoned clinician alike is management of the other interpersonal (such as attributes and manner of interaction; language) and intrapersonal (thoughts, feelings, beliefs; needs; satisfaction and rewards) factors. Indeed, as Walle (1974) stated, "Qualifying for therapeutic practice is one thing; suitability is another," and "It is easier to become a therapist than to be one" (p. 10). In other words, selecting and preparing for a profession is a labor-intensive endeavor in the short run. Helping clients and their families establish and realize communicative dreams while developing one's own personal and professional sense of self is a larger and dynamic challenge for the long run that lasts throughout one's professional life span.

Indeed, talking about aspects of one's personal intelligence, or development of one's professional self, "becomes a sensitive (as well as elusive) target to examine." Walle (1974) discussed the importance of the clinician's interpersonal and intrapersonal skills:

> If he [the clinician] projects the attitude that this [client] is one of God's finest creations, a human being, and this person is worthy of his best efforts, his genuine interest—not only because it is his job—then the patient will pick this up and think, "I too, must give my best efforts to help him help me." This is mutual reciprocation and a kind of love . . . that opens the gates of trust. (p. 11)

Furthermore, Walle (1974) discussed the importance of both the client and clinician being willing to take a personal risk; that is, to give something of themselves, something of value in the form of a personal belief about the client's capacity for change. He advised that, "If therapists can learn to care objectively and then sit still long enough to learn from the person who needs help, this—on a broad scale—could be the power to transform them both" (p. 11).

We began and now end this chapter by articulating the importance of the clinician and the client–clinician relationship to the change process. Argeropoulos (1974) presented a model depicting the relationship between one's self-concept and personal success or failure. The "tree of self-defeat" symbolizes the individual who has internalized negative qualities into his lifestyle, thus achieving little of a positive nature. In comparison, the "tree of self-realization" depicts the richness and fullness of life and positive achievement resulting from positive relationships of warmth and closeness. Argeropoulos likened the tree of self-defeat to a dormant tree of real life, stating, "Just as the dormant tree comes to life when the proper nurturant conditions of spring arrive, so can the defeated person come to life when the proper emotional climate is cultivated in his life" (p. 87). Such cultivation is within the domain of the effective clinician.

Many clients have a fund of positive, self-realizing forces within their communication environment (e.g., love, kindness, warmth, trust, hope, and mutual support) to which the clinician contributes by helping clients achieve their communication potential. These clients have internalized and retained an appropriate and positive personal construct, one focused on abilities, strengths, healing power, and self-actualization. Other clients, however, do not have such positive forces, or do not perceive such forces in a positive light. These clients have internalized feelings of negativity, insecurity, fear, self-pity, and dependency. In other words, these clients have formed a personal construct based on personal limitations rather than strengths, DISability rather than disABILITY, DISfluency rather than disFLUENCY. For both clients, the clinicians' role is formidable. Particularly for the latter, the clinician might serve as an "enlightened witness" (Miller, 1990), a singular person who significantly influences another by introducing sunshine to darkness, kindness to cruelty, positive movement to negative stagnation. Miller (1990) noted that a child who has known nothing but cruelty will accept and possibly gravitate toward, rather than resist, such an environment because he has no point of comparison. He will accept such a condition as normal behavior and often repeat it. An enlightened witness, Miller noted, is someone who offers him the experience of being loved, cherished, nurtured, and accepted, thus a window into a positive alternative.

The clinician can be that significant other, that change agent, who introduces the sweet taste of fluency freedom that ultimately yields communicative control and independence. The clinician creates opportunities for the client to experience fluency success, thus requiring the client to reexamine his personal construct, thereby redefining and reaffirming his internalized prognosis for positive change. To emphasize the importance of the affective elements of the change process (e.g., love, hope, trust, and nurture) minimizes neither the other interpersonal and intrapersonal factors discussed in this chapter nor the clinical procedures discussed in Chapters 8, 9, and 10. Clinical intervention is that client–clinician interaction that both targets and utilizes affective, behavioral, and cognitive dimensions of communication.

Within this and preceding chapters, we have discussed the clinician as participating in many different professional roles. Recently, Anderson, Lee-Wilkerson, and Chabon (1995) delineated the clinician's roles as including that of environmental planner and time manager, modeler/facilitator, observer/interactor/recorder, counselor/parent advisor, collaborator/team player, and guardian angel. While all of these roles are essential, I wish to address only the last one for our present purposes. The authors presented a touching vignette that I believe has import for working with people who stutter. When looking for a tutor for her child and after facing several dead ends, one of the authors contacted a teacher who had written a book about helping children to achieve in school while feeling good about themselves. During the conversation, the teacher gave the parent an opportunity to share her perceptions about her son's needs and to express her own concerns. The teacher agreed to work with the boy, adding that every child needs a guardian angel and that she would like to be his. The parent reported that the teacher's statement, unexpected and unusual, gave the parent a positive lift and an immediate feeling of hope and security. Anderson et al. (1995) suggested that it may be time for clinicians to assume quietly the role of guardian angels (not unlike Miller's, 1990, concept of the enlightened witness), as follows:

> As guardian angels, we may offer acceptance, protection, guidance, and inspiration, and expect our clients to make their contributions as well. This is truly the ultimate partnership. Our guardian angels believe in us and help us to believe in ourselves. This could perhaps be our greatest role as speech-language pathologists for, in this context, . . . intervention is at its most divine. (p. 59)

CHAPTER SUMMARY

This chapter, the first in Unit IV, addressed the clinician and the interpersonal relationship as the critical elements of effective intervention. This relationship is influenced by both intrapersonal and interpersonal factors. Once aware of and in control of such factors, clinicians can develop or improve their professional skills.

Interpersonal factors of effective clinicians include certain clinician behaviors, attributes, and features of language. Clinician behaviors refer to the goals, processes, and competencies for assessment, management, and transfer and maintenance with people who stutter that were presented in the "Guidelines for Practice in Stuttering Treatment" (ASHA, 1995; see Appendix A.3). Attributes of effective clinicians refer to a manner of interaction characterized by empathy; warmth; genuineness; personal magnetism; compatible friction; and realistic, focused optimism. Empathy is an authentic sensitivity for another person, being able to experience, and thereby understand, the experience of another person as if it were our own. Warmth is a composite of understanding, sincerity, friendliness, and respect that provides unconditional positive regard.

Genuineness refers to the ability to be one's true self as a person with a client while conveying professional competence and personal confidence. Personal magnetism reflects those qualities of the clinician that naturally are attractive, inviting, and arouse hope in the client. Compatible friction is the result of deliberately disturbing the client's equilibrium, which is necessary for change to occur, while the client experiences empathy, warmth, genuineness, and ongoing commitment from the clinician. Realistic, focused optimism refers to the creation of hope or faith that is centered on specific areas of the client's potential. Effective clinicians are aware of their language, or their verbal and nonverbal forms of communication, when working with people who stutter and their families.

Intrapersonal factors of effective clinicians include clinician thoughts, feelings, and beliefs; needs; and satisfaction and rewards. Effective clinicians understand their own personal constructs, monitor the potential impact of their attitudes toward stuttering and people who stutter, and are aware of the potential effects of their beliefs about the nature of stuttering and their own past experience with or observation of stuttering. Effective clinicians identify, acknowledge, and address their own needs related to the clinical process. Finally, effective clinicians identify their sources of internal satisfaction and personal reward in order to retain a sense of inherent meaning in their professional practice.

The chapter closed with an acknowledgment that it is easier to become a clinician than to be one, and that qualifying for clinical practice is not necessarily synonymous with suitability for clinical practice. In her unique capacity to facilitate change and to help people who stutter and their families realize their potential, the clinician was cast as enlightened witness and as a guardian angel.

Chapter 11 Study Questions

1. This chapter reviewed interpersonal and intrapersonal aspects of effective clinicians. What do you believe to be the ingredients of effective intervention? How might these elements be acquired? How might they be maintained? How do the factors you have identified relate to the concept of personal intelligence presented by Gardner (1983)?

2. We have discussed the multidimensionality of clinicians and clinical competence? What is clinical competence? What is the likelihood that a person who acquires the interpersonal and intrapersonal factors discussed necessarily will be clinically competent or effective as a clinician? What is meant by the distinction between qualification and suitability for clinical practice? Why is it more challenging to be a clinician than to become one?

3. Clinicians wear many different hats. In what ways might a clinician be an enlightened witness for a person who stutters and his family? How might a clinician serve as a guardian angel?

4. We reviewed the attitudes of clinicians about stuttering, people who stutter, and their feelings about themselves as potential change agents. We also reviewed several issues regarding current loopholes that exist in academic and clinical preparation of clinicians in the area of fluency and fluency disorders. How would you characterize both of these issues and what do you believe are their origins? Given your understanding of these issues, what recommendations do you have? What are your feelings about specialty certification in the area of fluency disorders and other areas of clinical practice?

5. In sharing my own personal construct, I distinguished between a desire to change the world and a desire to help clients and their families change their own worlds. How might each disposition influence the assessment and treatment processes? How might other personal constructs influence the processes of clinical intervention?

Unit IV

◆ ◆ ◆ ◆ ◆ ◆ ◆ ◆ ◆ ◆ ◆ ◆ ◆ ◆ ◆ ◆ ◆ ◆ ◆

The Clinician: A Paragon of Change

Chapter 11

The Clinician and the Client–Clinician Relationship

Chapter 12

Professional Preparation and Lifelong Learning: The Making of a Clinician

Chapter 12

Professional Preparation and Lifelong Learning: The Making of a Clinician

♦ ♦ ♦ ♦ ♦ ♦ ♦ ♦ ♦ ♦ ♦ ♦ ♦ ♦ ♦ ♦ ♦ ♦

Professional Preparation of Clinicians Who Work with People Who Stutter   476

Academic Process   477
  Academic Process Defined   477
  Revision in Training Standards   478
  Academic Knowledge   479

Clinical Process   480
  Clinical Process Defined   480
  Clinical Knowledge   480
  A Model for Clinician Development   481
  Clinical Process Components   483
    Understanding the Clinical Process   483
    Planning the Clinical Process   484
    Observing and Analyzing the Clinical Process   484
      Interaction Analysis Systems   484
      Nonverbal Analysis   485
      Individually Designed Procedures   486
    Integrating the Components of the Clinical Process   487

Supervisory Process   487
  Supervisory Process Defined   487
  Clinical Supervision Defined   488
  Supervisory Knowledge   489
  A Model for Supervisory Development   490
    Evaluation–Feedback Stage   492
    Transitional Stage   493
    Self-Supervision Stage   493
    Implications of the Continuum of Supervision   494
  Supervisory Process Components   495
    Understanding the Supervisory Process   495
    Planning the Supervisory Process   496
    Observing the Supervisory Process   497
      Interaction Analysis Systems   497
      Nonverbal Analysis   500
      Individually Designed Procedures   502
    Analyzing the Supervisory Process   502
    Integrating the Supervisory Process   503
  Avenues of Supervisory Preparation   504

Maintenance of Professional Competence 505

    Knowing and Internalizing the Desire To Learn 505

    Learning as a Lifelong Process 507

    Maintaining Parallels: Different Trees, Same Forest 508

        The Clinical and Supervisory Processes 508

        Developing, Maintaining, and Upgrading Professional Competence 509

        Back to the Beginning 509

Chapter Summary 510

Chapter 12 Study Questions 512

No man can reveal to you aught but that which already lies half asleep in the dawning of your own knowledge. The teacher who walks in the shadow of the temple, among his followers, gives not of his wisdom but rather of his faith and his lovingness. If he is indeed wise he does not bid you enter the house of his wisdom, but rather leads you to the threshold of your own mind.

(GIBRAN, 1923, P. 51)

How are good clinicians made? Are they born or are they cultivated? Walle (1974) distinguished between qualifications and suitability for therapeutic practice, noting that, "It is easier to become a therapist than to be one" (p. 10).

In the last chapter, we discussed the importance of the clinician and the client–clinician relationship to the change process, and the interpersonal and intrapersonal competencies that are among those necessary for clinicians to work effectively with people who stutter and their families. In the present chapter, we will address the academic, clinical, and supervisory processes by which such competencies are developed, and conclude with a discussion of three elements that are critical for maintaining and upgrading a clinician's competence across her professional career. In doing so, we will make the following points, among others:

- Professional preparation for clinicians who work with people who stutter must integrate experiences across the academic, clinical, and supervisory processes, and must impact the affective, behavioral, and cognitive domains.

- An explicit understanding of the academic, clinical, and supervisory processes enables its participants (i.e., namely clinicians) to contribute meaningfully to and thereby gain maximum benefit from the experience of professional preparation.

- Maintenance of professional competence requires internalizing the desire to learn, committing to learning as a lifelong process, and understanding and maintaining parallels in the nature and process of professional development over time.

- Professional preparation and lifelong learning provide an opportunity for learners to become teachers and teachers to become learners across the interactive and dynamic journey of life.

PROFESSIONAL PREPARATION OF CLINICIANS WHO WORK WITH PEOPLE WHO STUTTER

Discussing the education of speech–language pathologists and audiologists, Rassi and McElroy (1992) raised a most pertinent question for students and educators to consider: "Does received information translate into applied information?" (p. 443). Addressing learning and teaching from perspectives of frameworks, environments, methods, materials, contexts, and continua, the authors concluded, "Not necessarily. In some cases, it may be applied in a timely fashion; in others, not until years after it was obtained; and, in still others, it may never be applied" (p. 443). Indeed, the acquisition, application, creation, and thereby advancement of knowledge relevant to stuttering and people who stutter present a formidable challenge to all participants in the academic (i.e., students and professors), clinical (i.e., clients and clinicians), and supervisory (i.e., supervisees and supervisors) processes. All participants, in my view, are learners and teachers, whether learner/teacher or teacher/learner. All participants, while serving different roles in the respective processes, are working toward similar, if not the same, objectives—to learn and grow with and from our clients and their families in order to improve the communication world in which we all live. In this section, we will consider three distinct, albeit necessarily overlapping, instructional processes—academic, clinical, and supervisory—that help translate information received into information applied.

Traditionally, the academic process addresses the cognitive domain (i.e., thoughts and content) and the clinical and supervisory processes the behavioral domain (i.e., procedures and application). I have expressed my concern that professional preparation may be falling short, particularly in the area of student clinicians' affective knowledge. The three domains of knowledge (affective, behavioral, and cognitive) and the instructional processes by which they are acquired (academic, clinical, and supervisory) must be integrated. Furthermore, all processes within professional preparation must deliberately impact the affective domain (i.e., feelings, beliefs, and attitudes about stuttering and people who stutter). In light of the persistent negative stereotypes held by the general public, workers in professions allied to education and medicine, and speech–language pathologists, impacting clinicians' affective processes should be seen as a curricular imperative. To this end, each instructional process will be considered separately.

Most of you reading this chapter are student clinicians or professional speech–language pathologists. In either case, most of you are functioning both as a clinician within the clinical process (i.e., you are working with a client who stutters) and as a supervisee within the supervisory process (i.e., you are working with the support and direction of a supervisor, either in a graduate program of clinical education or within your employment setting). Some professional speech–language pathologists also may be functioning as a supervisor of other professionals. As you read and learn more about the processes in which many of you are currently engaged, consider how you might use your heightened knowledge to effect an even greater contribution on your part to your own professional development. It is often said that we reap what we sow. Professional preparation and lifelong learning should be no exception. Therefore, consider how the frameworks, methods, and materials discussed here might be useful to your own professional development now and later.

Academic Process

Academic Process Defined

The academic process typically begins upon one's entry into a program of professional preparation and continues until one's completion of that program. For purposes of discussion, the academic process will be assumed to be that which occurs within the classroom. Making such a general statement, I acknowledge that the dynamics of the classroom experience vary according to the uniqueness of and interaction among variables including the instructor, students, methods, materials, curricula, media, and so on, and that the classroom experience necessarily relates to and must overlap with the clinical and supervisory processes.

Revision in Training Standards

Recent changes by the American Speech–Language–Hearing Association (ASHA) resulted in the reduction in training standards, impacting significantly the academic and clinical processes. Prior to 1993, ASHA required a specified number of hours of supervised clinical experience (including evaluation and treatment) for each of the basic areas of disorder in speech–language pathology—articulation, language, voice, and fluency. ASHA also required that students complete the requisite coursework before engaging in the related clinical experiences. These two requirements necessitated that student clinicians receive both academic and clinical preparation across the spectrum of communication disorders before graduating and entering the professional arena. However, in 1993, the Council on Professional Standards (COPS) of ASHA revised its standards by deleting the number of hours specified in each disorder area, thus requiring only hours in more generic categories of "speech disorders" and "language disorders." In theory, this change allowed programs greater flexibility in designing the academic and clinical curriculum and in meeting ASHA standards. In practice, however, this meant that programs were free to cut back on clinical training in the areas where clients reportedly are hardest to find (e.g., stuttering and voice) and on academic training (coursework in fluency or voice was not required unless the student engaged in clinical practicum with clients demonstrating fluency or voice disorders, respectively).

While a standardized outcome measure continues to be required for all graduates of programs granting the masters degree in communication disorders (i.e., the National Examination in Speech–Language Pathology and Audiology, NESPA), individual programs now are more internally responsible for the nature and content of their curriculum. A survey conducted by Starkweather and Bishop (1994) one year after the new standards were put into effect revealed that two thirds of the programs surveyed had cut back either on the required academic coursework or clinical practicum in the area of stuttering (Starkweather & Givens-Ackerman, 1997). These results indeed are disturbing, particularly since clinical training in the area of stuttering according to earlier standards was considered insufficient (Mallard et al., 1988; Sommers & Caruso, 1995; St. Louis & Durrenberger, 1993; Williams, 1971), if not in violation of ASHA's Code of Ethics (ASHA, 1994a; see Appendix A.2).

Starkweather and Givens-Ackerman (1997) reviewed several positive consequences that have resulted from the reduction in the specification of requirements for clinical and academic training. Two positive outcomes were coordinated by ASHA's Special Interest Division #4 (Fluency and Fluency Disorders). First was the development of the Guidelines for Practice in Stuttering Treatment (ASHA, 1995; see Appendix A.3), referred to in the last chapter. Second was the establishment of criteria for specialty recognition in the area of fluency disorders, thus acknowledging clinicians who are especially equipped to work with people who stutter. As of this writing, Division #4's petition to establish a Commission on Fluency Disorders charged with implementing a fluency specialist recognition program has been reviewed by ASHA's Clinical Specialty Board. Once approved, the Commission could be appointed, functioning, and processing specialty recognition applications by late 1998 (Cooper, 1996, 1998). A third positive outcome was an increase in the public and political awareness of people who stutter and the clinicians who serve them. Several organizations became stronger and received increased public attention, including the International Fluency Association, ASHA's Special Interest Division #4, the Stuttering Foundation of America, and the National Stuttering Project (see Appendix B).

Academic Knowledge

Student clinicians acknowledge and professional speech–language pathologists recall that instructors have a significant responsibility for the design of academic courses and decisions related to objectives, content, process, and outcomes. It is important for clinicians, whether presently or previously engaged in the academic process, to understand the nature of the process and the origin of its content. Statements of general curricular guidelines are found in a variety of ASHA documents including Standards and Implementations for the Certificates of Clinical Competence (ASHA, 1994b), and Standards for Accreditation of Educational Programs in Speech–Language Pathology and Audiology (ASHA, 1992b). The most comprehensive framework for establishing objectives and content for coursework in fluency disorders is found in the section addressing Learned Attributes (p. 28) in the Guidelines for Practice in Stuttering Treatment (ASHA, 1995). These guidelines are instructive for all student clinicians and professional speech–language pathologists. The guidelines, abbreviated below and included in unedited form in Appendix A.3, address acquisition, understanding, integration, and application of knowledge in the following areas:

- Etiology and development of stuttering

- Phenomenology of stuttering (e.g., episodic variation, clustering, paradoxical intention, adaptation and consistency, spontaneous recovery, fluency enhancement, arousal effects)

- Normal and language-based (dis)fluency, rate, prosody, rhythm, and effort, and development of these speech characteristics

- Treatment planning from focused yet broad and dynamic perspectives (i.e., adjustable to accommodate new research findings and theoretical perspectives)

- Relations between a person's normal and abnormal speech behavior, and his beliefs, upbringing, and cultural background

- Processes of dynamic clinical interaction including transference, denial, grief, and victimization

- Communication about stuttering with clients and their families

- Psychopathology

- Cognitive and behavioral learning theory

Clinical Process

Clinical Process Defined

The clinical process is an interaction involving at least two sets of participants, the clinician and client (i.e., and family members). When the clinical process occurs within the supervisory framework as is typical for university training programs and other professional settings, the list of participants is extended to include the supervisor and the clinician who also fills the role of the supervisee (i.e., clinician/supervisee; Casey et al., 1988).

Clinical Knowledge

The Guidelines for Practice in Stuttering Treatment (ASHA, 1995) contain the most definitive statements of goals, processes, and competencies in the areas of assessment, management, and transfer and maintenance. As noted, this valuable document is printed in its entirety in Appendix A.3 and should be required reading for all providers (student clinicians, professional speech–language pathologists, clinical supervisors) and consumers (clients and their families) of fluency intervention services. Providers of clinical service should review the guidelines to build or verify their understanding of critical goals for intervention with people who stutter, procedures that have been found or are thought to be effective in reaching those goals, and necessary competencies for implementing the procedures. These guidelines also are useful to clinicians in self-assessment, helping them determine their own need for continued education in a particular area (Starkweather & Givens-Ackerman, 1997). Clinicians should be aware, however, that the guidelines emphasize acquisition and application of knowledge within the cognitive and behavioral domains. Additional self-assessment should be required with respect to one's affective knowledge (feelings, beliefs, and attitudes about stuttering and people who stutter). I emphasize this potential limitation within the guidelines to prevent clinicians from overlooking the importance of acquisition and application of affective knowledge. As discussed in the last chapter, all the emphasis on what is done within intervention (clinical procedures) and why it is done (clinical rationale) cannot replace the significance of how it is done (the manner with which the clinician communicates affectively her faith in the client's ability to improve and her confidence in the clinical process to achieve that change). People who stutter and their families should review the guidelines to build their understanding of intervention as a coherent process and to provide a framework to evaluate the services received. Cooper (1997) emphasized the importance of clients' satisfaction with clinicians' affective knowledge, advising clients as follows:

> If, from the very start, you don't like and respect your clinician, find another one. You need and deserve a clinician with whom you feel comfortable and with whom you can be open and honest about how you feel, think, and behave. If from the very first time you meet, your clinician doesn't make you feel good about being in therapy, find another. I am not saying everything should be sweetness and light in therapy. In fact, if it is, probably nothing is happening. But I am saying your clinician should make you feel good about being there. Research reveals that effective clinicians:
>
> - Express feelings openly—they let you know how they feel;
>
> - Are honest—they tell it like it is;

- Are positive in their attitudes—they see the good where many do not;
- Reflect feelings rather than direct feeling—they don't presume to tell others how they should feel;
- Are open minded—they are not judgmental;
- Are informative—they are perfectly clear about the purpose for each therapeutic activity;
- Are perseverative in their pursuit of goals—they hang in there;
- Are detail disciplined—they don't miss a thing. (pp. 164–165)

Furthermore, Cooper (1997) concluded that effective clinicians are: affectively verbal—viscerally vocal, affectively honest, primarily reflective—not affectively directive, devoid of dogma, noninterpretive, perseverative, informative, and detail disciplined. Indeed, clinical knowledge must include that which is affective and must be communicated to the client.

A Model for Clinician Development

The material presented in this section is directed toward the ongoing professional development of all clinicians who work with people who stutter and their families. Development of clinical competence is begun within professional preparation during the academic (student–professor interaction), clinical (client–clinician interaction), and supervisory (supervisee–supervisor interaction) processes, and is continued in renewal training, continued education, and self-study activities throughout one's career. Shapiro and Moses (1989) presented a model of clinician development (see Table 12.1), which contains a series of developmental phases in how clinicians organize and interpret information relevant to clinical planning, implementation, and problem solving. In other words, development of clinical expertise implies an observable and developmental sequence of skills. The model assumes that clinicians regularly engage in problem solving, which requires applying or constructing knowledge. Implicitly, construction of knowledge refers to creating ideas by reflecting on and making inferences about information and perceptions from goal-directed interaction. Explicitly, aspects of clinician development occur in four areas of problem solving, including orientation of perspective, dimensions of behavior conceptualized, possible solutions generated, and causal reasoning.

Clinicians functioning at an early developmental level, challenged by novel and complex problems encountered during clinical interaction with clients who stutter, typically reveal the following characteristics: centering on a personal point of view about communication, stuttering, and fluency intervention (i.e., viewing oneself as in control of a client's potential fluency improvement); considering relatively few variables when thinking about intervention strategies and causes of problems (i.e., focusing on only one aspect of a client's stuttering; e.g., behavior, thoughts, *or* feelings); generating relatively few problem solving procedures (i.e., intervention strategies; e.g., "We will do airflow therapy"), and failing to reflect on or modify causal assumptions after clinical intervention (e.g., "You're still too tense. That is why you stutter. We'll have to continue with airflow therapy").

At a more advanced level of clinical development, clinicians incorporate the client's perspective (i.e., viewing intervention and the change process as a

Table 12.1. Aspects of Development in Clinical Problem Solving

Aspect	From	To
Perspective	Identifies problems in the clinical interaction that affect self (i.e., that cause personal discomfort—clinician is major focus).	Identifies problems as seen from the perspective of others and self (client is major focus).
	Tends to think of problem resolution as caused by self or other authority figure.	Views problem resolution as being the result of active and shared client–clinician interaction (i.e., goal establishment and attainment).
	Evaluates the efficacy of problem-solving procedure from self-centered perspective.	Evaluates problem-solving procedure from multiple perspectives.
Dimensions of behavior conceptualized	Conceives of behavior as unidimensional. Views problem as affecting and affected by only one dimension of behavior.	Conceives of behavior as multidimensional. Views problem as affected by many dimensions of behavior.
Possible solutions generated	Thinks of one problem-solving procedure.	Generates and reflects upon multiple problem-solving strategies.
Causal concepts	Implements problem-solving strategy, but fails to reflect upon or modify causal theories.	Implements strategy and reflects upon and modifies, if appropriate, causal theories.

Note. From "Creative Problem Solving in Public School Supervision," by D. A. Shapiro & N. Moses, 1989, *Language, Speech, and Hearing Services in Schools, 20,* p. 323. Copyright 1989 by the American Speech–Language–Hearing Association. Reprinted with permission.

shared, interactive challenge); consider multiple variables related to intervention for and causes of stuttering (i.e., thinking about stuttering as a multidimensional problem that potentially impacts behaviors, thoughts, *and* feelings); generate multiple problem solving procedures (e.g., *Clinician:* "Why don't we consider building a foundation of fluency success so we can study and better understand all that you already are doing so well? From that we can get a handle on what we can get you to do even more often to increase your fluency. Then, we can study the remaining disfluencies and together decide which targets should receive focus. All the while, we can keep tabs on how you are feeling and what you are thinking as your fluency improves. What do you think about this preliminary plan? How does this relate to what you expressed you hoped to accomplish?"); and reflect on and modify causal assumptions after clinical intervention (e.g., *Clinician:* "I want to talk about your thoughts and feelings about stuttering and yourself as a communicator. This is what we call our personal construct about communication. Usually, what we think affects what we do and vice versa. Sometimes, one perpetuates the other, unless we address them directly";

Client, later: "I'm so glad you got me to think about my thoughts and feelings about stuttering and myself as a communicator. I had no idea that my thinking actually was working against me, maintaining the way I communicate, particularly how, when, and where I stutter.").

To verify that the developmental changes in problem-solving behavior indeed occur as clinicians acquire and integrate additional professional experience, Moses and Shapiro (1996) designed a taxonomy for assessing clinician development and applied it to a microanalysis of videotaped clinical sessions of three student clinicians. Independent raters analyzed 97 clinical problem episodes, which required a total of 3,589 classification decisions. Three developmental profiles of clinical problem solving were derived from the extensive analyses. The novice clinician ("Kitchen Sink Profile") was characterized by orienting to herself, attending to few dimensions of behavior, and generating a limited number of possible solutions to clinical problems. The intermediate clinician ("Map Reader Profile") was characterized by an emerging problem-solving ability reflecting inconsistency in assuming the client's perspective, referencing multiple dimensions of behavior, and generating multiple problem solutions. Finally, the more advanced clinician ("Air Traffic Controller Profile") was characterized by minimizing the number of problems encountered, approaching those that occurred from the dual perspectives of her client and herself, addressing multiple dimensions of behavior, and generating multiple problem solutions. The results supported the application of a developmental conceptualization to the assessment and facilitation of problem-solving skills in clinicians throughout the professional preparation experience including academic, clinical, and supervisory processes. Therefore, student clinicians and professional speech–language pathologists are encouraged to use the model presented to identify their own level of professional development when working with people who stutter and their families, and to monitor and facilitate their ongoing development over time.

Clinical Process Components

The components of the clinical process, as will be seen, are parallel to and compatible with those of the supervisory process. Casey et al. (1988) noted that the components constitute the tools of self-supervision, whereby clinicians at all levels and in all practice settings may assess, modify, and document changes that lead to establishment or maintenance of professional competence. The components of the clinical process (Casey et al., 1988), adapted from those described for the supervisory process (Anderson, 1988), include understanding, planning, observing, analyzing, and integrating the components of the clinical process. In order to help clinicians who are in graduate programs or in employment settings participate meaningfully and substantively within the clinical process, the components will be described now.

Understanding the Clinical Process. Understanding the clinical process of working with people who stutter and their family requires a familiarity with its other components, and the tasks and competencies required for each (ASHA, 1995). This familiarity is gained through coursework and continuing education related to communication and its disorders (specifically stuttering), instruction and dialogue about the clinical process including interpersonal and technical skills, and guided observation and supervised clinical practicum. Clinicians should become aware of the observation and analysis methods that are available for describing client and clinician behavior (Moses & Shapiro, 1996; Shapiro, 1985, 1987, 1994a; Shapiro & Anderson, 1988, 1989; Shapiro & Moses, 1989). To understand the client's communication behavior, clinicians may use standardized and nonstandardized instruments and procedures among others to develop short- and long-term goals and a related treatment plan. To understand the clinician's own communication behavior and intervention skills, she may analyze any of a number of baseline behaviors; use portions of the *Wisconsin Procedure for Appraisal of Clinical Competence* (W-PACC) (Shriberg et al., 1975) or the *UTD* (University of Texas–Dallas) *Competency Based Evaluation System* (Lougeay-Mottinger, Harris, Perlstein-Kaplan, & Felicetti, 1984); design individualized academic, clinical, and supervisory commitments with her supervisor (Shapiro & Anderson, 1988, 1989); or engage in any of the data collection and analysis procedures discussed in the Observing and Analyzing section, below.

Planning the Clinical Process. We discussed previously the importance of systematic planning in order for clients who stutter and their families to achieve maximum growth. The same should be said about planning for clinicians. Casey et al. (1988) listed six steps to achieve this mutual clinician and client growth, including identifying clinician and client needs and competencies related to clinical interaction, setting clinician and client short- and long-term goals, determining clinician and client baseline behaviors, identifying clinician behaviors to be used for assessing client functioning or influencing client growth, planning observation (i.e., identifying data to be collected on clinician and client, planning logistics of observation, identifying data collection procedures), and planning for data analysis and integration.

Observing and Analyzing the Clinical Process. The specific reasons for data collection, analysis, and interpretation will determine, or at least influence, the procedures or systems of analysis used. Casey et al. (1988) noted the following:

> Data collection, analysis, and interpretation regarding the clinical interaction are completed for a variety of reasons. Setting objectives, monitoring clinician and client change, planning for the [supervisory] conference interaction, checking perceptions, self-study, and research are some of the reasons that data are collected. Questions about the clinical process that are posed by the clinician, the client, or the supervisor can be answered in some way through the collection, analysis, and interpretation of clinical data. (p. 29)

Typically, data are collected during live clinician–client interaction or from audio- or videotape replay. Data collection procedures include verbatim recording, selected verbatim recording, rating, tally, interaction analysis, nonverbal analysis, and individually designed methods (Anderson, 1988; Casey et al., 1988; Shapiro, 1994a). For our discussion here, only interaction analysis, nonverbal analysis, and an individually designed method will be reviewed briefly.

INTERACTION ANALYSIS SYSTEMS. Interaction analysis systems are highly structured, low-inference instruments (Rosenshine & Furst, 1971, 1973) used for collecting, analyzing, and interpreting patterns of behavior occurring during the clinical (i.e., and supervisory) process (Shapiro, 1994a). Those available for the clinical process, each with unique categories and procedures, enable the clinician (i.e., or supervisor) to collect clinician and client data in order to analyze the interaction. Among the systems that I have found useful for heightening clinicians' understanding of the clinical process, particularly the language they use within it, are the Content and Sequence Analysis of Speech and Hearing Therapy (Boone & Prescott, 1972) and the Analysis of Behavior of Clinicians (ABC) System (Schubert, Miner, & Till, 1973). Both systems enable clinicians to become more aware of their own verbal behavior when interacting with people who stutter and their families. Once aware, clinicians may entertain changes in order to improve the effectiveness of the clinical interaction.

The "Boone-Prescott" (i.e., Content and Sequence Analysis of Speech and Hearing Therapy; Boone & Prescott, 1972) codes five clinician and five client categories of verbal behavior on a response grid and allows for analysis of individual verbal behaviors as well as patterns of verbal interaction between the client and clinician. Clinician behaviors include (a) explain/describe, (b) model/instruct, (c) good evaluative, (d) bad evaluative, and (e) neutral/social; client behaviors include (a) correct response, (b) incorrect response, (c) inappropriate social, (d) good self-evaluative, and (e) bad self-evaluative. A 5-minute segment is selected randomly from the middle portion of an audio- or videotape recorded clinical session or from live interaction. Each behavior is recorded as it occurs, thus making this system frequency-based, by marking a horizontal line on the Scoring Form, all of which are connected by vertical lines to show the sequence of interaction between the clinician and client. The quantitative summary of behaviors in each category and patterns of behavior are recorded on the Session Analysis Form.

The "ABC System" (i.e., Analysis of Behavior of Clinicians [ABC] System; Schubert, Miner, & Till, 1973) is a time-based, rather than frequency-based, system. Verbal behaviors are recorded every 3 seconds into any of eight clinician categories, three client categories, and a silence category. The clinician categories include: (a) observing and modifying lesson appropriately; (b) instruction and demonstration; (c–f) auditory or visual behaviors indicating: stimulation, positive reinforcement of client's correct response, negative reinforcement of client's incorrect response, or positive reinforcement of client's incorrect response; (g) relating irrelevant information or asking irrelevant questions; and (h) using authority or demonstrating disapproval. Client categories include: (a) responds correctly; (b) responds incorrectly; and (c) relating irrelevant information or asking irrelevant questions. The final category is silence. Data are collected from a 5-minute, randomly selected segment from an audio- or videotape recorded session or from live clinical interaction. The number of the category of behavior during each 3-second interval is recorded on the data collection grid, summarized on a Quick Analysis Form by counting the number of entries for each category, and then converted to percentages for comparison. Because this system is time-based, the duration of specified behaviors may be determined in addition to each participant's absolute and relative talk time.

NONVERBAL ANALYSIS. Collecting, analyzing, and interpreting nonverbal behaviors is important because of their potential influence on the communication in the clinical session. Nonverbal behaviors might include subtleties such as smiles, head nods, touches, leans, posture changes, eye contact, or vocal stress. Van Riper (1975) noted that he observed, tallied, and discussed with the clinician the following nonverbal behaviors believing that they provided valuable information about the clinical session: clinician's voice quality, inflection, and rate of speaking; appropriateness of interpersonal distance between clinician and client (e.g., number of times clinician physically withdrew from client); mobility of clinician and client (e.g., how fixated or stiff were their postures); ratio between smiles and frowns; number of mirrorings shown by clinician (e.g., When the client smiles, does the clinician smile too?); verbal (e.g., "What I mean is . . ."; "My point is . . .") and nonverbal (e.g., throat clearing, head scratching, sniffing, finger shaking) tics. Other categories of nonverbal behavior, described later under "Observing the Supervisory Process," are relevant to observing the clinical process as well.

INDIVIDUALLY DESIGNED PROCEDURES. A variety of procedures may be combined in order to tailor the observation and analysis of the clinical experience to the uniqueness of the clinician or client. What this means is that the methods used may be designed individually to highlight the clinician's entering level of skill, upon which individualized professional objectives are developed. The objectives may relate to any of the interpersonal or intrapersonal competencies discussed in Chapter 11. So, you are asking, "How does he do it?" The procedure I use for doing this is as follows. First, I determine with each clinician a handful of clinical skills that she feels are her relative strengths. Then, building on what the clinician already knows and can do, she and I identify one or two areas that might be targeted for improvement. Notice that the assessment of the clinician's skills is done *with* (i.e., to the extent possible and individually appropriate), rather than *for,* her and may involve use of the W-PACC, UTD, or other resources already discussed.

For each area identified for improvement, specific objectives and strategies are developed to facilitate her professional growth and are documented in writing. Furthermore, this process enables the clinician to focus on improving specific competencies—such as providing clients feedback regarding fluency and disfluency, expressing warmth and genuineness, using positive language, and controlling for nonverbal language—and enables me to provide focused, objective, and data-based feedback, rather than global feedback on her development. I have found this method to be particularly satisfying and effective with clinicians. They feel their uniqueness as people and as professionals is being not only considered but invited, and they are participating in their own professional growth from the outset.

This particular method resulted from an extensive descriptive and experimental analysis of commitments made during supervisory conferences and follow-through behaviors (Shapiro & Anderson, 1988, 1989). Individualized commitments made by clinicians/supervisees were documented in writing and carefully monitored for relative completion of each. Five different types of commitments served as the basis of the Commitment Classification System, including Clinical Procedures, Clinical Process Administration, Supervisory Procedures, Supervisory Process Information, and Academic Information/Teaching Function. The analysis addressed 1,389 commitments made by 64 student clinicians in 384 individual conferences at 12 universities. Results revealed that the greatest number of commitments made involved planning, analysis, and evaluation of the clinical process with particular attention on client behavior, and that the number of commitments completed was directly influenced by the written accountability in addition to other factors. Furthermore, clinicians completed more commitments when the written agreement was introduced early into and subsequently faded from supervisory conferences, and the written agreement was more beneficial for beginning clinicians than for experienced clinicians. Of particular importance was the demonstration that specific behaviors of clinicians/ supervisees can be followed and measured over time, and that certain behaviors of clinicians occur as a direct result of commitments made during conferences with their supervisors. Clinicians desiring more information on designing individualized commitments and monitoring each for completion may refer to the primary sources (Shapiro & Anderson, 1988, 1989).

Integrating the Components of the Clinical Process. Integrating the components requires understanding, planning, observing, and analyzing the clinical process. The supervisory conference is a catalyst for the process of integration. Casey et al. (1988) noted that for the advanced clinician who engages in self-supervision, "integration is accomplished through a 'conference' with one's self" (p. 43). In such conferences, the clinician considers the information acquired from each of the other components of the clinical process and how it may be integrated and applied to develop or maintain clinical competence or to facilitate self-study and ongoing professional growth.

Supervisory Process

We have discussed briefly the academic and clinical processes that are critical to clinicians' professional preparation. Why, then do we need to consider the supervisory process? In an earlier publication (Shapiro, 1987), I characterized as a "myth" the assumption that, "Academic coursework in human communication disorders prepares clinicians to enter the supervisory process" (p. 78). Supervisees typically enter supervision without knowledge of the supervisory process and, as a consequence, rely on and thereby become dependent upon individual supervisor's direction, without generalizing knowledge of the process to subsequent supervisory interactions. For this reason, clinicians need to be provided with an understanding of the supervisory process—distinct from the academic and clinical processes—and prepared to function meaningfully and proactively in the unique role of a supervisee. Therefore, we turn now to the supervisory process.

Supervisory Process Defined

The Committee on Supervision in Speech–Language Pathology and Audiology (ASHA, 1978, p. 479) defined the supervisory process as the "interaction that takes place between a supervisor and the clinician and may be related to the behavior of the clinician or the client or to the program in which the supervisor and clinician are employed," and defined supervisors as "individuals engaged in clinical teaching through observation, conferences, review of records, and other procedures, and which is related to the interaction between a clinician and a client and the evaluation or management of communication skills." The primary purposes of supervision are to ensure the highest quality of clinical service (i.e., by developing skills used to assess, treat, and otherwise manage the needs of people who demonstrate communication disorders), and to ensure ongoing professional self-study, understanding, and growth (i.e., career-long acquisition, integration, and application of information and skills necessary for quality clinical service) (ASHA, 1978, 1985; Casey et al., 1988; Shapiro, 1985, 1987, 1994a; Shapiro & Anderson, 1988, 1989).

Clinical Supervision Defined

While there are many models and procedures for supervision, most are compatible with, if not derivatives of, clinical supervision. Therefore, an understanding of clinical supervision is fundamental to understanding the supervisory process, knowledge, and components. Clinical supervision refers to "the tasks and skills of clinical teaching related to the interaction between a clinician and client" (ASHA, 1985, p. 57). Originally borrowed from the teacher education literature, clinical supervision refers to a "cycle" (Cogan, 1973) or "sequence" (Goldhammer, Anderson, & Krajewski, 1980) of supervision whereby primary emphasis is given to improvement of clinicians' professional (i.e., technical and interpersonal) skills. The procedures emphasize the importance of the conference as a critical component in the supervisory process. The cycle includes establishing the supervisee–supervisor relationship, planning with the supervisee (i.e., clinician), planning the strategy of observation, observing therapy, analyzing the clinical and supervisory processes, planning the strategy for the conference, conducting the conference, and renewed planning.

The word "clinical" conveys a face-to-face interaction between a supervisee (i.e., clinician) and supervisor who are engaged in objective, data-based observation and analysis of such "intensity of focus that binds the two together in a rather intimate professional relationship" (Goldhammer, 1969, p. 55). In fact, Van Riper (1965) acknowledged clinical supervision as "the most important of all staff functions" and indicated that it is in this personal interaction with student clinicians that supervisors "turn students into clinicians" (p. 75). The central theme of clinical supervision methodology is colleagueship, in which the supervisee and supervisor share in all phases of planning, observation, and objective analysis of data from the clinical and supervisory processes. This partnership reportedly leads to a more analytical, problem-solving, and self-supervising supervisee. Recently, this assumption was supported in that supervisees demonstrated changes in clinical and supervisory behavior when a form of commitment or written agreement is used (Shapiro & Anderson, 1988, 1989), and in clinical behavior when all aspects of supervision are jointly determined and data based (Gillam, Roussos, & Anderson, 1990).

On a number of occasions at invited workshops, conference presentations, and in publications (Shapiro, 1987), I have been invited to discuss my ideas about clinical supervision and specifically colleagueship, its central tenet. I have shared that I view clinical supervision as a dynamic, ongoing exchange in which the participants dialogue and shift perspective in order to consider alternative points of view (Moses & Shapiro, 1996; Shapiro & Moses, 1989). The supervisor provides the appropriate level of guidance to facilitate the supervisee's active role in establishing and monitoring specific objectives regarding the clinical and self-supervisory skills. The concept of colleagueship endorses the instructional process of clinical teaching as necessarily shared and interactive and a philosophy of teaching and learning by which we are all players, perhaps playing different but equally important roles. I also have defined colleagueship as a process in which each participant engages in unique and dynamic roles reflecting the individual needs and skill levels within a continuum.

On one such occasion, when I was nearing the end of a workshop presentation at a major university, a senior level faculty member stood and expressed cogently, "Like hell I'll consider a student a colleague!" It seemed to me that an outright rejection of the concept of colleagueship, before considering the process by which supervisees and supervisors strive to achieve professional equality, is incongruous with one of the central objectives of the supervisory process—to facilitate the supervisee's ability to think even more independently and creatively, to problem solve, and to self-supervise to the point where the supervisor's role becomes unnecessary. In fact, the objective of the supervisory process is parallel to that of the clinical process—to facilitate in the client improved communication skills (i.e., behaviors, thoughts, feelings), problem solving, and self-monitoring (i.e., internally generated feedback) and self-correction (i.e., implementation of correction in response to internal feedback). The assumptions that the faculty member and I held—our personal constructs regarding the process and product of clinical instruction and professional preparation—indeed were in contrast. He assumed colleagueship to be a dichotomy—that one either is or is not a colleague, and that skill level alone determines colleagueship. I believe he assumed that the supervisor's role was equivalent to a fountain of knowledge and the instructional process as one in which the supervisor continuously satiates the supervisee's professional thirst.

In contrast, I believe that clients, clinicians/supervisees, and supervisors all are partners, all comrades in the common struggle toward heightened understanding and improved communication. I do not believe that the participants must be of equal skill level in order to function as colleagues. What's more, I believe the roles and responsibilities of the participants necessarily must change with experience and skill improvement. By implication, the objectives for each supervisee (i.e., and supervisor) should be unique because each enters the continuum at a different skill level and will progress to a different point. The supervisee's strengths and needs are assessed and addressed individually, and evaluation is based on her own progress and potential from a shared perspective. A collegial context such as this also presents a vehicle for analysis and improvement of supervisors' skills. In fact, the more a supervisor becomes comfortable with and explicit about her efforts to improve her own professional skills, the more the supervisee will understand and commit to the process of ongoing and shared professional growth. Within such a dynamic, clinical, and collegial context, supervisees and supervisors learn with and from each other along the lifelong journey of professional growth.

Supervisory Knowledge

The concepts of clinical supervision and colleagueship within the context of the supervisory process were incorporated into a position statement by the ASHA Committee on Supervision in Speech–Language Pathology and Audiology (ASHA, 1985). The critical nature of self-guided study, analysis, and evaluation in supervision was expressed in this way:

> A central premise of supervision is that effective clinical teaching involves, in a fundamental way, the development of self-analysis, self-evaluation, and

problem-solving skills on the part of the individual being supervised. The success of clinical teaching rests largely on achievement of this goal. (p. 57)

Furthermore, the committee identified 13 tasks and supporting competencies for effective clinical supervision and presented guidelines for preparation of the supervisory participants. I noted earlier that the Guidelines for Practice in Stuttering Treatment (ASHA, 1995; see Appendix A.3) should be required reading for all participants in the clinical process, including providers and consumers of clinical service. Similarly, the Position Statement (i.e., Clinical Supervision in Speech–Language Pathology and Audiology; ASHA, 1985) should be required reading for all participants in the supervisory process, including clinicians/supervisees and supervisors. By being familiar with this document, supervisees can build their understanding of the supervisory process, of what is expected of them, and of what to expect of their supervisors. Supervisors can use the document for self-assessment, helping them evaluate their own supervisory skills, from which to develop professional growth plans for themselves. The position statement in its entirety, including the tasks, required competencies, and preparation guidelines for effective supervision, is reprinted in Appendix A.1. The required tasks follow:

1. Establishing and maintaining an effective working relationship with the supervisee

2. Assisting the supervisee in developing clinical goals and objectives

3. Assisting the supervisee in developing and refining assessment skills

4. Assisting the supervisee in developing and refining clinical management skills

5. Demonstrating for and participating with the supervisee in the clinical process

6. Assisting the supervisee in observing and analyzing assessment and treatment sessions

7. Assisting the supervisee in the development and maintenance of clinical and supervisory records

8. Interacting with the supervisee in planning, executing, and analyzing supervisory conferences

9. Assisting the supervisee in evaluation of clinical performance

10. Assisting the supervisee in developing skills of verbal reporting, writing, and editing

11. Sharing information regarding ethical, legal, regulatory, and reimbursement aspects of professional practice

12. Modeling and facilitating professional conduct

13. Demonstrating research skills in the clinical or supervisory processes

A Model for Supervisory Development

Clinical supervision emphasizes the importance of joint involvement and active participation of both supervisee and supervisor in all phases of the supervisory process. As originally conceived, however, clinical supervision (Cogan, 1973; Goldhammer et al., 1980) did not recognize or account for variation in the amount and type of supervision that may be needed by different participants who have different skills and needs or who may be at different stages of career development. Such a focus indeed is important because supervisors in speech–language pathology were found to behave in a consistently active, dominant manner, independent of supervisees' experience, competencies, needs, expectations, or desires. This means that supervisors behave the same from conference to conference throughout a practicum and do not exhibit significantly different behaviors from one supervisee to another (Blumberg, 1980; Brasseur, 1989; Culatta, Collucci, & Wiggins, 1975; Roberts & Smith, 1982; Shapiro, 1987, 1994a; Smith, 1978; Smith & Anderson, 1982a, 1982b).

One model of supervision, that presented by Anderson (1988), is consistent with the principles of clinical supervision and is particularly sensitive to the uniqueness and significance of what individual supervisees and supervisors bring to the supervisory interaction. That Continuum of Supervision, depicted in Figure 12.1, assumes that "supervision exists on a continuum which spans a professional career and that there are styles of interaction which are appropriate to each stage of the continuum" (p. 49). Furthermore, "It offers a structure for supervisors and supervisees to examine their own philosophies about supervision, identify their own behaviors, and determine what changes they wish to make, if any" (p. 50).

Other key features of the Continuum of Supervision are that the component stages, Evaluation–Feedback Stage, Transitional Stage, and Self-Supervision Stage, are not time bound. A supervisee may find herself at any point on the continuum at any time during her career. While clinicians beginning an initial practicum generally will enter the continuum at the Evaluation–Feedback Stage, other more experienced clinicians will find themselves at this beginning stage when they experience a different disorder category, type of client, work setting, technology, or procedure (Anderson, 1988; Brasseur, 1989; Casey et al., 1988). The relative dominance of the supervisor decreases, while that of the supervisee increases, as they move across the continuum. Both supervisee and supervisor share responsibility for recognizing their respective placements along the continuum, for identifying and effecting necessary growth-promoting changes, and for progressing along the continuum. The continuum is dynamic with respect to the supervisee's and supervisor's respective stages of supervision. Different styles of supervision are appropriate to each stage. The supervisee and supervisor must be able to adapt their individual styles as they move

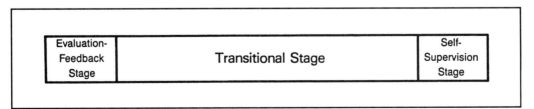

Figure 12.1. Stages of the Continuum of Supervision. *Note.* From *The Supervisory Process in Speech–Language–Pathology and Audiology* (p. 50), by J. L. Anderson, 1988, Boston, MA: Little Brown/College-Hill. Copyright 1988 by J. L. Anderson. Reprinted with permission.

back and forth along the continuum as different variables require. The stages, elaborated in Figure 12.2, are summarized as follows:

Evaluation–Feedback Stage. In this stage, the supervisor assumes a relatively dominant, controlling, superior role; the supervisee assumes a relatively passive, subordinate role. The supervisor provides direction, evaluation, and feedback; the supervisee serves as the receiver of information. As noted in Figure 12.2, the style of the supervisor's interaction is direct/active; that of the supervisee is passive. A novice clinician/supervisee or one who is engaging in a new type of disorder (e.g., neurogenic disfluency or psychogenic disfluency) or a new setting (e.g., school, hospital, or university) or a "marginal" clinician will find herself at this stage of the continuum. Anderson (1988) indicated that the marginal clinician, one "who is unknowledgable or clinically inept" (p. 51), may perseverate at this stage. "Unprepared for the clinical interaction, unable to problem-solve, overwhelmed by the dynamics of the situation, or accustomed to being told what to do, the supervisee at this stage assumes a very passive role" (p. 51). Innovative developments have been presented for working with clinicians who demonstrate sustained performance deficits and who are perseverating at the Evaluation–Feedback Stage (Shapiro et al., 1995). Anderson noted that supervisory dyads also may function at this stage because the supervisor does not perceive the supervisee as able to participate more independently, or because the supervisor's perception of his or her role is that of instructor or evaluator. Supervisors should be wary that in the latter case, the supervisee's needs are

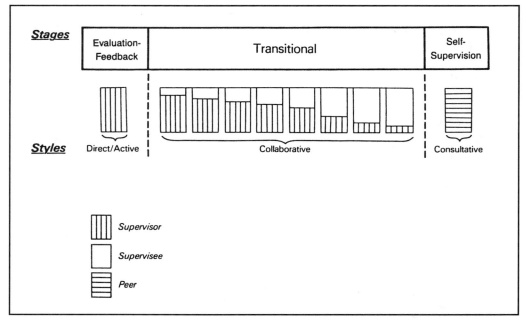

Figure 12.2. Composite of Stages of Supervision and Appropriate Styles for Each Stage. *Note.* From *The Supervisory Process in Speech–Language–Pathology and Audiology* (p. 62), by J. L. Anderson, 1988, Boston, MA: Little Brown/College-Hill. Copyright 1988 by J. L. Anderson. Reprinted with permission.

not likely being served. Anderson (1988) recommended that an objective for both supervisee and supervisor should be to move out of this stage as rapidly as possible, stating, "The purpose of supervision is not cloning" (p. 55).

Transitional Stage. The relative pattern of dominance shifts in the Transitional Stage. The supervisee has become increasingly knowledgeable and skillful and participates in planning, implementing, and evaluating both the clinical and supervisory processes. The supervisor recognizes the supervisee's emerging competence and is receptive to and encourages joint problem solving. The supervisor continues to provide some direction and feedback; however, the supervisee is moving increasingly toward independence and peer interaction, which characterize self-supervision. The supervisee may move back and forth within the Transitional Stage depending on related experiences, skills, and needs, as noted. For example, the clinician/supervisee may be relatively comfortable designing school-based treatment plans for children who stutter, but may need far more direction for a child who shows symptoms of Tourette Syndrome. Anderson (1988) noted that a collaborative style is appropriate in the Transitional Stage, in which "supervision is seen as a joint process where the supervisor and supervisee share responsibilities and interact as professionals to meet common objectives" (p. 58). In fact, there are times when the supervisee and supervisor may change roles within the Transitional Stage and within a collaborative style. Such a situation was described by Anderson (1988), as follows:

> For example, a student clinician, well-trained and with extensive experience in the clinical program and with a specific disorder area, may be working with a supervisor whose background in this area is different, limited, or not current. The supervisee might then assume a more active role in the collaboration, with the supervisor receiving the input about certain techniques or a differing philosophy. This requires openness on the part of the supervisor, and confidence, if not courage, on the part of the supervisee. (p. 59)

In other words, both the supervisee's and supervisor's skills and attitudes will influence the extent to which the Transitional Stage is characterized by joint participation, collaboration, and mutual professional growth.

Self-Supervision Stage. In the Self-Supervision Stage, the supervisee becomes even more actively involved in the clinical and supervisory processes and is relatively independent in developing and pursuing strategies for continued professional growth. Anderson (1988) noted as a cornerstone of this stage the supervisee's ability to self-analyze her own clinical behavior with accuracy and to alter it based on that analysis. She stated that the Self-Supervision Stage "denotes a level of independence in problem solving in which supervisees are no longer dependent upon supervisors for observation, analysis, and feedback about their clinical work" (p. 52). Nevertheless, the clinician/supervisee at this stage of development still desires collegial (i.e., peer or consultative) type of interaction. The supervisee now is and feels empowered to assess continually and make decisions about her own professional needs. This involves identifying strengths and weaknesses, making modifications, and seeking assistance or further knowledge as appropriate. This level of independent professional functioning is the terminal objective of the supervisory process. Some clinicians achieve this Self-Supervision Stage by the end of their graduate degree program; others do not. Some clinicians do not achieve this stage of independent functioning before many years of professional experience. This stage typically is characterized by a consultative style, a voluntary relationship emphasizing each participant's ability to help the other in using knowledge and skill to problem solve or in selecting and applying strategies for case management. The supervisor-peer in this stage is functioning as a consultant by listening, supporting, problem solving, and offering suggestions where appropriate. Anderson (1988) noted that if a true peer or consultant relationship exists, "these suggestions may be accepted, rejected, or built upon by the supervisee" (p. 61). Functioning as peers, the supervisee must be able, and the supervisor must be willing, to accept the supervisee's options, particularly that of rejecting suggestions.

Implications of the Continuum of Supervision. Determining at which stage the supervisee and supervisor are functioning, and therein which style of supervision is appropriate, is a challenging decision requiring insight and analysis of all participants. I noted earlier that most supervisors perceive that they are conceptualizing and using a continuum approach to facilitate their supervisees' development. In fact, most supervisors believe they treat supervisees differently, change their supervisory style based on each supervisee's level of expertise, and that their style most frequently is a collaborative one. In contrast, however, data collected on the supervisory conference indicate that most supervisors routinely use a direct/active style (which is appropriate only for the Evaluation–Feedback Stage), do not change this style over time (even when they perceive that they do), and use this same style with all supervisees. Anderson (1988) noted that some supervisors who become accustomed to the direct/active style may be unwilling or unable to change this style, a condition perpetuated by some supervisees' preference to remain dependent and passive. Shapiro (1987) advised supervisors to ask themselves the following questions to be sure that the dynamic needs of each supervisee are being addressed properly (i.e., that both the stage and style of supervision are appropriate for the supervisee):

> Do I give my experienced clinicians any different opportunities than I do beginning clinicians to establish a conference agenda, to problem solve, to observe and analyze? Do I encourage my clinicians to use "independent" judgment, but really hope they will conduct therapy my way—the right way? Do I provide opportunities for creativity, for initiation, for the application or development of knowledge? Do I support my clinicians by helping them understand the significance of their own cognitive disequilibrium—or healthy confusion—in order to approach and solve novel problems? In other words, what do I do and to what avail? (p. 81)

As presented, the Continuum of Supervision provides a framework within which to conceptualize professional growth and development throughout individual supervisory interactions and across one's career. Individuals may enter or exit the continuum at any point and may move back and forth on it, depending on different situational and experiential variables. It is the continuous movement among the continuum toward self-supervision and increasing professional independence that is the ultimate objective of the supervisory process.

Supervisory Process Components

Based on the model of clinical supervision in teacher education (Cogan, 1973; Goldhammer, 1969; Goldhammer et al., 1980), Anderson (1988) presented five components that are specific to supervision in speech–language pathology and audiology. These components are Understanding, Planning, Observing, Analyzing, and Integrating the Components of the Supervisory Process. She indicated that the components are inherent to the Collaborative Style, which is appropriate for the Transitional Stage on the continuum (see Figure 12.2). This transition is characterized by movement, change, and shifting roles by both the supervisee and supervisor. As Casey et al. (1988) pointed out, the components may serve as a framework of understanding for supervisees and supervisors functioning in the Evaluation–Feedback Stage and as a strategy for clinicians in the Self-Supervision Stage. Indeed, if participants—that is, clinicians/supervisees and supervisors—are going to emphasize development of clinical skills and professional self-growth across affective, behavioral, and cognitive domains, then they must understand and be able to analyze the components of the supervisory process. For this reason, what follows is a highlight of the components. Readers wanting more detail are encouraged to review the primary sources (Anderson, 1988; Cogan, 1973, Goldhammer, 1969; Goldhammer et al., 1980; Shapiro, 1985).

Understanding the Supervisory Process. The first component of the supervisory process, Understanding, is devoted to developing an explicit recognition of the entirety of supervision and its constituent elements. Participants in the supervisory process (that is, both supervisees and supervisors) have been found to hold different, if not contradictory, perceptions of the same event (e.g., involving conference interactions, written reports, clinician evaluations, and so forth) (Blumberg, 1980; Culatta et al., 1975; Roberts & Smith, 1982; Smith, 1978; Smith & Anderson, 1982a, 1982b). This should not seem surprising given that people in general who are not involved in supervision often hold different expectations for or perceptions of the same event. If the supervisor expects to use a collaborative style but the supervisee expects a direct/active style, however, conflict is sure to occur. Anderson (1988) noted the following:

> A period of discussion about the process into which the supervisor and supervisee are about to embark, preparation of the supervisee for his or her part in the experience, and sharing expectations and objectives should alleviate problems which might arise from such differences in perceptions. (p. 64)

Furthermore, Casey et al. (1988) suggested that when a supervisee fails to progress along the continuum, an early consideration should address whether or not the individual knows the continuum exists. Both the supervisee and supervisor need to understand what they are trying to accomplish and the process by which they are going about it. Such preparation may take the form of dialogue between supervisees and supervisors, or may be a component of clinical courses or others devoted to the supervisory process. This activity, however, is more than just an introductory phase. Discussion of the supervisory process should be ongoing because the needs and objectives are ever changing as are levels of experience—new insights are made and new problems arise.

Various topics have been recommended for inclusion in such discussions to facilitate understanding of the supervisory process (Anderson, 1988; Brasseur, 1989, Casey et al., 1988; Shapiro, 1987, 1994a). These include components of the supervisory process, supervisee's perceptions about supervision, goals and objectives for supervision, prior experiences in supervision, styles of supervision and supervisee's preferences, supervisee anxieties, and needs and competencies of the supervisee for placement on the continuum of supervision. Anderson (1988) noted that discussion of these topics allows the supervisee and supervisor to begin to establish their relationship, and that only then can they begin to focus on their client. Others (Culatta & Seltzer, 1976, 1977; McCrea, 1980; Pickering, 1984; Roberts & Smith, 1982) described conference interactions as typically structured and verbally dominated by the supervisor who provides information and suggestions without accompanying rationale or justification; supervisees recount what occurred in clinical session; and discussions are primarily cognitive rather than affective. When feelings are discussed, it is the client's feelings that receive attention; supervisees (and to a greater extent, supervisors) are loath to disclose or express their own feelings. Shapiro (1987) noted that rarely, if ever, do supervisors reveal their anxieties and fears about a clinical or supervisory situation, which might be viewed as necessary if a supervisor is to be truly genuine.

Planning the Supervisory Process. Clinicians generally are familiar with planning, particularly for their clients. It is indisputable that planning is critically linked to improvement of clients who stutter. It is just as important to plan for the supervisory process if clinician/supervisee (as well as supervisor) growth is considered to be an important outcome.

The purpose of planning is to isolate objectives for the clinical and supervisory interactions. For the clinical process, as reviewed earlier, plans are developed for the client and the clinician. For the supervisory process, plans are developed for the clinician/supervisee and the supervisor (Anderson, 1988, p. 65). Planning is a most critical component because it establishes a basis for all future activity. Initial data are collected in the Planning component (that is, if not already collected in the Understanding component) against which progress will be measured. From these data, long-term goals, short-term objectives, and related strategies are established for the clinical and supervisory processes. While it is not uncommon to plan for the client, planning for the clinician/supervisee and supervisor frequently is omitted. Planning implies priorities. I noted earlier that I engage each of my clinicians in self-assessment (including strengths and limitations) in order for her to design a professional development plan. In other words, a recognition of one's strengths should serve as a foundation to and point of departure for addressing identified limitations. You will notice that I recommend the same planning process for the supervisee (i.e., and supervisor) as I do for the client (Shapiro, 1987, 1994a).

Casey et al. (1988) noted that the following questions should guide the professional planning process: "Which goals are most important right now? How many objectives can reasonably be expected to be achieved in the current term and what are they? Do supervisor and supervisee have different priorities?" (pp. 17–18). If the supervisory participants have different priorities, then some negotiation will need to take place in order to determine the focus of subsequent interaction, observation, and feedback. Once the participants reach agreement, then the following foci will guide the planning of the Observation component: what will be observed (i.e., specific data to be collected), how will the observation be accomplished (methodology), how will the observational data be analyzed, how will the data be interpreted (criteria), how will the findings be integrated (future planning) (Casey et al., 1988). Additional factors to be considered include who will be responsible for each of the planning components noted, and how, when, and where each will take place. The planning is guided by the nature and characteristics of the situation and the characteristics of the individual participants and their respective placement along the continuum. Brasseur (1989) noted that the sincerity of the supervisor's intention to plan *with* a supervisee (not *for* her) can be seen in the extent to which the supervisee's ideas are accepted, developed, and implemented.

Observing the Supervisory Process. Observation occurs according to the objectives and procedures specified in the Planning component. A distinction is made between observation and evaluation. Observation is the collection and recording of objective and comprehensive data for subsequent analysis. Evaluation "implies a judgment or inference that is built upon a foundation of understanding, planning, objective observation, analysis, and integration" (Shapiro, 1994a, p. 72). Furthermore, observation requires application of the scientific process through systematic collection of accurate, objective, and reliable data. Observation, therefore, is not synonymous with watching. What's more, observation is not synonymous with supervision. Observation is only one component of supervision. Frequently I hear supervisors say, "I've got to go supervise my clinician" when they mean "I've got to go observe my clinician." Anderson (1988) noted that observation is "the place where real objectivity begins in the supervisory process, where data are collected and recorded by both supervisor and supervisee for further analysis and interpretation which then lead to the evaluation" (p. 65). The methods discussed earlier for observing the clinical process apply as well to the supervisory process (i.e., verbatim recording, selected verbatim recording, rating, tally, interaction analysis, nonverbal analysis, and individually designed methods). The specific methods to be used and each participant's respective role in the observation process are jointly determined in the Planing component. These methods are reviewed thoroughly elsewhere (Anderson, 1988; Brasseur, 1989; Casey et al., 1988; Dowling, 1992; Farmer & Farmer, 1989). Again, for our purposes, only interaction analysis, nonverbal analysis, and individually designed procedures will be addressed here.

INTERACTION ANALYSIS SYSTEMS. We defined interaction analysis systems earlier when discussing methods for observing the clinical process (i.e., client–clinician interaction). Other interaction analysis systems are available for the supervisory process (i.e., supervisee–supervisor interaction). Different systems are available to suit different purposes and specific questions being addressed. The systems code specific verbal behaviors that are objective, identifiable, and therefore, quantifiable. The systems yield descriptive frequency data, require few inferences on the part of the coder who analyzes one event at a time, and have numerous advantages and disadvantages (Anderson, 1980, 1988; Shapiro, 1987, 1994a). Among the interaction analysis systems I have found particularly useful for heightening supervisees' understanding of the supervisory process, and particularly the language they use within supervisory conferences, are the System for Analyzing Supervisor–Teacher Interaction (Blumberg, 1980), Underwood Category System for Analyzing Supervisor–Clinician Behavior (Seeley, 1973; Underwood, 1979), McCrea's Adapted Scales for the Assessment of Interpersonal Functioning in Speech Pathology Supervision Conferences (McCrea, 1980), and Smith's Adaptation of the Multidimensional Observational System for the Analysis of Interactions in Clinical Supervision (MOSAICS) (Smith, 1978). Recently, I used each of these instruments for interaction analysis and self-study involving one supervisee and one supervisor across 10 consecutive, individual supervisory conferences. Readers wishing to see how these instruments can be applied to identification and maintenance or change of supervisee and supervisor behavior or to review a thorough critique of these instruments are referred to "Interaction Analysis and Self-Study: A Single-Case Comparison of Four Methods of Analyzing Supervisory Conferences" (Shapiro, 1994a).

The System for Analyzing Supervisor–Teacher Interaction (Blumberg, 1980) originally was developed for use in education. It is time-based and records verbal behavior every 3 seconds or with a change of behavior, whichever occurs first. Only one category number is applied to a verbal behavior. It is based on the premise that learning is directly related to one's level of independence and that the supervisor's use of direct or indirect verbal behavior will influence the amount of independence demonstrated by the supervisee. There are 10 categories for the supervisor's verbal behavior: (a) demonstrates support-inducing communication behavior, (b) gives praise, (c) accepts or uses teacher's ideas, (d) asks for information, (e) gives information, (f) asks for opinions, (g) asks for suggestions, (h) gives opinions, (i) gives suggestions, and (j) gives criticism. Four supervisee verbal behaviors are categorized, including (a) asks for information, opinion, or suggestions; (b) gives information, opinion, or suggestions; (c) demonstrates positive social emotional behavior; and (d) demonstrates negative social emotional behavior. The final category is silence or confusion and applies to both participants. Quantitative and qualitative analysis is accomplished through an interaction matrix and focuses on the sequence of behaviors, not the content of the conference. Most categories address the cognitive domain, but some affective components can be interpreted from the matrix, which identifies "steady state" areas of behavior used in self-study. Blumberg's system is easy to learn, contains ground rules that are helpful in training for reliability in coding, and can be used for self-study, peer-study, or research. One significant weakness of this system is the lack of content validation.

The Underwood Category System for Analyzing Supervisor–Clinician Behavior (Seeley, 1973; Underwood, 1979) was adapted from Blumberg's system for use in speech–language pathology. The nine revised categories for supervisors' verbal behavior include: (a) supportive, (b) praise, (c) identifies problem, (d) uses clinician's ideas, (e) requests factual information, (f) provides factual information, (g) requests opinions/suggestions, (h) provides opinions/suggestions, and (i) criticism. Seven categories of supervisees' verbal behavior are used including: (a) identifies problem, (b) requests factual information, (c) provides factual information, (d) requests opinions/suggestions, (e) provides opinions/

suggestions, (f) positive social behavior, and (g) negative social behavior. Silence/confusion is the final category and applies to both participants. Definitions and procedures are clear, and the system is easy to learn. This system again relates to sequence of behaviors rather than conference content. Underwood provides a series of critical ratios that are useful for self-study and for summarizing and quantifying the data. As with Blumberg's system, the most critical weakness of Underwood's system is the lack of content validation, which limits application of this system for reliable research purposes. However, the system may be used for informal, descriptive self-analysis, peer-analysis, and joint supervisor–supervisee analysis.

McCrea's Adapted Scales for the Assessment of Interpersonal Functioning in Speech Pathology Supervision Conferences (McCrea, 1980) address exclusively the affective or interpersonal domain rather than the cognitive domain of the supervisory conference. The scales are based on the work of Carkhuff (1969a, 1969b), Gazda, Asbury, Balzer, Childers, and Walters (1977), and Rogers (1957). The basic premise is that if certain facilitative conditions are present within the supervisory interaction and if they are perceived by the supervisee, then the supervisee will experience positive changes. McCrea's system uses four categories for supervisors: (a) empathic understanding—sensitivity to and appreciation of the supervisee's feelings; (b) respect—unconditional, non-evaluative acceptance of the supervisee and the supervisee's ability to find solutions with proper guidance and experience; (c) facilitative genuineness—communicating one's own feelings and thoughts and conveying honesty, openness, and authenticity; and (d) concreteness of expression—specificity in order to demonstrate and facilitate understanding. Only one category, self-exploration—talking objectively about one's own behavior and related feelings and consequences—is used for supervisees. Operational definitions are specific, with clear procedures and ground rules for scoring. McCrea's Adapted Scales are frequency and rating based. That is, the particular verbal behavior is noted as being present or absent and then the behavior is rated on a facilitativeness scale from *1* to *7*. The higher ratings are interpreted as facilitative, number *5* is neutral, and the lower ratings are non-facilitative. The scales provide data about the interpersonal verbal behavior of the supervisor, the level of facilitativeness of these behaviors, the level of self-exploration of the supervisee, and the relationship of these behaviors to each other. Reliability and validity data are available and therefore support the use of this system for research as well as for self-study, peer-study, and joint supervisor–supervisee analysis.

Smith's Adaptation of the Multidimensional Observation System for the Analysis of Interactions in Clinical Supervision (MOSAICS) (Smith, 1978) is based on the work of Weller (1971), which analyzed the process of clinical supervision in teacher education (Cogan, 1973). The MOSAICS is multidimensional in that each unit of conversational discourse (i.e., pedagogical or conversational move) is coded in six category groups or dimensions. Each move first is categorized according to who is speaking—supervisor, supervisee, or observer. The same move then is coded according to type—structuring, soliciting, responding, reacting, or summarizing. The third coding looks at the content or topic of discussion. If the move is instructional, decisions are made under the headings of generality (general or specific), focus of the discussion (objectives, methods/materials, or execution), and domain of the move (cognitive, affective, or disciplinary/social interaction). If the move is not instructional, it is coded under related areas—subject matter, supervision, or general topics related or not related to speech–language pathology. The final category is substantive–logical meaning analysis where the move is coded to analyze the instructional process—including defining, interpreting, fact stating, explanation, evaluation, justification, suggestion, exploration of suggestion, opinion, and justification of opinion.

In Smith's Adaptation of the MOSAICS, five critical ratios are derived by combining parts of the coded data including the initiatory/reflexive ratio, an index describing the extent of initiation for each participant; the analytic/evaluative ratio, the extent to which each participant verifies by reference to one's own experiences (analytic) compared to a set of criteria or principles of judgment (evaluative); the diagnostic/prescriptive ratio, a dimension that distinguishes between processes that focus on analysis or evaluation of past or future instructional processes (diagnostic) and those that focus on actions or objectives that are recommended or assigned (prescriptive); the complex/simple ratio, a distinction between processes that relate statements, facts, evaluations, opinions, and suggestions to other factors, reasons, generalizations or principles (complex) and those processes that involve a single element (simple); and the participation membership ratio, the relative participation of each member compared to the total participation of all members in the conference. Smith's Adaptation of the MOSAICS is complex and provides in-depth information with unique attention to the content of the conference. The critical ratios and conversational pattern analysis provide a method for data manipulation and interpretation. The system can be used effectively in its entirety or in parts. All utterances by all participants are coded with equal attention, and both process and content are analyzed. Smith validated the adapted system, thus making it useful for correlational, descriptive, or experimental research.

NONVERBAL ANALYSIS. Verbal and nonverbal behaviors, whether occurring within the clinical or supervisory interaction, are functionally overlapping, interrelated, and interdependent. The distinction, however, is critical for training observation and interpersonal skills (Farmer & Farmer, 1989; McCready, Shapiro, & Kennedy, 1987). Farmer and Farmer (1989) noted that nonverbal behavior refers to communication events that transcend spoken or written words, and may account for as much as 80% of the meaning interpreted from an intended message. Furthermore, "Whereas verbal communication is the primary mode for conveying information, nonverbal communication is the primary mode for the affective component of the meaning. Nonverbal communication provides clues to help the listener interpret the verbal message" (Farmer & Farmer, 1989, p. 167). Nonverbal events, just like verbal events, may be interpreted differently by supervisory participants.

More experienced supervisees tend to use more frequent and positive nonverbal communication than those with less experience (Farmer & Farmer, 1989). In preparing for the supervisory process, both supervisees and supervisors should become aware of nonverbal behavior, gain academic information about nonverbal communication, and practice observing and managing nonverbal behavior in the clinical (i.e., client, clinician, and supervisor) and supervisory (i.e., supervisee and supervisor) interactions (Casey et al., 1988; Farmer & Farmer, 1989; McCready et al., 1987). Farmer and Farmer (1989, pp. 165–167) noted a number of areas in which supervisees and supervisors should gain familiarity and professional competence. Each of the following areas include nonverbal behavior that communicates a message:

- *Paralinguistics:* variations in voice quality or auditory nonverbal signals including prosody (vocal pitch, loudness, duration, quality, and timing), intonation (teasing, whining, and sarcasm), and distinctive sounds (yawning, crying, and laughing).

- *Kinesics:* movements including body movements, postures, gestures, facial expressions, and eye movements. Body movements and postures (i.e., position, shifts, and speed and rhythm of movements toward or away from someone) convey likes/dislikes, approval/disapproval, or other responses to another person. Gestures are expressive movements of the head or limbs (e.g., *yes* or *no* head shakes, hand clapping, nervous mannerisms) that may support or contradict the speaker's verbal message. Facial expressions and eye movements include facial posturing such as smiles, frowns, raised eyebrows, grimaces, winces, lip quivering, eye gaze, and change in pupil size, conveying whether the person is relaxed or tense, animated or stoic, concentrating or day dreaming, receptive or nonreceptive, directed or undirected, or in mutuality or avoiding.

- *Tactile communication:* touch of oneself or another person that communicates relaxation, calmness, warmth, protection, friendliness, anxiety, or fear.

- *Proxemics:* manipulating space by adjusting size or arrangement of room, setting, furniture, or interpersonal distance (e.g., intimate, social, public distances).

- *Chronemics:* time factors such as orientation, understanding, or structuring of time; reaction to time pressure; awareness of time; relative punctuality in arriving, starting, or ending sessions.

- *Color:* use of color in the setting (e.g., walls, floor, furniture), clothing, or other materials.

- *Olfactory sense:* smells, odors, or aromas within the environment or interpersonal context.

- *Gustatory sense:* tastes relevant to the interpersonal context.

- *Objects and artifacts:* clothing, jewelry, eyeglasses, hearing aids, personal possessions, or professional or personal markers that may support or distract from a message.

- *Atmosphere or ambiance:* overall communication through a setting, including and combining perceived attitudes, proxemics, colors, sounds or silence, olfactory messages, and object messages.

- *Silence:* oral quiet and body inactivity communicating listening, waiting, observing, gaining attention, thinking; anger, frustration, inability to talk or respond; boredom, discomfort, hostility, reverence, agreement, or grief.

- *Organismics:* physical attributes including height, weight, eye and skin color, body dimensions, gender, race, age; physically apparent characteristics of disability.

- *Situation or environment:* immediate setting characteristics of home, school, or work that influence perceived expectations and communication patterns.

Farmer and Farmer (1989) noted that all areas of nonverbal behavior may be intentional or unintentional and appropriate or inappropriate and are influenced by cultural, gender, and regional differences (see Chapter 6). Supervisees and supervisors should be familiar with the more hidden, albeit operative, dynamics (McCready et al., 1987) before initiating intervention that interprets or manipulates nonverbal communication.

INDIVIDUALLY DESIGNED PROCEDURES. We noted previously that there are many individually designed procedures for observing and analyzing the clinical process. Similarly, there are probably as many individually designed procedures for observing the supervisory process as there are supervisees and supervisors. I continue to design individual professional development plans with and for each clinician with whom I work. Identified and acknowledged strengths within the clinical process serve as a foundation for designing objectives, strategies, and observational data to be collected for monitoring professional growth. The same can be said about objectives, strategies, and data for the supervisory process. For example, a supervisee may wish to use observational data to target an increase in her active contribution to planning the supervisory conference agenda or in monitoring her follow-through behavior to commitments (related to the academic, clinical, or supervisory process) made in the supervisory conference. A supervisor may wish to collect verbal and nonverbal observational data to target an increase in her acknowledgment and use of supervisee's ideas and in her use of objective data to support justification and rationale provided to the supervisee (Shapiro, 1994a). Such an individualized methodology for studying and monitoring the behavior of supervisees and supervisors from the supervisory conference to later activities was presented by Shapiro and Anderson (1988, 1989). The methodology included a Commitment Documentation Form for listing and describing commitments made during the supervisory conference, a Commitment Classification System for analyzing the type of commitments made, and a Follow-Through Evaluation Form for documenting the subsequent behaviors (i.e., the observational data) relating to each commitment made in order to indicate relative completion or lack of completion. Readers wanting additional information regarding the design of individually designed procedures for establishing objectives and monitoring progress within the academic, clinical, and supervisory processes should refer to the primary sources (Shapiro, 1987, 1994a; Shapiro & Anderson, 1988, 1989).

Analyzing the Supervisory Process. The analysis component is a bridge between observation and evaluation. Analysis refers to logical interpretation of the objective data from events that have been planned and observed. Anderson (1988) noted that data are examined, categorized, summarized, organized, and interpreted in relation to the relative change in the client, clinician/supervisee, or supervisor. Analysis enables supervisees and supervisors to determine which objectives have been met and to identify salient individual and joint patterns of interaction. Analysis naturally follows the earlier components in which the supervisee and supervisor have determined which data are to be collected and what will be done with them. Furthermore, Anderson (1988) highlighted that the joint responsibility for interpretation of data is a critical component of Analysis. She indicated, "This is where supervisees, to whatever extent possible, begin to self-analyze, to problem-solve about their own behavior, and to look for the relationships between their behaviors and those of the client" (p. 66).

The supervisee's level of responsibility for analysis leading to self-evaluation and independent problem solving will increase as the she gains experience and progresses along the continuum of supervision. Just as analyzing data from clinical sessions helps the clinician/supervisee gain insights into relationships between clinician and client behavior, analyzing the supervisory conference helps its participants gain insights into the nature of their interaction that would not be possible without systematic and objective (i.e., scientific) study. Assisting supervisees with the ongoing, objective analysis and interpretation of objective observational data is one of the tasks of supervision (ASHA, 1985).

The questions addressed in the Analysis component depend upon the decisions made during the earlier components and the relative placement of both the supervisee and supervisor along the continuum of supervision. Brasseur (1989) concurred, noting that analysis and interpretation of the objective data may address any of the following questions, among others:

1. How many times did the clinician model, expand, and instruct?
2. What clinician behaviors preceded correct and incorrect responses?
3. What was the nature of the task(s) used to elicit responses?
4. What was the client's response rate (number of responses per minute)?
5. What was the content of directions and instructions?
6. What client behaviors follow certain clinician behaviors? (p. 285)

Casey et al. (1988) advised supervisory participants to be alert to the nature and types of data collected because of their import to future planning and observation. Specifically, they cautioned supervisees and supervisors to be wary to analyses that continually show only positive outcomes. While such data may show remarkably steady progress in some planned sequence, they also may indicate that planning is targeting objectives of insufficient challenge, thus failing to provide direction for future growth of the client, clinician/supervisee, or supervisor. Conversely, analyses that indicate continued failure to achieve the established objectives, whether addressing the clinical or supervisory process, may suggest that the target objectives or procedures are inappropriate to the individual's current level of functioning. They advised, "Either outcome implies a need for additional planning" (p. 21).

Integrating the Supervisory Process. Integrating the supervisory process, usually within the context of a supervisory conference, is an opportunity to merge the previous components of Understanding, Planning, Observing, and Analyzing. The supervisee and supervisor share and discuss the results of their analyses and reach shared conclusions. In my work in the field, I see too few supervisors scheduling regular conferences with their supervisees. The most frequent justification is a lack of time (Anderson, 1988; Casey et al., 1988; Shapiro, 1987). Attention to the earlier components, however, results in conferences that are focused, meaningful, and efficient. Casey et al. (1988) noted that, "Planning for observations, analysis, and integration itself provides a focus for the conference; presentation of objective, organized, and summary data precludes the time-consuming discussion of supervisor or supervisee perceptions about what took place" (p. 22). The recurrent findings that supervisory conferences frequently are characterized by recounting the chronology of what occurred in clinical sessions (Anderson, 1988; Brasseur, 1989; Shapiro, 1985, 1987; Smith, 1978) rather than by focusing on self-study and problem solving (Moses & Shapiro, 1996; Shapiro, 1994a; Shapiro & Moses, 1989) suggest a lack of planning or insufficient understanding or discussion of the respective roles and responsibilities of the supervisory participants. The extent to which planning for the supervisory conference is a shared activity again reflects the relative placement of each participant within the continuum of supervision. The events and objectives that were planned, observed, and analyzed are discussed with respect to the objective data collected. Interpretations are made according to the strategy to which the participants previously agreed.

As noted, the focus of the supervisory conference should be on problem solving. In fact, the purpose of the Integrating component, according to Anderson (1988), is operationalizing professional self-growth. This suggests that the objectives previously established for the supervisory interaction (i.e., those relating to supervisee and supervisor) should be handled with the same level of care in the conference as those specified for the clinical interaction (i.e., those relating to client and clinician). Casey et al. (1988) added that movement along the continuum requires increasing responsibility on the part of the supervisee for all aspects of the supervisory interaction. They recommended that the participants review periodically their respective responsibilities to ensure the appropriate incremental shifts in dominance. Furthermore, Brasseur (1989) reminded that advancement along the continuum requires a shift in supervisory style from direct/active (for the Evaluation–Feedback Stage) to collaborative (for the Transitional Stage) to consultative (for the Self-Supervision Stage). The periodic review should ensure that the components, responsibilities, and styles of supervision are ever changing and conducive to facilitating supervisee and supervisor growth. It is this necessarily dynamic quality of the supervisory process that has been described as "a process in progress" (Shapiro, 1985, p. 89).

Avenues of Supervisory Preparation

Before we began our discussion of the supervisory process, I underscored the need for student clinicians and professional speech–language pathologists to be provided with an understanding of the supervisory process and to be prepared for their unique role as supervisees within this process. This section addresses briefly various avenues of supervisory preparation that are available for supervisees (i.e., and supervisors) to gain specialized knowledge about supervision. Clinical supervision was distinguished as "a distinct area of expertise and practice" for which "competencies are developed by special preparation" (ASHA, 1985, p. 60). The preparation or specialized training, interpreted as "a viable area for specialized study" (ASHA, 1985, p. 60), was discussed within three avenues of implementation. These included specific curricular offerings from graduate programs, continuing educational experiences specific to the supervisory process, and research-directed activities. More recently, ASHA (1989) elaborated these avenues of preparation for the supervisory process.

Curricular offerings were addressed in terms of the objectives, content, and procedures of introductory courses, supervised practica, advanced seminars, and components in clinical management courses. Avenues for research as a form of supervisory preparation were discussed in terms of:

- *Levels of research*—independent research projects by individuals or groups of interested supervisees and supervisors, self-study, course projects or papers, and more advanced master's theses and doctoral dissertations;
- *Issues and foci of research*—activities and interactions of supervisees and supervisors, conference interaction, perceptions, affective variables, and effectiveness and preparation; and
- *Methodologies of research*—self-study, survey, case studies, descriptive/qualitative, correlational, and experimental designs.

Finally, avenues for continuing education as a form of supervisory preparation or renewal addressed formats of:

- *Continuing education*—lecture, panel discussions, videotape demonstrations, peer process formats, distance learning, teleconferences, independent study, practicum, and laboratory experience;
- *Dimensions of continuing education*—number and length of sessions, number of participants, practicum, and extent of direction provided;
- *Formal contexts of continuing education*—conventions, workshops, or sponsored programs; and
- *Informal contexts of continuing education*—study groups, staff meetings, personal networks, and independent or group self-assessment activities.

Content for continuing education activities may address a particular task and associated competencies from the position statement (ASHA, 1985) or a current issue in supervision (e.g., efficacy of supervision, evaluation of supervisees and supervisors, or supervision as a quality assurance mechanism), and must meet the needs of participants who may range in related experience from minimal or no formal preparation to extensive post-graduate education in the area of supervision. The three avenues of special preparation—curricular offerings, research, and continuing education—provide supervisees (i.e., and supervisors) with many and varied opportunities to access relevant models and resources for supervisory training.

MAINTENANCE OF PROFESSIONAL COMPETENCE

Our discussion of professional preparation has addressed the integration of academic, clinical, and supervisory processes in order to impact clinicians' affective, behavioral, and cognitive knowledge. We have implied that the processes of professional preparation must set in motion a generative pattern of internally motivated, lifelong learning. To conclude the discussion of professional development, we will explicate these points by addressing the importance of internalizing the desire to learn, committing to learning as a lifelong process, and understanding and maintaining parallels in the nature and processes of our professional development over time.

Knowing and Internalizing the Desire To Learn

Clinicians achieve tremendous strides in that period of formal professional development during which they complete their undergraduate and graduate education.

The mechanism for professional development, as it currently stands, is a good process and assumed to be effective in achieving its target objectives. Efficacy data, however, are needed to document the instructional effectiveness of what we do and what we require to determine the causal connections to developing professional competence. Nevertheless, like any good thing, there are a few inherent limitations. One such limitation is that what we do in professional preparation and how we do it may be lacking in ecological validity. In other words, some of the behaviors and attitudes being established in student clinicians may not be particularly suited for application to professional settings outside of academe.

Beukelman (1986) expressed similar concerns, stating that the experience of graduate education tends to develop in student clinicians behaviors that are "counterproductive," creating experts for the short-term rather than the long-term. Furthermore, he indicated that graduate education encourages learning only in structured contexts, rather than from the fire of internal motivation, thereby fostering deliberate and incomplete sharing of information, fear of losing power rather than being motivated by the sincere quest to learn and help, and feelings of territoriality and negative attitudes toward other professionals. Beukelman cautioned that the processes of professional preparation may be fostering "maladaptive" (p. 5) behaviors, thus developing "sprinters" rather than "long distance runners" (p. 8) and failing to engender sincere and professional questioning and problem-solving skills.

Adopting more of a student perspective based on her own personal experiences, Prutting (1985) described professional preparation as a "long battle for the light" (p. 5), a time during which "how you perceive yourself as an individual is a consequence of how you perform academically" (p. 5). She identified student clinicians' tendency to put themselves and their lives on hold while achieving relatively short-term objectives, often without realizing that they are missing the essence of the educational experience. She implored students to engage actively in the essential dailiness of their experiences, to immerse in the science and human value of what they are about, to nurture and embrace their own exuberance (i.e., "joie de vivre," p. 6), and to study how they conceptualize themselves and others within the world because that is at the core of the human spirit and how we approach all experiences within our lives. (Note the similarity here with the concept of understanding one's own personal construct, presented in Chapter 5.) These two articles (Beukelman, 1986; Prutting, 1985) should be required reading for all participants in professional preparation.

Do these observations and attendant suggestions mean that we should disparage the process of professional preparation? I do not believe so. They do mean, however, that there are unavoidably certain limitations about which we can become aware and thereby control, if not eliminate. The inherent limitations (e.g., semesters or quarters, mastery of whatever course we are currently taking or teaching, client-focus rather than communication system- and interdisciplinary-focus, and disorder rather than person emphasis) tend to foster clinicians who conceive of professional preparation as an end in itself, rather than a means to a beginning. Every day with every client provides a renewed beginning, an opportunity to integrate our skills to meet the strengths and needs of our clients and their families. This process enables us to grow and improve, with and from our clients, as people and as professionals. In other words, learning must be a lifelong, internally motivated process that brings us sincere joy and excitement in our quest to understand and help others. That concept of professional competence as lifelong pursuit will be addressed now.

Learning as a Lifelong Process

Just yesterday, my son who is 4 years old asked me, "What number is infinity?" Somewhat puzzled by the complexity of his question, I took him outside and, together, we looked up at the sky. I asked him to think about how far we could go into space. With little deliberation, we agreed that there was no limit. Infinity, I explained, is like that—without limit, forever, and always.

Learning as a lifelong process may be understood as similar to infinity— without limit, forever, and always. The notion of lifelong learning, which has been described as an "integration of person and process" (Rassi & McElroy, 1992, p. 443), refers to involving oneself in some form of continuing education in order to stay current in a field and upgrade one's skills, thereby maintaining professional competence. It is hard, if not impossible, to credential or regulate the exuberance or "joie de vivre" (Prutting, 1985, p. 6) that must innervate any sincere, internal, and long-term motivation to learn. Remaining current within one's chosen profession is a significant ethical commitment we make during our own professional preparation and upon entry into our career (ASHA, 1994a; see Appendix A.2). Kellum and Fagan (1992) noted that human service professionals, within 10 to 12 years of receiving their professional education, were found to be approximately half as competent as they were when they graduated. They noted, "With the explosion of new knowledge and technological advances occurring in the fields of speech–language pathology and audiology, degree half-life of two to three years may well be a reality" (p. 410). Furthermore, they indicated the following:

> It is imperative to recognize that today's degree merely marks the beginning of the education continuum. . . . Continuing one's professional education beyond the graduate training level is no longer a luxury but a necessity. The public's call for competent professionals demands it; our professional association's standards and ethical codes require it; and the individual professional's pride in his or her work should dictate it. (p. 410)

Clearly, the avenues of specialized training reviewed earlier, including curricular offerings, research, and continuing education, may be applied to lifelong learning within the academic, clinical, and supervisory domains. Self-study activity using interaction analysis instruments (Anderson, 1988; Casey et al., 1988; Shapiro, 1987, 1994a) was discussed as one mechanism for facilitating objective observations yielding heightened understanding and professional growth as clinical or supervisory participants. Rassi and McElroy (1992) summarized aptly when they stated, "Each professional is responsible for his/her own continued learning and application in each relevant area. This responsibility is critical to advancement of knowledge, to growth of a profession, and to ongoing development of every professional" (pp. 443–444).

Lifelong learning, a personal and professional commitment to oneself to be and remain the best one can be, must come from within. While certification (even specialty certification), licensure, and continuing education requirements are externally driven instructional mechanisms, integrating oneself with the process of lifelong professional growth requires internal motivation. Anyone can go through the motions. Only clinicians will care enough about past, present, and future clients to seek, find, and seize opportunities to stay current or upgrade their professional skills. The Continuum of Supervision (Anderson, 1988; see Figure 12.2), emphasizing professional growth leading to independent clinical functioning, self-evaluation, and consultative interactions with colleagues, is an ideal way of conceptualizing and monitoring one's development over time. Furthermore, the aspects of professional development in problem solving (Moses & Shapiro, 1996; Shapiro & Moses, 1989; see Table 12.1) relating to perspectives taken, dimensions of behavior conceptualized, solutions generated, and causal concepts, similarly may be applied to maintenance of professional competence. Models, methods, and materials are available to facilitate learning and to accommodate individual needs, circumstances, and learning styles. It is up to individual clinicians to persevere, for infinity.

Maintaining Parallels: Different Trees, Same Forest

The discussion of professional development will conclude by highlighting several pertinent and generative parallels.

The Clinical and Supervisory Processes

Historically, it has been assumed that the skills needed by supervisors are the same as those needed by clinicians. In fact, the Certificate of Clinical Competence continues to be the only credential issued by the American Speech–Language–Hearing Association for clinicians and supervisors. ASHA's Committee on Supervision in Speech–Language Pathology and Audiology (ASHA, 1978) acknowledged this assumption, as follows:

> Currently, to obtain the Certificate of Clinical Competence a Member must have completed the Clinical Fellowship Year under the supervision of a Member whose only qualification is the possession of the Certificate of Clinical Competence, which was attained in the same manner. The Member is then assumed to be qualified not only as a clinician but as a supervisor. In other words, in the eyes of the Association, to be a qualified clinician is also to be a qualified supervisor. (p. 482)

I have expressed my concern about this assumption (Shapiro, 1987). Furthermore, I fully support disciplined efforts to study and understand clinical supervision as a distinct area of expertise with unique tasks and related competencies (ASHA, 1985) and the avenues of preparation for acquiring such specialized training (ASHA, 1989). In making such statements, I am acknowledging the distinction between clinical and supervisory skills and training. Notwithstanding, I recognize a considerable area of overlap. Consider a number of clinical procedures reviewed in Chapters 8, 9, and 10 and their relevance to the supervisory process as well. These procedures include constructing a safe house in which learning happens, inviting objectives, creating opportunities for success, heightening the learner's awareness of such success, developing and transferring target skills, introducing and increasing levels of challenge systematically, modeling appropriate behaviors and skills, establishing or maintaining positive feelings about oneself as a learner, facilitating empowerment, and talking with learners in positive ways. The list could go on.

Similarly, consider the interpersonal and intrapersonal factors of effective clinicians reviewed in Chapter 11 and the relevance of these same factors to effective supervisees and supervisors. Those discussed include clinician attributes (such as empathy, warmth, genuineness, personal magnetism, compatible friction, and realistic and focused optimism), in addition to clinician behavior, language, needs, and satisfaction and rewards. Isn't the clinician as much the guardian angel to the client as the supervisor is to the supervisee? Couldn't Walle's (1974) observations about the clinical process—"Qualifying for therapeutic practice is one thing; suitability is another"—be applied to the supervisory process; and couldn't that about clinicians—"It is easier to become a therapist than to be one"—be applied to supervisors? While the clinical and supervisory processes are distinct and require unique skills, competencies, and forms of preparation, they nevertheless share a fund of knowledge that is necessary for effective practice in either endeavor.

Developing, Maintaining, and Upgrading Professional Competence

When considering learning and professional development as lifelong processes, we might recall and consider the usefulness of different models and procedures reviewed in this chapter for the purpose of developing clinical and supervisory skills. These included the Continuum of Supervision (Anderson, 1988), which is not time bound and therefore can be used to conceptualize professional development across one's professional life span. Similarly, the aspects of professional development (Shapiro & Moses, 1989) applied to clinician profiling (Moses & Shapiro, 1996) provide a mechanism for conceptualizing, observing, and monitoring continued development of problem solving skills over time. Finally, the methods reviewed for observing and analyzing the clinical and supervisory processes within professional preparation—interaction analysis, nonverbal analysis, and individually designed methods—could be applied again to maintaining or upgrading one's professional skills.

Back to the Beginning

Finally, the conceptual foundation built in Chapters 5, 6, and 7 for clinical intervention could as well be applied to the supervisory process and to lifelong learning. First, consider the importance of the personal construct. We emphasized that the client and clinician must understand the client's personal construct (i.e., thoughts and feelings about himself as a person and as a communicator and related assumptions and values) because it is the filter through which he interprets all events within his communicative world and by which he anticipates his future. Similarly, clinicians/supervisees and supervisors must understand their own personal constructs because of the interaction between their personal viewpoints and their effectiveness as change agents, and because of the potential for conflict of constructs. These statements imply at least two critical skills. One is ability to be honestly receptive to (by identifying, considering, respecting, and otherwise inviting) alternative points of view, particularly when they contrast with one's own. Another is the ability to initiate deliberate shifts from one's own perspective in order to consider alternative points of view (Moses & Shapiro, 1996; Shapiro, 1987; Shapiro & Moses, 1989). These skills will prove useful across instructional processes and over time in lifelong learning.

Second, we have emphasized that the family system is the most powerful communication network within which many of us will interact. Furthermore, communication occurs within systems and, therefore, should be addressed as such. Appreciating communication and communicators from the perspective of individual communication systems will help us understand those we serve, other helpers, and in so doing, ourselves.

Third, there is often strength in numbers, particularly when each person brings unique strengths and perspectives to the interdisciplinary team. Working effectively with interdisciplinary teams is consistent with the supervisory objective of achieving self-evaluation and lifelong professional independence through collaboration and eventual consultative relationships with professional colleagues (Anderson, 1988). Furthermore, such interdisciplinary interactions are conducive and facilitative to the aspects of lifelong professional development—perspectives considered, dimensions of behavior conceptualized, possible solutions generated, and causal concepts. These interactions, and the aspects of professional development they generate, contribute to maintaining and improving professional (academic, clinical, and supervisory) problem-solving skills (Moses & Shapiro, 1996; Shapiro & Moses, 1989) within the different domains of knowledge—affective, behavioral, and cognitive.

Finally, multicultural sensitivity and understanding provides but another opportunity to value people in their diverse and dynamic forms, thus enabling us to learn about others and, therefrom, ourselves. Again, such lessons are not time bound, and continue to contribute to our lifelong process of acquiring knowledge about communication and communicators within a most communicative world.

CHAPTER SUMMARY

Having discussed in the previous chapter the importance of clinicians as change agents within the clinical process, this chapter addressed the professional preparation of such persons who work with people who stutter and the process of lifelong learning. In addressing, "How are good clinicians made? Are they born or are they cultivated?" we emphasized four major points. First, professional preparation for clinicians who work with people who stutter must integrate experiences across academic, clinical, and supervisory processes, and must impact the affective, behavioral, and cognitive domains. Second, an explicit understanding of the academic, clinical, and supervisory processes enables clinicians to contribute meaningfully to and gain maximum benefit from the experience of professional preparation. Third, maintenance of clinical competence requires internalizing the desire to learn, committing to learning as a lifelong process, and understanding and maintaining parallels in the nature and process of professional development over time. Fourth, professional preparation and lifelong learning provide an opportunity for learners to become teachers and teachers to become learners across the interactive, dynamic journey of life.

Professional preparation of clinicians involves the academic, clinical, and supervisory processes, which are dynamically interrelated. The academic process is that which occurs within the classroom and has a significant impact on the clinical and supervisory processes. The clinical process is the interaction that occurs between the clinician and client (i.e., and family members). Comprehensive areas of critical academic and clinical knowledge are outlined within the Guidelines for Practice in Stuttering Treatment (ASHA, 1995; see Appendix A.3). The revised training standards that went into effect in 1993 have significant implications for professional preparation. Models for clinician development must recognize that development of clinical competence is begun within professional preparation during the academic (i.e., student–professor interaction), clinical (i.e., client–clinician interaction), and supervisory (i.e., supervisee–supervisor interaction) processes, and is continued in renewal training, continued education, and self-study activities throughout one's career. One such model (Shapiro & Moses, 1989) was presented containing a series of developmental phases in how clinicians organize and interpret information relevant to clinical planning, implementation, and problem solving. These phases address aspects of clinician development in four areas of problem solving, including orientation of perspective, dimensions of behavior conceptualized, possible solutions generated, and causal reasoning. The clinical process requires understanding, planning, observing, analyzing, and ultimately integrating all of the components inherent to the process.

The supervisory process refers to those necessarily interactive forms of clinical teaching between a supervisor and supervisee. Clinical supervision refers to "those tasks and skills of clinical teaching related to the interaction between a clinician and a client" (ASHA, 1985, p. 57), leading to improvement of the clinician's professional (i.e., technical and interpersonal) skills. Supervisory knowledge includes at least 13 tasks and supporting competencies for effective clinical supervision (ASHA, 1985). Emphasizing the importance of joint involvement and active participation of both the supervisee and supervisor in the phases of the supervisory process, the Continuum of Supervision (Anderson, 1988) is particularly sensitive to the uniqueness and significance of what individual supervisees and supervisors bring to the supervisory interaction. The continuum is not time bound, thus presenting a model of development across one's career and including three stages that require different styles of interaction—Evaluation–Feedback Stage (Direct/Active Style), Transitional Stage (Collaborative Style), and Self-Supervision Stage (Consultative Style). Parallel to the clinical process, the supervisory process requires understanding, planning, observing, analyzing, and integrating the dynamic components of the supervisory process. Various avenues for specialized preparation in the supervisory process are available including curricular offerings, continuing educational experiences, and research-directed activities.

The processes of professional preparation must set in motion a generative pattern of internally motivated, lifelong learning. In other words, maintenance of professional competence requires internalizing the desire to learn, committing to learning as a lifelong process, and understanding and maintaining parallels in the nature and process of our professional development over time.

Chapter 12 Study Questions

1. This chapter discussed professional preparation and lifelong learning as a composite of necessary processes for a career speech–language pathologist. In what ways do you feel the academic, clinical, and supervisory processes are interrelated? How do the knowledge, skills, and competencies within each process impact each other? How do the knowledge, skills, and competencies within each process impact that of the other processes?

2. We discussed two important documents—Guidelines for Practice in Stuttering Treatment (ASHA, 1995; see Appendix A.3) and the position statement titled Clinical Supervision in Speech–Language Pathology and Audiology (ASHA, 1985; see Appendix A.1). How is the necessary knowledge within the affective, behavioral, and cognitive domains addressed within each document? Which areas of knowledge do you feel are most critical to establishing and maintaining professional competence? How might these documents prove useful to professional preparation and to lifelong learning?

3. The components of the clinical and supervisory processes include understanding, planning, observing, analyzing, and integrating the respective and dynamic components. What are the similarities and differences between the components of learning across the academic, clinical, and supervisory processes? What implications are there in these similarities and difference to the processes of professional preparation and lifelong learning?

4. We reviewed a model of clinician development (Shapiro & Moses, 1989) that contains a series of developmental phases in how clinicians organize and interpret information relevant to clinical planning, implementation, and problem solving. Specifically, aspects of clinician development occur in four areas of problem solving, including orientation of perspective, dimensions of behavior conceptualized, possible solutions generated, and causal reasoning. What are the similarities and differences between this model and the Continuum of Supervision presented by Anderson (1988)? What is the relevance of the four aspects of development to the academic, clinical, and supervisory processes? Furthermore, what is the relevance of the four aspects to professional preparation and lifelong learning?

5. Maintenance of professional competence requires internalizing the desire to learn, committing to learning as a lifelong process, and understanding and maintaining parallels in the nature and process of our professional development over time. What do these processes mean to you? For student clinicians, how are these processes being set in motion during your professional preparation? For professional speech–language pathologists, how did your professional preparation set in motion the processes that are necessary for maintenance of professional competence? What is your plan at the present time to ensure lifelong learning and maintenance of professional competence?

Appendix A
Reprinted Publications

◆ ◆ ◆ ◆ ◆ ◆ ◆ ◆ ◆ ◆ ◆ ◆ ◆ ◆ ◆ ◆ ◆

Appendix A.1

**Clinical Supervision in Speech–Language
Pathology and Audiology**

Appendix A.2

Code of Ethics

Appendix A.3

Guidelines for Practice in Stuttering Treatment

Appendix A.4

Scope of Practice in Speech–Language Pathology

513

Position Statement

Clinical Supervision
in
Speech-Language Pathology
and
Audiology

The following position paper, developed by the Committee on Supervision, was adopted by the American Speech-Language-Hearing Association through its Legislative Council in November 1984 (LC 8-84). Members of the Committee included Elaine Brown-Grant, Patricia Casey, Bonnie Cleveland, Charles Diggs *(ex officio)*, Richard Forcucci, Noel Matkin, George Purvis, Kathryn Smith, Peggy Williams *(ex officio)*, Edward Wills, and Sandra Ulrich, Chair. Also contributing were the NSSLHA representatives Mary Kawell and Sheran Landis. The committee was under the guidance of Marianna Newton, Vice President for Professional and Governmental Affairs.

Contributions of members of the ASHA Committee on Supervision for the years 1976-1982 are acknowledged. The members of the 1978-1981 Subcommittee on Supervision (Noel Matkin, Chair) of the Council on Professional Standards in Speech-Language Pathology and Audiology are also acknowledged for their work from which the competencies presented herein were adapted.

WHEREAS, the American Speech-Language-Hearing Association (ASHA) needs a clear position on clinical supervision, and
WHEREAS, the necessity for having such a position for use in student training and in professional, legal, and governmental contexts has been recognized, and
WHEREAS, the Committee on Supervision in Speech-Language Pathology and Audiology has been charged to recommend guidelines for the roles and responsibilities of supervisors in various settings (LC 14-74), and
WHEREAS, a position statement on clinical supervision now has been developed, disseminated for both select and widespread peer review, and revised; therefore
RESOLVED, that the American Speech-Language-Hearing Association adopts "Clinical Supervision in Speech-Language Pathology and Audiology" as the recognized position of the Association.

Introduction

Clinical supervision is a part of the earliest history of the American Speech-Language-Hearing Association (ASHA). It is an integral part of the initial training of speech-language pathologists and audiologists, as well as their continued professional development at all levels and in all work settings.

ASHA has recognized the importance of supervision by specifying certain aspects of supervision in its requirements for the Certificates of Clinical Competence (CCC) and the Clinical Fellowship Year (CFY) (ASHA, 1982). Further, supervisory requirements are specified by the Council on Professional Standards in its standards and guidelines for both educational and professional services programs (Educational Standards Board, ASHA, 1980; Professional Services Board, ASHA, 1983). State laws for licensing and school certification consistently include requirements for supervision of practicum experiences and initial work performance. In addition, other regulatory and accrediting bodies (e.g., Joint Commission on Accreditation of Hospitals, Commission on Accreditation of Rehabilitation Facilities) require a mechanism for ongoing supervision throughout professional careers.

It is important to note that the term **clinical supervision,** as used in this document, refers to the tasks and skills of clinical teaching related to the interaction between a clinician and client. In its 1978 report, the Committee on Supervision in Speech-Language Pathology and Audiology differentiated between the two major roles of persons identified as supervisors: clinical teaching aspects and program management tasks. The Committee emphasized that although program management tasks relating to administration or coordination of programs may be a part of the person's job duties, the term **supervisor** referred to "individuals who engaged in clinical teaching through observation, conferences, review of records, and other procedures, and which is related to the interaction between a clinician and a client and the evaluation or management of communication skills" (*Asha,* 1978, p. 479). The Committee continues to recognize this distinction between tasks of administration or program management and those of clinical teaching, which is its central concern.

The importance of supervision to preparation of students and to assurance of quality clinical service has been assumed for some time. It is only recently, however, that the tasks of supervision have been well-defined, and that the special skills and competencies judged to be necessary for their effective application have been identified. This Position Paper addresses the following areas:

- tasks of supervision
- competencies for effective clinical supervision
- preparation of clinical supervisors

Tasks of Supervision

A central premise of supervision is that effective clinical teaching involves, in a fundamental way, the development of self-analysis, self-evaluation, and problem-solving skills on the part of the individual being supervised. The success of clinical teaching rests largely on the achievement of this goal. Further, the demonstration of quality clinical skills in supervisors is generally accepted as a prerequisite to supervision of students, as well as of those in the Clinical Fellowship Year or employed as certified speech-language pathologists or audiologists.

Outlined in this paper are 13 tasks basic to effective clinical teaching and constituting the distinct area of practice which comprises clinical supervision in communication disorders. The committee stresses that the level of preparation and experience of the supervisee, the particular work setting of the supervisor and supervisee, and client variables will influence the relative emphasis of each task in actual practice.

The tasks and their supporting competencies which follow are judged to have face validity as established by experts in the area of supervision, and by both select and widespread peer review. The committee recognizes the need for further validation and strongly encourages ongoing investigation. Until such time as more rigorous measures of validity are established, it will be particularly important for the tasks and competencies to be reviewed periodically through quality assurance procedures. Mechanisms such as Patient Care Audit and Child Services Review System appear to offer useful means for quality assurance in the supervisory tasks and competencies. Other procedures appropriate to specific work settings may also be selected.

The tasks of supervision discussed above follow:

1. establishing and maintaining an effective working relationship with the supervisee;
2. assisting the supervisee in developing clinical goals and objectives;
3. assisting the supervisee in developing and refining assessment skills;
4. assisting the supervisee in developing and refining clinical management skills;
5. demonstrating for and participating with the supervisee in the clinical process;
6. assisting the supervisee in observing and analyzing assessment and treatment sessions;
7. assisting the supervisee in the development and maintenance of clinical and supervisory records;
8. interacting with the supervisee in planning, executing, and analyzing supervisory conferences;
9. assisting the supervisee in evaluation of clinical performance;
10. assisting the supervisee in developing skills of verbal reporting, writing, and editing;
11. sharing information regarding ethical, legal, regulatory, and reimbursement aspects of professional practice;
12. modeling and facilitating professional conduct; and
13. demonstrating research skills in the clinical or supervisory processes.

Competencies for Effective Clinical Supervision

Although the competencies are listed separately according to task, each competency may be needed to perform a number of supervisor tasks.

1.0 Task: Establishing and maintaining an effective working relationship with the supervisee.

Competencies required:

1.1 Ability to facilitate an understanding of the clinical and supervisory processes.
1.2 Ability to organize and provide information regarding the logical sequences of supervisory interaction, that is, joint setting of goals and objectives, data collection and analysis, evaluation.
1.3 Ability to interact from a contemporary perspective with the supervisee in both the clinical and supervisory process.
1.4 Ability to apply learning principles in the supervisory process.
1.5 Ability to apply skills of interpersonal communication in the supervisory process.
1.6 Ability to facilitate independent thinking and problem solving by the supervisee.

1.7 Ability to maintain a professional and supportive relationship that allows supervisor and supervisee growth.
1.8 Ability to interact with the supervisee objectively.
1.9 Ability to establish joint communications regarding expectations and responsibilities in the clinical and supervisory processes.
1.10 Ability to evaluate, with the supervisee, the effectiveness of the ongoing supervisory relationship.

2.0 Task: Assisting the supervisee in developing clinical goals and objectives.

Competencies required:

2.1 Ability to assist the supervisee in planning effective client goals and objectives.
2.2 Ability to plan, with the supervisee, effective goals and objectives for clinical and professional growth.
2.3 Ability to assist the supervisee in using observation and assessment in preparation of client goals and objectives.
2.4 Ability to assist the supervisee in using self-analysis and previous evaluation in preparation of goals and objectives for professional growth.
2.5 Ability to assist the supervisee in assigning priorities to clinical goals and objectives.
2.6 Ability to assist the supervisee in assigning priorities to goals and objectives for professional growth.

3.0 Task: Assisting the supervisee in developing and refining assessment skills.

Competencies required:

3.1 Ability to share current research findings and evaluation procedures in communication disorders.
3.2 Ability to facilitate an integration of research findings in client assessment.
3.3 Ability to assist the supervisee in providing rationale for assessment procedures.
3.4 Ability to assist supervisee in communicating assessment procedures and rationales.
3.5 Ability to assist the supervisee in integrating findings and observations to make appropriate recommendations.
3.6 Ability to facilitate the supervisee's independent planning of assessment.

4.0 Task: Assisting the supervisee in developing and refining management skills.

Competencies required:

4.1 Ability to share current research findings and management procedures in communication disorders.
4.2 Ability to facilitate an integration of research findings in client management.
4.3 Ability to assist the supervisee in providing rationale for treatment procedures.
4.4 Ability to assist the supervisee in identifying appropriate sequences for client change.
4.5 Ability to assist the supervisee in adjusting steps in the progression toward a goal.
4.6 Ability to assist the supervisee in the description and measurement of client and clinician change.
4.7 Ability to assist the supervisee in documenting client and clinician change.
4.8 Ability to assist the supervisee in integrating documented client and clinician change to evaluate progress and specify future recommendations.

5.0 Task: Demonstrating for and participating with the supervisee in the clinical process.

Competencies required:

5.1 Ability to determine jointly when demonstration is appropriate.
5.2 Ability to demonstrate or participate in an effective client-clinician relationship.
5.3 Ability to demonstrate a variety of clinical techniques and participate with the supervisee in clinical management.
5.4 Ability to demonstrate or use jointly the specific materials and equipment of the profession.
5.5 Ability to demonstrate or participate jointly in counseling of clients or family/guardians of clients.

6.0 Task: Assisting the supervisee in observing and analyzing assessment and treatment sessions.

Competencies required:

6.1 Ability to assist the supervisee in learning a variety of data collection procedures.
6.2 Ability to assist the supervisee in selecting and executing data collection procedures.
6.3 Ability to assist the supervisee in accurately recording data.
6.4 Ability to assist the supervisee in analyzing and interpreting data objectively.
6.5 Ability to assist the supervisee in revising plans for client management based on data obtained.

7.0 Task: Assisting the supervisee in development and maintenance of clinical and supervisory records.

Competencies required:

7.1 Ability to assist the supervisee in applying record-keeping systems to supervisory and clinical processes.
7.2 Ability to assist the supervisee in effectively documenting supervisory and clinically related interactions.
7.3 Ability to assist the supervisee in organizing records to facilitate easy retrieval of information concerning clinical and supervisory interactions.
7.4 Ability to assist the supervisee in establishing and following policies and procedures to protect the confidentiality of clinical and supervisory records.
7.5 Ability to share information regarding documentation requirements of various accrediting and regulatory agencies and third-party funding sources.

8.0 Task: Interacting with the supervisee in planning, executing, and analyzing supervisory conferences.

Competencies required:

8.1 Ability to determine with the supervisee when a conference should be scheduled.
8.2 Ability to assist the supervisee in planning a supervisory conference agenda.
8.3 Ability to involve the supervisee in jointly establishing a conference agenda.
8.4 Ability to involve the supervisee in joint discussion of previously identified clinical or supervisory data or issues.
8.5 Ability to interact with the supervisee in a manner that facilitates the supervisee's self-exploration and problem solving.
8.6 Ability to adjust conference content based on the supervisee's level of training and experience.
8.7 Ability to encourage and maintain supervisee motivation for continuing self-growth.
8.8 Ability to assist the supervisee in making commitments for changes in clinical behavior.
8.9 Ability to involve the supervisee in ongoing analysis of supervisory interactions.

9.0 Task: Assisting the supervisee in evaluation of clinical performance.

Competencies required:

9.1 Ability to assist the supervisee in the use of clinical evaluation tools.
9.2 Ability to assist the supervisee in the description and measurement of his/her progress and achievement.
9.3 Ability to assist the supervisee in developing skills of self-evaluation.
9.4 Ability to evaluate clinical skills with the supervisee for purposes of grade assignment, completion of Clinical Fellowship Year, professional advancement, and so on.

10.0 Task: Assisting the supervisee in developing skills of verbal reporting, writing, and editing.

Competencies required:

10.1 Ability to assist the supervisee in identifying appropriate information to be included in a verbal or written report.
10.2 Ability to assist the supervisee in presenting information in a logical, concise, and sequential manner.
10.3 Ability to assist the supervisee in using appropriate professional terminology and style in verbal and written reporting.
10.4 Ability to assist the supervisee in adapting verbal and written reports to the work environment and communication situation.
10.5 Ability to alter and edit a report as appropriate while preserving the supervisee's writing style.

11.0 Task: Sharing information regarding ethical, legal, regulatory, and reimbursement aspects of the profession.

Competencies required:

11.1 Ability to communicate to the supervisee a knowledge of professional codes of ethics (e.g., ASHA, state licensing boards, and so on).
11.2 Ability to communicate to the supervisee an understanding of legal and regulatory documents and their impact on the practice of the profession (licensure, PL 94-142, Medicare, Medicaid, and so on).
11.3 Ability to communicate to the supervisee an understanding of reimbursement policies and procedures of the work setting.
11.4 Ability to communicate a knowledge of supervisee rights and appeal procedures specific to the work setting.

12.0 Task: Modeling and facilitating professional conduct.

Competencies required:

12.1 Ability to assume responsibility.
12.2 Ability to analyze, evaluate, and modify own behavior.
12.3 Ability to demonstrate ethical and legal conduct.
12.4 Ability to meet and respect deadlines.

12.5 Ability to maintain professional protocols (respect for confidentiality, etc.)

12.6 Ability to provide current information regarding professional standards (PSB, ESB, licensure, teacher certification, etc.).

12.7 Ability to communicate information regarding fees, billing procedures, and third-party reimbursement.

12.8 Ability to demonstrate familiarity with professional issues.

12.9 Ability to demonstrate continued professional growth.

13.0 Task: Demonstrating research skills in the clinical or supervisory processes.

Competencies required:

13.1 Ability to read, interpret, and apply clinical and supervisory research.

13.2 Ability to formulate clinical or supervisory research questions.

13.3 Ability to investigate clinical or supervisory research questions.

13.4 Ability to support and refute clinical or supervisory research findings.

13.5 Ability to report results of clinical or supervisory research and disseminate as appropriate (e.g., in-service, conferences, publications).

Preparation of Supervisors

The special skills and competencies for effective clinical supervision may be acquired through special training which may include, but is not limited to, the following:

1. Specific curricular offerings from graduate programs; examples include doctoral programs emphasizing supervision, other postgraduate preparation, and specified graduate courses.

2. Continuing educational experiences specific to the supervisory process (e.g., conferences, workshops, self-study).

3. Research-directed activities that provide insight in the supervisory process.

The major goal of training in supervision is mastery of the "Competencies for Effective Clinical Supervision." Since competence in clinical services and work experience sufficient to provide a broad clinical perspective are considered essential to achieving competence in supervision, it is apparent that most preparation in supervision will occur following the preservice level. Even so, positive effects of preservice introduction to supervision preparation have been described by both Anderson (1981) and Rassi (1983). Hence, the presentation of basic material about the supervisory process may enhance students' performance as supervisees, as well as provide them with a framework for later study.

The steadily increasing numbers of publications concerning supervision and the supervisory process indicate that basic information concerning supervision now is becoming more accessible in print to all speech-language pathologists and audiologists, regardless of geographical location and personal circumstances. In addition, conferences, workshops, and convention presentations concerning supervision in communication disorders are more widely available than ever before, and both coursework and supervisory practicum experiences are emerging in college and university educational programs. Further, although preparation in the supervisory process specific to communication disorders should be the major content, the commonality in principles of supervision across the teaching, counseling, social work, business, and health care professions suggests additional resources for those who desire to increase their supervisory knowledge and skills.

To meet the needs of persons who wish to prepare themselves as clinical supervisors, additional coursework, continuing education opportunities, and other programs in the supervisory process should be developed both within and outside graduate education programs. As noted in an earlier report on the status of supervision (ASHA, 1978), supervisors themselves expressed a strong desire for training in supervision. Further, systematic study and investigation of the supervisory process is seen as necessary to expansion of the data base from which increased knowledge about supervision and the supervisory process will emerge.

The "Tasks of Supervision" and "Competencies for Effective Clinical Supervision" are intended to serve as the basis for content and outcome in preparation of supervisors. The tasks and competencies will be particularly useful to supervisors for self-study and self-evaluation, as well as to the consumers of supervisory activity, that is, supervisees and employers.

A repeated concern by the ASHA membership is that implementation of any suggestions for qualifications of supervisors will lead to additional standards or credentialing. At this time, preparation in supervision is a viable area of specialized study. The competencies for effective supervision can be achieved and implemented by supervisors and employers.

Summary

Clinical supervision in speech-language pathology and audiology is a distinct area of expertise and practice. This paper defines the area of supervision, outlines the special tasks of which it is comprised, and describes the competencies for each task. The competencies are developed by special preparation, which may take at least three avenues of implementation. Additional coursework, continuing education opportunities and other programs in the supervisory process should be developed both within and outside of graduate education programs. At this time, preparation in supervision is a viable area for specialized study, with competence achieved and implemented by supervisors and employers. **Asha**

Bibliography

American Speech and Hearing Association. (1978). Current status of supervision of speech-language pathology and audiology [Special Report] *Asha, 20*, 478-486.

American Speech-Language-Hearing Association. (1980). *Standards for accreditation by the Education and Training Board*. Rockville, MD: ASHA.

American Speech-Language-Hearing Association. (1982). *Requirements for the certificates of clinical competence* (Rev.). Rockville, MD: ASHA.

American Speech-Language-Hearing Association. (1983). New standards for accreditation by the Professional Services Board. *Asha, 25*, 6, 51-58.

Anderson, J. (Ed.) (1980, July). *Proceedings: Conference on Training in the Supervisory Process in Speech-Language Pathology and Audiology*. Indiana University, Bloomington.

Anderson, J. (1981). A training program in clinical supervision. *Asha, 23*, 77-82.

Culatta, R., & Helmick, J. (1980). Clinical supervision: The state of the art—Part I. *Asha, 22*, 985-993.

Culatta, R., & Helmick, J. (1981). Clinical supervision: The state of the art—Part II. *Asha, 23*, 21-31.

Laney, M. (1982). Research and evaluation in the public schools. *Language, Speech, and Hearing Services in the Schools, 13*, 53-60.

Rassi, J. (1983, September). *Supervision in audiology*. Seminar presented at Hahnemann University, Philadelphia.

Appendix A
Reprinted Publications

◆ ◆ ◆ ◆ ◆ ◆ ◆ ◆ ◆ ◆ ◆ ◆ ◆ ◆ ◆ ◆ ◆ ◆ ◆ ◆

Appendix A.1

Clinical Supervision in Speech–Language
Pathology and Audiology

Appendix A.2

Code of Ethics

Appendix A.3

Guidelines for Practice in Stuttering Treatment

Appendix A.4

Scope of Practice in Speech–Language Pathology

Code of Ethics

Revised January 1, 1994

American Speech-Language-Hearing Association

Preamble

The preservation of the highest standards of integrity and ethical principles is vital to the responsible discharge of obligations in the professions of speech-language pathology and audiology. This Code of Ethics sets forth the fundamental principles and rules considered essential to this purpose.

Every individual who is (a) a member of the American Speech-Language-Hearing Association, whether certified or not, (b) a nonmember holding the Certificate of Clinical Competence from the Association, (c) an applicant for membership or certification, or (d) a Clinical Fellow seeking to fulfill standards for certification shall abide by this Code of Ethics.

Any action that violates the spirit and purpose of this Code shall be considered unethical. Failure to specify any particular responsibility or practice in this Code of Ethics shall not be construed as denial of the existence of such responsibilities or practices.

The fundamentals of ethical conduct are described by Principles of Ethics and by Rules of Ethics as they relate to responsibility to persons served, to the public, and to the professions of speech-language pathology and audiology.

Principles of Ethics, aspirational and inspirational in nature, form the underlying moral basis for the Code of Ethics. Individuals shall observe these principles as affirmative obligations under all conditions of professional activity.

Rules of Ethics are specific statements of minimally acceptable professional conduct or of prohibitions and are applicable to all individuals.

Principle of Ethics I

Individuals shall honor their responsibility to hold paramount the welfare of persons they serve professionally.

Rules of Ethics

A. Individuals shall provide all services competently.

B. Individuals shall use every resource, including referral when appropriate, to ensure that high-quality service is provided.

C. Individuals shall not discriminate in the delivery of professional services on the basis of race or ethnicity, gender, age, religion, national origin, sexual orientation, or disability.

D. Individuals shall fully inform the persons they serve of the nature and possible effects of services rendered and products dispensed.

E. Individuals shall evaluate the effectiveness of services rendered and of products dispensed and shall provide services or dispense products only when benefit can reasonably be expected.

F. Individuals shall not guarantee the results of any treatment or procedure, directly or by implication; however, they may make a reasonable statement of prognosis.

G. Individuals shall not evaluate or treat speech, language, or hearing disorders solely by correspondence.

H. Individuals shall maintain adequate records of professional services rendered and products dispensed and shall allow access to these records when appropriately authorized.

I. Individuals shall not reveal, without authorization, any professional or personal information about the person served professionally, unless required by law to do so, or unless doing so is necessary to protect the welfare of the person or of the community.

J. Individuals shall not charge for services not rendered, nor shall they misrepresent,[1] in any fashion, services rendered or products dispensed.

K. Individuals shall use persons in research or as subjects of teaching demonstrations only with their informed consent.

L. Individuals whose professional services are adversely affected by substance abuse or other health-related conditions shall seek professional assistance and, where appropriate, withdraw from the affected areas of practice.

---

[1] For purposes of this Code of Ethics, misrepresentation includes any untrue statements or statements that are likely to mislead. Misrepresentation also includes the failure to state any information that is material and that ought, in fairness, to be considered.

Principle of Ethics II

Individuals shall honor their responsibility to achieve and maintain the highest level of professional competence.

Rules of Ethics

A. Individuals shall engage in the provision of clinical services only when they hold the appropriate Certificate of Clinical Competence or when they are in the certification process and are supervised by an individual who holds the appropriate Certificate of Clinical Competence.

B. Individuals shall engage in only those aspects of the professions that are within the scope of their competence, considering their level of education, training, and experience.

C. Individuals shall continue their professional development throughout their careers.

D. Individuals shall delegate the provision of clinical services only to persons who are certified or to persons in the education or certification process who are appropriately supervised. The provision of support services may be delegated to persons who are neither certified nor in the certification process only when a certificate holder provides appropriate supervision.

E. Individuals shall prohibit any of their professional staff from providing services that exceed the staff member's competence, considering the staff member's level of education, training, and experience.

F. Individuals shall ensure that all equipment used in the provision of services is in proper working order and is properly calibrated.

Principle of Ethics III

Individuals shall honor their responsibility to the public by promoting public understanding of the professions, by supporting the development of services designed to fulfill the unmet needs of the public, and by providing accurate information in all communications involving any aspect of the professions.

Rules of Ethics

A. Individuals shall not misrepresent their credentials, competence, education, training, or experience.

B. Individuals shall not participate in professional activities that constitute a conflict of interest.

C. Individuals shall not misrepresent diagnostic information, services rendered, or products dispensed or engage in any scheme or artifice to defraud in connection with obtaining payment or reimbursement for such services or products.

D. Individuals' statements to the public shall provide accurate information about the nature and management of communication disorders, about the professions, and about professional services.

E. Individuals' statements to the public—advertising, announcing, and marketing their professional services, reporting research results, and promoting products—shall adhere to prevailing professional standards and shall not contain misrepresentations.

Principle of Ethics IV

Individuals shall honor their responsibilities to the professions and their relationships with colleagues, students, and members of allied professions. Individuals shall uphold the dignity and autonomy of the professions, maintain harmonious interprofessional and intraprofessional relationships, and accept the professions' self-imposed standards.

Rules of Ethics

A. Individuals shall prohibit anyone under their supervision from engaging in any practice that violates the Code of Ethics.

B. Individuals shall not engage in dishonesty, fraud, deceit, misrepresentation, or any form of conduct that adversely reflects on the professions or on the individual's fitness to serve persons professionally.

C. Individuals shall assign credit only to those who have contributed to a publication, presentation, or product. Credit shall be assigned in proportion to the contribution and only with the contributor's consent.

D. Individuals' statements to colleagues about professional services, research results, and products shall adhere to prevailing professional standards and shall contain no misrepresentations.

E. Individuals shall not provide professional services without exercising independent professional judgment, regardless of referral source or prescription.

F. Individuals shall not discriminate in their relationships with colleagues, students, and members of allied professions on the basis of race or ethnicity, gender, age, religion, national origin, sexual orientation, or disability.

G. Individuals who have reason to believe that the Code of Ethics has been violated shall inform the Ethical Practice Board.

H. Individuals shall cooperate fully with the Ethical Practice Board in its investigation and adjudication of matters related to this Code of Ethics.

Appendix A
Reprinted Publications

◆ ◆ ◆ ◆ ◆ ◆ ◆ ◆ ◆ ◆ ◆ ◆ ◆ ◆ ◆ ◆ ◆ ◆ ◆

Appendix A.1

Clinical Supervision in Speech–Language Pathology and Audiology

Appendix A.2

Code of Ethics

Appendix A.3

Guidelines for Practice in Stuttering Treatment

Appendix A.4

Scope of Practice in Speech–Language Pathology

• • • • • • • • • • ███ GUIDELINES ███ • • • • • • • • • •

Guidelines for Practice in Stuttering Treatment

Special Interest Division on Fluency and Fluency Disorders
American Speech-Language-Hearing Association

•••••••••••••••••••••••••••
These guidelines are an official statement of the American Speech-Language-Hearing Association (ASHA). They are guidelines for practice in stuttering treatment but are not official standards of the Association. They were developed by members of the Steering Committee of ASHA's Special Interest Division on Fluency and Fluency Disorders (Division 4): C. W. Starkweather, Kenneth St. Louis, Gordon Blood, Theodore Peters, Janice Westbrook, Hugo Gregory, Eugene Cooper, and Charles Healey, under the guidance of Crystal Cooper, vice president for professional practices. Lyn Goldberg provided support from the National Office. The Steering Committee acknowledges the assistance of Diane L. Eger, vice president for professional practices, 1991-1993.
•••••••••••••••••••••••••••

I. Introduction

The document that follows was developed by the Special Interest Division on Fluency and Fluency Disorders (Division 4) of ASHA in response to the affiliates' belief that the field lacked standards for the treatment of stuttering. It was felt too that the parallel move toward specialization made it necessary to define more clearly the role of nonspecialists. At the same time, the ASHA document, "Preferred Practice Patterns for the Professions of Speech-Language Pathology and Audiology" (*Asha* Supplement No. 11, March 1993), was published but addressed only Fluency

Assessment and only in the most general terms. The failure of this document to address the treatment of fluency disorders left a gap to be filled.

It should be noted that the Steering Committee felt that the state of knowledge in several key areas - specifically treatment efficacy and the measurement of stuttering - was not developed well enough to allow the promulgation of "standards." It was decided to provide less prescriptive "guidelines."

Another issue concerned the base of knowledge used to determine whether a goal is desirable or a practice appropriate to achieve a goal. The Steering Committee felt that a set of criteria for determining guidelines that was based entirely on empirical evidence would be too restrictive. Some treatment practices may be quite useful even though their efficacy has not yet been determined empirically. The committee felt that both common practice and published data should be considered.

Finally, the document does not take a position on stuttering theory or advocate a specific philosophy of treatment. Instead, it puts forward what is hoped to be an agreed upon set of goals and the procedures that are used to achieve them.

II. General Guidelines for Practice

Timing and Duration of Sessions

There is considerable variation in the timing and duration of treatment sessions and in the total duration of

treatment. Some residential programs treat clients very intensively, 6 or more hours each day for a number of weeks. Private clinicians may see clients one, two, or three times a week for a longer period of time. In the schools and hospitals, the timing and duration of sessions is restrained by overriding schedules. Intensive treatment may be expected to achieve more rapid change, but the intensive treatment alters the client's daily activity more extensively, creating a barrier to transfer that the clinician considers in planning treatment activities. Nonintensive treatment, on the other hand, disrupts the client's everyday life far less, but it may achieve change so slowly that the client becomes discouraged. Clinicians who see clients less frequently can sequence treatment activity for early success, or provide for other motivational activities that will keep the client interested in continuing treatment.

The Setting of Treatment

Clients are seen in a wide variety of settings. Some programs are residential, providing treatment, usually intensive, in a setting removed from the client's everyday life. Others treat clients in the communities where they live. Both residential and nonresidential treatment programs provide activities for effective transfer of new behaviors to the ordinary social situations of everyday life. Transfer can be achieved through carefully sequenced, monitored practice in real-life social situations. Programs that treat the client only in a limited setting and do not provide for monitored practice of newly learned behaviors in natural settings fall outside the guidelines of good practice. There are a number of ways to monitor a client's practice: (1) direct observation, in which the clinician is present during the practice session, (2) interviews with the client after practice sessions, and (3) listening, with the client, to audiotape recordings of practice sessions. In each case, monitoring should include opportunities for the clinician to discuss the practice session with the client so as to increase understanding, and opportunities to provide immediate feedback on the client's performance. Listening to audiotape recordings that are submitted by mail and responded to with written comments from the clinician falls outside the guidelines of good practice, if it is the only method of transfer. It should be recognized, however, that there are circumstances -- when a client lives in a remote area, for example -- where it may be impossible to provide service that is within the guidelines. The best practice, in these circumstances, is to make sure that both client and clinician are aware of any necessary limitations on treatment.

There is also variation in the duration of individual sessions. In general, clinicians plan sessions so that they are long enough to accomplish some stated objective, but not so long as to lose clients' attention through fatigue or boredom. The client's age and ability to attend are taken into consideration in determining the duration of sessions.

Duration of Treatment

The total duration of treatment is an important variable of practice. Clinicians want to be sure that treatment lasts long enough for effective change, but they do not want to continue to provide treatment when there is no longer any further benefit. Our field is in the process of researching the variables that affect treatment

duration, but we cannot yet say with certainty what these variables are. It seems clear that more intensive treatment produces more rapid change than nonintensive treatment (Prins, 1970). It also seems likely, but not yet demonstrated, that the complexity of a client's problem may influence the duration of treatment. People who stutter in a way that is unusually complex behaviorally, or who have other coexisting problems or disorders are likely to require considerable time in treatment. Those who are cognitively impaired, or who cannot attend easily, for example, would be expected to take longer in treatment. Also, the presence of a coexisting language or articulation disorder, or a psychoemotional disturbance, can lengthen treatment.

A client's personal level of motivation and commitment to the treatment process will also influence the duration of treatment. School-age, adolescent, and adult stutterers require longer durations of treatment than preschool children. In spite of the uncertainty that remains in this area, clinicians try to provide to clients and their families some sense of how long treatment may take, including the processes of maintenance and follow-up.

Complexity of Treatment

Stuttering is typically a complex problem. It may begin simply, but it usually, and sometimes quickly, becomes complex because of the reactions, defensive behaviors, and coping strategies of the person who stutters and the reactions of significant others in the listening environment. Furthermore, in older children and adults, the communicative difficulties that stuttering presents present barriers to social, educational, and vocational life that can greatly complicate the problem. In some cases, there can be serious emotional disturbance, such as depression or sociopathic behavior. These complexities create issues that clinicians help their clients deal with through treatment and referral. Stuttering treatments that do not address the complete problem in whatever complexity it presents are

not within the guidelines of good practice.

The Cost of Treatment

As independent professionals, clinicians working with stutterers have the responsibility of setting their own fees. In doing so, they consider a number of factors. People who stutter sometimes seek help with an intense longing for relief, and in some cases feel quite desperate. Clinicians, in setting their fees, do not exploit these feelings. In addition, the client's desire for help can be increased through statements by the clinician implying that the treatment is highly effective. The prohibition in the Code of Ethics of ASHA against misrepresentation in public statements has particular relevance for stuttering treatment. When clinicians make public statements about their own treatment programs, they are appropriately cautious about its effectiveness. It would seem well outside the guidelines of good practice for a clinician to make a public statement that a new technique could solve every stutterer's problem, and then charge far more than is the usual practice.

Typically, the amount of time the clinician spends in face-to-face contact with the client is the main yardstick by which the value of treatment is determined. Telephone contact, tape recordings, paper and electronic mail contact also have value, although not many clinicians charge for these services. The value of treatment for people who stutter lies in the supportive nature of the client-clinician relationship and in the clinician's ability to hear and see the stutterer's behavior and respond to it in a way that helps the client learn to talk more effectively.

III. Attributes of Clinicians Who Work With People Who Stutter

It is desirable for clinicians to have certain personal attitudes and qualities and a fund of certain information. The following list is an expanded version of the Texas Speech and Hearing Association Fluency Task Force's list of "Personal Clinician Competencies":

Personal Attributes

1. Is interested in and committed to the treatment of people with fluency disorders.
2. Is willing to develop as much knowledge and skill as possible related to diagnosis and treatment of stuttering and keeps abreast of current developments.
3. Is willing to refer clients when the need for more assistance is necessary.
4. Is willing to take an active role in the profession to know about specific services that are available both locally and nationally to clients who stutter.
5. Has good problem-solving skills and uses them when things do not go according to plan in evaluation and treatment.
6. Is flexible in thinking and planning.

Learned Attributes

7. Has a general understanding of the literature relative to the etiology and development of stuttering.
8. Has an adequate level of knowledge of the phenomenology of stuttering, particularly with regard to those phenomena that influence therapeutic practice, such as, episodic variation, clustering, paradoxical intention, adaptation and consistency, spontaneous recovery, fluency enhancement, arousal effects.
9. Has a general understanding of the literature on normal and language-based (dis)fluency, rate, prosody, rhythm, and effort, and the development of these speech characteristics and has the skill to gain new information from the literature as new findings are incorporated into it.
10. Has a view of stuttering that is focused enough to provide guidance in the planning of treatment but broad and adjustable enough to accommodate new research findings and theoretical perspectives.
11. Has an understanding and appreciation of the possible relations between a person's normal and

abnormal speech behavior on the one hand, and their beliefs, upbringing, and cultural background on the other.
12. Has an understanding and appreciation of the basic processes of dynamic clinical interaction, such as transference, denial, grief, victimization.
13. Can communicate relevant ideas about stuttering to clients and their families.
14. Has a general working knowledge of psychopathology.
15. Has a general working knowledge of cognitive and behavioral learning theory.

In addition, the specialist in fluency should meet the guidelines listed below:

IV. Specific Guidelines for Practice—Goals, Processes, and Competencies

This section contains three parts. First, a list of goals, appropriate to the treatment of fluency disorders, is described. The criterion for including goals is that they be acceptable and desirable for speech-language pathologists to try to reach with clients with fluency disorders. These goals follow from the nature of fluency disorders, and it is expected that few will disagree with the choice of goals. Indeed, peer review of the guidelines revealed a broad consensus on the goals.

The philosophy of treatment that a clinician believes in will, of course, strongly determine which goals are considered most important. This list is intended to include all goals that are considered appropriate by all philosophies of treatment currently held by speech-language pathologists who treat people who stutter. The order of goals presented in this document does not reflect their order of importance.

It is recognized that certain goals may be desirable for (some) clients to reach but are nevertheless outside the scope of practice for most speech-language pathologists, e.g., psychotherapeutic goals unrelated to fluency, or parenting issues unrelated to a child's fluency.

The second part lists processes

that are useful for achieving specific goals. The inclusion of processes in this list in no way mandates their use by clinicians. Some clinicians will rely exclusively on a few processes; others will combine many different processes. The list is an attempt to set down processes that are in widespread use by speech-language pathologists who treat stuttering.

The criteria for selecting processes combine empirical knowledge, theory, and common practice. For example, one goal is a reduction in the frequency of stuttering behaviors. Processes that have been shown empirically to reduce stuttering behaviors in a lasting way, for example, slowed parental speech rate for young stuttering children, have consequently been included. Another process, for example, instrumental extinction, might be included for more theoretical reasons. In some cases, either the empirical or the theoretical support is weak, and this weakness is pointed out in the document.

The third part identifies competencies -- skills and knowledge -- that clinicians can use to engage in the processes identified in part two. The criteria for inclusion in this list of competencies are simply logical. If the modification of cognitive structures that make it difficult for clients to think about their speech in a productive manner is a desirable goal, then cognitive restructuring is a useful process, and a competency in that technique is useful for clinicians to have. It is understood that not all clinicians will have all competencies, although it is expected that clinicians will continue to augment their current competencies through continuing education.

A. Assessment

Desirable goals in the assessment of fluency disorders:

Assessment Goal 1

Obtain a speech sample that is as representative as possible of the client's speech in everyday use.

Assessment Goal 2

Obtain a sample of the client's speech under circumstances that are constant from one client to the next.

Assessment Goal 3

Generate, from obtained speech samples and incidental observations, quantitative and qualitative descriptions of the client's fluent and disfluent speech behaviors that can be related where applicable to vocal tract physiology, and that are communicable to other interested professionals.

Assessment Goal 4

Obtain information about variables that affect the client's fluency level and apply this to treatment planning.

Assessment Goal 5

Obtain information about a client's early social, physical, behavioral, and speech development, including information about variables that might be related to the origin of the disorder or its course of development, and apply this information to treatment planning.

Assessment Goal 6

Obtain information about variables that might influence clinical outcome and/or the prognosis for treatment and apply this to treatment planning.

Assessment Goal 7

Obtain information about other communicative problems or disorders that may or may not be related to fluency.

Assessment Goal 8

Generate descriptions of the results of assessment that are communicable to other professional and lay persons.

Processes for achieving the goals of assessment

Processes for achieving Assessment Goal 1 -- achieving a representative sample

1. Observation and recording of the client's speech during an interview with the clinician about the client's stuttering disorder.
2. Observation and recording of the client talking to a relative or friend prior to meeting with the

clinician.
3. Observation and recording of a child playing with parents after instructions to the parents to play with the child as they normally would at home (Family Play Session).
4. Tape recordings made by the client of conversations during daily activities at work, home, or anywhere.

Processes for achieving Assessment Goal 2 -- a speech sample from a constant setting

1. Observation and recording of the client's speech in response to being asked to describe a standard stimulus picture.
2. Observation and recording of the client's speech while reading a standard passage aloud.
3. Observation and recording of the client's speech while the client plays a "barrier game"[1] with the clinician, or, preferably, with a third party.
4. Observation and recording of the client's speech during a structured interview, in which the clinician asks the same question of each client by referring to an interview form.
5. Observation and recording of the client's speech while performing a specific speech task, such as describing a job or a favorite activity or a school subject.

Processes for achieving Assessment Goal 3 -- quantitative and qualitative description of the client's fluency level

1. Administering any of a variety of published tests of fluency, stuttering severity, attitudes toward stuttering and speech, self-efficacy as a speaker, situational fears, and avoidance behavior.
2. Administering any of a variety of systematic protocols for coding speech sample(s) so as to reflect

[1]In the barrier game, the client and another person sit opposite each other at a table. A barrier is erected across the table so that the two cannot see each other. The client has to direct the other person in the assembly of, for instance, a puzzle, piece of equipment or toy.

the categories of disfluency, and the extent of fluency or nonfluency, and the presence and type of secondary behaviors.
3. Transcribing a speech sample verbatim in such a way as to accurately reflect all fluent and nonfluent speech behavior.
4. Identifying and counting the frequency of primary and secondary stuttering behaviors.
5. Measuring the duration of discontinuous and continuous speech elements.
6. Measuring speech rate (syllables per second with pauses included) and articulatory rate (syllables per second with pauses excluded).
7. Observing and recording behavioral and/or physiological measurements of oral, laryngeal, and respiratory behavior so as to relate specifically identified stuttering behaviors to possible vocal tract events and to assess the capacity for fluent speech production.
8. Describing qualitatively any of the nonmeasurable aspects of fluency, such as apparent level of muscular tension, emotional reactivity to speech or stuttering behaviors, coping behaviors, nonverbal aspects of stuttering behavior, or anomalies of social interaction such as poor eye contact, generalized low muscle tonus, poor body posture.

Processes for achieving Assessment Goal 4 -- assessing variables that affect fluency

1. Developing and systematically testing hypotheses about variables that might affect fluency level, for example, talking slowly to a stuttering child to see if a measurable improvement in fluency can be obtained.
2. Interviewing the client or the client's family about social circumstances, words, listeners, sentence types, speech sounds, that improve or exacerbate fluency.
3. Playing videotapes or audiotapes of parent-child interactions to the parents of a child who presents

with a potential or actual fluency disorder.

4. Conducting a variety of brief trial treatment procedures, such as delayed auditory feedback, whispering, rate modification.

Processes for achieving Assessment Goal 5 -- getting and using a developmental history

1. Developing questionnaires or other written materials (e.g., fluency autobiography) designed to obtain potentially relevant background information.

2. Interviewing the client, the client's family, or others about developmental milestones of motor control, social-emotional behavior, speech and language, and cognitive level.

Processes for achieving Assessment Goal 6 -- getting and using prognostic information and information that will optimize treatment planning

1. Administering tests or reading reports of others who have administered formal tests of intelligence, attitudes, motivation, comprehension, ability to take direction, or other prognostic indicators.

2. Making informal tests and observations related to intelligence, attitudes, motivation, comprehension, ability to take direction, or other prognostic indicators.

Processes for achieving Assessment Goal 7 -- getting and using information about coexisting problems

1. Administering tests or reading reports of others who have administered formal tests of language, voice, articulation, psycho-emotional function, learning disability, cognitive level, or auditory or visual deficits and using this information to plan for treatment and to provide prognostic information.

2. Making informal observations of language, voice, articulation, psycho-emotional function, learning disability, cognitive level, or auditory or visual deficits, and using this information to plan for treat-

ment and to provide prognostic information.

Processes for achieving Assessment Goal 8 -- communicating the results of assessment

1. Writing reports of assessment processes designed to be read by physicians, psychologists, and other non-speech-language pathology professionals.

2. Writing comprehensive reports of assessment processes designed to be read by the current or subsequent clinicians.

3. Reporting the results of assessment processes, formally or informally, to the client and/or the client's family/significant others.

Clinician competencies related to assessment [2]

1. Can differentiate between a child's normally disfluent speech, language-based disfluency, the speech of a child at risk for stuttering, and the speech of a child who has already begun to stutter.

2. Can distinguish cluttered from stuttered speech and understands the potential relationship between these two disorders.

3. Can relate the findings of language, articulation, voice, and hearing tests to the development of stuttering.

4. Can obtain a thorough case history from an adult client or the family of a child client.

5. Can obtain a useful speech sample and evaluate it for stuttering severity both informally by subjective impression and formally by calculating relevant measures such as the frequency of disfluency, duration of disfluency, speaking rate.

6. Is familiar with the available diagnostic tests for stuttering that serve to objectify aspects of the client's communication pattern (secondary features, avoidance patterns, attitudes, etc.) that may

---

[2]This list of competencies is an expanded and revised version of a list prepared originally by the Texas Speech and Hearing Association Fluency Task Force.

---

not be readily observed.

7. Is able to identify, and measure where feasible, environmental variables (i.e., aspects, such as time pressure, emotional reactions, interruptions, nonverbal behavior, demand speech, or the speech of significant others) that may be related to the onset, development, and maintenance of stuttering and to fluctuations in the severity of stuttering.

8. Can identify disfluencies by type (prolongation, repetition, etc.) and, in addition, can describe qualitatively the fluency of a person's speech.

9. Can relate, to the extent possible, what stuttered speech sounds like to the vocal tract behavior that is producing it (for example, recognizing the subtle acoustic cues that signal vocal straining).

10. Can, in appropriate consultation with the client or parents, construct a treatment program, based on the results of comprehensive testing, on the client's personal emotional and attitudinal development, and on past treatment history, that fits the unique needs of each client's disorder(s).

11. Can administer predetermined programs in a diagnostic way so that decisions with regard to branching and repeating of parts of the program reflect the unique needs of each client's disorder(s).

12. Can explain clearly to clients or their families/significant others what treatment options, including the various types of speech treatment, medication, devices, self-help groups, and other forms of treatment are available, why they may or may not be appropriate to a specific case, and what outcomes can be expected from each, based on knowledge of the available literature.

B. Management

Desirable goals in the management of fluency disorders

Management Goal 1

Reduce the frequency with which stuttering behaviors occur without increasing the use of other behaviors that are not a part of normal speech production.

Management Goal 2

Reduce the severity, duration, and abnormality of stuttering behaviors until they are or resemble normal speech discontinuities.

Management Goal 3

Reduce the use of defensive behaviors.[3]

Note that when clients use avoidance behaviors that are successful (in that they avoid stuttering behavior) they will appear to have made progress toward Management Goal 1, but in fact will have done so by including some additional, and abnormal, behavior. For example, clients who are able to change words so as to avoid saying a word that they will stutter on will have a reduced frequency of stuttering behavior, but they will also have an increased frequency of cognitive behaviors involved in the search for and retrieval of substitute words.

Management Goal 4

Remove or reduce processes serving to create, exacerbate, or maintain stuttering behaviors.

In children, this might entail modification of the child's parents' behavior so as to reduce maladaptive reactions to the child's stuttering behavior. In adults it might include teaching the client how to change his or her listeners' behavior. In some cases, there may be reinforcement for stuttering, such as excuses for failure, or getting attention that is otherwise not forthcoming. In other cases, denial may prevent an adult from perceiving the extent to which stuttering affects his or her life.

---

[3]Defensive behaviors are behaviors performed so as to prevent, avoid, escape from, or minimize aversive events, real or imagined (Bandura, 1969). A somewhat broader category than avoidance behaviors, defensive behaviors include also struggled stuttering behavior, trying to force a word or sound out, rushing through a phrase so as to "get past" the stuttering.

Management Goal 5

Help the person who stutters make treatment (e.g., adaptive) decisions about how to handle speech and social situations in everyday living.

This includes such things as helping the client learn how to respond to people who try to talk for him or her, or helping the client learn not to use behaviors that avoid, rather than confront, specific social situations such as using the telephone, ordering in a restaurant, or helping the client learn that changing words costs something in personal self-esteem. This also includes teaching the client how to politely influence listeners' behavior so that the client's fluency can be improved.

Management Goal 6

Increase the frequency of social activity and speaking.

Clients who have adopted reticence as a strategy to deal with stuttering will need help in regaining a normal amount of social speech.

Management Goal 7

Reduce attitudes, beliefs, and thought processes that interfere with fluent speech production or that hinder the achievement of other treatment goals.

In some adults this might involve modifying their attitude toward very brief stuttering behaviors so as to prevent stuttering from returning at a later date. Similarly, certain attitudes toward fluency and disfluency, or beliefs about these attitudes, can maintain stuttering behaviors, for example, perfectionist fluency, abhorrence of normal disfluency, rigidity in speech behavior. Some clients may have attitudes toward themselves that serve to exacerbate or maintain stuttering behaviors, for example, low self-esteem, lack of confidence, or feelings of worthlessness.

Management Goal 8

Reduce emotional reactions to

specific stimuli when these have a negative impact on stuttering behavior or on attempts to modify stuttering behavior.

For example, fear of specific social situations, word fears, a sense of intimidation by specific categories of listeners, a sense of helplessness or fear of specific speech tasks, such as answering the telephone or asking questions in class, or a fear of the embarrassment of stuttering in public. This should not be confused with the reduction of defensive behavior, which is one kind of reaction to these fears. Both fear reduction and defensive behavior reduction can be appropriate.

Management Goal 9

Where necessary, seek helpful combinations and sequences of treatments, including referral, for problems other than stuttering that may accompany the fluency disorder, such as, cluttering, learning disability, language/phonological disorder, voice disorder, psycho-emotional disturbance.

Management Goal 10

Provide information and guidance to clients, families, and other significant persons about the nature of stuttering, normal fluency and disfluency, and the course of treatment and prognosis for recovery.

In addition, help clients and families/significant others understand the nature of past treatment and the availability and possible utility of other options, including other forms of treatment, devices, and self-help groups.

Processes for achieving the goals of management

It is not the intention of this document to assert that all processes should be used with all clients. A process for reducing excitement is useful only with a client whose fluency is adversely influenced by excitement. For each client, clinicians choose a set of appropriate goals, based on a careful evaluation of the client. Having established what are appropriate goals for a client, a selection of processes to achieve these goals is made. At times during treatment, both goals and processes should be re-evaluated, and after treatment, it is likewise appropriate to review the selection of goals and processes and evaluate them with regard to the outcome of treatment.

Note that processes are not exactly the same as techniques. There might be several techniques for engaging in a particular process. For example, one process mentioned below is "Identify reinforcers for stuttering." A clinician could engage in this process by interviewing clients and asking what happens after they stutter, or spend some time with clients, observing them in real speaking situations, or interview people who know the clients well, such as parents, siblings, or partners. Each of these techniques would or could result in the identification of reinforcers that are contingent on stuttering behavior.

Note that referral and consultation are processes that may be used to achieve goals.

Processes for achieving Management Goal 1–Reducing the frequency of stuttering behaviors

1. Fluency-shaping approach:
   a. Slowed rate of speech movements.
      • typically taught in stages of speed (e.g., Rate I, Rate II, and Slow-Normal Rate)
   b. Easy onset of voicing.
      • slow inhalation
      • soft but true voice changing to full voice before vowel initiation
      • practice in order to shorten the time taken up by the onset of voicing period
   c. Blending, or continuous voicing.
   d. Light articulatory contacts.
   e. Smooth, slow speech movements.
   f. Use of computer-assisted feedback to train clients in fluency -- producing coordinated speech production movements.
2. Vocal control treatment approach.
   a. Better vocal tone, breath support,

full resonance, efficient and relaxed voice, adequate loudness.
   b. Typically accompanied by systematic desensitization.
3. Contingency management:
   a. Combined reinforcement for fluent speech and mild, nonaversive punishment for stuttering behaviors.
   b. Successive approximation (shaping) toward fluent speech.
   c. Practice in a systematically sequenced series of steps from where fluent speech is easiest to achieve toward where fluency is more difficult to achieve, for example, through gradually increasing the length and complexity of an utterance, or through a hierarchy of feared social situations.
   d. Use of fluency-enhancement, in the clinic, or via a wearable device, may be a useful way to establish the behavior in the first place.
   e. Use of computer-assisted devices to ensure rapid and consistent feedback.
   f. Systematically administered reinforcement for more natural-sounding speech.
4. Reduction of speech-associated anxiety:
   a. Systematic desensitization to social situations.
   b. Desensitization to the experience of stuttering (confrontation).
   c. Pseudostuttering (voluntary stuttering, or faking).
   d. With children, through counseling parents, reduction or removal of as many anxiety-producing events as possible.
5. Reduction of speech-associated excitement:
   a. With children, through counseling parents, reduction of as many exciting events as practical and reasonable.
6. In prevention, training parents to speak more slowly but with normal intonation, timing, and stress patterns.
7. In prevention, training parents to talk less often, and with simpler language, to interrupt less often, and to ask fewer questions requir-

ing long complex answers.

Processes for achieving Management Goal 2–reducing the abnormality, severity, or duration of stuttering behaviors

1. Disfluency shaping:
   a. Help the client learn ways to be disfluent in a more normal way.
   b. Remove, through modeling and practice, one behavior at a time until disfluencies are normal in type.
2. Muscle tension reduction:
   a. Reduction of oral and vocal muscular tension during speech.
      • slowed rate and rate control
      • direct suggestion to reduce muscle tension in specific parts of the vocal tract
      • referrals for the possible use of medication to achieve muscle relaxation
      • attitude modification via techniques described below
3. Repair treatment:
   a. Teach client the various types of speech sounds and how they are fluently produced.
   b. Teach client the types of stuttering behaviors used by client.
   c. Teach client types of repairs -- ways of changing from the stuttered to the nonstuttered type of production.
   d. Practice repairs in different environments.
   e. Work on one or two specific sounds or sound category at a time.
4. Stuttering modification sequence:
   a. Post-block modification, or cancellation.
   b. In-block modification, or pull-out.
   c. Pre-block modification, or preparatory set.
5. Counterconditioning techniques:
   a. Associating stuttering with pleasant events, for example, "reinforcement" for stuttering, or tag game.
   b. Voluntary stuttering.
6. Confrontational (nonavoidance) techniques:
   a. Discussion with the client of specific behaviors, the circumstances under which they occurred, and

the variables that may have influenced them.

b. Listening to or watching with clients audio or videotapes of themselves while speaking and discussing specific behaviors and reactions with them.

Processes for achieving Management Goal 3–reducing defensive behaviors

1. Extinction of defensive behavior:
   a. For secondary (avoidance) behavior:
      - direct instructions to stop performing the secondary behavior, accompanied by an alternative to stuttering behavior, for example, in-block modification (pull-outs), or slowed speech, or monitored vocalization
      - punishment (time-out, response cost or other nonaversive punishment only) accompanied by an alternative to stuttering behavior
   b. For primary (escape) behavior, that is, struggled disfluency:
      - stuttering modification sequence of post-block, in-block, pre-block modification
      - modeling stuttering that is easy and free of struggle, then reinforcing the client for disfluency that is less struggled
      - direct suggestions, accompanied by cuing and reminders
      - discussions about the client's stuttering pattern, approaching feared situations, to toughen attitudes toward stuttering
2. In prevention, training parents in the relaxed production of occasional disfluencies that are normal for their child's age.

Processes for achieving Management Goal 4–removing processes that may be maintaining stuttering behaviors

1. Instrumental (operant) conditioning:
   a. Identify reinforcers for stuttering.
   b. Remove conditions in the environment, including in the client's "internal environment" that are reinforcing stuttering or defensive behavior.
2. Defensive counterconditioning:
   a. Identify aversive consequences

for stuttering.
   b. Identify stimuli, or constellations of stimuli (situations) associated with or predictive of aversive consequences, as in a hierarchy of speech situations.
   c. Identify behaviors that terminate or avoid the aversive consequences.
   d. Provide experiences for the client in which the conditioned stimuli occur, but the avoidance behaviors are NOT performed and no aversive consequences follow.
   e. Help client learn how to handle pressure situations while still using newly learned fluency skills.
3. Vicarious conditioning:
   a. Identify speech models who are reinforced for stuttering, or who avoid stuttering or try to avoid stuttering (i.e., use defensive behavior), or who demonstrate negative emotional reactions to disfluency.
   b. Counsel, train, or modify the behavior of these models so as to remove or reduce the occurrence of vicarious conditioning.
4. Environmental manipulation:
   a. Alter the client's environment, external or internal, so as to remove any conditioning process that is exacerbating or maintaining stuttering behavior:
      - by counseling significant others
      - by counseling the client
      - by providing for experiences that will alter attitudes or beliefs that result in deleterious conditioning processes.

Processes for achieving Management Goal 5–helping clients learn how to make decisions about everyday speaking situations

1. Identification of specific decisions about social behavior that may affect fluency, for example, deciding to let a colleague answer the phone even though the client is closer to it.
2. Counseling, including sensitive explanations about how decisions based on defensive reactions serve to increase fear and decrease self-confidence.
3. Identify, with the client's help,

attainable behavioral goals for more effective decision-making.
4. Plan activities that will provide opportunities for the client to make better decisions.
5. Reinforce client for making decisions that are more conducive to speaking fluently and with confidence.
6. Help clients foresee the natural consequences of their decisions to use or not use learned treatment techniques in day-to-day activities.
7. Attendance in a support group with other people who stutter.

Processes for achieving Management Goal 6–increasing social activity and speaking behavior

1. Provide reinforcement for entering speech situations previously feared.
2. Encouragement and reinforcement for talking more often and in and in a wider variety of situations, structured hierarchically from least to most stressful or intimidating.
3. Encourage client to participate in a self-help group.
4. Use of a fluency-enhancing device to make possible social activity that would otherwise be too intimidating for the client.

Processes for achieving Management Goal 7–improving self esteem or revising a perfectionist attitude toward speech

1. Counsel the client so as to provide for successful experiences of any kind.
2. Counsel the client so as to provide for successful speech experiences.

3. Validation of the client as a person and speaker:
   a. Listen to the client and demonstrate appreciation of the client as a person.
   b. Listen to the client and validate aspects of speech that are unrelated to fluency, through expressed appreciation for aspects of the client's speech that are normal or superior, e.g., voice quality, expressiveness, word choice, articulation.
   c. Listen to the client and validate fluency, where appropriate, by

expressed appreciation for stuttering behaviors that are less struggled or less abnormal.

d. Transfer similar listening skills to client (self-listening).

4. Provide for increased attention from significant others.

5. Help client attain better identification of self through support group or other activities.

6. Provide for increased tolerance of failings through counseling, modeling.

7. Positive self-talk and affirmation training.

Processes for achieving Management Goal 8–reducing negative reactions to stuttering and social situations that have included stuttering in the past

1. Confrontational desensitization to stuttering events:

   a. Talk about stuttering with the client in an objective way.

   b. Have clients learn, through self-demonstration, that speech improves when they "give permission to stutter" or stutter on purpose.

   c. Stuttering on purpose in the clinical setting.

   d. Stuttering on purpose in real situations.

   e. Keep a record of situations in which clients have stuttered on purpose or allowed themselves to stutter.

2. Desensitization to anxiety-provoking speech situations:

   a. Traditional systematic desensitization:

   • constructing a hierarchy of feared words, listeners, and situations

   • inducing a physically and emotionally relaxed state

   • imagining feared situations while in a relaxed state

   • imagining oneself talking to feared listeners while in a relaxed state

   • imagining oneself producing feared words while in a relaxed state

   • imagining oneself stuttering while in a relaxed state

   • testing the effects of these experiences in real situations

b. in vivo systematic desensitization:

   • .....feared words, listeners, and situations

   • systematically talking in real life situations, starting with the easiest elements in the hierarchy, and gradually increasing the level of difficulty. A fluency-enhancing device may provide a place to begin this process, although it will be important to wean the client from the device so as not to create a dependency on it.

Processes for achieving Management Goal 9–dealing with coexisting problems:

1. Referral to other professionals with regard to psycho-emotional or learning disability problems.

2. Team treatment with other speech-language pathologists so as to work simultaneously on language, phonological, or voice problems.

3. Sequencing treatment so as to deal with one problem at a time. Usually this means postponing work on language, voice, or articulation until fluency is under control, but sometimes it means postponing work on fluency until some progress is made on the other disorder, for example, improved intelligibility.

4. Designing treatment plans that deal simultaneously with stuttering and coexisting problems.

Processes for achieving Management Goal 10–providing information to significant others:

1. Direct counseling of parents, spouses, siblings, and others.

2. Bibliotherapy for parents, spouses, physicians, psychologists, and others.

3. Use of audio and videotape to present to clients and the parents of clients examples of specific behaviors and reactions.

4. Provide information about other treatment approaches, treatment devices, self-help and consumer advocate groups.

5. Provide information about third-party payment options.

Clinic competencies related to management

1. Is familiar with the appropriate goals of treatment and the processes for achieving them and can engage these processes, choosing techniques that are best for the client, and administer them with an attitude that balances the goal of normal speech with a tolerance for abnormal speech.

2. Has flexibility in choosing and changing the level of difficulty of tasks based on fluency level of the client.

3. Can teach clients to produce vocal tract behaviors that result in normal sounding speech production.

4. Has sufficient counseling skills so as to interact with clients of all ages and develop a reasonable set of expectations in the client.

5. Has a thorough understanding of, and knows how to put into practice, the principles of conditioning and learning so as to achieve a successful and appropriate modification of speech behavior.

6. Understands the relations between stuttering and other related disorders of fluency, such as cluttering, neurogenic and psychogenic stuttering, as well as disorders of language, articulation, learning, and so on, and can with flexibility identify sequences and combinations of treatment options that are helpful to the client.

7. Understands the dimensions of normal fluency and the relation of normal fluency to speech situations and is able to work toward normal speech, with an awareness of the compromises among effort, fluency, and natural-sounding communication.

8. Understands that some stuttering behaviors may be reactions to other stuttering behaviors and knows how to plan treatment to account for this.

9. Can evaluate available treatment programs with regard to treatment application for a wide variety of clients.

10. Is able to decide, based on objective progress, motivational level, and cost in time and money when

it is appropriate to terminate treatment.

11. Is aware of the continuous nature of fluency and can identify subtle changes in speech or other behaviors related to treatment change and explain their importance to the client.

12. Can explain stuttering and treatment for stuttering to lay persons, such as day care workers, teachers, baby sitters, grandparents, and others who may influence the life of children who stutter.

13. Knows how to develop a plan for assessing objectively the efficacy of treatment in an ongoing way.

14. Can recognize problems that are treated by professionals other than speech-language pathologists and can guide a client to acceptance of an appropriate referral.

C. Transfer and Maintenance

Desirable goals in the transfer and maintenance of acquired fluency behaviors

Transfer and Maintenance Goal 1
Generalization of the behavioral changes learned in the treatment setting to speech situations in the client's everyday life.

Transfer and Maintenance Goal 2
A sense of committed interest and self-reliance on the part of clients in managing their own speech behavior, balanced against an awareness of the need for occasional help (professional or otherwise) as needed.

Transfer and Maintenance Goal 3
Ability on the client's part at recognizing the earliest signs of returning emotional reactions and/or stuttering behaviors and knowledge and skill for dealing with these occurrences.

Transfer and Maintenance Goal 4
In parents, knowledge and skills needed to facilitate their child's further development of fluency.

Processes for achieving transfer and maintenance goals

Processes for achieving Transfer and Maintenance Goal 1 -- **generalization of behavior to external settings.**

1. Variation of speech use within the treatment setting.
2. Role-playing of social interactions while using new behaviors.
3. Hierarchically structured practice in the client's everyday life, monitored by the clinician via tape recordings and/or interviews.
4. Continued practice in the treatment setting.
5. Use of self-help and support groups.

Process for achieving Transfer and Maintenance Goal 2 -- **self-reliance and commitment.**

1. Counseling clients to assist themselves in taking over the process of decision making in treatment.
2. Providing exercises for the client designed to increase skills at self-evaluation and self-treatment planning.
3. Gradually reducing the clinician's input in making decisions about treatment.
4. Gradually decreasing the frequency of contact between clinician and client.
5. Use of self-help and support groups.

Processes for achieving Transfer and Maintenance Goal 3 -- **self-monitored maintenance.**

1. Practice at self-listening and identification of stuttering behaviors, even brief or barely noticeable ones.
2. Counseling and training in the modification of brief and barely noticeable stuttering behaviors.
3. Counseling and training at recognizing changes in client's attitude, specifically increasing tendency to avoid speech situations and/or stuttering.
4. Use of self-help and support groups.

Processes for achieving Transfer and Maintenance Goal 4 -- **parent facilitation of child's fluency development**

1. Counseling and training families in recognition of subtle signs of returning struggle.
2. Desensitization and empowerment of parents so as to reduce anxious reactions to signs of returning struggle behavior.
3. Training parents and other family members in skills useful in providing a fluency-enhancing atmosphere.
4. Use of family support groups.

Clinician competencies related to transfer and maintenance

1. Is aware of the principles of stimulus generalization and response transfer.
2. Has knowledge of, and can implement a variety of procedures to achieve transfer and maintenance of behavior changes achieved in the clinical setting.
3. Can, through guidance and counseling, help clients develop an attitude toward maintenance that includes an understanding of their own responsibility for their speech yet permits occasional booster session (e.g., the dental model) and that tolerates failure yet appreciates success.
4. Can help the client develop an awareness of the subtler forms of (returning) abnormality and know how to deal with them in a variety of ways, such as the use of home practice, graded hierarchical practice in social situations, and support groups.
5. Knows how to counsel parents regarding changes they can make at home that will facilitate their child's fluency development or encourage the generalization of gains made in treatment.

Appendix A
Reprinted Publications

◆ ◆ ◆ ◆ ◆ ◆ ◆ ◆ ◆ ◆ ◆ ◆ ◆ ◆ ◆ ◆ ◆ ◆ ◆

Appendix A.1
Clinical Supervision in Speech–Language Pathology and Audiology

Appendix A.2
Code of Ethics

Appendix A.3
Guidelines for Practice in Stuttering Treatment

Appendix A.4
Scope of Practice in Speech–Language Pathology

AMERICAN
SPEECH-LANGUAGE-
HEARING
ASSOCIATION

Scope of Practice in Speech-Language Pathology

*Ad Hoc Committee on Scope of Practice
in Speech-Language Pathology*

This scope of practice in speech-language pathology statement is an official policy of the American Speech-Language-Hearing Association (ASHA). It was developed by the Ad Hoc Committee on Scope of Practice in Speech-Language Pathology: Sarah W. Blackstone, chair; Diane Paul-Brown, ex officio; David A. Brandt; Rhonda Friedlander; Luis F. Riquelme; and Mark Ylvisaker. Crystal S. Cooper, vice president for professional practices in speech-language pathology, served as monitoring vice-president. The contributions of the editor, Jude Langsam, and select and widespread peer reviewers are gratefully acknowledged. This statement supersedes the Scope of Practice, Speech-Language Pathology and Audiology statement (LC 6-89), Asha, April 1990, 1-2.

Scope of Practice in Speech-Language Pathology

Preamble

The purpose of this statement is to define the scope of practice of speech-language pathology in order to:

(1) delineate areas of services and supports provided by ASHA members and certificate holders in accordance with the ASHA Code of Ethics. Services refer to clinical services for individuals with speech, voice, language, communication, and swallowing disorders, aimed at the amelioration of difficulties stemming from such disorders. Supports refer to environmental modifications, assistive technology, and guidance for communication partners to help persons with these disorders;

Index terms: Scope, speech-language pathology; scope of practice, speech-language pathology; practice guidelines, speech-language pathology; standards of practice, speech-language pathology

(2) educate health care, education, and other professionals, consumers, payers, regulators, and members of the general public about treatment and other services and supports offered by speech-language pathologists as qualified providers;

(3) assist members and certificate holders in their efforts to provide appropriate and high quality speech-language pathology services and supports to persons across the life span with speech, voice, language, communication, and swallowing disabilities;

(4) establish a reference for curriculum review of education programs in speech-language pathology.

The scope of practice defined here and the areas specifically set forth are part of an effort to describe the broad range of services and supports offered within the profession. It is recognized, however, that levels of experience, skill, and proficiency with respect to the activities identified within this scope of practice vary among the individual providers. It may not be possible for speech-language pathologists to practice in all areas of the field. As the ASHA Code of Ethics specifies, individuals may only practice in areas where they are competent based on their education, training, and experience (American Speech-Language-Hearing Association, 1994). However, nothing limits speech-language pathologists from expanding their current level of expertise. Certain clients or practice settings may necessitate that speech-language pathologists pursue additional education or training to expand their personal scope of practice.

This scope of practice statement does not supersede existing state licensure laws or affect the interpretation or implementation of such laws. It may serve, however, as a model for the development or modification of licensure laws.

The schema in Figure 1 depicts the relationship of the scope of practice to ASHA's policy documents of the Association that address current and emerging speech-language pathology practice areas; that is, preferred practice patterns, guidelines, and position statements.

Finally, it is recognized that speech-language pathology is a dynamic and continuously developing practice area. Listing specific areas within this scope of practice does not necessarily exclude other, new, or emerging areas. Indeed, changes in service delivery systems, the increasing numbers of persons who need communication services, and technological and scientific advances have mandated that a scope of practice for the profession of speech-language pathology be a dynamic statement. For these reasons this document will undergo periodic review and possible revision.

Statement

The goal of the profession of speech-language pathology and its members is provision of the highest quality treatment and other services consistent with the fundamental right of those served to participate in decisions that affect their lives.

Speech-language pathologists hold the master's or doctoral degree, the Certificate of Clinical Competence of the American Speech-Language-Hearing Association, and state licensure where applicable.

These professionals serve individuals, families, groups, and the general public through their involvement in a broad range of professional activities. They work to prevent speech, voice, language, communication, swallowing, and related disabilities. They screen, identify, assess, diagnose, refer, and provide treatment and intervention, including consultation and follow-up services, to persons of all ages with, or at risk for, speech, voice, language, communication, swallowing, and related disabilities. They counsel individuals with these disorders, as well as their families, caregivers, and other service providers, related to the disorders and their management. Speech-language pathologists select, prescribe, dispense, and provide services supporting the effective use of augmentative and alternative communication devices and other communication prostheses and assistive devices.

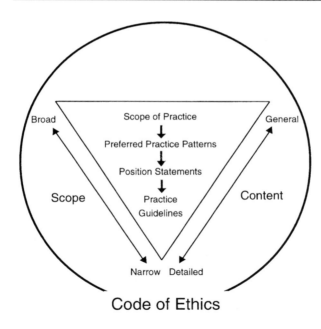

Figure 1. Conceptual Framework of ASHA Policy Statements

Speech-language pathologists are autonomous professionals who identify, assess, diagnose, prevent, and treat speech, voice, language, communication, and swallowing disorders.

The documents depicted in this diagram together serve as a guide to professional practice in speech-language pathology.

Speech-language pathologists also teach, supervise, and manage clinical and educational programs, and engage in program development, program oversight, and research activities related to communication sciences and disorders, swallowing, and related areas.

They measure treatment outcomes, evaluate the effectiveness of their practices, modify services in relation to their evaluations, and disseminate these findings. They also serve as case managers and expert witnesses. As an integral part of their practice, speech-language pathologists work to increase public awareness and advocate for the people they serve.

Speech-language pathologists provide services in settings that are deemed appropriate, including but not limited to health care, educational, community, vocational, and home settings. Speech-language pathologists serve diverse populations. The client population includes persons of different race, age, gender, religion, national origin, and sexual orientation. Speech-language pathologists' caseloads include persons from diverse ethnic, cultural, or linguistic backgrounds, and persons with disabilities. Although speech-language pathologists are prohibited from discriminating in the provision of professional services based on these factors, in some cases such factors may be relevant to the development of an appropriate treatment plan. These factors may be considered in treatment plans only when firmly grounded in scientific and professional knowledge.

As primary care providers of communication treatment and other services, speech-language pathologists are autonomous professionals; that is, their services need not be prescribed by another. However, in most cases individuals are best served when speech-language pathologists work collaboratively with other professionals, individuals with disabilities, and their family members. Similarly, it is recognized that related fields and professions may have some knowledge, skills, and experience that could be applied to some areas within this scope of practice. Defining the scope of practice of speech-language pathologists is not meant to exclude members of other professions or related fields from rendering services in common practice areas.

The practice of speech-language pathology includes:

(1) Providing screening, identification, assessment, diagnosis, treatment, intervention (i.e., prevention, restoration, amelioration, compensation) and follow-up services for disorders of:

• speech: articulation, fluency, voice (including respiration, phonation, and resonance)

• language (involving the parameters of phonology, morphology, syntax, semantics, and pragmatics; and including disorders of receptive and expressive communication in oral, written, graphic, and manual modalities)

• oral, pharyngeal, cervical esophageal, and related functions (e.g., dysphagia, including disorders of swallowing and oral function for feeding; orofacial myofunctional disorders)

• cognitive aspects of communication (including communication disability and other functional disabilities associated with cognitive impairment)

• social aspects of communication (including challenging behavior, ineffective social skills, lack of communication opportunities);

(2) Providing consultation and counseling, and making referrals when appropriate;

(3) Training and supporting family members and other communication partners of individuals with speech, voice, language, communication, and swallowing disabilities;

(4) Developing and establishing effective augmentative and alternative communication techniques and strategies, including selecting, prescribing, and dispensing of aids and devices and training individuals, their families, and other communication partners in their use;

(5) Selecting, fitting, and establishing effective use of appropriate prosthetic/adaptive devices for speaking and swallowing (e.g., tracheoesophageal valves, electrolarynges, speaking valves);

(6) Using instrumental technology to diagnose and treat disorders of communication and swallowing (e.g., videofluoroscopy, nasendoscopy, ultrasonography, stroboscopy);

(7) Providing aural rehabilitation and related counseling services to individuals with hearing loss and to their families;

(8) Collaborating in the assessment of central auditory processing disorders in cases in which there is evidence of speech, language, and/or other cognitive-communication disorders; providing intervention for individuals with central auditory processing disorders.

(9) Conducting pure-tone air conduction hearing screening and screening tympanometry for the purpose of the initial identification and/or referral of individuals with other communication disorders or possible middle ear pathology.

(10) Enhancing speech and language proficiency and communication effectiveness, including but not

limited to accent reduction, collaboration with teachers of English as a second language, and improvement of voice, performance, and singing;

(11) Training and supervising support personnel;

(12) Developing and managing academic and clinical programs in communication sciences and disorders;

(13) Conducting, disseminating, and applying research in communication sciences and disorders;

(14) Measuring outcomes of treatment and conducting continuous evaluation of the effectiveness of practices and programs to improve and maintain quality of services.

Refer to the Reference List for the most recent ASHA documents on these topics.

Reference List

General

American Speech-Language-Hearing Association. (1993). Definition of communication disorders and variations. *Asha, 35* (Suppl. 10), 40-41.

American Speech-Language-Hearing Association. (1993). Preferred practice patterns for the professions of speech-language pathology and audiology. *Asha, 35* (Suppl. 11), 1-100.

American Speech-Language-Hearing Association. (1994). Code of ethics. *Asha, 36* (Suppl. 13), 1-2.

Speech: Articulation, Fluency, Voice

American Speech-Language-Hearing Association. (1992). Position statement and guidelines for evaluation and treatment for tracheoesophageal fistulization/puncture. *Asha, 34* (Suppl. 7), 17-21.

American Speech-Language-Hearing Association. (1992). Position statement and guidelines for vocal tract visualization and imaging. *Asha, 34* (Suppl. 7), 31-40.

American Speech-Language-Hearing Association. (1993). Position statement and guidelines for oral and oropharyngeal prostheses. *Asha, 35* (Suppl. 10), 14-16.

American Speech-Language-Hearing Association. (1993). Position statement and guidelines on the use of voice prostheses in tracheotomized persons with or without ventilatory dependence. *Asha, 35* (Suppl. 10), 17-20.

American Speech-Language-Hearing Association. (1995, March). Guidelines for practice in stuttering treatment. *Asha, 37* (Suppl. 14), 26-35.

Language

American Speech-Language-Hearing Association. (1975). Meeting the needs of children and adults with disorders of language: the role of the speech-language pathologist and audiologist. *Asha, 17* (4), 273-277.

American Speech-Language-Hearing Association. (1982). Definition of language. *Asha, 24* (6), 44.

American Speech-Language-Hearing Association. (1982). Position statement on language learning disorders. *Asha, 24* (11), 937-944.

American Speech-Language-Hearing Association. (1989). Issues in determining eligibility for language intervention. *Asha, 31* (3), 113-118.

American Speech-Language-Hearing Association. (1991). Guidelines for speech-language pathologists serving persons with language, socio-communicative and/or cognitive-communicative impairments. *Asha, 33* (Suppl. 5), 21-28.

American Speech-Language-Hearing Association Task Force on Central Auditory Processing Consensus Development. (1995). *Central auditory processing: Current status of research and implications for clinical practice.* Rockville, MD: ASHA.

Oral, Pharyngeal, Cervical Esophageal, and Related Functions

American Speech-Language-Hearing Association. (1987). Ad hoc committee on dysphagia report. *Asha, 29* (4), 57-58.

American Speech-Language-Hearing Association. (1989). Report: Ad hoc committee on labial-lingual posturing function. *Asha, 31* (11), 92-94.

American Speech-Language-Hearing Association. (1990). Knowledge and skills needed by speech-language pathologists providing services to dysphagic patients/clients. *Asha, 32* (Suppl. 2), 7-12.

American Speech-Language-Hearing Association. (1991). The role of the speech-language pathologist in assessment and management of oral myofunctional disorders. *Asha, 33* (Suppl. 5), 7.

American Speech-Language-Hearing Association. (1992). Position statement and guidelines for instrumental diagnostic procedures for swallowing, *Asha, 34* (Suppl. 7), 25-33.

American Speech-Language-Hearing Association. (1993). Orofacial myofunctional disorders: knowledge and skills. *Asha, 35* (Suppl. 10), 21-23.

Cognitive Aspects of Communication

American Speech-Language-Hearing Association. (1982). Serving the communicatively handicapped mentally retarded individual. *Asha, 24* (8), 547-553.

American Speech-Language-Hearing Association. (1987). The role of speech-language pathologists in the habilitation and rehabilitation of cognitively impaired individuals. *Asha, 29* (6), 53-55.

American Speech-Language-Hearing Association. (1988). The role of speech-language pathologists in the identification, diagnosis, and treatment of individuals with cognitive-communicative impairments. *Asha, 30* (3), 79.

American Speech-Language-Hearing Association. (1989). Report: Interdisciplinary approaches to brain damage. *Asha, 31* (10), 238-239.

American Speech-Language-Hearing Association. (1990). Interdisciplinary approaches to brain damage. *Asha, 32* (Suppl. 2), 3.

American Speech-Language-Hearing Association. (1991). Guidelines for speech-language pathologists serving persons with language, socio-communicative and/or cognitive-communicative impairments. *Asha, 33* (Suppl. 5), 21-28.

American Speech-Language-Hearing Association (1995). Guidelines for the structure and function of an interdisciplinary team for persons with brain injury. *Asha, 37* (Suppl. 14), 23.

Social Aspects of Communication

American Speech-Language-Hearing Association. (1990). Interdisciplinary approaches to brain damage. *Asha, 32* (Suppl. 2), 3.

American Speech-Language-Hearing Association. (1991). Guidelines for speech-language pathologists serving persons with language, socio-communicative and/or cognitive-communicative impairments. *Asha, 33* (Suppl. 5), 21-28.

Augmentative and Alternative Communication

American Speech-Language-Hearing Association. (1989). Competencies for speech-language pathologists providing services in augmentative communication. *Asha, 31* (3), 107-110.

American Speech-Language-Hearing Association. (1991). Augmentative and alternative communication. *Asha, 33* (Suppl. 5), 8.

American Speech-Language-Hearing Association. (1991). Report: Augmentative and alternative communication. *Asha, 33* (Suppl. 5), 9-12.

(See also prosthetic/adaptive devices)

Prosthetic/Adaptive Devices

American Speech-Language-Hearing Association. (1992). Position statement and guidelines for evaluation and treatment for tracheoesophageal fistulization/puncture. *Asha, 34* (Suppl. 7), 17-21.

American Speech-Language-Hearing Association. (1992). Position statement and guidelines for vocal tract visualization and imaging. *Asha, 34* (Suppl. 7), 31-40.

American Speech-Language-Hearing Association. (1993). Position statement and guidelines for oral and oropharyngeal prostheses. *Asha, 35* (Suppl. 10), 14-16.

American Speech-Language-Hearing Association. (1993). Position statement and guidelines on the use of voice prostheses in tracheotomized persons with or without ventilatory dependence. *Asha, 35* (Suppl. 10), 17-20.

(See also augmentative and alternative communication)

Instrumental Technology

American Speech-Language-Hearing Association. (1992). Position statement and guidelines for instrumental diagnostic procedures for swallowing. *Asha, 34* (Suppl. 7), 25-30.

American Speech-Language-Hearing Association. (1992). Position statement and guidelines for vocal tract visualization and imaging. *Asha, 34* (Suppl. 7), 31-40.

Aural Rehabilitation

American Speech-Language-Hearing Association. (1984). Competencies for aural rehabilitation. *Asha, 26* (5), 37-41.

American Speech-Language-Hearing Association. (1990). Aural rehabilitation: an annotated bibliography. *Asha, 32* (Suppl. 1), 1-12.

Hearing Screening

American National Standards Institute. (1989). *Specifications for audiometers* (ANSI S3.6.-1989). New York: Acoustical Society of America.

American Speech-Language-Hearing Association. (1990). Guidelines for screening for hearing impairments and middle-ear disorders. *Asha, 32* (Suppl. 2), 17-24.

American Speech-Language-Hearing Association. (1991). Issues in ethics: clinical practice by certificate holders in the profession in which they are not certified. *Asha, 33* (12), 51.

American National Standards Institute. (1991). *Maximum permissible ambient noise levels for audiometric test rooms* (ANSI S3.1-1991). New York: Acoustical Society of America.

Communication Instruction

American Speech-Language-Hearing Association. (1979). Standards for effective oral communication programs. *Asha, 21* (12), 1002.

American Speech-Language-Hearing Association. (1983). Social dialects (and implications). *Asha, 25* (9), 23-27.

American Speech-Language-Hearing Association. (1993). The role of the speech-language pathologist and teacher of voice in the remediation of singers with voice disorders. *Asha, 35* (1), 63.

Supervision

American Speech-Language-Hearing Association. (1985). Clinical supervision in speech-language pathology and audiology. *Asha, 28* (6), 57-60.

American Speech-Language-Hearing Association. (1989). Preparation models for the supervisory process in speech-language pathology and audiology. *Asha, 32* (3), 97-106.

American Speech-Language-Hearing Association. (1992). Supervision of student clinicians. *Asha, 34* (Suppl. 9), 8.

American Speech-Language-Hearing Association. (1992). Clinical fellowship supervisor's responsibilities. *Asha, 34* (Suppl. 9), 16-17.

Research

American Speech-Language-Hearing Association. (1992). Ethics in research and professional practice. *Asha, 34* (Suppl. 9), 11-12.

Appendix B

Resources:
Materials and Organizations

◆　◆　◆　◆　◆　◆　◆　◆　◆　◆　◆　◆　◆　◆　◆　◆　◆　◆

MATERIALS FOR GENERAL USE ABOUT CHILDREN WHO STUTTER

Booklets

If Your Child Stutters: A Guide for Parents (Publication 11, 3rd revised edition, 1989, by S. Ainsworth and J. Fraser, published by the Stuttering Foundation of America, 56 pages). Practical suggestions are given for parents to help a young child who stutters or is beginning to stutter. Also available in Spanish and French.

Stuttering and Your Child: Questions and Answers (Publication 22, 1989, E. G. Conture and J. Fraser [Eds.], Stuttering Foundation of America, 64 pages). Written for parents, teachers, day-care providers, and others, this book addresses commonly asked questions about stuttering and people who stutter.

Understanding Stuttering: Information for Parents (Revised edition, 1990, by E. B. Cooper, National Easter Seal Society [70 East Lake Street, Chicago, IL 60601], 30 pages). This book addresses the nature, causes, and diagnostic indicators of stuttering; provides suggestions for parents; and reviews critical elements of treatment programs.

A Guide for Parents of Children Who Stutter (National Stuttering Project, 16 pages). This booklet reviews the nature of stuttering and provides suggestions for parents of young children who are beginning to stutter.

Brochures (from the Stuttering Foundation of America)

"If You Think Your Child is Stuttering"

"The Child Who Stutters at School: Notes to the Teacher"

"National Stuttering Awareness Week"

"How to React When Speaking With Someone Who Stutters"

"Did You Know . . ." (Fact Sheet)

Brochure (from the National Stuttering Project)

"What the Teacher Can Do To Help the Child Who Stutters"

Videotapes

Prevention of Stuttering [Part 1]: Identifying the Danger Signs (1976, by E. L. Walle, Stuttering Foundation of America, 33 minutes). This video illustrates characteristics of early stuttering in young children and distinguishes between normal disfluency and incipient stuttering.

Childhood Stuttering: A Videotape for Parents (1994; by E. G. Conture, J. Fraser, B. E. Guitar, and D. E. Williams; Stuttering Foundation of America; 29 minutes). This video reviews the nature of stuttering in young children and provides useful suggestions for interacting with children who are beginning to stutter.

Therapy in Action: The School-Age Child Who Stutters (1997–1998, by E. G. Conture, B. E. Guitar, J. Fraser, J. H. Campbell, H. H. Gregory, P. R. Ramig, and P. M. Zebrowski; Stuttering Foundation of America; 38 minutes). This video addresses strategies to help school-age children who stutter and presents segments of therapy in action.

MATERIALS FOR CHILDREN WHO STUTTER

Stories

A Way Through the Forest: One Boy's Story With a Happy Ending (1995, by D. A. Shapiro, published by Aaron's Associates; see Chapter 9). This story presents one boy's personal experiences in dealing with stuttering and the ultimate joy in gaining communication freedom. In so doing, suggestions are provided for parents and speech–language pathologists in how to interact with children who stutter.

Booklets

The Adventures of Phil Carrot: The Forest of Discord (1995, by M. Sugarman and K. C. Swain, published by M. G. Sugarman [7626 Valentine Street, Oakland, CA, 94605], 41 pages). This book presents the summer adventures of a group of friends including Phil, a boy who stutters. Encountering fun, fear, and frustration, Phil ultimately discovers that friendship begins inside by liking and accepting oneself.

► **Note:** A critical review of 20 works of children's fiction was presented by T. Bushey and R. Martin (1988, Stuttering in Children's Literature, *Language, Speech, and Hearing Services in Schools, 19*, 235–250). This review is recommended for those who are interested in children's fiction involving a character who stutters (i.e., particularly how the authors portray symptoms, causes, and treatment of stuttering).

MATERIALS FOR PHYSICIANS ABOUT CHILDREN WHO STUTTER

Booklets

The Child Who Stutters: To the Pediatrician (Publication 23, 1991, by B. Guitar and E. G. Conture, Stuttering Foundation of America, 16 pages). This book explains the difference between normal disfluency and stuttering and presents suggestions for counseling and referral.

The Child Who Stutters: To the Family Physician (Publication 24, 1992). This book is a duplicate of Publication 23, with a different cover directed to the family physician.

MATERIALS FOR GENERAL USE ABOUT AND FOR ADULTS WHO STUTTER

Booklets

To the Stutterer (Publication 9, 1972, S. B. Hood [Ed.], Stuttering Foundation of America, 114 pages). This book provides practical advice written by 24 men and women speech–language pathologists who have stuttered, advising what helped them and what they believe will help other people to control their speech disfluency.

Self-Therapy for the Stutterer (Publication 12, 8th edition, 1993, by M. Fraser, Stuttering Foundation of America, 192 pages). Written for adults who cannot obtain direct treatment, this book describes self-therapy activities.

Do You Stutter: A Guide for Teens (Publication 21, 1987, J. Fraser and W. H. Perkins [Eds.], Stuttering Foundation of America, 80 pages). Written by seven speech–language pathologists, this book gives practical advice to teens on coping with stuttering.

A Stutterer's Story: An Autobiography (Publication 61, 1980 [2nd revised printing, 1994], by F. P. Murray and S. G. Edwards, Stuttering Foundation of America, 168 pages). This book presents a personal account of one man's experiences in coping with life as a person who stutters and reviews a basic knowledge base in adult stuttering and childhood stuttering.

Tangled Tongue: Living With a Stutter (1985, by J. A. Carlisle, University of Toronto Press, 258 pages). This autobiographical account traces one man's experiences and observations in living as a person who stutters, and ultimately conveys an inner world of frustration, courage, and determination.

Stuttering: A Life Bound Up in Words (1997, by M. Jezer, Basic Books/Harper Collins, 266 pages). This book presents the memories and observations of one person who stutters and, in so doing, conveys a personal story of fear, coping, and persistence, ultimately giving way to triumph and success.

Brochures (from the Stuttering Foundation of America)

"Turning on to Therapy"

"Using The Telephone: A Guide for People Who Stutter"

"National Stuttering Awareness Week"

"How to React When Speaking With Someone Who Stutters"

"Did You Know . . . " (Fact Sheet)

Videotapes

Do You Stutter: Straight Talk For Teens (1996; by B. E. Guitar, E. G. Conture, J. Fraser, H. H. Gregory, and P. Ramig; Stuttering Foundation of America,

35 minutes). Presenting interactions between several teens who stutter and their clinicians, this video addresses the nature of stuttering, thoughts and feelings associated with stuttering, and personal and clinical strategies for addressing stuttering.

OTHER MATERIALS FOR PROFESSIONAL USE

Booklets (from the Stuttering Foundation of America)

Stuttering Words (Publication 2, 3rd edition, 1997, S. B. Hood [Ed.], 72 pages). This glossary addresses terms associated with fluency and fluency disorders.

Stuttering: Treatment of the Young Stutterer in the School (Publication 4, 1964, C. Van Riper [Ed.], 62 pages). Raising and addressing questions frequently asked by school clinicians, various authorities discuss the challenges of school-based treatment for young children who stutter.

Stuttering: Successes and Failures in Therapy (Publication 6, 1968, H. L. Luper [Ed.], 148 pages). Nine speech–language pathologists present case histories of clinical successes and failures, describing and analyzing the procedures used and results attained.

Therapy for Stutterers (Publication 10, 1974, C. W. Starkweather [Ed.], 120 pages). Specialists in speech–language pathology outline a program of treatment for working with adolescents and adults who stutter.

Treating the School Age Stutterer: A Guide for Clinicians (Publication 14, 1979, by C. W. Dell, 110 pages). This book describes a variety of clinical procedures for working with children who stutter.

Stuttering: An Integration of Contemporary Therapies (Publication 16, 1980, by B. Guitar and T. J. Peters, 79 pages). Treatment strategies based on stuttering modification and fluency shaping are discussed and integrated for clients of all ages.

Counseling Stutterers (Publication 18, 1983, J. F. Gruss [Ed.], 80 pages). This book addresses the counseling aspect of treatment with adults and with parents of children who are receiving fluency intervention.

Stuttering Therapy: Transfer and Maintenance (Publication 19, 1984, J. F. Gruss [Ed.], 109 pages). This book addresses the importance of transfer and maintenance procedures during and following direct intervention.

Stuttering Therapy: Prevention and Intervention With Children (Publication 20, 1985, H. H. Gregory [Ed.], 151 pages). Prevention and early intervention techniques with young children are presented.

Videotapes

Adult Stuttering Therapy (1977, by C. Van Riper, Stuttering Foundation of America). In a series of eight videotapes (ranging from 28 to 52 minutes each),

Van Riper demonstrates assessment and stuttering modification treatment with Jeff, a young adult who stutters. Seven consecutive weekly treatment sessions illustrate diagnosis, identification, desensitization, variation, modification (including cancellation and monitoring), and stabilization, followed by a session 1 year later. A ninth tape (*Adult Stuttering Therapy: A Twenty Year Follow-up With Jeff,* 1995, 36 minutes) was added recently. Its contains an interview with Jeff about the long-term effectiveness of his treatment.

ORGANIZATIONS FOR PEOPLE INTERESTED IN STUTTERING

Within the United States

American Speech–Language–Hearing Association (ASHA, 10801 Rockville Pike, Rockville, MD 20852, Phone: 301-897-5700). ASHA is the credentialling organization of speech–language pathologists and audiologists and the largest advocacy body for people with communication disorders and their families. Also, ASHA is the umbrella organization for Special Interest Division #4 (i.e., Fluency and Fluency Disorders), which is spearheading specialty certification in fluency disorders for speech–language pathologists.

International Fluency Association (IFA, c/o Howard D. Schwartz, Chair, Membership Committee, Department of Communicative Disorders, Northern Illinois University, DeKalb, IL 60115, Phone: 815-753-1429). IFA brings together proponents of the major approaches to stuttering (i.e., theoretical, empirical, and clinical) from different disciplines and cultures and fosters collaboration between professionals, people who stutter, and support groups. IFA sponsors the *Journal of Fluency Disorders* as its official publication and holds an international convention every 3 years.

National Stuttering Project (NSP, 5100 East La Palma Avenue, Suite 208, Anaheim Hills, CA 92807, Phone: 800-364-1677). NSP is the largest self-help organization for people who stutter. Approximately 20% of its 4,000 members are speech–language pathologists. It sponsors a monthly newsletter ("Letting Go") and an annual convention.

Speak Easy International Foundation (233 Concord Drive, Paramus, NJ 07652, Phone: 201-262-0895). Speak Easy is a self-help organization for people who stutter. It sponsors a newsletter and an annual convention.

Stuttering Foundation of America (SFA, 3100 Walnut Grove, Suite 603, P. O. Box 11749, Memphis, TN 38111-0749, Phone: 800-992-9392). SFA publishes low-cost materials about stuttering for people who stutter, their families, speech–language pathologists, and others. Also, it sponsors conferences and other training opportunities for speech–language pathologists.

Outside of the United States

There are many organizations outside of the United States addressing self-help and consumer affairs in addition to others committed to therapy and research.

In the interest of conserving space, and because addresses and phone numbers tend to change, the individual organizations outside of the United States are not listed here. However, listings of international organizations located throughout North America, South America, Europe, Asia, Australia, and Africa can be found in Carlisle (1985, *Tangled Tongue: Living With a Stutter,* pp. 239–255), Starkweather and Givens-Ackerman (1997, *Stuttering,* pp. 205–208), and The Stuttering Home Page (See Websites, below).

ELECTRONIC NETWORK SYSTEMS
Discussion Forums

- Stutt-L:

  Listserv Address: LISTSERV@VM.TEMPLE.EDU
  List Address: STUTT-L@VM.TEMPLE.EDU
  Owner: C. W. Starkweather

- Stut-Hlp:

  Listproc Address: LISTPROC2@ECNET.NET
  List Address: STUT-HLP@ECNET.NET
  Owner: Bob Quesal

- Stutt-X:

  Listserv Address: LISTSERV@ASUVM.INRE.ASU.EDU
  List Address: STUTT-X@ASUVM.INRE.ASU.EDU
  Owner: Don Mower

- UseNet Discussion Group:

  ALT.SUPPORT.STUTTERING

- Web Sites

  American Speech-Language-Hearing Association
  http://www.asha.org

  National Stuttering Project
  http://www.nspstutter.org

  Stuttering Foundation of America
  http://www.stuttersfa.org

  The Stuttering Home Page. This site is maintained by Judith Maginnis Kuster at Minnesota State University, Mankato.
  http://www.mankato.msus.edu/dept/comdis/kuster/stutter.html

References

◆ ◆ ◆ ◆ ◆ ◆ ◆ ◆ ◆ ◆ ◆ ◆ ◆ ◆ ◆ ◆ ◆ ◆

Adler, S. (1993). *Multicultural communication skills in the classroom.* Needham Heights, MA: Allyn & Bacon.

Ainsworth, S., & Fraser, J. (1989). *If your child stutters: A guide for parents* (3rd ed.). [Publication 11]. Memphis, TN: Stuttering Foundation of America.

Ambrose, N. G., Yairi, E., & Cox, N. (1993). Genetic aspects of early childhood stuttering. *Journal of Speech and Hearing Research, 36,* 701–706.

American Speech and Hearing Association, Committee on Supervision in Speech Pathology and Audiology. (1978). Current status of supervision of speech–language pathology and audiology. [Special report]. *Asha, 20,* 478–486.

American Speech–Language–Hearing Association, Committee on Supervision in Speech–Language Pathology and Audiology. (1985). Clinical supervision in speech–language pathology and audiology. [Position statement]. *Asha, 27* (6), 57–60.

American Speech–Language–Hearing Association, Committee on the Status of Racial Minorities. (1987). *Multicultural professional education in communication disorders: Curriculum approaches.* Rockville, MD: American Speech–Language–Hearing Association.

American Speech–Language–Hearing Association, Committee on Supervision in Speech–Language Pathology and Audiology. (1989). Preparation models for the supervisory process in speech–language pathology and audiology. [Tutorial]. *Asha, 31*(3), 97–106.

American Speech–Language–Hearing Association, Committee on the Status of Racial Minorities. (1991, May). Multicultural action agenda 2000. *Asha, 33,* 39–41.

American Speech–Language–Hearing Association [Long-Range Strategic Planning Board]. (1992a, May). ASHA's proposed long-range strategic plan 1994–1999. *Asha, 34,* 32–36.

American Speech–Language–Hearing Association [Educational Standards Board]. (1992b). Standards for accreditation of educational programs in speech–language pathology and audiology [Chapter III]. In Educational Standards Board, *1992 Accreditation Manual* (pp. 13–22). Rockville, MD: American Speech–Language–Hearing Association.

American Speech–Language–Hearing Association. (1994a). Code of ethics. *Asha, 36* (March, Suppl. 13), pp. 1–2.

American Speech–Language–Hearing Association [Clinical Certification Board]. (1994b). Standards and implementations for the certificates of clinical competence [Chapter III]. In Clinical Certification Board, *Membership and certification handbook: Speech–Language Pathology—1995* (pp. 7–17). Rockville, MD: American Speech–Language–Hearing Association.

American Speech–Language–Hearing Association. (1995, March). Guidelines for practice in stuttering treatment. *Asha, 37* (Suppl. 14, pp. 26–35).

American Speech–Language–Hearing Association. (1996a, Spring). Guidelines for the training, credentialing, use, and supervision of speech–language pathology assistants. *Asha, 38* (Suppl. 16, pp. 21–34).

American Speech–Language–Hearing Association. (1996b, Spring). Scope of practice in speech–language pathology. *Asha, 38* (Suppl. 16, pp. 16–20).

American Speech–Language–Hearing Association. (1996c, September). *Task force on educational standards for coordinated levels of service delivery.* [Draft, Special Interest Division #4: Fluency and Fluency Disorders]. Rockville, MD: American Speech–Language–Hearing Association.

Anderson, D. (1995). Historical perceptions of stuttering as reflected in the arts. In C. W. Stark-weather & H. F. M. Peters (Eds.), *Stuttering: Proceedings of the First World Congress on Fluency Disorders, Munich, Germany, August 8–11, 1994* (pp. 567–570) [Vol. II]. Nijmegen, The Netherlands: University of Nijmegen Press.

Anderson, J. L. (Ed.). (1980). *Conference on training in the supervisory process in speech–language pathology and audiology* [Proceedings]. Bloomington: Indiana University.

Anderson, J. L. (1988). *The supervisory process in speech–language pathology and audiology.* Boston, MA: Little, Brown/College-Hill.

Anderson, N. B., Lee-Wilkerson, D., & Chabon, S. (1995). *Preschool language disorders.* [Clinical Series #12]. Rockville, MD: National Student Speech Language Hearing Association.

Andrews, G. (1984). Epidemiology of stuttering. In R. F. Curlee & W. H. Perkins (Eds.), *Nature and treatment of stuttering: New directions* (pp. 1–12). San Diego, CA: College-Hill.

Andrews, G., Craig, A., Feyer, A., Hoddinott, S., Howie, P., & Neilson, M. (1983). Stuttering: A review of research findings and theories circa 1982. *Journal of Speech and Hearing Disorders, 48,* 226–246.

Andrews, G., Guitar, B., & Howie, P. (1980). Meta-analysis of the effects of stuttering treatment. *Journal of Speech and Hearing Disorders, 45,* 287–307.

Andrews, G., & Ingham, R. J. (1971). Stuttering: Considerations in the evaluation of treatment. *British Journal of Disorders of Communication, 6,* 129–138.

Andrews, J. R., & Andrews, M. A. (1990). *Family based treatment in communicative disorders: A systemic approach.* Sandwich, IL: Janelle Publications.

Argeropoulos, J. (1974). Self-concept and the client–clinician relationship. In L. L. Emerick & S. B. Hood (Eds.), *The client–clinician relationship: Essays on interpersonal sensitivity in the therapeutic transaction* (pp. 84–91). Springfield, IL: Charles C. Thomas.

Arnold, G. E. (1965). Physiology and pathology of speech and language. In R. Luchsinger & G. E. Arnold, *Voice–Speech–Language, Clinical communicology: Its physiology and pathology* (pp. 335–791). Belmont, CA: Wadsworth.

Aronson, A. E. (1973). *Psychogenic voice disorders: An interdisciplinary approach to detection, diagnosis, and therapy.* Philadelphia, PA: W. B. Saunders.

Aronson, A. E. (1990). *Clinical voice disorders: An interdisciplinary approach* (3rd ed.) New York: Thieme Medical Publishers.

Attanasio, J. S. (1987a). A case of late-onset or acquired stuttering in adult life. *Journal of Fluency Disorders, 12,* 287–290.

Attanasio, J. S. (1987b). The dodo was Lewis Carroll, you see: Reflections and speculations. *Journal of Fluency Disorders, 12,* 107–118.

Battle, D. E. (1993). Introduction. In D. E. Battle (Ed.), *Communication disorders in multicultural populations* (pp. xv–xxiv). Stoneham, MA: Andover Medical Publishers/Butterworth-Heinemann.

Beasley, D. S., & Davis, G. A. (1981). Preface. In D. S. Beasley & G. A. Davis (Eds.), *Aging: Communication processes and disorders* (pp. xv–xvi). New York: Grune & Stratton.

Benecken, J. (1995). On the nature and psychological relevance of a stigma: The "stutterer" or: What happens, when "Grace Fails"? In C. W. Starkweather & H. F. M. Peters (Eds.), *Stuttering: Proceedings of the First World Congress on Fluency Disorders, Munich, Germany, August 8–11, 1994* (pp. 548–550) [Vol. II]. Nijmegen, The Netherlands: University of Nijmegen Press.

Bengtson, V. L., & Schaie, K. W. (1989). Preface. In V. L. Bengtson & K. W. Schaie (Eds.), *The course of later life: Research and reflections* (pp. vii–xi). New York: Springer.

Benjamin, B. J. (1988). Changes in speech production and linguistic behavior with aging. In B. B. Shadden (Ed.), *Communication behavior and aging: A sourcebook for clinicians* (pp. 162–181). Baltimore, MD: Williams & Wilkins.

Bess, F. H., Clark, B. S., & Mitchell, H. R. (Eds.). (1986). *Concerns for minority groups in communication disorders* [ASHA Reports 16]. Rockville, MD: American Speech–Language–Hearing Association.

Beukelman, D. R. (1986). The transition from graduate student to speech–language pathologist in a hospital setting. *National Student Speech Language Hearing Association Journal, 14,* 5–10.

Bjerkan, B. (1980). Word fragmentations and repetitions in the spontaneous speech of 2–6-yr-old children. *Journal of Fluency Disorders, 5,* 137–148.

Blood, G. W. (1995a). A behavioral-cognitive therapy program for adults who stutter: Computers and counseling. *Journal of Communication Disorders, 28,* 165–180.

Blood, G. W. (1995b). POWER²: Relapse management with adolescents who stutter. *Language, Speech, and Hearing Services in Schools, 26,* 169–179.

Bloodstein, O. (1958). Stuttering as an anticipatory struggle reaction. In J. Eisenson (Ed.), *Stuttering: A symposium* (pp. 1–69). New York: Harper & Row.

Bloodstein, O. (1960). The development of stuttering: II. Developmental phases. *Journal of Speech and Hearing Disorders, 25,* 366–376.

Bloodstein, O. (1975). Stuttering as tension and fragmentation. In J. Eisenson (Ed.), *Stuttering: A second symposium* (pp. 1–95). New York: Harper & Row.

Bloodstein, O. (1981). *A handbook on stuttering* (3rd ed.). Chicago, IL: National Easter Seal Society.

Bloodstein, O. (1984). Stuttering as an anticipatory struggle disorder. In R. F. Curlee & W. H. Perkins (Eds.), *Nature and treatment of stuttering: New directions* (pp. 171–186). San Diego, CA: College-Hill.

Bloodstein, O. (1986). Semantics and beliefs. In G. H. Shames & H. Rubin (Eds.), *Stuttering then and now* (pp. 130–139). Columbus, OH: Charles E. Merrill.

Bloodstein, O. (1988). Verification of stuttering in a suspected malingerer. *Journal of Fluency Disorders, 13,* 83–88.

Bloodstein, O. (1990). On pluttering, skivering, and floggering: A commentary. *Journal of Speech and Hearing Disorders, 55,* 392–393.

Bloodstein, O. (1993). *Stuttering: The search for a cause and cure.* Needham Heights, MA: Allyn & Bacon.

Bloodstein, O. (1995). *A handbook on stuttering* (5th ed.). San Diego, CA: Singular.

Bluemel, C. S. (1932). Primary and secondary stammering. *Quarterly Journal of Speech, 18,* 187–200.

Bluemel, C. S. (1935). *Stammering and allied disorders.* New York: Macmillan.

Bluemel, C. S. (1957). *The riddle of stuttering.* Danville, IL: Interstate Publishing.

Blumberg, A. (1980). *Supervisors and teachers: A private cold war* (2nd ed.). Berkeley, CA: McCutchan.

Boberg, E. (1981). Maintenance of fluency: An experimental program. In E. Boberg (Ed.), *Maintenance of fluency: Proceedings of the Banff Conference* [Banff, Alberta, June, 1979] (pp. 71–112). New York: Elsevier.

Boberg, E. (1984). Behavioral transfer and maintenance programs for adolescent and adult stutterers. In J. F. Gruss (Ed.), *Stuttering therapy: Transfer and maintenance* [Publication 19] (pp. 41–61). Memphis, TN: Stuttering Foundation of America.

Boberg, E., & Kully, D. (1985). *Comprehensive stuttering treatment program.* San Diego, CA: College-Hill.

Boone, D. R., & Prescott, T. E. (1972). Content and sequence analysis of speech and hearing therapy. *Asha, 14,* 58–62.

Botterill, W., & Cook, F. (1987). Personal construct theory and the treatment of adolescent dysfluency. In L. Rustin, H. Purser, & D. Rowley (Eds.), *Progress in the treatment of fluency disorders* (pp. 147–165). London, England: Taylor & Francis.

Bowen, M. (1976). Theory in the practice of psychotherapy. In P. J. Guerin, Jr. (Ed.), *Family therapy: Theory and practice* (pp. 42–90). New York: Gardner.

Brady, J. P. (1991). The pharmacology of stuttering: A critical review. *American Journal of Psychiatry, 148*(10), 1309–1316.

Brasseur, J. (1989). The supervisory process: A continuum perspective. *Language, Speech, and Hearing Services in Schools, 20,* 274–295.

Brutten, G. J. (1975). Stuttering: Topography, assessment, and behavior-change strategies. In J. Eisenson (Ed.), *Stuttering: A second symposium* (pp. 199–262). New York: Harper & Row.

Brutten, G. J. (Ed.). (1993). Proceedings of the NIDCD Workshop on Treatment Efficacy Research in Stuttering [September 21–22, 1992]. *Journal of Fluency Disorders, 18,* 121–361.

Brutten, G. J., & Shoemaker, D. J. (1971). A two-factor learning theory of stuttering. In L. E. Travis (Ed.), *Handbook of speech pathology and audiology* (pp. 1035–1072). Englewood Cliffs, NJ: Prentice-Hall.

Bruun, R. D., & Bruun, B. (1994). *A mind of its own. Tourette's Syndrome: A story and a guide.* New York: Oxford University Press.

Bushey, T., & Martin, R. (1988). Stuttering in children's literature. *Language, Speech, and Hearing Services in Schools, 19,* 235–250.

Byrne, A., Byrne, M. K., & Zibin, T. O. (1993). Transient neurogenic stuttering. *International Journal of Eating Disorders, 14*(4), 511–514.

Campbell, L. R. (1985). *A study of comparability of master's level training and certification requirements and needs of speech–language pathologists (competencies, duties, employment, continuing education).* Unpublished doctoral dissertation, Howard University.

Canter, G. J. (1971). Observations on neurogenic stuttering: A contribution to differential diagnosis. *British Journal of Disorders of Communication, 6*(2), 139–143.

Carkhuff, R. R. (1969a). *Helping and human relations: A primer for lay and professional helpers* (Vol. I). New York: Holt, Rinehart & Winston.

Carkhuff, R. R. (1969b). *Helping and human relations: A primer for lay and professional helpers* (Vol. II). New York: Holt, Rinehart & Winston.

Carlisle, J. A. (1985). *Tangled tongue: Living with a stutter.* Toronto: University of Toronto Press.

Carter, E. A., & Orfanidis, M. M. (1976). Family therapy with one person and the family therapist's own family. In P. J. Guerin, Jr. (Ed.), *Family therapy: Theory and practice* (pp. 193–219). New York: Gardner.

Casey, P. L., Smith, K. J., & Ulrich, S. R. (1988). *Self-supervision: A career tool for audiologists and speech–language pathologists.* [Clinical Series No. 10]. Rockville, MD: National Student Speech Language Hearing Association.

Clark, R. M. (1964). Our enterprising predecessors and Charles Sydney Bluemel. *Asha, 6,* 107–114.

Clark, R. M., & Murray, F. P. (1965). Alterations in self-concept: A barometer of progress in individuals undergoing therapy for stuttering. In D. A. Barbara (Ed.), *New directions in stuttering: Theory and practice* (pp. 131–158). Springfield, IL: Charles C. Thomas.

Cogan, M. L. (1973). *Clinical supervision.* Boston, MA: Houghton Mifflin.

Colburn, N., & Mysak, E. D. (1982a). Developmental disfluency and emerging grammar I. Disfluency characteristics in early syntactic utterances. *Journal of Speech and Hearing Research, 25,* 414–420.

Colburn, N., & Mysak, E. D. (1982b). Developmental disfluency and emerging grammar II. Co-occurrence of disfluency with specified semantic-syntactic structures. *Journal of Speech and Hearing Research, 25,* 421–427.

Cole, L. (1989). E pluribus pluribus: Multicultural imperatives for the 1990s and beyond. *Asha, 31*(9), 65–70.

Cole, L. (1992, May). We're serious. *Asha, 34,* 38–39.

Colligan, N. (1989, December). Recognizing Tourette Syndrome in the classroom. *School Nurse* [Reprinted by Tourette Syndrome Association, 42–40 Bell Blvd., Bayside, NY 11361].

Comings, D. E. (1995). Tourette's syndrome: A behavioral spectrum disorder. In W. J. Weiner & A. E. Lang (Eds.), *Behavioral Neurology of Movement Disorders* [Advances in Neurology Series, Vol. 65] (pp. 293–303). New York: Raven Press.

Conture, E. G. (1990a). Childhood stuttering: What is it and who does it? In J. A. Cooper (Ed.), *Research needs in stuttering: Roadblocks and future directions* [ASHA Reports 18] (pp. 2–14). Rockville, MD: American Speech–Language–Hearing Association.

Conture, E. G. (1990b). *Stuttering* (2nd ed.). Englewood Cliffs, NJ: Prentice-Hall.

Conture, E. G. (1997). Evaluating childhood stuttering. In R. F. Curlee & G. M. Siegel (Eds.), *Nature and treatment of stuttering: New directions* (2nd ed.) (pp. 239–256). Needham Heights, MA: Allyn & Bacon.

Conture, E. G., & Fraser, J. (Eds.). (1989). *Stuttering and your child: Questions and Answers.* [Publication 22]. Memphis, TN: Stuttering Foundation of America.

Conture, E. G., & Guitar, B. E. (1993). Evaluating efficacy of treatment of stuttering: School-age children. *Journal of Fluency Disorders, 18,* 253–287.

Conture, E. G., Louko, L. J., & Edwards, M. L. (1993). Simultaneously treating stuttering and disordered phonology in children: Experimental treatment, preliminary findings. *American Journal of Speech–Language Pathology, 2*(3), 72–81.

Cooper, E. B. (1976). *Personalized fluency control therapy: An integrated behavior and relationship therapy for stutterers.* Austin, TX: Learning Concepts.

Cooper, E. B. (1977). Controversies about stuttering therapy. *Journal of Fluency Disorders, 2,* 75–86.

Cooper, E. B. (1979). Intervention procedures for the young stutterer. In H. H. Gregory (Ed.), *Controversies about stuttering therapy* (pp. 63–96). Baltimore, MD: University Park Press.

Cooper, E. B. (1987a). The chronic perseverative stuttering syndrome: Incurable stuttering. *Journal of Fluency Disorders, 12,* 381–388.

Cooper, E. B. (1987b). The Cooper Personalized Fluency Control Therapy. In L. Rustin, H. Purser, & D. Rowley (Eds.), *Progress in the treatment of fluency disorders* (pp. 124–146). London, England: Taylor & Francis.

Cooper, E. B. (1990a). Stuttering nuggets from a perennially perplexed but persevering prospector. *The Clinical Connection, 4*(1), 1–4.

Cooper, E. B. (1990b). *Understanding stuttering: Information for parents* (Revised ed.). Chicago, IL: National Easter Seal Society.

Cooper, E. B. (1993a). Chronic perseverative stuttering syndrome: A harmful or helpful construct? *American Journal of Speech–Language Pathology, 2*(3), 11–15.

Cooper, E. B. (1993b). Chronic perseverative stuttering syndrome: Cooper responds to Ham. *American Journal of Speech–Language Pathology, 2*(3), 21–22.

Cooper, E. B. (1993c). Red herrings, dead horses, straw men, and blind alleys: Escaping the stuttering conundrum. *Journal of Fluency Disorders, 18,* 375–387.

Cooper, E. B. (1996, October). Coordinator's corner. *Special Interest Divisions: Fluency and Fluency Disorders, 6*(3), 1–2. [Division 4 Newsletter; Rockville, MD: American Speech–Language–Hearing Association].

Cooper, E. B. (1997). Fluency disorders. In T. A. Crowe (Ed.), *Applications of counseling in speech–language pathology and audiology* (pp. 145–166). Baltimore, MD: Williams & Wilkins.

Cooper, E. B. (1998, January). Coordinator's column. *Special Interest Division 4: Fluency and Fluency Disorders, 8*(1), 1–3. [Division 4 Newsletter; Rockville, MD: American Speech–Language–Hearing Association].

Cooper, E. B., & Cooper, C. S. (1985a). Clinician attitudes toward stuttering: A decade of change (1973–1983). *Journal of Fluency Disorders, 10,* 19–33.

Cooper, E. B., & Cooper, C. S. (1985b). The effective clinician [Chapter 3]. In E. B. Cooper & C. S. Cooper, *Cooper Personalized Fluency Control Therapy–Revised* [handbook]. Allen, TX: DLM Teaching Resources.

Cooper, E. B., & Cooper, C. S. (1991). A fluency disorders prevention program for preschoolers and children in the primary grades. *American Journal of Speech–Language Pathology, 1*(1), 28–31.

Cooper, E. B., & Cooper, C. S. (1993). Fluency disorders. In D. E. Battle (Ed.), *Communication disorders in multicultural populations* (pp. 189–211). Stoneham, MA: Andover Medical Publishers/Butterworth-Heinemann.

Cooper, E. B., & Cooper, C. S. (1995). Treating fluency disordered adolescents. *Journal of Communication Disorders, 28,* 125–142.

Cooper, E. B., & Cooper, C. S. (1996). Clinician attitudes towards stuttering: Two decades of change. *Journal of Fluency Disorders, 21,* 119–135.

Cooper, E. B., & Rustin, L. (1985). Clinician attitudes toward stuttering in the United States and Great Britain: A cross-cultural study. *Journal of Fluency Disorders, 10,* 1–17.

Costello, J. M. (1980). Operant conditioning and the treatment of stuttering. In W. Perkins (Ed.), *Seminars in Speech, Language and Hearing* [Strategies in Stuttering Therapy, Vol. 1, No. 4] (pp. 311–325), New York: Thieme-Stratton.

Costello, J. M. (1983). Current behavioral treatments for children. In D. Prins, & R. J. Ingham (Eds.), *Treatment of stuttering in early childhood: Methods and issues* (pp. 69–112). San Diego, CA: College-Hill.

Cox, M. D. (1986). The psychologically maladjusted stutterer. In K. O. St. Louis (Ed.), *The atypical stutterer: Principles and practices of rehabilitation* (pp. 93–122). Orlando, FL: Academic Press.

Cox, N. J. (1988). Molecular genetics: The key to the puzzle of stuttering? *Asha, 30*(4), 36–40.

Cox, N. J. (1993). Stuttering: A complex behavioral disorder for our times? *American Journal of Medical Genetics (Neuropsychiatric Genetics), 48,* 177–178.

Crowe, T. A., & Walton, J. H. (1981). Teacher attitudes toward stuttering. *Journal of Fluency Disorders, 6,* 163–174.

Culatta, R., Colucci, S., & Wiggins, E. (1975, March). Clinical supervisors and trainees: Two views of a process. *Asha, 17,* 152–157.

Culatta, R., & Goldberg, S. A. (1995). *Stuttering therapy: An integrated approach to theory and practice.* Needham Heights, MA: Allyn & Bacon.

Culatta, R., & Leeper, L. (1987). Disfluency in childhood: It's not always stuttering. *Journal of Childhood Communication Disorders, 10*(2), 95–106.

Culatta, R., & Leeper, L. (1988). Dysfluency isn't always stuttering. *Journal of Speech and Hearing Disorders, 53,* 486–488.

Culatta, R., & Leeper, L. H. (1989–1990). The differential diagnosis of disfluency. *National Student Speech Language Hearing Association Journal, 17,* 59–64.

Culatta, R., & Seltzer, H. (1976). Content and sequence analysis of the supervisory session. *Asha, 18,* 8–12.

Culatta, R., & Seltzer, H. (1977). Content and sequence analysis of the supervisory session: A report of clinical use. *Asha, 19,* 523–526.

Curlee, R. F. (1993). Preface. In R. F. Curlee (Ed.), *Stuttering and related disorders of fluency* (pp. xi–xiv). New York: Thieme Medical Publishers.

Curlee, R. F., & Perkins, W. H. (Eds.). (1984). *Nature and treatment of stuttering: New directions.* San Diego, CA: College-Hill.

Curlee, R. F., & Siegel, G. M. (Eds.). (1997). *Nature and treatment of stuttering: New directions* (2nd ed.). Needham Heights, MA: Allyn & Bacon.

Dalton, P., & Hardcastle, W. J. (1989). *Disorders of fluency* (2nd ed.). London, England: Whurr Publishers.

Daly, D. A. (1986). The clutterer. In K. O. St. Louis (Ed.), *The atypical stutterer: Principles and practices of rehabilitation* (pp. 155–192). Orlando, FL: Academic Press.

Daly, D. A. (1988). A practitioner's view of stuttering. *Asha, 30*(4), 34–35.

Daly, D. A. (1993). Cluttering: Another fluency syndrome. In R. F. Curlee (Ed.), *Stuttering and related disorders of fluency* (pp. 179–204). New York: Thieme Medical Publishers.

Daly, D. A. (1996). *The source for stuttering and cluttering.* Moline, IL: LinguiSystems.

Daly, D. A., Simon, C. A., & Burnett-Stolnack, M. (1995). Helping adolescents who stutter focus on fluency. *Language, Speech, and Hearing Services in Schools, 26,* 162–168.

Deal, J. L. (1982). Sudden onset of stuttering: A case report. *Journal of Speech and Hearing Disorders, 47,* 301–304.

Deal, J. L., & Doro, J. M. (1987). Episodic hysterical stuttering. *Journal of Speech and Hearing Disorders, 52,* 299–300.

De Buck, A. (1970). *Egyptian readingbook: Exercises and Middle Egyptian texts* (3rd ed.). Leiden, Holland: Nederlands Instituut Voor Het Nabije Oosten.

Dell, C. W. (1979). *Treating the school age stutterer: A guide for clinicians.* [Publication 14]. Memphis, TN: Stuttering Foundation of America.

Dell, C. W. (1993). Treating school-age stutterers. In R. F. Curlee (Ed.), *Stuttering and related disorders of fluency* (pp. 45–67). New York: Thieme Medical Publishers.

Dempsey, G. L., & Granich, M. (1978). Hypno-behavioral therapy in the case of a traumatic stutterer: A case study. *International Journal of Clinical and Experimental Hypnosis, 26,* 125–133.

Diedrich, W. M. (1984). Cluttering: Its diagnosis. In H. Winitz (Ed.), *Treating articulation disorders: For clinicians by clinicians* (pp. 307–323). Baltimore, MD: University Park Press.

Diehl, C. F. (1958). *A compendium of research and theory on stuttering.* Springfield, IL: Charles C. Thomas.

Douglass, E., & Quarrington, B. (1952). The differentiation of interiorized and exteriorized secondary stuttering. *Journal of Speech and Hearing Disorders, 17,* 377–385.

Dowling, S. (1992). *Implementing the supervisory process: Theory and practice.* Englewood Cliffs, NJ: Prentice-Hall.

Downes, J. J., Sharp, H. M., Costall, B. M., Sagar, H. J., & Howe, J. (1993). Alternating fluency in Parkinson's disease. *Brain, 116,* 887–902.

Duchin, S. W., & Mysak, E. D. (1987). Disfluency and rate characteristics of young adult, middle-aged, and older males. *Journal of Communication Disorders, 20,* 245–257.

Duffy, J. R. (1995). *Motor speech disorders: Substrates, differential diagnosis, and management.* St. Louis, MO: Mosby.

Eisenson, J. (1958). A perseverative theory of stuttering. In J. Eisenson (Ed.), *Stuttering: A symposium* (pp. 223–271). New York: Harper & Row.

Eisenson, J. (1975). Stuttering as perseverative behavior. In J. Eisenson (Ed.), *Stuttering: A second symposium* (pp. 401–452). New York: Harper & Row.

Emerick, L. L. (1966). Bibliotherapy for stutterers: Four case histories. *Quarterly Journal of Speech, 52*(1), 74–79.

Emerick, L. L. (1974a). Mea Culpa: Failures with stutterers. In L. L. Emerick & S. B. Hood (Eds.), *The client–clinician relationship: Essays on interpersonal sensitivity in the therapeutic transaction* (pp. 109–115). Springfield, IL: Charles C. Thomas.

Emerick, L. L. (1974b). Stuttering therapy: Dimensions of interpersonal sensitivity. In L. L. Emerick & S. B. Hood (Eds.), *The client–clinician relationship: Essays on interpersonal sensitivity in the therapeutic transaction* (pp. 92–102). Springfield, IL: Charles C. Thomas.

Emerick, L. L., & Haynes, W. O. (1986). *Diagnosis and evaluation in speech pathology* (3rd ed.). Englewood Cliffs, NJ: Prentice-Hall.

Emerick, L. L., & Hood, S. B. (1974). Preface. In L. L. Emerick & S. B. Hood (Eds.), *The client–clinician relationship: Essays on interpersonal sensitivity in the therapeutic transaction* (pp. vii–viii). Springfield, IL: Charles C. Thomas.

Epstein, N. B., & Bishop, D. S. (1981). Problem-centered systems therapy of the family. In A. S. Gurman & D. P. Kniskern (Eds.), *Handbook of family therapy* (pp. 444–482). New York: Brunner/Mazel.

Fairbanks, G. (1954). Systematic research in experimental phonetics: 1. A theory of the speech mechanism as a servosystem. *Journal of Speech and Hearing Disorders, 19,* 133–139.

Fairbanks, G. (1960). *Voice and articulation drillbook* (2nd ed.). New York: Harper & Row.

Fantry, L. (1990, January 5). Stuttering and Acquired Immunodeficiency Syndrome. [Letter]. *Journal of the American Medical Association, 263*(1), 38.

Farmer, S. S., & Farmer, J. L. (1989). *Supervision in communication disorders*. Columbus, OH: Merrill.

Felsenfeld, S. (1996). Progress and needs in the genetics of stuttering. *Journal of Fluency Disorders, 21,* 77–103.

Felsenfeld, S. (1997). Epidemiology and genetics of stuttering. In R. F. Curlee & G. M. Siegel (Eds.), *Nature and treatment of stuttering: New directions* (2nd ed.) (pp. 3–23). Needham Heights, MA: Allyn & Bacon.

Fey, M. E. (1986). *Language intervention with young children*. Austin, TX: PRO-ED.

Finkelstein, S. (1968). *Sense and nonsense of McLuhan*. New York: International Publishers.

Finn, P., Ingham, R. J., Yairi, E., & Ambrose, N. (1994, November). *Unassisted recovery from stuttering in preschool children: A perceptual study*. Paper presented at the Annual Convention of the American Speech–Language–Hearing Association, New Orleans, LA. [Abstract published in *Asha, 36* (October), p. 52].

Florance, C. L. (1986, Fall). Predicting prognosis in stuttering therapy. *Hearsay: Journal of the Ohio Speech and Hearing Association,* 70–73.

Fransella, F. (1972). *Personal change and reconstruction: Research on a treatment of stuttering*. London, England: Academic Press.

Freund, H. (1966). *Psychopathology and the problems of stuttering: With special consideration of clinical and historical aspects*. Springfield, IL: Charles C. Thomas.

Friend, M., & Cook, L. (1996). *Interactions: Collaboration skills for school professionals* (2nd ed.). White Plains, NY: Longman.

Froeschels, E. (1955). Contribution to the relationship between stuttering and cluttering. *Logopaedie en Phoniatrie, 4,* 1–6.

Froeschels, E. (1956). [Untitled contribution]. In E. F. Hahn & E. S. Hahn (Eds.), *Stuttering: Significant theories and therapies* (2nd ed.) (pp. 41–47). Stanford, CA: Stanford University Press.

Froeschels, E. (1964). *Selected papers of Emil Froeschels, 1940–1964*. Amsterdam, The Netherlands: North-Holland Publishing Co.

Gardner, H. (1983). *Frames of mind: The theory of multiple intelligences.* New York: Basic Books/ Harper Collins.

Garner, H. S., Uhl, M., & Cox, A. W. (1992). *Interdisciplinary teamwork training guide.* Richmond, VA: Virginia Institute for Developmental Disabilities.

Garrard, K. R. (1990–1991). A guide for assessing young children's expressive language skills through language sampling. *National Student Speech Language Hearing Association Journal, 18,* 87–95.

Gazda, G. M., Asbury, F. R., Balzer, F. J., Childers, W. C., & Walters, R. P. (1977). *Human relations development—A manual for educators* (2nd ed.). Boston, MA: Allyn & Bacon.

Gibran, K. (1923). *The prophet.* New York: Alfred A. Knopf.

Gillam, R. B., Roussos, C. S., & Anderson, J. L. (1990). Facilitating changes in supervisees' clinical behaviors: An experimental investigation of supervisory effectiveness. *Journal of Speech and Hearing Disorders, 55,* 729–739.

Glauber, P. (1958). The psychoanalysis of stuttering. In J. Eisenson (Ed.), *Stuttering: A symposium* (pp. 71–119). New York: Harper & Row.

Goldberg, B. (1989, June/July). Historic treatments for stuttering: From pebbles to psychoanalysis. *Asha, 31,* 71.

Goldhammer, R. (1969). *Clinical supervision: Special methods for the supervision of teachers.* New York: Holt, Rinehart & Winston.

Goldhammer, R., Anderson, R. H., & Krajewski, R. J. (1980). *Clinical supervision: Special methods for the supervision of teachers* (2nd ed.). New York: Holt, Rinehart & Winston.

Goldiamond, I. (1965). Stuttering and fluency as manipulable operant responses classes. In L. Krasner & L. P. Ullmann (Eds.), *Research in behavior modification: New developments and implications* (pp. 106–156). New York: Holt, Rinehart & Winston.

Gordon, P. A., & Luper, H. L. (1992a). The early identification of beginning stuttering I: Protocols. *American Journal of Speech–Language Pathology, 1*(3), 43–53.

Gordon, P. A., & Luper, H. L. (1992b). The early identification of beginning stuttering II: Problems. *American Journal of Speech–Language Pathology, 1*(4), 49–55.

Gottwald, S. R., & Starkweather, C. W. (1984, November). *Stuttering prevention: Rationale and method.* Short course presented at the Annual Convention of the American Speech–Language–Hearing Association, San Francisco, CA. [Abstract published in *Asha, 26* (10), p. 169].

Gottwald, S. R., & Starkweather, C. W. (1995). Fluency intervention for preschoolers and their families in the public schools. *Language, Speech, and Hearing Services in Schools, 26,* 117–126.

Gouge, C. G., & Shapiro, D. A. (1989–1990). A concurrent approach to fluency treatment. *National Student Speech Language Hearing Association Journal, 17,* 72–76.

Gregory, H. H. (1979). Controversial issues: Statement and review of the literature. In H. H. Gregory (Ed.), *Controversies about stuttering therapy* (pp. 1–62). Baltimore, MD: University Park Press.

Gregory, H. H. (1984). Prevention of stuttering: Management of early stages. In R. F. Curlee & W. H. Perkins (Eds.), *Nature and treatment of stuttering: New directions* (pp. 335–355). San Diego, CA: College-Hill.

Gregory, H. H. (1986a). Environmental manipulation and family counseling. In G. H. Shames & H. Rubin (Eds.), *Stuttering then and now* (pp. 271–291). Columbus, OH: Charles E. Merrill.

Gregory, H. H. (1986b). *Stuttering: Differential evaluation and therapy.* Austin, TX: PRO-ED.

Gregory, H. H. (1989). What is involved in therapy? In E. G. Conture & J. Fraser (Eds.), *Stuttering and your child: Questions and answers* [Publication 22] (pp. 43–54). Memphis, TN: Stuttering Foundation of America.

Gregory, H. H. (1995). Analysis and commentary. *Language, Speech, and Hearing Services in Schools, 26,* 196–200.

Guitar, B. (1976). Pretreatment factors associated with the outcome of stuttering therapy. *Journal of Speech and Hearing Research, 19,* 590–600.

Guitar, B. (1997). Therapy for children's stuttering and emotions. In R. F. Curlee & G. M. Siegel (Eds.), *Nature and treatment of stuttering: New directions* (2nd ed.) (pp. 280–291). Needham Heights, MA: Allyn & Bacon.

Guitar, B., & Bass, C. (1978). Stuttering therapy: The relation between attitude change and long-term outcome. *Journal of Speech and Hearing Disorders, 43,* 392–400.

Guitar, B., & Peters, T. J. (1980). *Stuttering: An integration of contemporary therapies.* [Publication 16]. Memphis, TN: Stuttering Foundation of America.

Guyette, T. W., & Baumgartner, J. M. (1988). Stuttering in the adult. In N. J. Lass, L. V. McReynolds, J. L. Northern, & D. E. Yoder (Eds.), *Handbook of speech–language pathology and audiology* (pp. 640–654). Toronto: B. C. Decker.

Hahn, E. F., & Hahn, E. S. (1956). *Stuttering: Significant theories and therapies* (2nd ed.). Stanford, CA: Stanford University Press.

Hall, D. E., Wray, D. F., & Conti, D. M. (1986, Fall). The language-disfluency relationship: A case study. *Hearsay: Journal of the Ohio Speech and Hearing Association,* 110–113.

Hall, P. K. (1977). The occurrence of disfluencies in language-disordered school-age children. *Journal of Speech and Hearing Disorders, 42,* 364–369.

Ham, R. (1986). *Techniques of stuttering therapy.* Englewood Cliffs, NJ: Prentice-Hall.

Ham, R. E. (1990). *Therapy of stuttering: Preschool through adolescence.* Englewood Cliffs, NJ: Prentice-Hall.

Hamayan, E. V., & Damico, J. S. (Eds.). (1991). *Limiting bias in the assessment of bilingual students.* Austin, TX: PRO-ED.

Hartke, R. J. (Ed.). (1991). Introduction. In R. J. Hartke (Ed.), *Psychological aspects of geriatric rehabilitation* (pp. 1–8). Gaithersburg, MD: Aspen.

Hartman, A., & Laird, J. (1983). *Family-centered social work practice.* New York: Free Press/Macmillan.

Haynes, W. O., Pindzola, R. H., & Emerick, L. L. (1992). *Diagnosis and evaluation in speech pathology* (4th ed.). Englewood Cliffs, NJ: Prentice-Hall.

Healey, E. C., & Scott, L. A. (1995). Strategies for treating elementary school-age children who stutter: An integrative approach. *Language, Speech, and Hearing Services in Schools, 26,* 151–161.

Helm, N. A., Butler, R. B., & Canter, G. J. (1980). Neurogenic acquired stuttering. *Journal of Fluency Disorders, 5,* 269–279.

Helm-Estabrooks, N. (1986). Diagnosis and management of neurogenic stuttering in adults. In K. O. St. Louis (Ed.), *The atypical stutterer: Principles and practices of rehabilitation* (pp. 193–217). Orlando, FL: Academic Press.

Helm-Estabrooks, N. (1993). Stuttering associated with acquired neurological disease. In R. F. Curlee (Ed.), *Stuttering and related disorders of fluency* (pp. 205–219). New York: Thieme Medical Publishers.

Helm-Estabrooks, N., Yeo, R., Geschwind, N., Freedman, M., & Weinstein, C. (1986, August). Stuttering: Disappearance and reappearance with acquired brain lesions. *Neurology, 36,* 1109–1112.

Hood, S. B. (1974). Clients, clinicians and therapy. In L. L. Emerick & S. B. Hood (Eds.), *The client–clinician relationship: Essays on interpersonal sensitivity in the therapeutic transaction* (pp. 45–59). Springfield, IL: Charles C. Thomas.

Hooper, C. R. (1996, Winter). Forming a therapeutic alliance with older adults. *Asha, 38*(1), 43–45.

Jewish Publication Society of America. (1965). *The Holy Scriptures* (rev. ed.). Philadelphia, PA: Jewish Publication Society of America/World Publishing.

Jezer, M. (1997). *Stuttering: A life bound up in words.* New York: Basic Books/Harper & Row.

Johnson, B. A., & Mata-Pistokache, T. (1996). Introduction to multicultural issues: Identifying, assessing, and treating children of various cultural backgrounds. In B. A. Johnson, *Language disorders in children: An introductory clinical perspective* (pp. 265–339). Albany, NY: Delmar.

Johnson, E., Sickels, E. R., & Sayers, F. C. (1970). *Anthology of children's literature* (4th ed.). Boston, MA: Houghton Mifflin.

Johnson, W. (1930). *Because I stutter.* New York: D. Appleton & Co.

Johnson, W. (1939). The treatment of stuttering. *The Journal of Speech Disorders, 4,* 170–172.

Johnson, W. (1942). A study of the onset and development of stuttering. *Journal of Speech Disorders, 7,* 251–257.

Johnson, W. (1944). The Indians have no word for it. I. Stuttering in children. *Quarterly Journal of Speech, 30,* 330–337.

Johnson, W. (1958a). Introduction: The six men and the stuttering. In J. Eisenson (Ed.), *Stuttering: A symposium* (pp. xi–xxiv). New York: Harper & Row.

Johnson, W. (1958b). *Toward understanding stuttering.* Chicago, IL: National Society for Crippled Children and Adults.

Johnson, W., & Associates. (1959). *The onset of stuttering: Research findings and implications.* Minneapolis, MN: University of Minnesota Press.

Johnson, W. (1961). *Stuttering and what you can do about it.* Danville, IL: Interstate.

Johnston, J. R. (1983). What is language intervention? The role of theory [Discussion to Part I]. In J. Miller, D. E. Yoder, & R. Schiefelbusch (Eds.), *Contemporary issues in language intervention* [ASHA Reports 12] (pp. 52–57). Rockville, MD: American Speech–Language–Hearing Association.

Karniol, R. (1992). Stuttering out of bilingualism. *First Language, 12,* 255–283.

Kauffman, J. M., & Hallahan, D. P. (Eds.). (1995). *The illusion of full inclusion: A comprehensive critique of a current special education bandwagon.* Austin, TX: PRO-ED.

Kellum, G. D., & Fagan, E. C. (1992). Continuing education. In J. A. Rassi & M. D. McElroy (Eds.), *The education of audiologists and speech–language pathologists* (pp. 409–420). Timonium, MD: York Press.

Kelly, E. M., & Conture, E. G. (1992). Speaking rates, response time latencies, and interrupting behaviors of young stutterers, nonstutterers, and their mothers. *Journal of Speech and Hearing Research, 35,* 1256–1267.

Kelly, G. A. (1955a). *The psychology of personal constructs. Volume One: A theory of personality.* New York: W. W. Norton.

Kelly, G. A. (1955b). *The psychology of personal constructs. Volume Two: Clinical diagnosis and psychotherapy.* New York: W. W. Norton.

Kent, R. D. (1983). Facts about stuttering: Neuropsychologic perspectives. *Journal of Speech and Hearing Disorders, 48,* 249–255.

Kent, R. D. (1989–1990). Fragmentation of clinical service and clinical science in communication disorders. *National Student Speech Language Hearing Association Journal, 17,* 4–16.

Keys, W. T., & Ruder, K. F. (1992, September). A review of commercialized fluency treatment programs (CFTPS). *ECHO* [Official journal of the National Black Association for Speech–Language and Hearing, NBASLH], 14–24.

Kidd, K. K. (1984). Stuttering as a genetic disorder. In R. F. Curlee & W. H. Perkins (Eds.), *Nature and treatment of stuttering: New directions* (pp. 149–169). San Diego, CA: College-Hill.

Klein, H. B., & Moses, N. (1994). *Intervention planning for children with communication disorders: A guide for clinical practicum and professional practice.* Englewood Cliffs, NJ: Prentice-Hall.

Klein, H. B., & Moses, N. (in press). *Intervention planning for adults with communication disorders.* Needham Heights, MA: Allyn & Bacon.

Klingbeil, G. M. (1939). The historical background of the modern speech clinic. *The Journal of Speech Disorders, 4,* 115–132.

Kuhn, T. S. (1970). *The structure of scientific revolutions* (2nd ed.). Chicago, IL: University of Chicago Press [*International Encyclopedia of Unified Science, 2*(2)].

Lass, N. J., Ruscello, D. M., Pannbacker, M. D., Schmitt, J. F., & Everly-Myers, D. S. (1989). Speech–language pathologists' perceptions of child and adult female and male stutterers. *Journal of Fluency Disorders, 14,* 127–134.

Lass, N. J., Ruscello, D. M., Pannbacker, M., Schmitt, J. F., Kiser, A. M., Mussa, A. M., & Lockhart, P. (1994). School administrators' perceptions of people who stutter. *Language, Speech, and Hearing Services in Schools, 25*(2), 90–93.

Lass, N. J., Ruscello, D. M., Schmitt, J. F., Pannbacker, M. D., Orlando, M. B., Dean, K. A., Ruziska, J. C., & Bradshaw, K. H. (1992). Teachers' perceptions of stutterers. *Language, Speech, and Hearing Services in Schools, 23*(1), 78–81.

Lazarus, A. A., & Fay, A. (1975). *I can if I think I can.* New York: Warner Books.

Leith, W. R. (1986). Treating the stutterer with atypical cultural influences. In K. O. St. Louis (Ed.), *The atypical stutterer: Principles and practices of rehabilitation* (pp. 9–34). Orlando, FL: Academic Press.

Lew, E. (1995, July/August). My stuttering saved my life. *Letting Go.* Anaheim Hills, CA: National Stuttering Project.

Lewis, G. A. (1899). *The origin and treatment of stammering.* Detroit, MI: Phono-Meter Press.

Lichtheim, M. (1973). *Ancient Egyptian literature: A book of readings* (Vol. I: The old and middle kingdoms). Berkeley: University of California Press.

Liles, B. Z., Lerman, J., Christensen, L., & St. Ledger, J. (1992). A case description of verbal and signed disfluencies of a 10-year-old boy who is retarded. *Language, Speech, and Hearing Services in Schools, 23,* 107–112.

Lohr, J. B., & Wisniewski, A. A. (1987). *Movement disorders: A neuropsychiatric approach.* New York: Guilford Press.

Lopez, O. L., Becker, J. T., Dew, M. A., Banks, G., Dorst, S. K., & McNeil, M. (1994, November). Speech motor control disorder after HIV infection. *Neurology, 44,* 2187–2189.

Lougeay-Mottinger, J., Harris, M. R., Perlstein-Kaplan, K. E., & Felicetti, T. (1984). UTD competency based evaluation system. *Asha, 26* (11), 39–43.

Louko, L. J., Edwards, M. L., & Conture, E. G. (1990). Phonological characteristics of young stutterers and their normally fluent peers: Preliminary observations. *Journal of Fluency Disorders, 15,* 191–210.

Ludlow, C. L., & Braun, A. (1993). Research evaluating the use of neuropharmacological agents for treating stuttering: Possibilities and problems. *Journal of Fluency Disorders, 18,* 169–182.

Luper, H. L. (Ed.). (1968). *Stuttering: Successes and failures in therapy.* [Publication 6]. Memphis, TN: Stuttering Foundation of America.

Luper, H. L., & Mulder, R. L. (1964). *Stuttering: Therapy for children.* Englewood Cliffs, NJ: Prentice-Hall.

Luterman, D. M. (1996). *Counseling persons with communication disorders and their families* (3rd ed.). Austin, TX: PRO-ED.

MacFarlane, W. B., Hanson, M., Walton, W., & Mellon, C. D. (1991). Stuttering in five generations of a single family: A preliminary report including evidence supporting a sex-modified mode of transmission. *Journal of Fluency Disorders, 16,* 117–123.

MacNeil, R. D., & Teague, M. L. (1987). *Aging and leisure: Vitality in later life.* Englewood Cliffs, NJ: Prentice-Hall.

Mahr, G., & Leith, W. (1992). Psychogenic stuttering of adult onset. *Journal of Speech and Hearing Research, 35,* 283–286.

Mallard, A. R., Gardner, L. S., & Downey, C. S. (1988). Clinical training in stuttering for school clinicians. *Journal of Fluency Disorders, 13,* 253–259.

Manning, W. H. (1991). Making progress during and after treatment. In W. H. Perkins (Ed.), *Seminars in Speech and Language, 12* (pp. 349–354). New York: Thieme Medical Publishers.

Manning, W. H. (1996). *Clinical decision making in the diagnosis and treatment of fluency disorders.* Albany, NY: Delmar.

Manning, W. H., Dailey, D., & Wallace, S. (1984). Attitude and personality characteristics of older stutterers. *Journal of Fluency Disorders, 9,* 207–215.

Manning, W. H., & Monte, K. L. (1981). Fluency breaks in older speakers: Implications for a model of stuttering throughout the life cycle. *Journal of Fluency Disorders, 6,* 35–48.

Manning, W. H., & Shirkey, E. A. (1981). Fluency and the aging process. In D. S. Beasley & G. A. Davis (Eds.), *Aging: Communication processes and disorders* (pp. 175–189). New York: Grune & Stratton.

May, H. G., & Metzger, B. M. (1962). *The Holy Bible: Revised standard version containing the Old and New Testaments.* New York: Oxford University Press.

McCarthy, M. M. (1981). Speech effect of theophylline. [Letter]. *Pediatrics, 68*(5), 749–750.

McCrea, E. S. (1980). Supervisee ability to self-explore and four facilitative dimensions of supervisor behavior in individual conferences in speech–language pathology (Doctoral dissertation, Indiana University, 1980). *Dissertation Abstracts International, 41,* 2134B.

McCready, V., Shapiro, D., & Kennedy, K. (1987). Identifying hidden dynamics in supervision: Four scenarios. In M. B. Crago & M. Pickering (Eds.), *Supervision in human communication disorders: Perspectives on a process* (pp. 169–201). Boston, MA: Little, Brown/College-Hill.

McGoldrick, M., & Carter, E. A. (1982). The family life cycle. In F. Walsh (Ed.), *Normal family processes* (pp. 167–195). New York: Guilford Press.

McGonigel, M. J., & Garland, C. W. (1988). The individualized family service plan and the early intervention team: Team and family issues and recommended practices. *Infants and Young Children, 1*(1), 10–21.

McLuhan, M. (1964). *Understanding media: The extensions of man.* New York: McGraw-Hill.

McLuhan, M., & Fiore, Q. (1967). *The medium is the massage.* New York: Random House.

Meltzer, A. (1992). Horn stuttering. *Journal of Fluency Disorders, 17,* 257–264.

Merrill, J. C., & Lowenstein, R. L. (1971). *Media, messages, and men: New perspectives in communication.* New York: David McKay.

Messick, S. (1980). Test validity and the ethics of assessment. *American Psychologist, 35*(11), 1012–1027.

Meyers, S. C., & Freeman, F. J. (1985a). Interruptions as a variable in stuttering and disfluency. *Journal of Speech and Hearing Research, 28,* 428–435.

Meyers, S. C., & Freeman, F. J. (1985b). Mother and child speech rates as a variable in stuttering and disfluency. *Journal of Speech and Hearing Research, 28,* 436–444.

Miller, A. (1990). *Banished knowledge: Facing childhood injuries.* [Translation]. New York: Doubleday.

Minuchin, S. (1974). *Families and family therapy.* Cambridge, MA: Harvard University Press.

Minuchin, S., & Fishman, H. C. (1981). *Family therapy techniques.* Cambridge, MA: Harvard University Press.

Montgomery, B. M., & Fitch, J. L. (1988). The prevalence of stuttering in the hearing-impaired school age population. *Journal of Speech and Hearing Disorders, 53,* 131–135.

Moscicki, E. K. (1984, August). The prevalence of 'incidence' is too high. *Asha, 26*(8), 39–40.

Moses, N., & Shapiro, D. A. (1992). Assessing and facilitating clinical problem solving in the supervisory process. In S. Dowling (Ed.), *Total quality supervision: Effecting optimal performance.* [Proceedings of the 1992 national conference on supervision]. (pp. 70–77). Houston, TX: University of Houston.

Moses, N., & Shapiro, D. A. (1996). A developmental conceptualization of clinical problem solving. *Journal of Communication Disorders, 29,* 199–221.

Muma, J. (1978). Connell, Spradlin, & McReynolds: Right but wrong! [Letter]. *Journal of Speech and Hearing Disorders, 43,* 549–552.

Murphy, A. T. (1974). The quiet hyena: Two monologues in search of a dialogue. In L. L. Emerick & S. B. Hood (Eds.), *The client–clinician relationship: Essays on interpersonal sensitivity in the therapeutic transaction* (pp. 29–44). Springfield, IL: Charles C. Thomas.

Murphy, A. T., & FitzSimons, R. M. (1960). *Stuttering and personality dynamics: Play therapy, projective therapy, and counseling.* New York: Ronald Press.

Murray, F. P., & Edwards, S. G. (1980). *A stutterer's story.* Danville, IL: Interstate.

Myers, J. E., & Schwiebert, V. L. (1996). *Competencies for gerontological counseling.* Alexandria, VA: American Counseling Association.

Nellum-Davis, P. (1993). Clinical practice issues. In D. E. Battle (Ed.), *Communication disorders in multicultural populations* (pp. 306–316). Stoneham, MA: Andover Medical/Butterworth-Heinemann.

Nichols, K. (1987). *Feelings of Western Carolina University students toward stutterers and stuttering.* Unpublished manuscript. Cullowhee, NC: Western Carolina University.

Nicolosi, L., Harryman, E., & Kresheck, J. (1996). *Terminology of Communication Disorders: Speech–Language–Hearing* (4th ed.). Baltimore, MD: Williams & Wilkins.

Nippold, M. A. (1990). Concomitant speech and language disorders in stuttering children: A critique of the literature. *Journal of Speech and Hearing Disorders, 55,* 51–60.

Nurnberg, H. G., & Greenwald, B. (1981). Stuttering: An unusual side effect of phenothiazines. *American Journal of Psychiatry, 138*(3), 386–387.

Ogletree, B. T., & Daniels, D. B. (1995). Communication-based assessment and intervention for prelinguistic infants and toddlers: Strategies and issues. In J. A. Blackman (Ed.), *Identification and assessment in early intervention* (pp. 222–234). Gaithersburg, MD: Aspen.

Ogletree, B. T., Saddler, Y. N., & Bowers, L. S. (1995). Speech–language pathology. In B. A. Thyer & N. P. Kropf (Eds.), *Developmental disabilities: A handbook for interdisciplinary practice* (pp. 217–233). Cambridge, MA: Brookline Books.

Parker, G. (1979). Parental characteristics in relation to depressive disorders. *British Journal of Psychiatry, 134,* 138–147.

Paul, R. (1995). *Language disorders from infancy through adolescence: Assessment and intervention.* St. Louis, MO: Mosby.

Pauls, D. L., Leckman, J. F., & Cohen, D. J. (1993). Familial relationship between Gilles de la Tourette's Syndrome, attention deficit disorder, learning disabilities, speech disorders, and stuttering. *Journal of the American Academy of Child and Adolescent Psychiatry, 32*(5), 1044–1050.

Peacher, W. G., & Harris, W. E. (1946). Speech disorders in World War II: VIII. Stuttering. *Journal of Speech Disorders, 11,* 303–308.

Perkins, W. H. (1973a). Replacement of stuttering with normal speech: I. Rationale. *Journal of Speech and Hearing Disorders, 38,* 283–294.

Perkins, W. H. (1973b). Replacement of stuttering with normal speech: II. Clinical procedures. *Journal of Speech and Hearing Disorders, 38,* 295–303.

Perkins, W. H. (1978). *Human perspectives in speech and language disorders.* St. Louis, MO: Mosby.

Perkins, W. H. (1979). From psychoanalysis to discoordination. In H. H. Gregory (Ed.), *Controversies about stuttering therapy* (pp. 97–127). Baltimore, MD: University Park Press.

Perkins, W. H. (1983). Stuttering vs. fluency. In J. F. Gruss (Ed.), *Counseling stutterers* [Publication 18] (pp. 59–68). Memphis, TN: Stuttering Foundation of America.

Perkins, W. H. (1984). An alternative to automatic fluency. In J. F. Gruss (Ed.), *Stuttering therapy: Transfer and maintenance* [Publication 19] (pp. 63–74). Memphis, TN: Stuttering Foundation of America.

Perkins, W. H. (1990a). What is stuttering? *Journal of Speech and Hearing Disorders, 55,* 370–382.

Perkins, W. H. (1990b). Gratitude, good intentions, and red herrings: A response to commentaries. *Journal of Speech and Hearing Disorders, 55,* 402–404.

Perkins, W. H., Rudas, J., Johnson, L., Michael, W. B., & Curlee, R. F. (1974). Replacement of stuttering with normal speech: III. Clinical effectiveness. *Journal of Speech and Hearing Disorders, 39,* 416–428.

Peters, H. F. M., & Starkweather, C. W. (1989). Development of stuttering throughout life. *Journal of Fluency Disorders, 14,* 303–321.

Peters, T. J., & Guitar, B. (1991). *Stuttering: An integrated approach to its nature and treatment.* Baltimore, MD: Williams & Wilkins.

Pickering, M. (1984). Interpersonal communication in speech–language pathology supervisory conferences: A qualitative study. *Journal of Speech and Hearing Disorders, 49,* 189–195.

Pindzola, R. H., Jenkins, M. M., & Lokken, K. J. (1989). Speaking rates of young children. *Language, Speech, and Hearing Services in Schools, 20*(2), 133–138.

Pindzola, R. H., & White, D. T. (1986). A protocol for differentiating the incipient stutterer. *Language, Speech, and Hearing Services in Schools, 17*(1), 2–15.

Post, J. G., & Leith, W. R. (1983). I'd rather tell a story than be one. *Asha, 25* (4), 23–26.

Prins, D. (1993). Management of stuttering: Treatment of adolescents and adults. In R. F. Curlee (Ed.), *Stuttering and related disorders of fluency* (pp. 115–138). New York: Thieme Medical Publishers.

Prutting, C. A. (1985). The long battle for the light. *National Student Speech Language Hearing Association Journal, 13,* 5–9.

Quader, S. E. (1977). Dysarthria: An unusual side effect of tricyclic antidepressants. *British Medical Journal, 2,* 97.

Quinn, P. T., & Andrews, G. (1977). Neurological stuttering—A clinical entity? *Journal of Neurology, Neurosurgery, and Psychiatry, 40,* 699–701.

Quinn, P. T., & Peachey, E. C. (1973). Haloperidol in the treatment of stutterers. [Letter]. *British Journal of Psychiatry, 123,* 247–248.

Ragsdale, J. D., & Ashby, J. K. (1982). Speech–language pathologists' connotations of stuttering. *Journal of Speech and Hearing Research, 25,* 75–80.

Rakowski, W., & Pearlman, D. N. (1995). Demographic aspects of aging: Current and future trends. In W. Reichel (Ed.), *Care of the elderly: Clinical aspects of aging* (4th ed.) (pp. 488–495). Baltimore, MD: Williams & Wilkins.

Ramig, P. R. (1993). Parent–clinician–child partnership in the therapeutic process of the preschool- and elementary-aged child who stutters. *Seminars in Speech and Language, 14*(3), 226–237.

Ramig, P. R., & Bennett, E. M. (1995). Working with 7- to 12-year-old children who stutter: Ideas for intervention in the public schools. *Language, Speech, and Hearing Services in Schools, 26,* 138–150.

Rassi, J. A., & McElroy, M. D. (1992). Epilogue: Integration of person and process. In J. A. Rassi & M. D. McElroy (Eds.), *The education of audiologists and speech–language pathologists* (pp. 443–445). Timonium, MD: York Press.

Ratner, N. B. (1995). Treating the child who stutters with concomitant language or phonological impairment. *Language, Speech, and Hearing Services in Schools, 26,* 180–186.

Ratner, N. B., & Benitez, M. (1985). Linguistic analysis of a bilingual stutterer. *Journal of Fluency Disorders, 10,* 211–219.

Riley, G. D. (1994). *Stuttering severity instrument for children and adults* (3rd ed.) [SSI–3, Test Record and Frequency Computation Form]. Austin, TX: PRO-ED.

Ripich, D. N. (1991). Preface. In D. N. Ripich (Ed.), *Handbook of geriatric communication disorders* (pp. xi–xii). Austin, TX: PRO-ED.

Rivara, J. B., Jaffe, K. M., Fay, G. C., Polissar, N. L., Martin, K. M., Shurtleff, H. A., & Liao, S. (1993). Family functioning and injury severity as predictors of child functioning one year following traumatic brain injury. *Archives of Physical Medicine and Rehabilitation, 74,* 1047–1055.

Roberts, J. E., & Smith, K. J. (1982). Supervisor-supervisee role differences and consistency of behavior in supervisory conferences. *Journal of Speech and Hearing Research, 25,* 428–434.

Rogers, C. R. (1957). The necessary and sufficient conditions of therapeutic personality change. *Journal of Consulting Psychology, 21,* 95–103.

Rogers, C. R. (1961). *On becoming a person.* Boston, MA: Houghton Mifflin.

Rokusek, C. (1995). An introduction to the concept of interdisciplinary practice. In B. A. Thyer & N. P. Kropf (Eds.), *Developmental disabilities: A handbook for interdisciplinary practice* (pp. 1–12). Cambridge, MA: Brookline Books.

Rollin, W. J. (1987). *The psychology of communication disorders in individuals and their families.* Englewood Cliffs, NJ: Prentice-Hall.

Rosenbek, J. C. (1984). Stuttering secondary to nervous system damage. In R. F. Curlee & W. H. Perkins (Eds.), *Nature and treatment of stuttering: New directions* (pp. 31–48). San Diego, CA: College-Hill.

Rosenbek, J. C., McNeil, M. R., Lemme, M. L., Prescott, T. E., & Alfrey, A. C. (1975). Speech and language findings in a chronic hemodialysis patient: A case report. *Journal of Speech and Hearing Disorders, 40,* 245–252.

Rosenbek, J., Messert, B., Collins, M., & Wertz, R. T. (1978). Stuttering following brain damage. *Brain and Language, 6,* 82–96.

Rosenfield, D. B., & Nudelman, H. B. (1991). Fluency, dysfluency, and aging. In D. N. Ripich (Ed.), *Handbook of geriatric communication disorders* (pp. 227–238). Austin, TX: PRO-ED.

Rosenshine, B., & Furst, N. (1971). Research on teacher performance criteria. In B. O. Smith (Ed.), *Research in teacher education: A symposium* (pp. 37–72). Englewood Cliffs, NJ: Prentice-Hall.

Rosenshine, B., & Furst, N. (1973). The use of direct observation to study teaching. In R. M. W. Travers (Ed.), *Second handbook of research on teaching* (pp. 122–183). Chicago, IL: Rand McNally & Co.

Roth, C. R., Aronson, A. E., & Davis, L. J., Jr. (1989). Clinical studies in psychogenic stuttering of adult onset. *Journal of Speech and Hearing Disorders, 54,* 634–646.

Rubin, I. L. (1995). Forward. In B. A. Thyer & N. P. Kroph (Eds.), *Developmental disabilities: A handbook for interdisciplinary practice* (pp. v–viii). Cambridge, MA: Brookline Books.

Ruscello, D. M., Lass, N. J., & Brown, J. (1988). College students' perceptions of stutterers. *National Student Speech Language Hearing Association Journal, 16,* 115–120.

Rush, W. L., & The League of Human Dignity. (not dated). *Write with dignity: Reporting on people with disabilities.* Lincoln, NE: Hitchcock Center.

Rustin, L. (1987). The treatment of childhood dysfluency through active parental involvement. In L. Rustin, H. Purser, & D. Rowley (Eds.), *Progress in the treatment of fluency disorders* (pp. 166–180). London, England: Taylor & Francis.

Rustin, L., Botterill, W., & Kelman, E. (1996). *Assessment and therapy for young dysfluent children: Family interaction.* San Diego, CA: Singular.

Rustin, L., & Purser, H. (1991). Child development, families, and the problem of stuttering. In L. Rustin (Ed.), *Parents, families, and the stuttering child* (pp. 1–24). San Diego, CA: Singular.

Ryan, B. P. (1974). *Programmed therapy for stuttering in children and adults.* Springfield, IL: Charles C. Thomas.

Ryan, B. P. (1992). Articulation, language, rate, and fluency characteristics of stuttering and non-stuttering preschool children. *Journal of Speech and Hearing Research, 35,* 333–342.

Ryan, B. P., & Van Kirk, B. (1971). *Programmed conditioning for fluency: Program book.* Monterey, CA: Behavioral Sciences Institute.

Satir, V. (1967). *Conjoint family therapy: A guide to theory and technique* (Revised ed.). Palo Alto, CA: Science and Behavior Books.

Scahill, L., Lynch, K. A., & Ort, S. I. (1995). Tourette Syndrome: Update and review. *Journal of School Nursing, 11*(2), 26–32.

Scheuerle, J. (1992). *Counseling in speech–language pathology and audiology.* New York: Merrill/Macmillan.

Schubert, G. W., Miner, A. L., & Till, J. A. (1973). *The analysis of behavior of clinicians (ABC) system.* Unpublished manuscript, University of North Dakota, Grand Forks.

Schulz, J. B. (1993). Heroes in disguise. In A. P. Turnbull, J. M. Patterson, S. K. Behr, D. L. Murphy, J. G. Marquis, & M. J. Blue-Banning (Eds.), *Cognitive coping, families, and disability* (pp. 31–41). Baltimore, MD: Brookes.

Schwartz, H. D. (1993). Adolescents who stutter. *Journal of Fluency Disorders, 18,* 289–302.

Schwartz, H. D., & Conture, E. G. (1988). Subgrouping young stutterers: Preliminary behavioral observations. *Journal of Speech and Hearing Research, 31,* 62–71.

Schwartz, H. D., Zebrowski, P. M., & Counture, E. G. (1990). Behaviors at the onset of stuttering. *Journal of Fluency Disorders, 15,* 77–86.

Screen, R. M., & Anderson, N. B. (1994). *Multicultural perspectives in communication disorders.* San Diego, CA: Singular.

Seeley, J. U. (Underwood). (1973). Interaction analysis between the supervisor and the speech and hearing clinician (Doctoral dissertation, University of Denver, 1973). *Dissertation Abstracts International, 34,* 2995B.

Shadden, B. B. (1988). Communication and aging: An overview. In B. B. Shadden (Ed.), *Communication behavior and aging: A sourcebook for clinicians* (pp. 3–11). Baltimore, MD: Williams & Wilkins.

Shames, G. H. (1975). Operant conditioning and stuttering. In J. Eisenson (Ed.), *Stuttering: A second symposium* (pp. 263–332). New York: Harper & Row.

Shames, G. H., & Florance, C. L. (1980). *Stutter-free speech: A goal for therapy.* Columbus, OH: Charles E. Merrill.

Shames, G. H., & Rubin, H. (Eds.). (1986). *Stuttering then and now.* Columbus, OH: Charles E. Merrill.

Shapiro, D. A. (1985). Clinical Supervision: A process in progress. *National Student Speech Language Hearing Association Journal, 13,* 89–108.

Shapiro, D. A. (1987, Fall). Myths in the method to the madness of supervision. *Hearsay: Journal of the Ohio Speech and Hearing Association,* 78–83.

Shapiro, D. A. (1994a). Interaction analysis and self-study: A single-case comparison of four methods of analyzing supervisory conferences. *Language, Speech, and Hearing Services in Schools, 25,* 67–75

Shapiro, D. A. (1994b). Tender gender issues. *Asha, 36*(11), 46–49.

Shapiro, D. A. (1995, March). A way through the forest: One boy's story with a happy ending. *The Staff,* pp. 2, 7. (Available from Aaron's Associates, 6114 Waterway, Garland, TX 75043; Reprinted from *Letting Go Jr.,* 1988, *2*(3), pp. 4, 7).

Shapiro, D. A. (in press). Stuttering and spider stories: Intervention planning with adults who stutter. In H. B. Klein & N. Moses (Eds.), *Intervention planning for adults with communication disorders.* Needham Heights, MA: Allyn & Bacon.

Shapiro, D. A., & Anderson, J. L. (1988). An analysis of commitments made by student clinicians in speech–language pathology and audiology. *Journal of Speech and Hearing Disorders, 53,* 202–210.

Shapiro, D. A., & Anderson, J. L. (1989). One measure of supervisory effectiveness in speech–language pathology and audiology. *Journal of Speech and Hearing Disorders, 54,* 549–557.

Shapiro, D. A., Brotherton, W. D., & Ogletree, B. T. (1995). The graduate student with marginal abilities in communication disorders: Concept and intervention strategies. *The Supervisors' Forum, 2,* 64–70.

Shapiro, D. A., & Moses, N. (1989). Creative problem solving in public school supervision. *Language, Speech, and Hearing Services in Schools, 20,* 320–332.

Sheehan, J. (1958). Conflict theory of stuttering. In J. Eisenson (Ed.), *Stuttering: A symposium* (pp. 121–166). New York: Harper & Row.

Sheehan, J. G. (1970). *Stuttering: Research and therapy.* New York: Harper & Row.

Sheehan, J. G. (1975). Conflict theory and avoidance-reduction therapy. In J. Eisenson (Ed.), *Stuttering: A second symposium* (pp. 97–198). New York: Harper & Row.

Sheehy, G. (1976). *Passages: Predictable crises of adult life.* New York: E. P. Dutton & Co.

Shine, R. E. (1980). Direct management of the beginning stutterer. In W. Perkins (Ed.), *Seminars in Speech, Language and Hearing* [Strategies in Stuttering Therapy, Vol. 1, No. 4] (pp. 339–350). New York: Thieme-Stratton.

Shine, R. E. (1984). Assessment and fluency training with the young stutterer. In M. Peins (Ed.), *Contemporary approaches in stuttering therapy* (pp. 173–216). Boston, MA: Little, Brown.

Shipley, K. G., & McAfee, J. G. (1992). *Assessment in speech–language pathology: A resource manual.* San Diego, CA: Singular.

Shirkey, E. A. (1987). Forensic verification of stuttering. *Journal of Fluency Disorders, 12,* 197–203.

Shriberg, L. D., Filley, F. S., Hayes, D. M., Kwiatkowski, J., Schatz, J. A., Simmons, K. M., & Smith, M. E. (1975). The Wisconsin procedure for appraisal of clinical competence (W–PACC): Model and data. *Asha, 17,* 158–165.

Siegel, G. M. (1990). Moses the stutterer: An interpretation of Deuteronomy 3:23. In J. Albach (Ed.), *To say what is ours: The best of ten years of Letting Go* (pp. VII-7–VII-12). San Francisco, CA: National Stuttering Project.

Silverman, E.-M. (1982). Speech–language clinicians' and university students' impressions of women and girls who stutter. *Journal of Fluency Disorders, 7,* 469–478.

Silverman, F. H. (1988). The "monster" study. *Journal of Fluency Disorders, 13,* 225–231.

Silverman, F. H. (1996). *Stuttering and other fluency disorders* (2nd ed.). Needham Heights, MA: Allyn & Bacon.

Silverman, F. H., & Bohlman, P. (1988). Flute stuttering. *Journal of Fluency Disorders, 13,* 427–428.

Silverman, F. H., & Silverman, E.-M. (1971, August). Stutter-like behavior in the manual communication of the deaf. *Perceptual and Motor Skills, 33,* 45–46.

Smith, K. J. (1978). Identification of perceived effectiveness components in the individual supervisory conference in speech pathology and an evaluation of the relationship between ratings and content in the conferences (Doctoral dissertation, Indiana University, 1977). *Dissertation Abstracts International, 39,* 680B.

Smith, K. J., & Anderson, J. L. (1982a). Development and validation of an individual supervisory conference rating scale for use in speech–language pathology. *Journal of Speech and Hearing Research, 25,* 243–251.

Smith, K. J., & Anderson, J. L. (1982b). Relationship of perceived effectiveness to verbal interaction/content variables in supervisory conferences in speech–language pathology. *Journal of Speech and Hearing Research, 25,* 252–261.

Sokoly, M. M., & Dokecki, P. R. (1992). Ethical perspectives on family-centered early intervention. *Infants and Young Children, 4*(4), 23–32.

Sommers, R. K., & Caruso, A. J. (1995). Inservice training in speech–language pathology: Are we meeting the needs for fluency training? *American Journal of Speech–Language Pathology, 4*(3), 22–28.

Starkweather, C. W. (1984). On fluency. *National Student Speech Language Hearing Association Journal, 12,* 30–37.

Starkweather, C. W. (1985). The development of fluency in normal children. In H. H. Gregory (Ed.), *Stuttering therapy: Prevention and intervention with children* [Publication 20] (pp. 67–100). Memphis, TN: Stuttering Foundation of America.

Starkweather, C. W. (1987). *Fluency and stuttering.* Englewood Cliffs, NJ: Prentice-Hall.

Starkweather, C. W. (1993). Issues in the efficacy of treatment for fluency disorders. *Journal of Fluency Disorders, 18,* 151–168.

Starkweather, C. W. (1997). Therapy for younger children. In R. F. Curlee & G. M. Siegel (Eds.), *Nature and treatment of stuttering: New directions* (2nd ed.) (pp. 257–279). Needham Heights, MA: Allyn & Bacon.

Starkweather, C. W., & Bishop, J. (1994). *Required practicum hours in fluency: A survey of training supervisors.* [Report to the Council on Professional Standards]. Rockville, MD: American Speech–Language–Hearing Association.

Starkweather, C. W., & Givens-Ackerman, J. (1997). *Stuttering.* Austin, TX: PRO-ED.

Starkweather, C. W., Gottwald, S. R., & Halfond, M. M. (1990). *Stuttering prevention: A clinical method.* Englewood Cliffs, NJ: Prentice-Hall.

St. Louis, K. O. (Ed.). (1996). Research and opinion on cluttering: State of the art and science. *Journal of Fluency Disorders, 21,* 171–371.

St. Louis, K. O., & Durrenberger, C. H. (1993, December). What communication disorders do experienced clinicians prefer to manage? *Asha, 35,* 23–31.

St. Louis, K. O., & Hinzman, A. R. (1986). Studies of cluttering: Perceptions of cluttering by speech–language pathologists and educators. *Journal of Fluency Disorders, 11,* 131–149.

St. Louis, K. O., Hinzman, A. R., & Hull, F. M. (1985). Studies of cluttering: Disfluency and language measures in young possible clutterers and stutterers. *Journal of Fluency Disorders, 10,* 151–172.

St. Louis, K. O., & Lass, N. J. (1981). A survey of communicative disorders students' attitudes toward stuttering. *Journal of Fluency Disorders, 6,* 49–79.

St. Louis, K. O., & Myers, F. L. (1997). Management of cluttering and related fluency disorders. In R. F. Curlee & G. M. Siegel (Eds.), *Nature and treatment of stuttering: New directions* (2nd ed.) (pp. 313–332). Needham Heights, MA: Allyn & Bacon.

Stoneman, Z., & Malone, D. M. (1995). The changing nature of interdisciplinary practice. In B. A. Thyer & N. P. Kropf (Eds.), *Developmental disabilities: A handbook for interdisciplinary practice* (pp. 234–247). Cambridge, MA: Brookline Books.

Tapia, F. (1969). Haldol in the treatment of children with tics and stutterers—and an incidental finding. *Psychiatric Quarterly, 43,* 647–649.

Taylor, O. L. (1986). Historical perspectives and conceptual framework. In O. L. Taylor (Ed.), *Treatment of communication disorders in culturally and linguistically diverse populations* (pp. 3–19). San Diego, CA: College-Hill.

Taylor, O. L. (1993). Forward. In D. E. Battle (Ed.), *Communication disorders in multicultural populations* (pp. xii–xiii). Stoneham, MA: Andover Medical Publishers/Butterworth-Heinemann.

Taylor, O. L., & Clarke, M. G. (1994). Culture and communication disorders: A theoretical framework. *Seminars in Speech and Language, 15*(2), 103–113.

Terry, W. (1994). When his sound was silenced. *Parade Magazine,* December 25, 12–13.

Thyer, B. A., & Kropf, N. P. (1995). Preface. In B. A. Thyer & N. P. Kropf (Eds.), *Developmental disabilities: A handbook for interdisciplinary practice* (pp. i–iii). Cambridge, MA: Brookline Books.

Tiger, R. J., Irvine, T. L., & Reis, R. P. (1980). Cluttering as a complex of learning disabilities. *Language, Speech, and Hearing Services in Schools, 11*(1), 3–14.

Tillis, M., & Wagner, W. (1984). *Stutterin' boy.* New York: Rawson Associates.

Tolchard, B. (1995). Treatment of Gilles de la Tourette Syndrome using behavioural psychotherapy: A single case example. *Journal of Psychiatric and Mental Health Nursing, 2*(4), 233–236.

Travis, L. E. (1971). The unspeakable feelings of people with special reference to stuttering. In L. E. Travis (Ed.), *Handbook of Speech Pathology and Audiology* (pp. 1009–1033). Englewood Cliffs, NJ: Prentice-Hall.

Travis, L. E. (1978). The cerebral dominance theory of stuttering: 1931–1978. *Journal of Speech and Hearing Disorders, 43,* 278–281.

Tudor, M. (1939). *An experimental study of the effect of evaluative labeling on speech fluency.* Unpublished master's thesis, University of Iowa.

Turnbaugh, K. R., Guitar, B. E., & Hoffman, P. R. (1979). Speech clinicians' attribution of personality traits as a function of stuttering severity. *Journal of Speech and Hearing Research, 22,* 37–45.

Turnbull, A. P., Patterson, J. M., Behr, S. K., Murphy, D. L., Marquis, J. G., & Blue-Banning, M. J. (Eds.). (1993). *Cognitive coping, families, and disability.* Baltimore, MD: Brookes.

Turnbull, A. P., & Turnbull, H. R., III. (1990). *Families, professionals, and exceptionality: A special partnership* (2nd ed.). Columbus, OH: Merrill.

Underwood, J. K. (1979). *Underwood category system for analyzing supervisor–clinician behavior.* Unpublished manuscript, University of Northern Colorado, Greeley.

United States Bureau of the Census. (1990). *Statistical abstract of the United States—1990: The national data book* (110th ed.). Washington, DC: United States Department of Commerce/Government Printing Office.

Van Riper, C. (1965). Supervision of clinical practice. *Asha, 7,* 75–77.

Van Riper, C. (1972). *Speech correction: Principles and methods* (5th ed.). Englewood Cliffs, NJ: Prentice-Hall.

Van Riper, C. (1973). *The treatment of stuttering.* Englewood Cliffs, NJ: Prentice-Hall.

Van Riper, C. (1974). Success and failure in speech therapy. In L. L. Emerick & S. B. Hood (Eds.), *The client–clinician relationship: Essays on interpersonal sensitivity in the therapeutic transaction* (pp. 103–106). Springfield, IL: Charles C. Thomas. [Reprinted from *Journal of Speech and Hearing Disorders,* 1966, *31,* pp. 276–279].

Van Riper, C. (1975). The stutterer's clinician. In J. Eisenson (Ed.), *Stuttering: A second symposium* (pp. 453–492). New York: Harper & Row.

Van Riper, C. (1982). *The nature of stuttering* (2nd ed.). Englewood Cliffs, NJ: Prentice-Hall.

Van Riper, C. (1991). Some ancient history. *Journal of Fluency Disorders, 17,* 25–28.

Van Riper, C., & Erickson, R. L. (1996). *Speech correction: An introduction to speech pathology and audiology* (9th ed.). Needham Heights, MA: Allyn & Bacon.

Villa, R. A., & Thousand, J. S. (Eds.). (1995). *Creating an inclusive school.* Alexandria, VA: Association for Supervision and Curriculum Development.

Vinnard, R. T. (1990a, January). AIDS-related acquired stuttering. *Quo Vadis, 2*(2), 6. [Newsletter of the Center for Fluent Speech, 42388 Avenue Eleven, Madera, CA 93638, phone: 209-439-2533].

Vinnard, R. T. (1990b, September). Dr. Comings writes on Tourette's [Editorial comment]. *Quo Vadis, 2*(5), 1, 3. [Newsletter of the Center for Fluent Speech, 42388 Avenue Eleven, Madera, CA 93638, phone: 209-439-2533].

Wall, M. J., & Myers, F. L. (1995). *Clinical management of childhood stuttering* (2nd ed.). Austin, TX: PRO-ED.

Walle, E. L. (1974). A journey in experiences in interpersonal relations with sociopathic criminals. In L. L. Emerick & S. B. Hood (Eds.), *The client–clinician relationship: Essays on interpersonal sensitivity in the therapeutic transaction* (pp. 3–28). Springfield, IL: Charles C. Thomas.

Walle, E. L. (1976). Prevention of stuttering [Part 1]: Identifying the danger signs. [Film/Videotape]. Memphis, TN: Stuttering Foundation of America.

Wallen, V. (1961). Primary stuttering in a 28-year-old adult. *Journal of Speech and Hearing Disorders, 26,* 394–395.

Wand, R. R., Matazow, G. S., Shady, G. A., Furer, P., & Staley, D. (1993). Tourette Syndrome: Associated symptoms and most disabling features. *Neuroscience and Biobehavioral Reviews, 17*(3), 271–275.

Watson, J. B. (1995). Exploring the attitudes of adults who stutter. *Journal of Communication Disorders, 28,* 143–164.

Webster, E. J. (1977). *Counseling with parents of handicapped children: Guidelines for improving communication.* New York: Grune & Stratton.

Webster, R. L. (1979). Empirical considerations regarding stuttering therapy. In H. H. Gregory (Ed.), *Controversies about stuttering therapy* (pp. 209–239). Baltimore, MD: University Park Press.

Weiner, A. E. (1981). A case of adult onset of stuttering. *Journal of Fluency Disorders, 6,* 181–186.

Weiss, D. A. (1964). *Cluttering.* Englewood Cliffs, NJ: Prentice-Hall.

Weller, R. H. (1971). *Verbal communication in instructional supervision: An observational system for and research study of clinical supervision in groups.* New York: Teachers College Press, Columbia University.

Wells, P. G., & Malcolm, M. T. (1971). Controlled trial of the treatment of 36 stutterers. *British Journal of Psychiatry, 119,* 603–604.

West, R. (1958). An agnostic's speculations about stuttering. In J. Eisenson (Ed.), *Stuttering: A symposium* (pp. 167–222). New York: Harper & Row.

Westby, C. E. (1994). Multicultural issues. In J. B. Tomblin, H. L. Morris, & D. C. Spriestersbach (Eds.), *Diagnosis in speech–language pathology* (pp. 29–51). San Diego, CA: Singular.

Wexler, K. B. (1982). Developmental disfluency in 2-, 4-, and 6-year-old boys in neutral and stress situations. *Journal of Speech and Hearing Research, 25,* 229–234.

Whitaker, C. (1976). A family is a four-dimensional relationship. In P. J. Guerin, Jr. (Ed.), *Family therapy: Theory and practice* (pp. 182–192). New York: Gardner Press.

Wiggins, M. E. (1994). The Black Caucus of the American Speech and Hearing Association: A history. In R. M. Screen & N. B. Anderson, *Multicultural perspectives in communication disorders* (pp. 31–42). San Diego, CA: Singular.

Wilcox, M. J. (1989). Delivering communication-based services to infants, toddlers, and their families: Approaches and models. *Topics in Language Disorders, 10*(1), 68–79.

Williams, D. E. (1957). A point of view about 'stuttering.' *Journal of Speech and Hearing Disorders, 22*(3), 390–397.

Williams, D. E. (1971). Stuttering therapy for children. In L. E. Travis (Ed.), *Handbook of speech pathology and audiology* (pp. 1073–1093). Englewood Cliffs, NJ: Prentice-Hall.

Williams, D. E. (1978). Differential diagnosis of disorders of fluency. In F. L. Darley & D. C. Spriestersbach (Eds.), *Diagnostic methods in speech pathology* (2nd ed.) (pp. 409–438). New York: Harper & Row.

Williams, D. E. (1979). A perspective on approaches to stuttering therapy. In H. H. Gregory (Ed.), *Controversies about stuttering therapy* (pp. 241–268). Baltimore, MD: University Park Press.

Williams, D. E. (1983). Talking with children who stutter. In J. F. Gruss (Ed.), *Counseling stutterers* [Publication 18] (pp. 35–45). Memphis, TN: Stuttering Foundation of America.

Williams, D. E. (1984). Working with children in the school environment. In J. F. Gruss (Ed.), *Stuttering therapy: Transfer and maintenance* [Publication 19] (pp. 29–40). Memphis, TN: Stuttering Foundation of America.

Williams, D. E., Darley, F. L., & Spriestersbach, D. C. (1978). Appraisal of rate and fluency. In F. L. Darley & D. C. Spriestersbach (Eds.), *Diagnostic methods in speech pathology* (2nd ed.) (pp. 256–283). New York: Harper & Row.

Wingate, M. E. (1964). A standard definition of stuttering. *Journal of Speech and Hearing Disorders, 29*, 484–489.

Wingate, M. E. (1969). Sound and pattern in "artificial" fluency. *Journal of Speech and Hearing Research, 12*, 677–686.

Wingate, M. E. (1976). *Stuttering: Theory and treatment.* New York: Irvington Publishers/Halsted Press.

Wingate, M. E. (1983). Speaking unassisted: Comments on a paper by Andrews et al. *Journal of Speech and Hearing Disorders, 48*, 255–263.

Wingate, M. E. (1988). *The structure of stuttering: A psycholinguistic analysis.* New York: Springer-Verlag.

Winslow, M., & Guitar, B. (1994). The effects of structured turn-taking on disfluencies: A case study. *Language, Speech, and Hearing Services in Schools, 25*, 251–257.

Wischner, G. J. (1950). Stuttering behavior and learning: A preliminary theoretical formulation. *Journal of Speech and Hearing Disorders, 15*, 324–335.

Wischner, G. J. (1952). An experimental approach to expectancy and anxiety in stuttering behavior. *Journal of Speech and Hearing Disorders, 17*, 139–154.

Woods, C. L., & Williams, D. E. (1971). Speech clinicians' conceptions of boys and men who stutter. *Journal of Speech and Hearing Disorders, 36*, 225–234.

Woods, C. L., & Williams, D. E. (1976). Traits attributed to stuttering and normally fluent males. *Journal of Speech and Hearing Research, 19*, 267–278.

World Health Organization. (1977). *Manual of the international statistical classification of diseases, injuries, and causes of death* [Vol. 1]. Geneva: World Health Organization.

Yairi, E. (1981). Disfluencies of normally speaking two-year-old children. *Journal of Speech and Hearing Research, 24*, 490–495.

Yairi, E. (1993). Epidemiologic and other considerations in treatment efficacy research with preschool age children who stutter. *Journal of Fluency Disorders, 18*, 197–219.

Yairi, E. (1997). Disfluency characteristics of childhood stuttering. In R. F. Curlee & G. M. Siegel (Eds.), *Nature and treatment of stuttering: New directions* (2nd ed.) (pp. 49–78). Needham Heights, MA: Allyn & Bacon.

Yairi, E., & Ambrose, N. (1992a). A longitudinal study of stuttering in children: A preliminary report. *Journal of Speech and Hearing Research, 35,* 755–760.

Yairi, E., & Ambrose, N. (1992b). Onset of stuttering in preschool children: Selected factors. *Journal of Speech and Hearing Research, 35,* 782–788.

Yairi, E., Ambrose, N. G., & Niermann, R. (1993). The early months of stuttering: A developmental study. *Journal of Speech and Hearing Research, 36,* 521–528.

Yairi, E., & Carrico, D. M. (1992). Early childhood stuttering: Pediatricians' attitudes and practices. *American Journal of Speech–Language Pathology, 1*(3), 54–62.

Yairi, E., & Clifton, N. F., Jr. (1972). Disfluent speech behavior of preschool children, high school seniors, and geriatric persons. *Journal of Speech and Hearing Research, 15,* 714–719.

Yairi, E., & Williams, D. E. (1970). Speech clinicians' stereotypes of elementary-school boys who stutter. *Journal of Communication Disorders, 3,* 161–170.

Yairi, E., & Williams, D. E. (1971). Reports of parental attitudes by stuttering and by nonstuttering children. *Journal of Speech and Hearing Research, 14,* 596–604.

Yeakle, M. K., & Cooper, E. B. (1986). Teacher perceptions of stuttering. *Journal of Fluency Disorders, 11,* 345–359.

Young, M. A. (1985). Increasing the frequency of stuttering. *Journal of Speech and Hearing Research, 28,* 282–293.

Zarski, J. J., DePompei, R., & Zook, A. II (1988). Traumatic head injury: Dimensions of family responsivity. *Journal of Head Trauma Rehabilitation, 3*(4), 31–41.

Zebrowski, P. M. (1994). Stuttering. In J. B. Tomblin, H. L. Morris, & D. C. Spriestersbach (Eds.), *Diagnosis in Speech–Language Pathology* (pp. 215–245). San Diego, CA: Singular.

Zebrowski, P. M. (1995). The topography of beginning stuttering. *Journal of Communication Disorders, 28,* 75–91.

Zebrowski, P. M. (1997). Assisting young children who stutter and their families: Defining the role of the speech–language pathologist. *American Journal of Speech–Language Pathology, 6*(2), 19–28.

Zimmermann, G. (1980a). Articulatory dynamics of fluent utterances of stutterers and nonstutterers. *Journal of Speech and Hearing Research, 23,* 95–107.

Zimmermann, G. (1980b). Stuttering: A disorder of movement. *Journal of Speech and Hearing Research, 23,* 122–136.

Zimmermann, G. (1984). Articulatory dynamics of stutterers. In R. F. Curlee & W. H. Perkins (Eds.), *Nature and treatment of stuttering: New directions* (pp. 131–147). San Diego, CA: College-Hill.

Zimmermann, G., Liljeblad, S., Frank, A., & Cleeland, C. (1983). The Indians have many terms for it: Stuttering among the Bannock-Shoshoni. [Research Note]. *Journal of Speech and Hearing Research, 26,* 315–318.

Zimmermann, G. N., Smith, A., & Hanley, J. M. (1981). Stuttering: In need of a unifying conceptual framework. *Journal of Speech and Hearing Research, 24,* 25–31.

Author Index

Adler, S., 166, 173
Ainsworth, S., 114, 262, 542
Alfrey, A. C., 106
Ambrose, N., 45, 49, 245, 260, 272, 287
Anderson, D., 23, 24
Anderson, J. L., 424, 460, 483, 484, 486–488, 491–498, 502–504, 507–512
Anderson, N. B., 166, 173, 470
Anderson, R. H., 488
Andrews, G., 17, 21, 35, 46, 47, 48, 50, 51, 53, 73, 77, 78, 79, 106, 310, 319, 368, 395, 396, 414, 451
Andrews, J. R., 125–126, 128, 141, 369
Andrews, M. A., 125–126, 128, 141, 369
Argeropoulos, J., 450, 469
Arnold, G. E., 97, 108
Aronson, A. E., 110
Asbury, F. R., 452, 499
Ashby, J. K., 20, 461
Attanasio, J. S., 47, 61, 108

Balzer, F. J., 452, 499
Bass, C., 401
Battle, D. E., 164–167, 174, 176
Baumgartner, J. M., 47, 48, 50, 51
Baxley, B., 330, 455
Beasley, D. S., 372
Benecken, J., 23, 24
Bengtson, V. L., 374
Benitez, M., 114
Benjamin, B. J., 373
Bennett, E. M., 329, 331, 348
Bess, F. H., 173
Beukelman, D. R., 506
Bishop, D. S., 125, 128
Bishop, J., 478
Bjerkan, B., 47
Blood, G. W., 6, 420, 421, 422
Bloodstein, O., 6, 9, 11, 35, 36, 42–44, 46, 50–54, 65, 74–77, 86, 109, 110, 123, 134, 135, 168, 183, 236, 337, 340, 369, 370, 373, 399

Bluemel, C. S., 37, 54, 65, 70, 86, 108
Blumberg, A., 491, 495, 498
Boberg, D., 184
Bohlman, P., 115
Boone, D. R., 424, 485
Botterill, W., 120, 124, 244
Bowen, M., 125
Bowers, L. S., 156
Brady, J. P., 113
Brasseur, J., 491, 496, 497, 503, 504
Braun, A., 113
Brotherton, W. D., 466
Brown, J., 20
Brutten, G. J., 78, 450, 451
Bruun, B., 111, 113
Bruun, R. D., 111, 113
Burnett-Stolnack, M., 368
Bushey, T., 23–24, 543
Butler, R. B., 106
Byrne, A., 107
Byrne, M. K., 107

Campbell, J. H., 543
Canter, G. J., 103, 106
Carkhuff, R. R., 450, 452, 499
Carlisle, J. A., 86, 407, 544
Carrico, D. M., 20
Carter, E. A., 125, 140, 141, 145, 146, 147–148
Caruso, A. J., 461, 478
Casey, P. L., 424, 460, 480, 483, 484, 487, 488, 491, 495–497, 500, 503, 504, 507
Chabon, S., 470
Childers, W. C., 452, 499
Christensen, L., 115
Clark, B. S., 173
Clark, R. M., 61, 62, 65
Clarke, M. G., 166
Cleeland, C., 166
Clifton, N. F., Jr., 373
Cogan, M. L., 488, 491, 495, 499
Cohen, D. J., 113
Colburn, N., 113, 114
Cole, L., 165–166, 172
Colligan, N., 111–113
Collins, M., 102
Collucci, S., 491

Comings, D. E., 111, 113
Conti, D. M., 113
Conture, E. G., 14, 16, 44, 47, 183, 227, 229, 239, 244, 245, 247, 249–250, 262, 273, 277, 294, 295, 301, 340–343, 368, 369, 373, 388, 397, 462, 542–545
Cook, F., 120, 124
Cook, L., 156, 159
Cooper, C. S., 20, 21, 134, 168, 169, 172, 236, 348, 370, 402, 403, 415, 421, 450, 451, 461–463
Cooper, E. B., 8, 13–14, 20, 21, 134, 165, 168, 169, 172, 236, 262, 334, 337, 348, 370, 397, 402–404, 415, 421, 450, 451, 461–463, 479–481, 542
Corcoran, L. H., 61, 62
Costall, B. M., 105
Costello, J. M., 184
Cox, A. W., 162
Cox, M. D., 108
Cox, N., 49
Crowe, T. A., 20
Culatta, R., xix, 9, 11, 65, 97, 99, 102–104, 106, 108–110, 113, 114, 134, 168, 169, 172, 173, 193, 491, 495, 496
Curlee, R. F., 46, 61, 62, 183, 184

Dailey, D., 373
Dalton, P., 97
Daly, D. A., 22, 97–101, 119, 316, 330–331, 368, 369, 373, 397, 399, 400–402, 414–415, 421, 422, 454, 461
Damico, J. S., 173
Daniels, D. B., 159–160
Darley, F. L., 46
Davis, G. A., 372
De Buck, A., 61
Deal, J. L., 108–109
Dell, C. W., 183, 316, 327, 328, 332, 344, 346–349, 351, 352, 545

Dempsey, G. L., 108
DePompei, R., 131–132
Diedrich, W. M., 97
Diehl, C. F., 65
Dokecki, P. R., 155, 159
Doro, J. M., 108, 109
Douglass, E., 123, 135
Dowling, S., 497
Downes, J. J., 105
Downey, C. S., 301
Duchin, S. W., 395
Duffy, J. R., 389
Durrenberger, C. H., 21, 461, 478

Edwards, M. L., 340
Edwards, S. G., 65, 407, 544
Eisenson, J., 79–80
Emerick, L. L., 36, 47–49, 61, 70, 71, 449, 451–453, 457–459, 461, 467
Epstein, N. B., 125, 128
Everly-Myers, D. S., 461

Fagan, E. C., 507
Fairbanks, G., 80, 389
Fantry, L., 106–107
Farmer, J. L., 497, 500–502
Farmer, S. S., 497, 500–502
Fay, A., 415
Felicetti, T., 484
Felsenfeld, S., 49
Fey, M. E., 113, 229, 230
Finkelstein, S., 331
Finn, P., 45, 245, 287
Fiore, Q., 331
Fishman, H. C., 139
Fitch, J. L., 115
FitzSimons, R. M., 450, 454
Florance, C. L., 184, 397–400, 402
Frank, A., 166
Fransella, F., 123
Fraser, J., 114, 262, 542–545
Fraser, M., 544
Freedman, M., 105
Freeman, F. J., 81
Freund, H., 65, 108, 109, 372
Friend, M., 156, 159
Froeschels, E., 37, 54, 97
Furer, P., 111
Furst, N., 484

Gardner, H., 467, 468, 471
Gardner, L. S., 301
Garland, C. W., 159
Garner, H. S., 162
Garrard, K. R., 227, 229
Gazda, G. M., 452, 499

Geschwind, N., 105
Gibran, K., 476
Gillam, R. B., 488
Givens-Ackerman, J., 301, 463, 478, 480
Glauber, P., 11
Goldberg, B., 64, 69–70
Goldberg, S. A., xix, 9, 11, 65, 97, 99, 102–104, 106, 108–110, 134, 168, 169, 172, 173, 193
Goldhammer, R., 488, 491, 495
Goldiamond, I., 184
Golenischeff, W., 62
Gordon, P. A., 76, 114, 236, 237
Gottwald, S. R., 81
Gouge, C. G., 413
Granich, M., 108
Greenwald, B., 106
Gregory, H. H., 11, 134, 183, 270, 349, 544–545
Gregory, P. R., 543
Gruss, J. F., 545
Guitar, B., 13, 17, 20, 35, 47–51, 53, 75, 81, 82, 84, 87, 88, 182–193, 202, 224, 227, 232–233, 239, 245, 247, 250, 260, 270–273, 294, 295, 298, 302, 309, 315, 325, 328, 332, 333, 340, 344, 368–370, 373, 384–386, 396, 398, 401, 402, 408, 418, 425, 456, 542–545
Guyette, T. W., 47, 48, 50, 51

Hahn, E. F., 65
Hahn, E. S., 65
Halfond, M. M., 81
Hall, D. E., 113, 114
Hall, P. K., 113
Hallahan, D. P., 161
Ham, R. E., 8, 10, 36, 47, 193
Hamayan, E. V., 173
Hanley, J. M., 80
Hanson, M., 373
Hardcastle, W. J., 97
Harris, M. R., 484
Harris, W. E., 108
Harryman, E., 12–13
Hartke, R. J., 371
Hartman, A., 141
Haynes, W. O., 36, 47–49, 70–72, 108, 217, 218, 223–225, 229, 235, 251, 257–259, 294, 295, 309, 310, 369, 370, 374–375, 382, 396–399, 410
Healey, E. C., 301
Helm, N. A., 106

Helm-Estabrooks, N., 99, 102–108
Hinzman, A. R., 97
Hoffman, P. R., 20
Hood, S. B., 451, 544, 545
Hooper, C. R., 375, 376, 409
Howe, J., 105
Howie, P., 53
Hull, F. M., 97

Ingham, R. J., 45, 395, 396
Irvine, T. L., 97

Jenkins, M. M., 250
Jezer, M., 407, 544
Johnson, B. A., 164, 167, 172
Johnson, E., 218
Johnson, L., 184
Johnson, W., 28, 34, 35, 56, 60, 74, 78, 166
Johnson, W., & Associates, 74, 247
Johnston, J. R., 10, 119

Karniol, R., 114
Kauffman, J. M., 161
Kellum, G. D., 507
Kelly, E. M., 249–250
Kelly, G. A., 119–122, 124, 150
Kelman, E., 244
Kennedy, K., 500
Kent, R. D., 10, 15, 102
Keys, W. T., 173
Kidd, K. K., 48, 49
Klein, H. B., 10, 123, 156–157, 158
Klingbeil, G. M., 65
Krajewski, R. J., 488
Kresheck, J., 12–13
Kropf, N. P., 156
Kuhn, T., 155, 177
Kully, D., 184

Laird, J., 141
Lass, N. J., 20, 461
Lazarus, A. A., 415
Leckman, J. F., 113
Leeper, L. H., 106, 113, 114
Lee-Wilkerson, D., 470
Leith, W. R., 22, 47, 108, 109, 168–174
Lemme, M. L., 106
Lerman, J., 115
Lew, E., 52, 109
Lewis, G. A., 65
Lichtheim, M., 62–63
Liles, B. Z., 115
Liljeblad, S., 166
Lohr, J. B., 111
Lokken, K. J., 250

Lopez, O. L., 107
Lougeay-Mottinger, J., 484
Louko, L. J., 340
Lowenstein, R. L., 331
Ludlow, C. L., 113
Luper, H. L., 76, 114, 183, 236, 237, 451, 545
Luterman, D. M., 125, 128–131, 139, 141, 142
Lynch, K. A., 111

MacFarlane, W. B., 373
MacNeil, R. D., 371, 372
Mahr, G., 47, 108, 109
Malcolm, M. T., 113
Mallard, A. R., 301, 461, 478
Malone, D. M., 159–163
Manning, W. H., 21, 61, 62, 301, 328–330, 333–335, 338–341, 343, 344, 348, 349, 351–354, 369, 370, 372–373, 392, 397, 418, 419, 422, 423, 425, 450–451, 453, 458, 459, 461–464, 547
Martin, R., 23–24, 543
Mata-Pistokache, T., 164, 167, 172
Matazow, G. S., 111
May, H. G., 63, 64
McAfee, J. G., 389
McCarthy, M. M., 106
McCrea, E. S., 496, 498, 499
McCready, V., 500, 502
McElroy, M. D., 476–477, 507
McGoldrick, M., 145, 146, 147–148
McGonigel, M. J., 159
McLuhan, M., 331
McNeil, M. R., 106
Mellon, C. D., 373
Meltzer, A., 115
Merrill, J. C., 331
Messert, B., 102
Messick, S., 119
Metzger, B. M., 63, 64
Meyers, S. C., 81
Michael, W. B., 184
Michel, J., 166
Miller, A., 469, 470
Miner, A. L., 424, 485
Minuchin, S., 139
Mitchell, H. R., 173
Monte, K. L., 373
Montgomery, B. M., 115
Moscicki, E. K., 47
Moses, N., xx, 10, 123, 156–158, 163, 170, 279, 313, 428–429, 458, 481–484, 488, 504, 508–512

Mulder, R. L., 183
Muma, J., 230
Murphy, A. T., 450, 451, 454
Murray, F. P., 61, 62, 65, 407, 544
Myers, F. L., 7, 36, 44, 97, 113, 193, 340
Myers, J. E., 371, 372
Mysak, E. D., 113, 114, 395

Nellum-Davis, P., 172
Nichols, K., 21
Nicolosi, L., 12–13, 70–72, 77–79, 110, 256
Niermann, R., 45, 245
Nippold, M. A., 340
Nudelman, H. B., 370, 373
Nurnberg, H. G., 106

Ogletree, B. T., 156, 159–160, 466
Orfanidis, M. M., 125, 140, 141
Ort, S. I., 111

Pannbacker, M., 461
Parker, G., 74
Paul, R., 173
Pauls, D. L., 113
Peacher, W. G., 108
Peachey, E. C., 113
Pearlman, D. N., 371–372
Perkins, W. H., 9–10, 12, 46, 97, 146–147, 183, 184, 334, 401, 544
Perlstein-Kaplan, K. E., 484
Peters, H. F. M., 373
Peters, T. J., 13, 17, 20, 35, 47–51, 75, 82, 84, 87, 88, 182–193, 202, 224, 227, 232–233, 239, 245, 247, 250, 260, 270–273, 294, 298, 302, 309, 315, 325, 328, 332, 333, 340, 344, 368–370, 373, 384–386, 396, 398, 402, 408, 418, 425, 545
Pickering, M., 496
Pindzola, R. H., 47, 114, 237, 240–242, 250
Post, J. G., 22
Prescott, T. E., 106, 424, 485
Prins, D., 397, 399, 401
Prutting, C. A., 506, 507
Purser, H., 133

Quader, S. E., 106
Quarrington, B., 123, 135
Quinn, P. T., 106, 113

Ragsdale, J. D., 20, 461
Rakowski, W., 371–372
Ramig, P. R., 329, 331, 344, 348, 544–545
Rassi, J. A., 476–477, 507
Ratner, N. B., 114, 340–344
Reis, R. P., 97
Riley, G. D., 251, 252–253
Ripich, D. N., 374
Rivara, J. B., 131
Roberts, J. E., 491, 495, 496
Rogers, C. R., 452–455, 499
Rokusek, C., 155, 156, 158–162, 177
Rollin, W. J., 132–133, 141, 146
Rosenbek, J. C., 102–104, 106
Rosenfield, D. B., 370, 373
Rosenshine, B., 484
Roth, C. R., 109
Roussos, C. S., 488
Rubin, H., 65, 134, 193
Rubin, I. L., 156
Rudas, J., 184
Ruder, K. F., 173
Ruscello, D. M., 20, 461
Rush, W. L., 15–16
Rustin, L., 20, 133, 244, 461
Ryan, B. P., 183–184, 193, 203–210, 234, 250

Saddler, Y. N., 156
Sagar, H. J., 105
Satir, V., 141
Sayers, F. C., 218
Scahill, L., 111
Schaie, K. W., 374
Scheuerle, J., 371
Schmitt, J. F., 461
Schubert, G. W., 424, 485
Schulz, J. B., 139
Schwartz, H. D., 44, 247, 369
Schwiebert, V. L., 371, 372
Scott, L. A., 301
Screen, R. M., 166, 173
Seeley, J. U., 498
Seltzer, H., 496
Shadden, B. B., 372
Shady, G. A., 111
Shames, G. H., 65, 77–78, 134, 184, 193
Shapiro, D. A., xx, 27, 123, 163, 170, 172, 257, 274, 279, 299–300, 312, 313, 375, 413, 424, 428–429, 452, 458, 460, 466, 467, 481–484, 486–488, 491, 492, 494–498, 500, 502–504, 507–512, 543
Sharp, H. M., 105
Sheehan, J., 77, 183, 369

Sheehy, G., 408
Shine, R. E., 134, 184
Shipley, K. G., 389
Shirkey, E. A., 52, 109, 110,
    370, 372–373
Shoemaker, D. J., 78
Shriberg, L. D., 484
Sickels, E. R., 218
Siegel, G. M., 46, 64
Silverman, E.-M., 20, 47, 115
Silverman, F. H., 9, 10, 23, 35,
    47, 48, 51, 52, 60, 65,
    70–72, 74–75, 82, 85,
    97, 103, 104, 108–111,
    115–116, 134, 301, 397,
    462
Simon, C. A., 368
Smith, A., 80
Smith, K. J., 424, 491, 495,
    496, 498–500, 504
Sokoly, M. M., 155, 159
Sommers, R. K., 461, 478
Spriestersbach, D. C., 46
St. Ledger, J., 115
St. Louis, K. O., 20, 21, 97,
    461, 478
Staley, D., 111
Starkweather, C. W., 6–8, 22,
    26, 51, 81, 82, 87, 88,
    239, 248, 271, 272, 275,
    301, 328, 340, 341, 373,
    380, 418–419, 463, 478,
    480, 545
Stoneman, Z., 159–163
Sugarman, M., 543
Swain, K. C., 543

Tapia, F., 111, 113
Taylor, O. L., 166, 167
Teague, M. L., 371, 372
Terry, W., 61
Thousand, J. S., 161
Thyer, B. A., 156
Tiger, R. J., 97, 99
Till, J. A., 424, 485
Tillis, M., 61
Tolchard, B., 113
Travis, L. E., 11, 79

Tudor, M., 74–75
Turnbaugh, K. R., 20, 461
Turnbull, A. P., 127, 131,
    134–137, 139, 142, 143,
    147–149, 164, 165, 172
Turnbull, H. R., III, 127,
    134–137, 139, 142, 143,
    147–149, 164, 165, 172

Uhl, M., 162
Ulrich, S. R., 424
Underwood, J. K., 498–499
U.S. Bureau of the Census, 167

Van Kirk, B., 183–184, 193,
    203, 205–208, 234
Van Riper, C., 3, 4, 11–13,
    16–18, 20, 25, 26, 29,
    35–42, 45–49, 52, 54,
    60, 65, 74, 76–77, 79,
    80, 87–88, 114, 115,
    134, 166, 168, 183, 184,
    193–201, 203, 210, 211,
    230, 231, 237, 238, 251,
    255, 261, 270, 273, 277,
    324–325, 332, 333, 337,
    372, 373, 398, 408, 416,
    418, 450, 451, 453–467,
    485–486, 488, 545–546
Villa, R. A., 161
Vinnard, R. T., 107, 111, 113

Wagner, W., 61
Wall, M. J., 7, 36, 44, 113, 193,
    340
Wallace, S., 373
Walle, E. L., 114, 239, 243, 451,
    466–469, 476, 509, 542
Wallen, V., 108
Walters, R. P., 452, 499
Walton, J. H., 20
Walton, W., 373
Wand, R. R., 111
Watson, J. B., 399–400, 414,
    416
Webb, A., 62
Webster, E. J., 270
Webster, R. L., 184

Weiner, A. E., 108
Weinstein, C., 105
Weiss, D. A., 97–98
Weller, R. H., 499
Wells, P. G., 113
Wertz, R. T., 102
West, R., 79, 457
Westby, C. E., 173
Wexler, K. B., 113
Whitaker, C., 125
White, D. T., 114, 237,
    240–242
Wiggins, E., 491
Wiggins, M. E., 166
Wilcox, M. J., 159
Williams, D. E., 7, 15, 17, 20,
    26, 35, 46, 74, 135, 183,
    216, 226, 232–234, 249,
    251, 254, 256, 297, 298,
    301–304, 320–321,
    332–333, 351, 383–385,
    395, 461, 478, 542–543
Wingate, M. E., 9, 11, 12, 44,
    45, 47, 48, 50, 53, 65, 74,
    86, 184
Winslow, M., 81
Wischner, G. J., 78
Wisniewski, A. A., 111
Woods, C. L., 20, 461
World Health Organization, 12,
    102
Wray, D. F., 113

Yairi, E., 20, 45, 48, 49, 74,
    129, 135, 245–247, 260,
    272, 287, 373, 461
Yeakle, M. K., 20
Yeo, R., 105
Young, M. A., 52

Zarski, J. J., 131–132
Zebrowski, P. M., 44, 236, 239,
    244, 245, 247, 248, 256,
    272, 273
Zibin, T. O., 107
Zimmermann, G., 80, 166
Zook, A. II, 131–132

Subject Index

◆ ◆ ◆ ◆ ◆ ◆ ◆ ◆ ◆ ◆ ◆ ◆ ◆ ◆ ◆ ◆ ◆ ◆ ◆ ◆

Aaron and Moses, 63–64
ABC System, 485
Academic process
  academic knowledge, 479
  definition of, 477–478
  in professional preparation, 477–479
  revised training standards, 478–479
  summary on, 510–511
Acceptable stuttering, 186
Accountability, 161
Acquired disfluency following laryngectomy, 110–111
Active listening, 423
ADA (Americans with Disabilities Act), 16, 161
Adaptability of families, 140
Adaptation
  in adolescents, adults, and senior adults, 396
  definition of, 51, 251
  measurement of, 256
  with negative suggestion, 198
  in preschool children, 251, 256
  in school-age children, 309
  to stress, 198
  in stuttering modification, 198
Adapted Scales for Assessment of Interpersonal Functioning in Speech Pathology Supervision conferences, 498, 499
Adductor spasmodic dysphonia, 110
Adolescents
  active role in maintenance of speech fluency, 424–425
  assessment procedures for, 382–394, 443
  audio- and videotape recording of, 376
  awareness and study of speech fluency by, 414–415
  benchmarking and, 426
  case history form, 375–379
  chronic perseverative stuttering (CPS) syndrome, 402–405
  client and family interview, 383–392
  clinical portrait of, 434–442
  communication hierarchies of, 418
  diagnosis of, 397
  direct fluency challenge for, 418
  Disfluency Frequency Index (DFI), 395
  Disfluency Type Index (DTI), 395
  extrafamily considerations for, 409–410, 441–442
  feelings and attitudes of, 396, 399–400, 416–417, 424
  fluency facilitating techniques for, 415–416
  fluency shaping for, 392–393

  general precepts on, 368–370, 442–443
  informational materials for, 407, 542–546
  intrafamily considerations for, 408–409, 441
  and maintenance of fluency-inducing effects of treatment, 424–433
  opportunities created for fluency success, 412–414
  personal constructs of, 427–430
  positive feelings about communication and about oneself as communicator, 420–424
  post-assessment interview of, 405–407
  post-assessment procedures for, 394–407, 443
  preassessment conference for, 376, 380–381
  preassessment procedures for, 375–381
  preliminary phone call to, 376
  prognosis and recommendations for, 397–405
  relapse and, 418–422
  resistance to potential fluency disrupters for, 417–420
  and revisiting past stuttering behaviors, 426–427
  "safe house" for, 411–412
  significant others/conversational partners of, 376, 431–433
  speech analysis of, 395–396, 434–435
  speech–language sample with communicative pressure, 391–392
  speech–language sample without communicative pressure, 387–389
  structured activities with communicative pressure, 391–392
  structured activities without communicative pressure, 389–391
  stuttering modification for, 393–394
  summary on, 442–444
  and transfer of fluency facilitating techniques, 417
  treatment goals for, 407, 436–437, 444
  treatment objectives for, 407–408, 412, 437–438
  treatment of, 407–433, 436–440, 444
  treatment procedures for, 410–433
  treatment rationale for, 408–410, 438
  trial management for, 392–394, 435–436
Adult Stuttering Therapy, 545–546
Adults. *See also* People who stutter; Senior adults
  active role in maintenance of speech fluency, 424–425
  assessment procedures for, 382–394, 443
  audio- and videotape recording of, 376

awareness and study of speech fluency by, 414–415

benchmarking and, 426

case history form, 375–379

chronic perseverative stuttering (CPS) syndrome, 402–405

client and family interview, 383–392

clinical portrait of, 434–442

communication hierarchies of, 418

comparison of people who stutter and those who do not, 49–51

diagnosis of, 397

direct fluency challenge for, 418

Disfluency Frequency Index (DFI), 395

Disfluency Type Index (DTI), 395

extrafamily considerations for, 409–410, 441–442

feelings and attitudes of, 396, 399–400, 416–417, 424

fluency facilitating techniques for, 415–416

fluency shaping for, 392–393

general precepts on, 368, 370, 442–443

historical and contemporary people who stutter, 60–61

increase and transfer of fluent speech, 411–417

informational materials for, 407, 542–546

intrafamily considerations for, 408–409, 441

and maintenance of fluency-inducing effects of treatment, 424–433

opportunities created for fluency success, 412–414

personal constructs of, 427–430

positive feelings about communication and about oneself as communicator, 420–424

post-assessment interview of, 405–407

post-assessment procedures for, 394–407, 443

preassessment conference for, 376, 380–381

preassessment procedures for, 375–381, 443

preliminary phone call to, 376

prognosis and recommendations for, 397–405

relapse and, 418–422

resistance to potential fluency disrupters for, 417–420

and revisiting past stuttering behaviors, 426–427

"safe house" for, 411–412

significant others/conversational partners of, 376, 431–433

speech analysis of, 395–396, 434–435

speech–language sample with communicative pressure, 391–392

speech–language sample without communicative pressure, 387–389

structured activities with communicative pressure, 391–392

structured activities without communicative pressure, 389–391

stuttering modification for, 393–394

summary on, 442–444

and transfer of fluency facilitating techniques, 417

treatment goals for, 407, 436–437, 444

treatment objectives for, 407–408, 412, 437–438

treatment of, 407–433, 436–440, 444

treatment procedures for, 410–433

treatment rationale for, 408–410, 438

trial management for, 392–394, 435–436

"Advanced stutterers", 368. *See also* Adolescents; Adults; Senior adults

Adventures of Phil Carrott (Sugarman and Swain), 543

Affirmation training, 422

African Americans, 138, 166, 371–372. *See also* Ethnic minorities

Age at onset of stuttering, 47, 83

Aging. *See* Senior adults

AIDS, 106–107

Airflow therapy, 325

Alzheimer's-type dementia, 106

American Speech–Language–Hearing Association (ASHA), 22, 29, 119, 166–168, 398, 451, 452, 462–463, 465, 470, 478–480, 483, 487–490, 504, 505, 507, 508, 511, 512, 514–540, 546–547

Americans with Disabilities Act (P.L. 101-336), 16, 161, 466

Amitriptyline, 106

Analysis of Behavior of Clinicians (ABC) System, 485

Anatomical defect, stuttering as, 65

Anticipation, definition of, 51

Anticipatory struggle behavior, 74–77

Antidepressants, 106

Approximation/modification, in stuttering modification, 200–201, 202

Articulation, 25

Articulation disorder, stuttering as, 66–67

ASHA, 22, 29, 119, 166–168, 398, 451, 452, 462–463, 465, 470, 478–480, 483, 487–490, 504, 505, 507, 508, 511, 512, 514–540, 546–547

ASHA Black Caucus, 166

ASHA Code of Ethics, 398, 478, 520–521

ASHA Commission on Fluency Disorders, 479

ASHA Committee on Supervision in Speech–Language Pathology and Audiology, 489–490, 508

ASHA Council on Professional Standards (COPS), 478

ASHA "Guidelines for Practice in Stuttering," 452, 470, 478, 479, 480, 511, 512, 524–533

ASHA Position Statement on Clinical Supervision in Speech–Language Pathology and Audiology, 490, 512, 514–517

ASHA Scope of Practice in Speech–Language Pathology, 536–540

ASHA Standards and Implementations for the Certificates of Clinical Competence, 479

ASHA Standards for Accreditation of Educational Programs in Speech–Language Pathology and Audiology, 479
Asians/Pacific Islanders, 167. *See also* Ethnic minorities
Assessment
    of adolescents, 382–394, 443
    of adults, 382–394, 443
    child interview, 298–305
    client and family interview for adolescents and adults, 383–392
    parent interviews, 224–227, 296–297
    parent–preschool child interaction, 227–228
    of preschool children, 223–235, 285
    preschool child–clinician interaction, 229–234
    of school-age children, 296–307, 360
    of senior adults, 382–394, 443
    speech–language sample with communicative pressure, 234
    speech–language sample without communicative pressure, 229–233
    structured activities with communicative pressure, 234
    structured activities without communicative pressure, 233–234
    teacher interview, 297–298
Associated (or secondary) behaviors
    adolescents, adults, and senior adults, 396
    bizarre characteristics of, 19
    definition of, 15
    fluency tricks and, 18–19
    hierarchical development of, 19–20
    preschool children, 250
    school-age children, 309
Assumptions about stuttering, 34–35, 88–89. *See also* Attitudes; Stereotypes of stuttering
Attitude, positive pretreatment attitude, 399–400
Attitudes
    of adolescents, 396, 399–400, 416–417, 424
    of adults, 396, 399–400, 416–417, 424
    change of, in stuttering modification, 200
    of clinicians, 21–22, 401–402, 458–460, 461–464
    of parents, 270–272, 346–347
    of preschool children, 278–279
    of school-age children, 309, 329–333
    of senior adults, 396, 399–400, 416–417, 424
    treatment outcome and, 21–22, 399–402
Audiotape recording during assessment, 218, 223, 376
Avoidance reduction, 77
Avoidance response, stuttering as, 77–78, 91

Behavioral phenomena, stuttering as interaction of, 78–79
Benchmarking, 336, 426
Biases toward stuttering, 20–24, 169–170, 270–272, 461–464

Bible accounts, 63–64
Bilateral masking noise, 17
Bilingualism, 83, 114
Biochemical theory and dysphemia, 79, 92
"Boone-Prescott" codes, 485
Brain, compared to computer, 84
Brain injury, 83, 104–105, 131
Brain lesion, 80, 92
Brain tumor, 106
Breakdown theories, 79–80
Broncho dialator, 106
"Buddy system," 328–329

Cancellation, 200–201, 202, 325
Case history forms, 218, 219–222, 375–379
Central nervous system, 50–51
Cerebral dominance, incomplete, 79, 92
Change
    clinicians' importance to change process, 450–452
    in family life cycle, 145–149
    and family patterns, 140–142
    friction necessary for, 458
Chaos within families, 140
Checklists
    cluttering, 100
    CPS syndrome, 404
    Tourette Syndrome, 111–113
Child interview, 298–305
Childhood Stuttering: A Videotape for Parents, 262, 282, 542–543
Children. *See* Adolescents; Preschool children; School-age children
Children's books, 23–24, 299–300, 543
Choice Corollary, of constructive alternativism, 121
Choral reading, 17
Chronic illness in childhood, 131
Chronic perseverative stuttering (CPS) syndrome, 402–405
Classical conditioning, 78, 92
Client–clinician relationship. *See* Clinicians
Clinical portraits
    adolescents, adults, and senior adults, 434–442
    preschool children, 280–285
    school-age children, 355–359
Clinical process
    clinical knowledge, 480–481
    components of, 483–487
    continuing education for, 508–509
    definition of, 480
    individually designed procedures for analysis of, 486–487
    interaction analysis systems for, 484–485
    model for clinician development, 481–483
    nonverbal analysis of, 485–486
    observation and analysis of, 484–487
    planning, 484

in professional preparation, 480–487
summary on, 511
understanding, 483–484
Clinical supervision. *See* Supervisory process
Clinical Supervision in Speech–Language
Pathology and Audiology (ASHA), 490,
512, 514–517
Clinicians
attitudes of, 21–22, 401–402, 458–460,
461–464
attributes and manner of interaction, 452–460
cautions against elitism, 349–350
change process and, 450–452
compatible friction and, 458
as comrades, xix
continuing education for, 505–510, 511
and desire to learn, 505–507
empathy of, 453–454
and errors, 459–460
genuineness of, 455–457
as guardian angels, 468–470
interpersonal factors of effective clinicians,
452–460, 470–471
intrapersonal factors of effective clinicians,
460–468, 471
language used by, 460
needs of, 464–466
optimism of, 458–460
origin of therapist as term, xix
parents and, 344–348
personal constructs of, 460–461
personal magnetism of, 457–458
preschool children and, 229–234
professional effectiveness of, 450–451
professional preparation of, 462–463,
476–505, 510–511
satisfaction and rewards of, 466–468
student clinicians, 334–335
summary on, 470–471
teachers and, 348–355
warmth of, 454–455
Closed head injury, 104–105
Cluttering, 97–101
Code of Ethics (ASHA), 398, 478, 520–521
Cognitive restructuring, 325
Cohesion within families, 139–140
Commission on Fluency Disorders (ASHA), 479
Commonality Corollary, of constructive
alternativism, 122
Communication hierarchies, 328, 418
Communicative failure, stuttering as, 74–77, 91
Compatible friction, and clinicians, 458
Comrades, author's use of term, xix
Concomitant disorders, 340–343
Conflict theory of stuttering, 77, 91
Consistency
in adolescents, adults, and senior adults, 396
definition of, 51, 251, 256
measurement of, 256

in preschool children, 251, 256
in school-age children, 309
Constitutional factors, 87
Construction Corollary, of constructive
alternativism, 121
Constructive alternativism, 120, 121–122
Constructs. *See* Personal constructs
Contemporary figures who stutter, 60–61
Content and Sequence Analysis of Speech and
Hearing Therapy, 485
Continuing education for clinicians, 505–510, 511
Continuity hypothesis, 75–76, 91
Continuum of Supervision, 490–495
Controlled fluency, 185–186
COPS. *See* Council on Professional Standards
(COPS)
Cost containment, 161
Council on Professional Standards (COPS), 478
CPS syndrome, 402–405
Creating an Inclusive School (Villa and
Thousand), 161
Creek analogy, 276, 325
Cultural awareness. *See* Multicultural awareness
Cybernetic theory of stuttering, 80, 92

DAF (Delayed Auditory Feedback), 17, 184, 205,
206–207
Delayed Auditory Feedback (DAF), 17, 184, 205,
206–207
Demand speech, 81, 269
Demands and capacities model, 81–82, 89–90, 92
Dementia, 106
Desensitization phase of stuttering modification,
194–195, 197–199
Development of stuttering, 35–45
Developmental factors, 84, 88
DFI. *See* Disfluency Frequency Index (DFI)
Diagnosis
of adolescents, 397
of adults, 397
origin of term, 257
of preschool children, 235, 257–258, 286
of school-age children, 309–310, 360
of senior adults, 397
stuttering modification and, 194
Diagnosogenic theory, 74–75, 91
Dichotomy Corollary, of constructive
alternativism, 121
Disfluency. *See also* Stuttering
acquired disfluency following laryngectomy,
110–111
adductor spasmodic dysphonia, 110
frequency of, 239, 243–246, 308
linguistic disfluency, 113–114
in manual communication, 115
molecular description of speech disfluency,
247–248, 308, 395
neurogenic disfluency, 99, 102–108

normal developmental disfluency, 114,
216–217, 236–243
during playing wind instrument, 115–116
psychogenic disfluency, 108–109
and rate of speech, 248–250, 308
secondary characteristics and, 250
in senior adults, 372–374
severity rating of, 250–255
types of, 14–15, 46, 246–247, 308
versus dysfluency, 8
Disfluency Frequency Index (DFI), 239, 243–246,
308, 395
Disfluency Type Index (DTI), 246–247, 308, 395
Disturbed feedback, as cause of stuttering, 80, 92
Diversity among families, 134
Do You Stutter: A Guide for Teens (Fraser and
Perkins), 544
Do You Stutter: Straight Talk for Teens, 407,
544–545
DTI. *See* Disfluency Type Index (DTI)
Duration of stuttering, 14
Dysfluency versus disfluency, 8. *See also*
Disfluency
Dysphemia and biochemical theory, 79, 92
Dysphonia, spastic, 110

Education of All Handicapped Children Act
(P.L. 94-142), 158, 161, 175
Egyptian hieroglyphics, 61–63
Electrolarynx, 110–111
Electronic network systems, 547
Elitism, 349–350
Empathy of clinicians, 423, 453–454
Encouragement, 423
Environmental factors in stuttering, 48–49, 89–90
Errors, and clinicians, 459–460
Escape behaviors, 200
Esophageal speech, 110–111
Ethical dilemmas, 275
Ethics Code (ASHA), 398, 478, 520–521
Ethnic minorities, 138, 166–168, 371–372. *See
also* Multicultural awareness
Etiology of neurogenic disfluency, 102–108
Etiology of stuttering
as avoidance response, 77–78, 91
brain lesion, 80, 92
breakdown theories, 79–80
as communicative failure and anticipatory
struggle behavior, 74–77, 91
conflict theory of stuttering and avoidance
reduction, 77, 91
constitutional factors, 87
continuity hypothesis, 75–76, 91
cybernetic theory of stuttering, 80, 92
definition of, 70–73
demands and capacities model, 81–82,
89–90, 92
developmental factors, 84, 88
diagnosogenic theory, 74–75, 91

disturbed feedback, 80, 92
dysphemia and biochemical theory, 79, 92
incomplete cerebral dominance, 79, 92
instrumental avoidance act theory, 78, 91
as interaction of behavioral phenomena, 78–79
as learned behavior, 69, 77–79, 78–79, 91–92
as neurotic response, 68, 73–74, 91
operant conditioning and stuttering, 77–78, 91
perpetuating factors, 72–73, 85–86, 91
perseveration theory, 79–80, 92
as physiological deficit, 79–80, 92
precipitating factors, 71–72, 88–91
predisposing factors, 70–72, 82–83, 87–88, 91
preparatory set, 76–77, 91
primary stuttering theory, 76–77, 91
Shapiro's theoretical perspectives, 86–91, 92
theoretical explanations, 73–92
two-factor learning theory of stuttering, 78–79,
91–92
Evaluation–Feedback Stage of supervision, 491,
492–493
Exceptionality, characteristics of, 135
Exodus, book of, 63–64
Experience Corollary, of constructive
alternativism, 121
Exploration of self, 199
Extrapyramidal diseases, 105

Families
access to parents, 344
adaptability of, 140
of adolescents, adults, and senior adults who
stutter, 408–409, 441
and assessment of preschool children, 223–235
attitude of parents toward stuttering, 270–272,
346–347
chaos within, 140
characteristics of, 134–138
cohesion within, 139–140
development and change in, 147–149
diversity among, 134
functions of, 142–145
informational materials for, 262, 282, 542–546
interactions within, 138–142
life cycle of, 145–149
multicultural considerations toward, 169–172
needs of parents, 346–348
optimal families, 128–129
parent intervention for preschool children,
263–272, 281, 282, 286
parent interviews, 224–227, 259–262,
296–297, 311–312
parent–preschool child interaction, 227–228
as partners with professionals, 127–128
patterns of, and change, 140–142
respect for primary role of parents, 345–346
rigidity within, 140
roles in, 145–146
of school-age children, 313–314, 358

special challenges of, 137–138
stress in, 146–147
successful families, 129–130
Family based treatment. *See also* Family systems
theory
effectiveness of, 130–132
families and professionals as partners in,
127–128
fluency disorders and, 132–134
modeling characteristics of optimal families,
128–129
modeling characteristics of successful families,
129–130
multicultural considerations in, 169–175, 176
school-age children and, 344–348
summary on, 149
Family systems theory. *See also* Families
characteristics of families, 134–138
diversity among families, 134
family based treatment and, 127–134, 149
focus on systems rather than behaviors in, 127
functions of families, 142–145
importance of, 510
interactions within family, 138–142
life cycle of families, 145–149
as paradigm shift, 125–127
polyocular perspective of, 125–126
summary on, 150
understanding rather than labeling in, 126–127
Female–male ratio for stuttering, 48
Fiddler on the Roof, 86
Fluency. *See also* Disfluency; Fluency shaping
conditions inducing, 17, 51
conditions inhibiting, 52
controlled fluency, 185–186
definition of, 6–8, 28
facilitating controls versus tricks, 16–20
language fluency, 7, 28
phonologic fluency, 7
pragmatic fluency, 7
semantic fluency, 7
speech fluency, 7
spontaneous fluency, 184–185
syntactic fluency, 7
Fluency disrupters, 268–270, 277–278, 327–329,
417–420
Fluency-inducing conditions, 17, 51
Fluency-inhibiting conditions, 52
Fluency shaping
for adolescents, 392–393
for adults, 392–393
advantages and disadvantages of, 189
affective treatment goals of, 185, 187
behavioral treatment goals of, 184–186,
208–209
combined with stuttering modification
approach, 192
counting, charting, timing in, 205
criterion test in, 205
DAF, 205, 206–207

definition of, 183
diagnostic indicators for treatment design, 190,
191
distinguished from stuttering modification,
184–188
establishment programs, 205–207
GILCU, 205–206
maintenance phase of, 208
premise of, 184, 185
for preschool children, 235
Programmed Conditioning for Fluency, 183,
203
*Programmed Therapy for Stuttering in
Children and Adults,* 183–184, 203, 204
for senior adults, 392–393
structure of treatment, 185, 188
stuttering interview, 203, 205
summary on, 210
transfer phase of, 207–208
treatment procedures, 185, 188
Fluent stuttering, 7
Frequency of stuttering
in adolescents, adults, and senior adults, 395
definition of, 14
Disfluency Frequency Index (DFI), 239,
243–246, 308, 395
in preschool children, 239, 243–246
in school-age children, 308
Friction and change, 458
Functioning in society, 26–27

Gender differences in stuttering, 48, 83
Genuineness of clinicians, 455–457
GILCU (Gradual Increase in Length and
Complexity of Utterance), 184, 205–206
Gradual Increase in Length and Complexity of
Utterance (GILCU), 184, 205–206
Guide for Parents of Children Who Stutter, 542
"Guidelines for Practice in Stuttering" (ASHA),
452, 470, 478, 479, 480, 511, 512, 524–533

Head injury, 131–132
Head trauma, 104–105
Heredity
cluttering and, 99
stuttering and, 48–49, 83
Hieroglyphics, 61–63
Hispanics, 167, 371. *See also* Ethnic minorities
Historical figures who stutter, 60–61
History of stuttering
Bible accounts, 63–64
Egyptian hieroglyphics, 61–63
historical and contemporary people who
stutter, 60–61
professional medical literature, 64–70
stuttering as anatomical defect, 65
stuttering as articulation disorder, 66–67
stuttering as disorder of neuroanatomy/motor
speech dysfunction, 67–68
stuttering as learned behavior, 69